ENEDIYNE ANTIBIOTICS AS ANTITUMOR AGENTS

ENEDIYNE ANTIBIOTICS AS ANTITUMOR AGENTS

EDITED BY

DONALD B. BORDERS

BioSource Pharm, Inc.
Suffern, New York

TERRENCE W. DOYLE

OncoRx, Inc.
New Haven, Connecticut

Marcel Dekker, Inc.   New York • Basel • Hong Kong

Library of Congress Cataloging-in-Publication Data

Enediyne antibiotics as antitumor agents / edited by Donald B. Borders, Terrence W.
  Doyle.
        p.   cm.
      Includes bibliographical references and index.
      ISBN 0-8247-8938-5 (acid-free paper)
      1. Antineoplastic antibiotics.   I. Borders, Donald B.   II. Doyle, Terrence W.
  RC271.A65.E54   1994
  616.99'2061—dc20   94-37776
                                                                              CIP

The publisher offers discounts on this book when ordered in bulk quantities.
For more information, write to Special Sales/Professional Marketing at the
address below.

This book is printed on acid-free paper.

MARCEL DEKKER, INC.
270 Madison Avenue, New York, New York 10016

Current printing (last digit):
10 9 8 7 6 5 4 3 2 1

PRINTED IN THE UNITED STATES OF AMERICA

Preface

The discovery, isolation, and structure elucidation of biologically active natural products have frequently played a very important role in the development of new commercially important compounds for medical and agricultural applications. Antibiotic research is an excellent example of this type of approach which has resulted in one of the largest and most successful product areas for the pharmaceutical industry. Natural products are a valuable resource for diverse chemical structures with selected stereochemistry. Frequently, even the simplest structures derived from nature can be a challenge to the synthetic chemist due to functionality and stereochemistry.

Antitumor antibiotics are active against bacteria and certain types of tumor cells. The mechanism for antibacterial and antitumor activity is apparently the same and is frequently the result of DNA damage. The reason for selectivity toward tumor cells rather than normal cells is probably the rapid proliferation of cancer cells, with a higher probability of toxic effects for these faster growing cells.

Enediyne antitumor antibiotics represent a novel chemical class of antibiotics with remarkable biological properties. As a class, they are the most potent, highly active antitumor agents ever discovered. Some members are over 1000 times more potent than adriamycin, one of the most effective clinically used antitumor antibiotics. The unusual biological properties of these compounds are a consequence of equally unique chemical features: molecules with cyclic enediynes within 9- and 10-member rings; novel sugars, including an hydroxylamino sugar; and an allylic methyl trisulfide group. When calicheamicin and esperamicin interact with DNA, a fragile trisulfide group acts as a trigger to initiate the formation of a diradical from the enediyne. This free radical portion of the interacting molecule performs as a warhead to induce DNA damage which is frequently a double-strand cleavage. This type of damage is usually nonrepairable for the cell, with a single event being lethal. This unique property may explain the extreme potency of the enediyne antibiotics. Because of these remarkable chemical and biological properties, there has been an intense effort by the pharmaceutical industry and academia over the last several years to study these substances with the hope of developing fundamentally new, clinically useful antitumor agents.

This text will provide a comprehensive and up-to-date view of enediyne antitumor antibiotics. The chapters cover the discovery of these compounds and various aspects of their development through preclinical and clinical studies. The text is interdisciplinary, covering microbiology, chemistry, biochemistry, and biology and should allow scientists with an interest in any one phase of this work to also be able to gain a broad overview of the field. The microbiologist will find extensive treatments of the fermentation development, the biosyntheses, the isolation of blocked mutants, and factors that have led to yield improvements of 2-4 orders of magnitude such as the unique iodide effect. For the chemist, there is detailed information covering product isolation and structural elucidation using the full armamentarium of instrumental techniques, including proton and carbon nuclear magnetic resonance, mass spectrometry, circular dichroism, x-ray crystallography and electron spectroscopy for chemical analysis. The very selective chemical degradations for these complex, sensitive molecules are reviewed and provide an insight into how structures were established. Once the structures of the calicheamicins, esperamicins, dynemicins, and neocarzinostatin were published, an astonishing burst of activity resulted in the organic synthesis community, which is reviewed in Chapter 18. The total synthesis of calicheamicin γ_1^I is fully detailed. The realization that these unique molecules were theoretically capable of unrepairable double-strand cleavage of DNA has led to intense efforts to establish their mechanisms of action, which is presented in three of the chapters. Theoretical studies of the Bergman cyclization reaction and the molecular dynamics of drug-DNA complexes are covered. The preclinical biology of the enediyne antibiotics is reviewed in several chapters. Because of the toxicity of these agents, the preparation of monoclonal antibody conjugates to calicheamicin was pursued. The very successful use of these targeted agents to treat tumors in mice is reviewed. Information on clinical studies of esperamicin and the polymer conjugates of neocarzinostatin are presented along with preclinical data for monoclonal antibody conjugates of calicheamicin, one of which is expected to enter clinical trials soon.

The information on discovery of calicheamicin and esperamicin is presented in a form not available in standard journal papers, and should not only bring various aspects of the work together in one text but also provide an insight into factors that led to the discovery of these most unusual compounds. In addition, it is hoped that the many descriptions of novel procedures, approaches, and observations of unexplained effects mentioned throughout the text will stimulate the development of new areas of research.

Donald B. Borders
Terrence W. Doyle

Contents

Contents

Part V.   Synthetic Methodologies

Contributors

Donald B. Borders, Ph.D. President, BioSource Pharm, Inc., Suffern, New York

Anna Maria Casazza, Ph.D. Executive Director, Department of Experimental Therapeutics, Bristol-Myers Squibb Pharmaceutical Research Institute, Princeton, New Jersey

Wei-Dong Ding, Ph.D. Senior Research Scientist, Natural Products Research Section, Medical Research Division, Lederle Laboratories, American Cyanamid Company, Pearl River, New York

Terrence W. Doyle, Ph.D. Vice President of Research, OncoRx, Inc., New Haven, Connecticut

Frederick E. Durr, Ph.D. Associate Director, Oncology Technologies, Oncology and Immunology Research, Medical Research Division, Lederle Laboratories, American Cyanamid Company, Pearl River, New York

George A. Ellestad, Ph.D. Research Fellow, Natural Products Research Section, Medical Research Division, Lederle Laboratories, American Cyanamid Company, Pearl River, New York

Amedeo A. Fantini, Ph.D.*   Principal Research Microbiologist, Infectious Disease Research Division, Lederle Laboratories, American Cyanamid Company, Pearl River, New York

Salvatore Forenza, Ph.D.   Director, Natural Products Research, Bristol-Myers Squibb Pharmaceutical Research Institute, Wallingford, Connecticut

Irving H. Goldberg, M.D., Ph.D.   Professor, Department of Biological Chemistry and Molecular Pharmacology, Harvard Medical School, Boston, Massachusetts

Jerzy Golik, Ph.D.   Principal Scientist, Department of Antitumor Chemistry, Bristol-Myers Squibb Pharmaceutical Research Institute, Wallingford, Connecticut

Michael Greenstein, Ph.D.   Head, Department of Microbiology and Automated Technology, Medical Research Division, Lederle Laboratories, American Cyanamid Company, Pearl River, New York

Randall L. Halcomb, Ph.D.   Assistant Professor, Department of Chemistry and Biochemistry, University of Colorado, Boulder, Colorado

Philip R. Hamann, Ph.D.   Project Leader, Medical Research Division, Lederle Laboratories, American Cyanamid Company, Pearl River, New York

Lois M. Hinman, Ph.D.   Assistant Director, International Registration, Medical Research Division, Lederle Laboratories, American Cyanamid Company, Pearl River, New York

Lizzy S. Kappen, Ph.D.   Principal Associate, Department of Biological Chemistry and Molecular Pharmacology, Harvard Medical School, Boston, Massachusetts

Susan L. Kelley, M.D.   Immunology Clinical Research, Bristol-Myers Squibb Pharmaceutical Research Institute, Wallingford, Connecticut

Masataka Konishi, Ph.D.   Director, Drug Research Department, Zenyaku Kogyo Company Ltd., Tokyo, Japan

---

**Present Affiliation*: Fermentation Consulting Services, New City, New York.

Nydia A. Kuck, M.S. Group Leader, Infectious Disease Research, Medical Research Division, Lederle Laboratories, American Cyanamid Company, Pearl River, New York

Kin Sing Lam, Ph.D. Principal Scientist, Natural Products Research, Bristol-Myers Squibb Pharmaceutical Research Institute, Wallingford, Connecticut

David R. Langley, Ph.D. Senior Research Investigator I, Department of Computerated Drug Design (Antitumor Research), Bristol-Myers Squibb Pharmaceutical Research Institute, Wallingford, Connecticut

May D. Lee, Ph.D. Associate Director, Department of Molecular Diversity, Microcide Pharmaceuticals, Inc., Mountain View, California

Hiroshi Maeda, Ph.D., M.D. Professor and Chairman, Department of Microbiology, Kumamoto University School of Medicine, Kumamoto, Japan

William M. Maiese, Ph.D. Director, Natural Products Research, Medical Research Division, Lederle Laboratories, American Cyanamid Company, Pearl River, New York

William J. McGahren, Ph.D.* Senior Research Chemist, Natural Products Research Section, Medical Research Division, Lederle Laboratories, American Cyanamid Company, Pearl River, New York

Toshikazu Oki, Ph.D. Professor, Bioindustrial Research Center, Toyama Prefectural University, Toyama, Japan

David M. Rothstein, Ph.D. Senior Scientist, Department of Drug Discovery, Myco Pharmaceuticals, Inc., Cambridge, Massachusetts

Raymond T. Testa, Ph.D. Section Director, Infectious Disease Research, Medical Research Division, Lederle Laboratories, American Cyanamid Company, Pearl River, New York

Craig A. Townsend, Ph.D Professor, Department of Chemistry, Johns Hopkins University, Baltimore, Maryland

---

*Retired

Janis Upeslacis, Ph.D.   Head, Department of Oncology and Immunology Research, Medical Research Division, Lederle Laboratories, American Cyanamid Company, Pearl River, New York

Judith A. Veitch   Research Scientist I, Natural Products Research, Bristol-Myers Squibb Pharmaceutical Research Institute, Wallingford, Connecticut

Roslyn E. Wallace, B.S.*   Senior Research Scientist, Oncology and Immunology Research, Medical Research Division, Lederle Laboratories, American Cyanamid Company, Pearl River, New York

Mary Jo Wildey, Ph.D.   Group Leader, Microbiology and Automated Technology, Medical Research Division, Lederle Laboratories, American Cyanamid Company, Pearl River, New York

Nada Zein, Ph.D.   Senior Research Investigator, Oncology Drug Discovery, Bristol-Myers Squibb Pharmaceutical Research Institute, Princeton, New Jersey

---

*Retired

Enediyne Antitumor Antibiotics

Terrence W. Doyle
OncoRx, Inc., New Haven, Connecticut

Donald B. Borders
BioSource Pharm, Inc., Suffern, New York

I. NEW CLASS OF ANTIBIOTICS

The enediyne antibiotics are extremely potent antitumor agents with a unique molecular architecture. These compounds represent a new chemical structure class for antibiotics in which all members contain a unit sometimes referred to as a warhead, which consists of two acetylenic groups conjugated to a double bond or incipient double bond within a nine- or 10-membered ring. At room temperature in the presence of DNA, the warhead of an enediyne antibiotic undergoes a remarkable reaction yielding sp^2 carbon-centered diradicals as the biologically active species. Thus far, there have been three basic families within the enediyne antibiotic class. These are defined as the (1) calicheamicin/esperamicin, (2) dynemicin, and (3) chromoprotein types. The first recognized members of this new class were calicheamicin and esperamicin (1–4). Both antibiotics occur as complexes of many closely related components.

During the structure studies for calicheamicin γ_1^I and esperamicin A_1 it became apparent that the enediynes could be triggered to aromatize via cleavage of the trisulfide with formation of a diradical intermediate and that this diradical species was probably responsible for the DNA-damaging properties of the molecule. From this observation it was also speculated that neocarzinostatin might undergo a similar aromatization process (2) since it was previously known that the neocarzinostatin DNA-damaging mechanism involved free radicals when activated by thiols. Neocarzinostatin consists of a nonpeptidic chromophore, which is complexed with a protein that acts as a carrier and stabilizer for the chromophore. Since the mechanism of action for neocarzinostatin chromophore seemed similar to that of calicheamicin and esperamicin and it contained two acetylenic units in a nine-membered ring, the neocarzinostatin chromophore was then considered as another member of the new enediyne class of antibiotics. Prior to that time, the proposed structure for the neocarzinostatin chromophore was somewhat difficult to accept and neocarzinostatin seemed unrelated to all other structurally defined antibiotics. The structure elucidation of the neocarzinostatin chromophore had been completed 2 years before that of calicheamicin and esperamicin, and elegant studies of the mechanism of action were well underway (see Chapter 16). The family of enediynes represented by neocarzinostatin is now designated as the chromoproteins.

Calicheamicin γ_1^I is one of the major components of the calicheamicin complex and is over 1000 times more potent than adriamycin against tumor models in mice. Most of the other enediyne antibiotics have similar biological potencies. Adriamycin is clinically one of the most useful antitumor agents. The chemistry, biology, and mechanism of action of the enediyne antibiotics have been the topics of several recent reviews (5–10).

All of the enediyne antibiotics were originally derived by fermentation of microorganisms. The organisms found to produce the different enediyne complexes include various species of *Micromonospora, Actinomadura,* and *Streptomyces.* The unique chemistry, extremely potent biological effects, and clinical potential of the enediyne antibiotics have stimulated intense efforts to synthesize the antibiotics and simplified variants of the enediyne warhead. The total syntheses of calicheamicin γ_1^I and di- and tri-*O*-methyl dynemicin A were recently reported by Nicolaou (11–13) and Schreiber (14), respectively.

II. CALICHEAMICIN AND ESPERAMICIN

It was not until the initial structure communications appeared (1–4) in the same issue of the *Journal of the American Chemical Society* that scientists at American Cyanamid and Bristol-Myers Squibb realized that both pharmaceutical firms were exploring related antitumor agents in the same novel structure class. The calicheamicins from American Cyanamid were produced by *Micromonospora echinospora* spp. *calichensis* and the esperamicins from Bristol-Myers Squibb were produced by *Actinomadura verrucosospora.* Since the producing organisms were significantly different and the components of the calicheamicin complex were unique in having a halogen atom, the relationship between the calicheamicin and esperamicin complexes was not obvious from the initial characterization data.

However, when the total structures were revealed, it was surprizing to find the same enediyne unit and unique amino sugars in both structure families. Previous communications by the Warner-Lambert and Fujisawa pharmaceutical companies on preliminary characterization of other potent antitumor agents produced by various species of *Actinomadura* suggested that these antibiotics were very similar or identical to esperamicin (15).

Initially the enediyne complex discovered by American Cyanamid was called calichemicin after the name of the producing organism, *M. echinospora* spp. *calichensis,* which was isolated from caliche soil in Texas. This name was immediately changed after the appearance of the structure publication, since another company protested about this toxic substance (all antitumor agents are toxic) having a name that sounded and looked too much like the name of their company. To resolve this problem the name was changed to calicheamicin to destroy the "chem" in the original name and yet relate as much as possible to previous published work. The esperamicins were discovered as metabolites of a strain of *A. verrucosospora* isolated from a soil sample collected at Pto Esperanza, Misiones, Argentina. Accordingly, they were named esperamicins to reflect the origin of the sample and the hope that this powerful new agent acting by a previously undescribed mechanism might be useful as a clinical antitumor drug.

Calicheamicin γ_1^1 **(1)** and esperamicin **(2)** have the same amino sugars, thio sugar, and enediyne chromophore with a methyl trisulfide group. However, there is a difference in substitution adjacent to the keto group of the chromophore, the substitution of the aromatic groups, and the arrangement of substituent sugar and aromatic units off the chromophore. Although both molecules cleave DNA by the same free radical mechanism, these differences in structure lead to a different DNA sequence cutting specificity, which will be discussed in subsequent chapters. For both calicheamicin and esperamicin, the event that triggers the reaction sequence leading to the formation of the diradical species is the cleavage of the methyl trisulfide group. Glutathione is the most prevalent thiol in mammalian cells, and recent studies suggest that under physiologically relevant conditions, it may react with calicheamicin bound to DNA to trigger the sequence of events leading to DNA damage (16). The calicheamicin γ_1^1 is stable in the presence of DNA as long as exogenous thiol is excluded (17). In this same study the binding of calicheamicin to DNA was studied by nuclear magnetic resonance (NMR) spectroscopy (17), which showed preferential binding of calicheamicin to specific DNA sites with some distortion of the DNA.

With small molecule mimetics of calicheamicin and esperamicin not having a methyl trisulfide group, alternative triggering groups have been designed such as the simple α,β-unsaturated ketone of Magnus and co-workers (18a) and the enol-keto trigger of Semmelhack et al. (18b). The synthetic potential of the enediyne chemistry, derived from the studies of the free radical generation by the antibiotics, has been applied to the construction of multicyclic ring systems by utilization of tandem enediyne radical cyclizations (19).

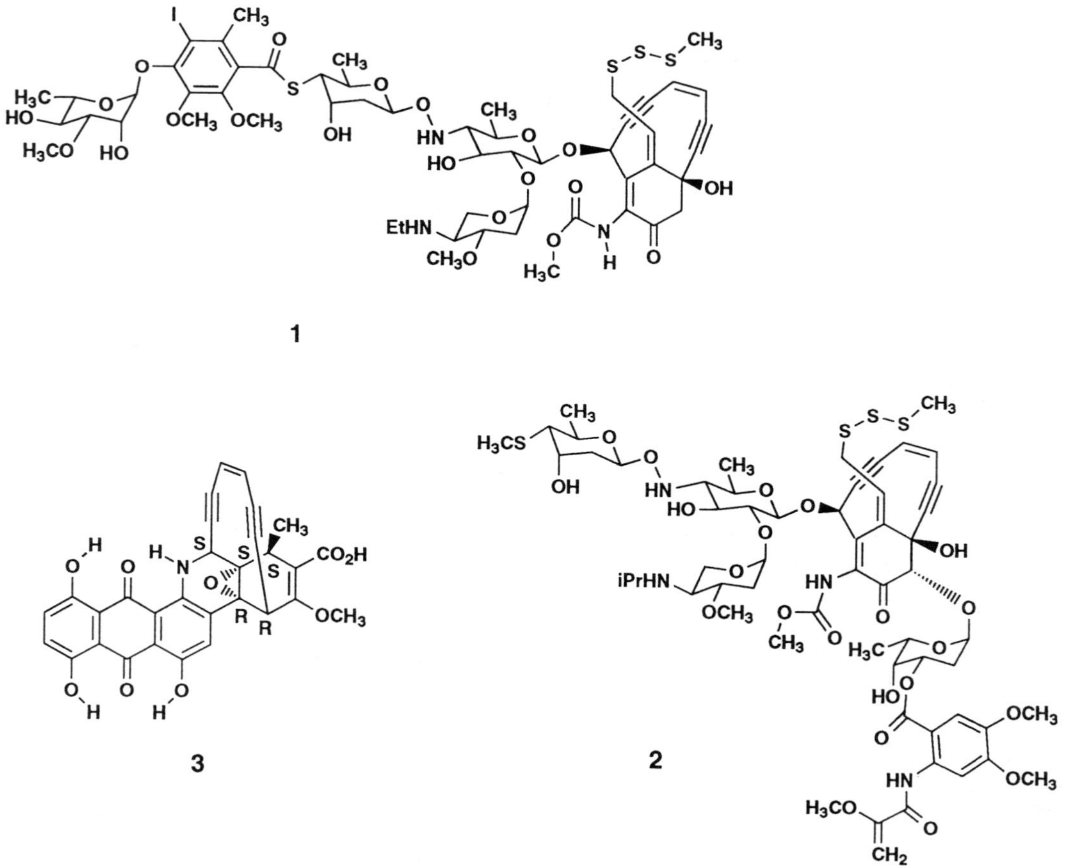

Figure 1 Structural formulae for calichaemicin γ_1^I (1), esperamicin A_1 (2) and dynemicin (3).

From the initial studies, which defined the new structure class of the enediynes and established these compounds as the most potent antitumor agents known, came a greatly expanded effort on the part of industry and academia to explore the chemistry, the biology at the molecular level, and the commercial potential of these compounds. Bristol-Myers Squibb advanced esperamicin A_1 into clinical trials, but an unpredicted toxicity required withdrawal of the drug from phase II clinical efficacy trials as described in Chapter 14. Because of the extreme potency of calicheamicin γ_1^1 and its potential for toxicity, American Cyanamid explored the possibility of conjugating the drug to monoclonal antibodies to obtain a targeted antitumor agent. These studies proved to be very encouraging (Chapter 6), and it was anticipated that a monoclonal antibody conjugate of calicheamicin would go into clinical trials near the end of 1994.

III. DYNEMICIN

Two years after the structure papers appeared on calicheamicin and esperamicin, a new enediyne-type antibiotic complex was reported by the Bristol-Myers Squibb group (see Chapter 15). This new, extremely potent antitumor antibiotic had an enediyne unit associated with the hydroxyanthraquinone chromophore of the classical anthracycline antibiotics. The major component of the complex was called dynemicin A **(3).** This molecule became the target of a number of synthetic studies and within 4 years of the structure publication the total synthesis of O-methyl analogs were reported (14).

IV. CHROMOPROTEINS

The chromoproteins are a group of potent antitumor antibiotics that consist of a nonpeptidic chromophore complexed with an apoprotein that acts as a carrier. These antibiotics generally possess broad-spectrum antitumor activity against solid-tumor cell lines both in vitro and in vivo. Excellent activity against resistant cell lines has also been observed. The highly acidic protein imparts stability to the chromophore, makes it water soluble, aids in export of the chromophore from the producing organism, and probably acts to protect the organism from DNA damage; e.g., when the kedarcidin-producing organism was exposed to kedarcidin in an attempt to improve production, significant up-regulation of apoprotein production (10-20-fold) was the result (20). Consequently there has been considerable interest in determining the tertiary structure of both the apoproteins and the holoproteins.

This effort has received some impetus from the observation that the apoproteins of auromomycin (macromomycin) and actinoxanthin (ACX) showed considerable homology to that of neocarzinostatin (NCS) and that the single crystal X-ray structures of both macromomycin (MCM) (21) and apoactinoxanthin (22) display close similarities to one another, both being Greek-key β-barrel structures. Subsequent X-ray work has demonstrated that the neocarzinostatin apo- (23,24) and holoproteins (24) are closely related to the apoproteins of auromomycin and actinoxanthin as well. Based on their primary sequence, the apoproteins of both kedarcidin (25) and C1027 (26) are also closely related to the other three (see Fig. 2 for the primary sequences of all five proteins). Homology mapping of the kedarcidin (27), neocarzinostatin (27,28), and C1027 (27) apoproteins on the crystal structures of macromomycin/actinoxanthin followed by molecular dynamics energy minimization predicts very similar solution structures for all five apoproteins. In the case of kedarcidin and neocarzinostatin, the predicted solution structures agree closely with those determined by 3-D NMR studies (29,30) (Fig. 3).

The NCS holoprotein consists of seven antiparallel β-strands forming two β-sheets. The alignment of these β-strands results in an elongated β-barrel, which contains a cavity consisting of residues from a four-β-stranded sheet and a shorter β-segment. The chromophore binds in the hydrophobic cavity at the base of the cleft, with the enediyne ring being sandwiched between two phenylalnine side chains (residues 52 and 78) (24). The amino sugar of the neocarzinostatin chromophore (NCS-CHR) projects out of the pocket in a position to salt-bridge to acidic residues. Myers notes that while "the binding pockets of NCS, ACX and MCM have similar overall shapes . . . the locations of side chains around the pockets are quite different" and that each chromoprotein appears adapted to bind a specific chromophore.

In addition to the properties described above, the apoproteins of macromomycin, kedarcidin, and C1027 have been shown to possess activity as peptidases. Based on the 10-fold potency increase observed for kedarcidin holoprotein versus the chromophore itself, Zein and co-workers compared the activity of carefully purified apoprotein and the intact kedarcidin against a variety of targets including both DNA and proteins. The apoprotein had no activity as a DNA-active agent. Because of the acidic nature of the apoprotein, its activity against basic histones was evaluated. It was found that kedarcidin apoprotein is an efficient cleaver of histones with histone H_1 being the preferred target. Similar activity was noted for both kedarcidin itself and neocarzinostatin. It is interesting to speculate that the apoprotein may play a role in exposing the DNA to attack by the chromophore (31). An examination of the molecular dynamics model of kedarcidin reveals two potential sites for serine protease activity involving Asp15, Arg69, and Ser71 or Asp54, His53, and Ser65 (32). Earlier Montgomery and co-workers had shown that macromomycin has aminopeptidase activity (33).

The elucidation of the structure of NCS-CHR by Edo and co-workers in 1985 was a critical event in the history of the enediyne antibiotics (34). This achievement was especially significant given the relative instability of NCS-CHR, the difficulties in extracting it from the holoprotein, and the state of the art in NMR

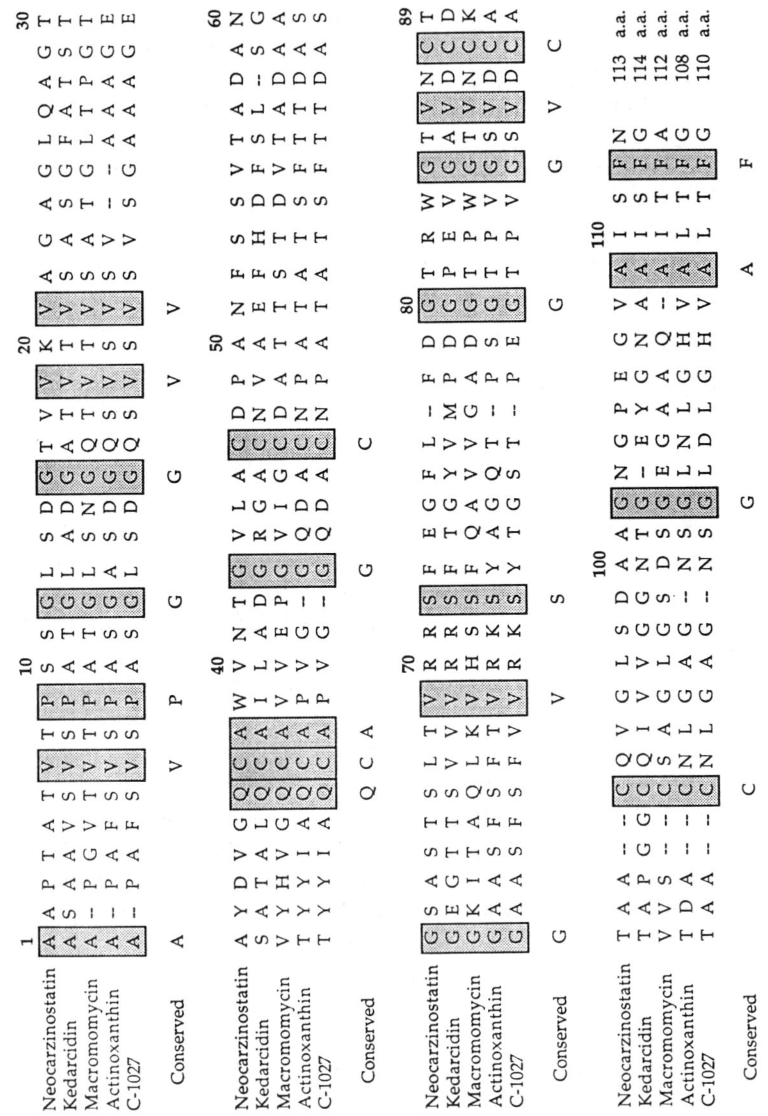

Figure 2 Primary sequences of the apoproteins of neocarzinostatin, kedarcidin, macromomycin (auromomycin), actinoxanthin, and C1027.

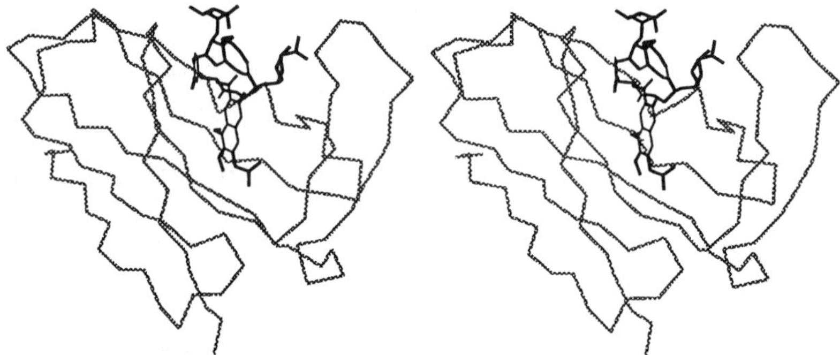

Figure 3 Stereoview of kedarcidin chromophore bound in the cleft of the apoprotein as determined by molecular modeling.

spectroscopy at the time. The structure elucidation of NCS-CHR, its mechanism of action, and its use as a paradigm for the synthesis of DNA-cleaving diradical generators are adequately reviewed elsewhere in this volume. More recently, the structures of the chromophores of kedarcidin (35), C1027 (36), and maduropeptin (37) have been reported (Fig. 4).

Kedarcidin was initially detected in cytotoxicity assays as a water-soluble compound having properties similar but not identical to those of neocarzinostatin (38). It is an acidic chromoprotein (pI = 3.65) of apparent molecular weight of 12,400 Daltons (35). Initial attempts to isolate the chromophore were unsuccessful owing to its poor stability in most organic solvents. Considerable substructural information was obtained by selective methanolysis experiments from which the structures of the two carbohydrate residues and the bridging azatyrosine residue could be deduced (39,40). Reduction of the crude chromophore fraction followed by isolation of the major products gave critical information concerning the structure of the enediyne core and the attachment of the carbohydrate and bridging amino acid residues (Fig. 5) as well as important clues regarding its activation (35,40). Biological evaluation of kedarcidin showed it to be capable of highly selective DNA single-strand breakage following bioreductive activation (41). Despite the structural similarity of the chromophores of kedarcidin and neocarzinostatin, the pattern of DNA strand cleavage by the latter was similar to that seen for calicheamicin $\gamma_1{}^1$. In vivo kedarcidin chromophore as well as the intact complex exhibits excellent activity in murine and human tumor xenograft models (see Chapter 14).

The discovery, isolation, and antitumor activity of C1027 were reported in 1988–1989 by Otani and co-workers (42). Like both neocarzinostatin and kedarcidin, the compound was an acidic chromoprotein (pI = 3.5–3.7) of apparent

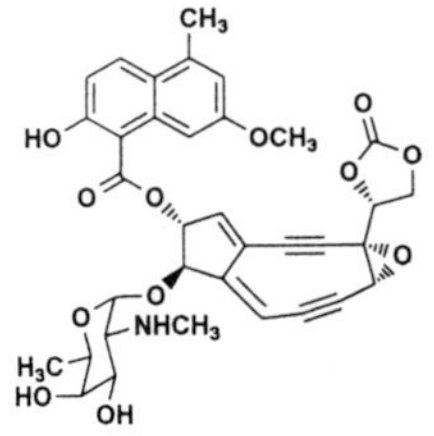

Figure 4 Structural formulae for the chromophores of neocarzinostatin (**4**), kedarcidin (**5**), C1027 (**6**), and maduropeptin (**7**).

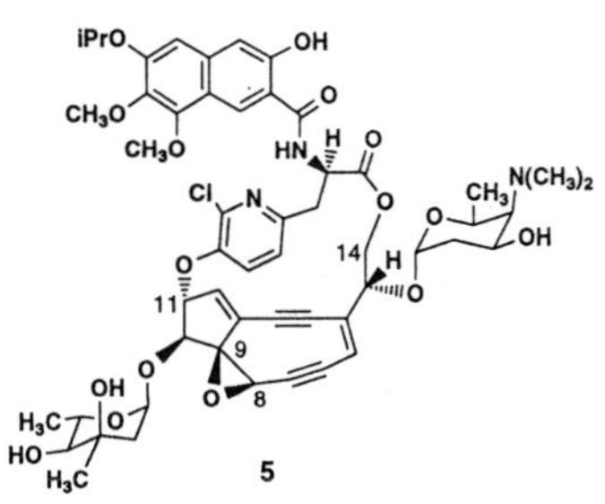

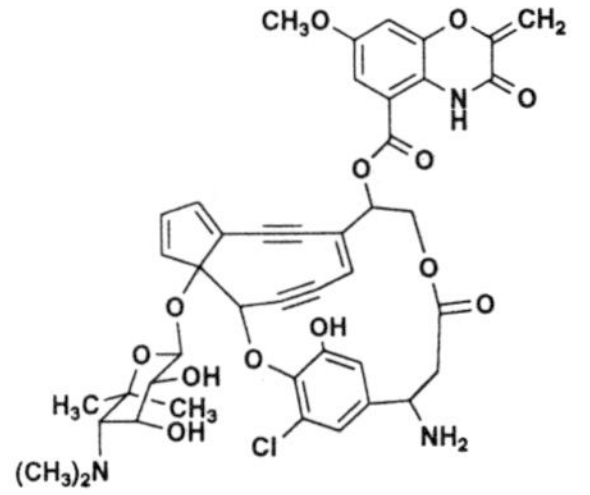

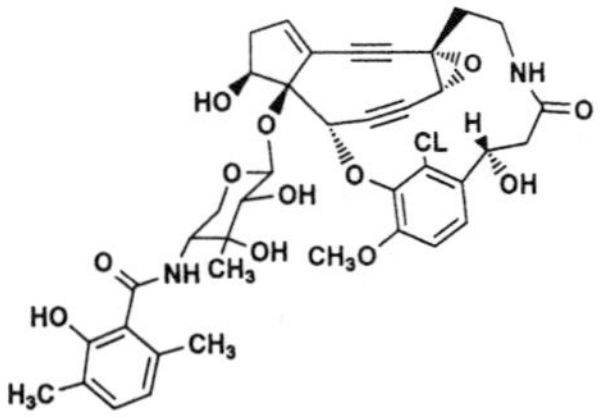

molecular weight 15,000 Daltons. Its mechanism of action was shown to involve single-strand DNA cleavage (43). The separation of the chromophore and apoprotein (C1027 AG) permitted sequencing of the apoprotein and initial characterization of a degradation product of the chromophore (44). Interestingly, this degradation product was almost identical to that reported from attempts to isolate the chromophore of auromomycin (Fig. 6) (45). Given the high degree of homology between the genes for the apoproteins of C1027 and auromomycin (57%), it is possible that the structures of the chromophores may also be closely related (46). The structure of the C1027 chromophore was reported as shown in Figure 4 (38). More recently, the absolute configuration of the aminosugar portion of the structure has been confirmed by synthesis (47). While both kedarcidin and C1027 are closely related to neocarzinostatin biogenetically, they differ in that they are both bridged structures. In the former case the bridge is between C14 and C11 of the core while in the latter the bridge is shorter, spanning from C14 to C8. Kedarcidin is protected from Bergman cyclization by the C9–C8 epoxide, which imparts sufficient ring strain. It is less clear why the C1027 chromophore has sufficient stability to permit isolation. Sugiura and Matsumoto (43c) report

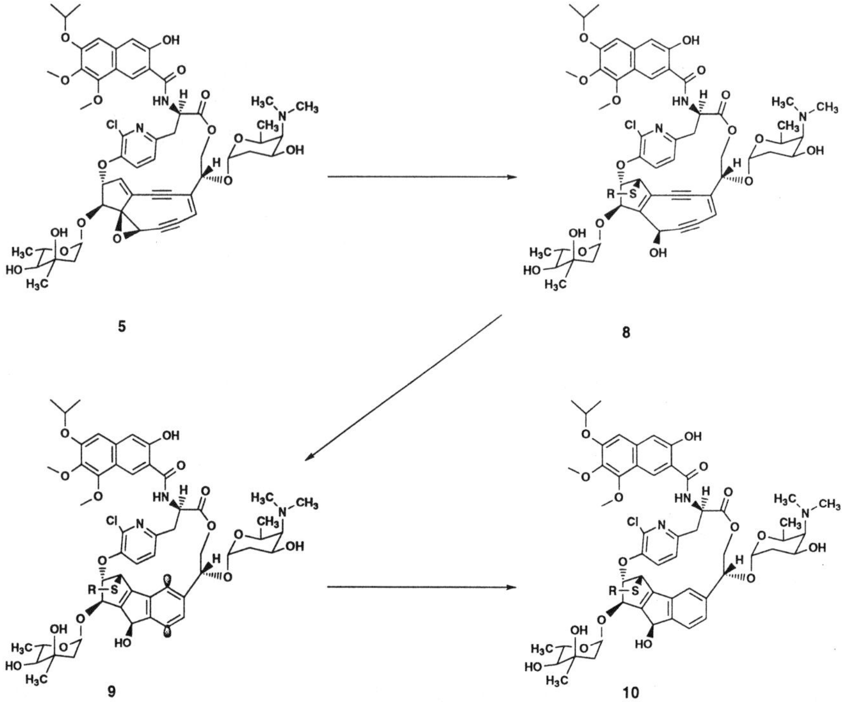

Figure 5 Activation cascade for the kedarcidin in the presence of thiols.

DNA cleavage even in the absence of thiols or reductants, which is consistent with the reported structure.

The most recent of the chromoproteins to be reported is maduropeptin (37,48). The apoprotein in this case, while acidic, has an apparent molecular weight of 32,000 Daltons. Initial amino acid sequencing indicates no homology with the

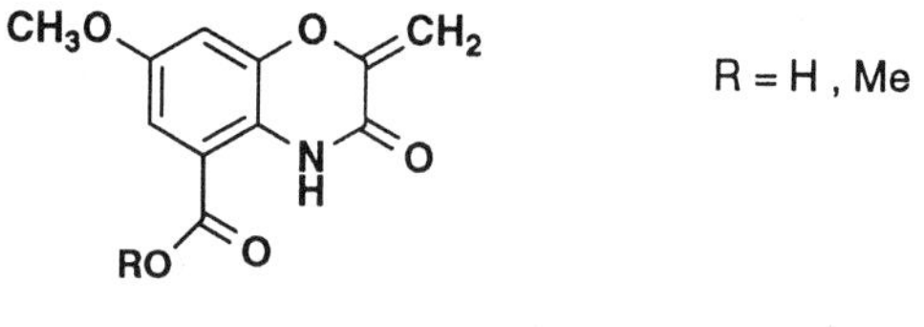

Figure 6 Degradation products of auromomycin and C1027 chromophores.

known chromoproteins (49). Preliminary mechanistic studies with maduropeptin chromophore indicated that the compound causes single-strand DNA breaks without requiring reductive activation (50). Comparison of the proposed structure of maduropeptin chromophore with that of C1027 shows many similarities including carbohydrate substitution at the C9 position and a bridge between C8 and C14. In the case of C1027, the question is how the enediyne is protected from Bergman cyclization through complexation with the apoprotein. With maduropeptin the question is twofold: how is the molecule activated for Bergman cyclization and how does the highly strained epoxide with a bridge extending from one face of the C_9 ring to the other face survive? The answer to the latter question is that it does not survive outside the protection of the apoprotein. To date the intact maduropeptin chromophore has not been isolated and alternatives to the proposed structure **12** are possible (e.g., **15**). Depending on the method used to decomplex the chromophore from the apoprotein, a series of degradation products have been isolated which in turn undergo further reaction, ultimately alkylating the DNA as well as cleaving it via Bergman cyclization and radical abstraction from the backbone of the DNA. These pathways are outlined in Figure 7. The evidence supporting this pathway is as follows. Based on the experience gained with kedarcidin, the holoprotein of maduropeptin was absorbed onto an anion exchange resin,

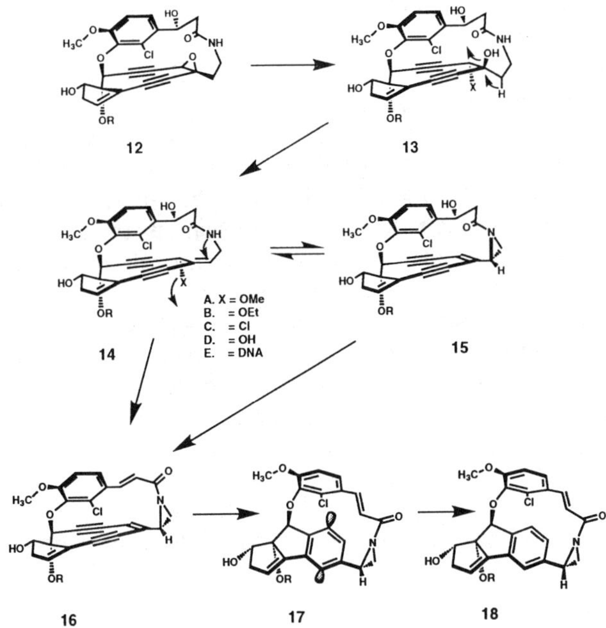

Figure 7 Activation cascade for maduropeptin chromophore.

washed, and dried. This stabilized the holoprotein and permitted a series of desorption experiments to be carried out to release the chromophore. Desorption using methanol gave a mixture of three compounds: **14a, 14c,** and **18**. When the resin was warmed prior to desorption, the primary product was **18**. Desorption of the chromophore using ethanol in place of methanol gave **14b** rather than **14a**. Prolonged exposure of the resin to NaCl gave higher amounts of **14b** as well as an additional solvolysis product **14d**. The structures of **14a, 14c,** and **17** were rigorously established using NMR and HRMS. Thus it is proposed that maduropeptin chromophore **12** undergoes solvolysis of the highly unstable epoxide to yield **13** (not isolated), which loses water to yield **14**. The possibility of direct DNA alkylation to yield **14e** cannot be ruled out. Compound **14a** is an active DNA-cleaving agent. Participation of the amide nitrogen in the displacement of the methoxy group with concomitant loss of water would yield the α,β-unsaturated acylaziridinyl enediyne **16**. This would in turn undergo Bergman cyclization and cleave the DNA leaving the reactive aziridinyl compound **18**, which also possesses antitumor activity in its own right. One could also propose that the maduropeptin alternative structure **15** undergoes ready solvolysis to yield **14a–d** or that **15** could dehydrate to give **16** directly.

The chromoproteins are in many ways the most fascinating members of the enediyne family. It is likely that new discoveries will continue to be made. Areas of obvious scientific interest that are as yet unresolved are the structures of the chromophores from auromomycin and actinoxanthin and whether or not the producing organisms for esperamicin, calicheamicin, and dynemicin also coproduce protective apoproteins. The relative stability of these latter compounds permitted their direct extraction from the broth. The success of production improvement studies for esperamicin (see Chapter 10), however, implies that the mutant strains have some method of protecting their DNA from the markedly increased level of drug (50–100-fold). This may be due to more efficient drug efflux, but it is also possible that transport protein up-regulation is involved. It is also interesting to speculate on the evolutionary role of the apoproteins in prokaryotes. The neocarzinostatin, C1027, auromomycin, and actinoxanthin producers are all *Streptomyces* species and produce apoproteins with high structural homology. Kedarcidin, on the other hand, is produced by an unusual organism with characteristics intermediate between *Streptoalloteichus* and *Saccharothrix*. Maduropeptin is produced by *Actinomadura madurae*. Its apoprotein is larger and shows little homology to the apoproteins discussed above. The mechanisms by which these simple organisms have evolved the ability to synthesize apoproteins adapted to binding specific secondary metabolites and, at least in the case of kedarcidin to up-regulate its production, are certainly worthy of further study.

REFERENCES

1. M. D. Lee, T. S. Dunne, M. M. Siegel, C. C. Chang, G. O. Morton, and D. B. Borders, *J. Am. Chem. Soc., 109,* 3464 (1987).

2. M. D. Lee, T. S. Dunne, C. C. Chang, G. A. Ellestad, M. M. Siegel, G. O. Morton, W. J. McGahren, and D. B. Borders, *J. Am. Chem. Soc., 109*, 3466 (1897).

3. J. Golik, J. Clardy, G. Dubay, G. Groenewold, H. Kawaguchi, M. Konishi, B. Krishnan, H. Ohkuma, K. Saitoh, and T. W. Doyle, *J. Am. Chem. Soc., 109*, 3461 (1987).

4. J. Golik, J. Clardy, G. Dubay, G. Groenewold, H. Kawaguchi, M. Konishi, B. Krishnan, H. Ohkuma, K. Saitoh, and T. W. Doyle, *J. Am. Chem. Soc., 109*, 3462 (1987).

5. M. D. Lee, G. A. Ellestad, and D. B. Borders, *Acc. Chem. Res., 24*, 235 (1991).

6. K. C. Nicolaou, and W-M. Dai, *Agnew. Chem. Int. Ed. Engl., 30*, 1387 (1991).

7. K. C. Nicolaou, and A. L. Smith, *Acc. Chem. Res., 25*, 497 (1992).

8. K. C. Nicolaou, *Chem. Britain, 30*, 33 (1994).

9. G. A. Ellestad, N. Zein, and W-D. Ding, *Adv. DNA Sequence Specific Agents, 1*, 293 (1992).

10. M. D. Lee, F. E. Durr, L. M. Hinman, P. R. Hamann, and G. A. Ellestad, *Adv. Med. Chem., 2*, 31 (1993).

11. R. D. Groneberg, T. Miyazaki, N. A. Stylianides, T. J. Schulze, W. Stahl, E. P. Schreiner, T. Suzuki, Y. Iwabuchi, A. L. Smith, and K. C. Nicolaou, *J. Am. Chem. Soc., 115*, 7593 (1993).

12. A. L. Smith, E. N. Pitsinos, C-K. Hwang, Y. Mizuno, H. Saimoto, G. R. Scarlato, T. Suzuki, and K. C. Nicolaou, *J. Am. Chem. Soc., 115*, 7612 (1993).

13. K. C. Nicolaou, C. W. Hummel, M. Nakada, K. Shibayama, E. N. Pitsinos, H. Saimoto, Y. Mizuno, K-U. Baldenius, and A. L. Smith, *J. Am. Chem. Soc., 115*, 7625 (1993).

14. J. Taunton, J. L. Wood, and S. L. Schreiber, *J. Am. Chem. Soc., 115*, 10378 (1993).

15. K. S. Lam, and S. Forenza, This volume, Chapter 10.

16. A. G. Myers, C. B. Cohen, and B. M. Kwon, *J. Am. Chem. Soc., 116*, 1255 (1994).

17. S. Walker, J. Murnick, D. Kahne, *J. Am. Chem. Soc., 115*, 7954 (1993).

18. (a) P. Magnus, S. Fortt, T. Pitterna, J. P. Snyder, *J. Am. Chem. Soc., 112*, 4986 (1990). (b) M. F. Semmelhack, J. J. Gallagher, T. Minami, and T. Date, *J. Am. Chem. Soc., 115*, 11618 (1993).

19. J. W. Grissom, T. L. Calkins, and M. Egan, *J. Am. Chem. Soc., 115*, 11744 (1993).

20. K. S. Lam, and S. Forenza, unpublished observations.

21. P. Van Roey, and T. A. Beerman, *Proc. Natl Acad. Sci. USA, 86*, 6587 (1989).

22. V. Z. Pletnev, A. P. Kuzin, S. D. Trakhanov, and P. V. Kostetsky, *Biopolymers, 21*, 287 (1982).

23. A. Teplyakov, G. Oblomova, K. Wilson, and K. Kuromizu, *Eur. J. Biochem., 213*, 737 (1993).

24. K-H. Kim, B-M. Kwon, A. G. Myers, and D. C. Rees, *Science, 262*, 1042 (1993).

25. S. J. Hofstead, J. A. Matson, A. R. Malacko, and H. Marquardt, *J. Antibiotics, 45*, 1250 (1992).

26. T. Otani, T. Yasuhara, Y. Minami, T. Shimazu, R. Zhang, and M. Y. Xie, *Agric. Biol. Chem., 55*, 407 (1991).

27. D. R. Langley, unpublished observations.

28. M. Ishiguro, S. Imajo, and M. Hirama, *J. Med. Chem., 34,* 2366 (1991).

29. For kedarcidin: K. L. Constantine, K. L. Colson, M. Wittekind, M. S. Friedricks, N. Zein, J. Tuttle, D. R. Langley, J. E. Leet, D. R. Schroeder, K. S. Lam, B. Farmer, W. J. Metzler, II, R. E. Bruccoleri, and L. Mueller, submitted to *Biochemistry.*

30. For neocarzinostatin: (a) H. Takashima, S. Amiya, and Y. Kobayashi, *J. Biochem., 109,* 807 (1991). (b) T. Tanaka, M. Hirama, M. Ueno, S. Imajo, M. Ishiguro, M. Mizugaki, K. Edo, and H. Komatsu, *Tetrahedron Lett, 32,* 3175 (1991). (c) E. Adjadj, E. Quiniou, J. Mispelter, V. Favaudon, and J-M Lhoste, *Eur. J. Biochem., 210,* 305 (1992). (d) X. Gao, *J. Mol. Biol., 225,* 125 (1992).

31. N. Zein, A. M. Casazza, T. W. Doyle, J. E. Leet, D. R. Schroeder, W. Solomon, and S. G. Nadler, *Proc. Natl Acad. Sci. USA, 90,* 8009 (1993).

32. D. R. Langley, unpublished results.

33. A. Zaheer, S. Zaheer, and R. Montgomery, *J. Biol. Chem., 260,* 11787 (1985).

34. K. Edo, M. Mizagaki, Y. Koide, H. Seto, K. Furihata, N. Otake, and N. Ishida, *Tetrahedron Lett, 26,* 331 (1985).

35. J. E. Leet, D. R. Schroeder, D. R. Langley, K. L. Colson, S. Huang, S. E. Klohr, M. S. Lee, J. Golik, S. J. Hofstead, T. W. Doyle, and J. A. Matson, *J. Am. Chem. Soc., 115,* 8432 (1993).

36. (a) Y. Minami, K. Yoshida, R. Azuma, M. Saeki, and T. Otani, *Tetrahedron Lett, 34,* 2633 (1993). (b) K-I. Yoshida, Y. Minami, R. Azuma, M. Saeki, and T. Otani, *Tetrahedron Lett., 34,* 2637 (1993).

37. D. R. Schroeder, presented at 3rd International Conference on the Biotechnology of Microbial Products, Society for Industrial Microbiology, Rohnert Park, CA, April 1993, paper S4, manuscript submitted to *J. Am. Chem. Soc.*

38. K. S. Lam, G. A. Hesler, D. R. Gustavson, A. R. Crosswell, J. M. Veitch, S. Forenza, and K. Tomita, *J. Antibiotics, 44,* 472 (1991).

39. J. E. Leet, J. Golik, S. J. Hofstead, J. A. Matson, A. Y. Lee, and J. Clardy, *Tetrahedron Lett., 33,* 6107 (1992).

40. J. E. Leet, D. R. Schroeder, S. J. Hofstead, J. Golik, K. L. Colson, S. Huang, S. E. Klohr, T. W. Doyle, and J. A. Matson, *J. Am. Chem. Soc., 114,* 7946 (1992).

41. N. Zein, K. L. Colson, J. E. Keet, D. R. Schroeder, W. Solomon, T. W. Doyle, and A. M. Casazza, *Proc. Natl Acad. Sci. USA, 90,* 2822 (1993).

42. (a) J. Hu, Y-C. Xue, M-Y. Xie, R. Zhang, T. Otani, Y. Minami, Y. Yamada, and T. Marunaka, *J. Antibiotics, 41,* 1575 (1988). (b) T. Otani, Y. Minami, T. Marunaka, R. Zhang, and M-Y. Xie, *J. Antibiotics, 41,* 1580 (1988). (c) Y-S. Zhen, X-Y. Ming, B. Yu, T. Otani, H. Saito, and Y. Yamada, *J. Antibiotics, 42,* 12494 (1989).

43. (a) Y. Sugimoto, Y. Otani, S. Oie, K. Wierzba, and Y. Yamada, *J. Antibiotics, 43,* 417 (1990). (b) Y-J. Xu, D-D. Li, and Y. S. Zhen, *Cancer Chemother. Pharmacol., 27,* 41 (1990). (c) Y. Sugiura and T. Matsumoto, *Biochemistry, 32,* 5548 (1993).

44. T. Otani, Y. Minami, K. Sakawa, and K-I. Yoshida, *J. Antibiotics, 44,* 564 (1993).

45. Y. Kumada, T. Miwa, N. Naoi, K. Watanabe, H. Nagawana, T. Takita, H. Umezawa, H. Nakamura, and Y. Iitaka, *J. Antibiotics, 36,* 200 (1983).
46. N. Sakata, S. Ikeno, M. Hori, M. Hamada, and T. Otani, *Biosci. Biotechnol. Biochem., 56,* 1592 (1992).
47. K-I. Iida, T. Ishii, M. Hirama, T. Otani, Y. Minami, and K. I. Yoshida, *Tetrahedron Lett., 34,* 4079 (1993).
48. M. Hanada, H. Ohkuma, T. Yonemoto, K. Tomita, M. Ohbayashi, H. Kamei, T. Miyaki, M. Konishi, H. Kawaguchi, and S. Forenza, *J. Antibiotics, 44,* 403 (1991).
49. H. Marquardt, unpublished observations.
50. N. Zein, unpublished observations.

2

The Biochemical Induction Assay and Its Application in the Detection of the Calicheamicins

Michael Greenstein, Mary Jo Wildey, and William M. Maiese
Lederle Laboratories, American Cyanamid Company, Pearl River, New York

I. INTRODUCTION

Descriptions of the disease process known in the modern era as cancer date back to the days of antiquity. As the earliest natural products scientists, the healers of many ancient civilizations ranging from the most advanced to the most primitive developed various herbal remedies for this disease on the basis of empirical observation. The details regarding these treatments and their effectiveness are for the most part poorly documented. During the past century, however, an understanding of the mechanisms by which the growth of cancer cells can be selectively arrested has begun to evolve. In fact, during the initial half of the twentieth century, high-energy irradiation and chemical agents such as nitrogen mustard were first found to retard the progression of a variety of cancers, and early in the second half of the century it became evident that their effects must be mediated through a specific mechanism of DNA damage. In natural products screening, where one is dealing with complex mixtures frequently containing the active ingredient of choice in submicrogram quantities, this mechanistic handle has ultimately led to the rational design of highly sensitive, selective in vitro prescreens that can predict which samples and components within those samples should have the greatest potential for in vivo anticancer activity.

In 1953, Andre Lwoff (1) elegantly reviewed the phenomenon of lysogeny, in which bacterial strains carry a bacteriophage genome as a latent, repressed unit,

17

called the *prophage,* that is faithfully transmitted to all progeny cells. In his dissertation, Lwoff cited information demonstrating that the prophage could be induced to enter an active lytic cycle leading to a release of mature, infectious phage particles upon treatment with DNA damagers such as radiation and nitrogen mustard. He subsequently suggested that this lysogenic induction phenomenon might be applied as an assay for carcinogenic or carcinostatic treatments. Over the next 10 years, it was shown that a number of natural products with antitumor activity, including azaserine (2) and mitomycin C (3), in fact induce lysogenic phage production.

In the early 1960s, the first serious efforts to apply lysogenic induction as a prescreen for DNA-damaging antitumor antibiotics were described (4–7). The test systems involved the incubation of log phase *Escherichia coli* (λ) lysogenic cultures together with the test compound or sample for as long as 3 hours. After this treatment period, released phage particles and induced bacteria were quantitated in an agar plate plaque assay requiring an additional overnight incubation. The utility of the approach was demonstrated by the observation that one of the antibiotics active in the induction assay, phleomycin, was subsequently effective in a number of mouse tumor model systems (4). It was also clear that compounds indirectly initiating DNA damage, such as the antimetabolite aminopterin, would induce phage development, and that certain categories of compounds interacting with DNA were not active (6).

The versatility of the lysogenic induction assay was significantly enhanced with the development of the biochemical induction assay (BIA) by Elespuru and Yarmolinsky (8). The genetically constructed *E. coli* (λ) lysogen employed in this test system, strain BR513, carries a *lacZ* reporter gene, which encodes the enzyme β-galactosidase, fused to the λ P_L promoter (Fig. 1). In addition, the prophage was made defective in various genes required for complete phage particle

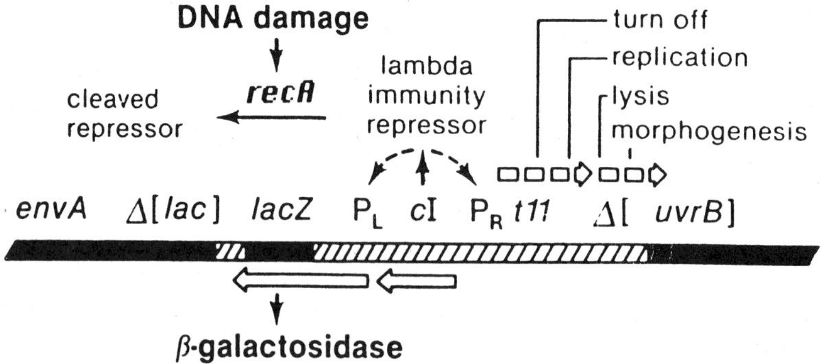

Figure 1   The genotype of *E. coli* BR513 and the properties of this strain related to its production of β-galactosidase in response to DNA damage. (Adapted from Ref. 8.)

development. As a result, exposure to DNA-damaging agents resulted in the induction of β-galactosidase, which is readily assayed in a short time period with a variety of chromogenic substrates. The host strain also has mutations in the *envA* and *uvrB* genes to enhance outer membrane permeability to chemicals and sensitivity to DNA-damaging treatments, respectively. The BIA was developed as both a quantitative, liquid and a versatile, semiquantitative, agar plate assay, which could be completed in only 3–4 hours. At the time of the development of these assays, the agar plate BIA (Fig. 2) was best suited for screening applications and also fulfilled the special needs associated with microbial products programs, including microbial strain and fermentation modification and the tracking of active components during chemical isolation procedures (9). The liquid BIA, originally designed as a somewhat cumbersome test tube assay, was well suited to quantitative enzyme-induction measurements but was not especially practical for screening (Fig. 3). Our enhancement of these procedures was instrumental to our discovery of the calicheamicin family of antitumor antibiotics.

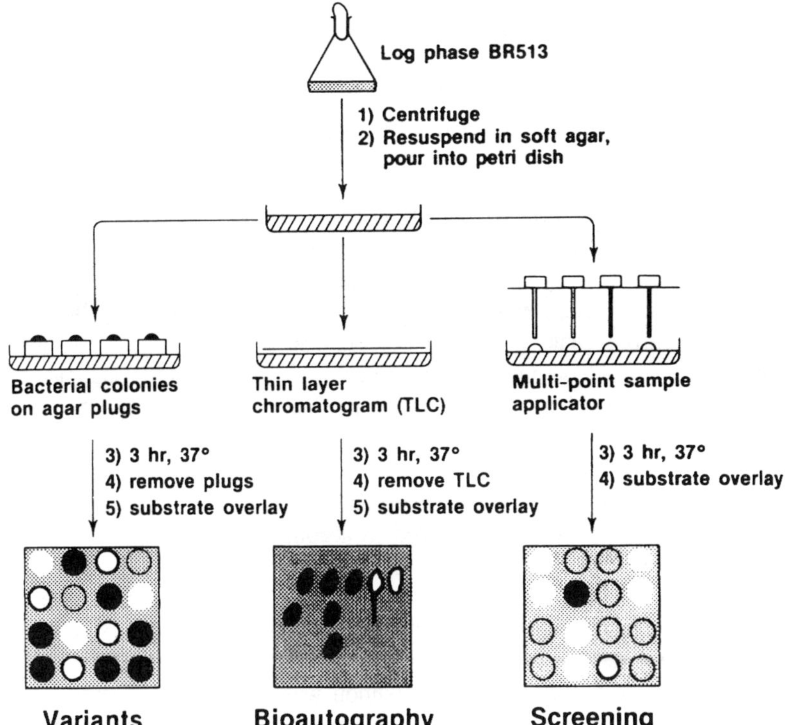

Figure 2 The agar plate BIA and its versatility in natural products research. (From Ref. 9.)

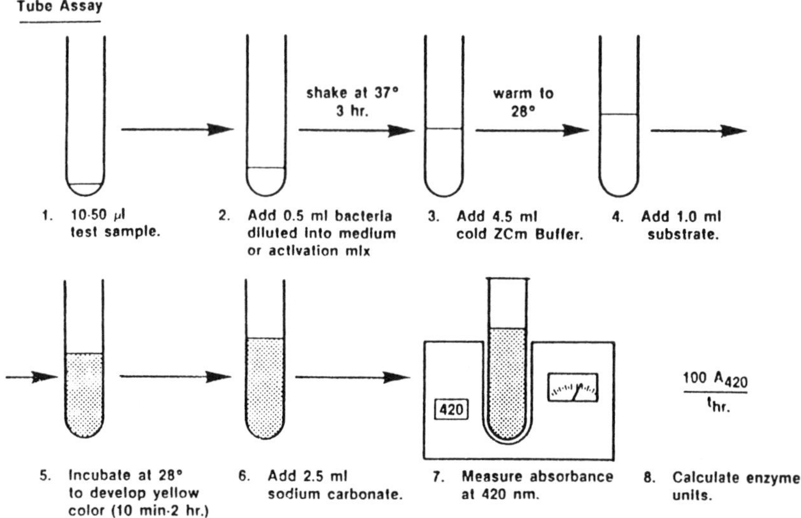

Figure 3   The liquid test tube BIA. (From Ref. 12.)

II. SCREENING WITH THE MICROTITER BIA

In the early 1980s, developments in liquid assay technology were introduced that would revolutionize the drug-screening process. Advances included the introduction of 96-well microtiter (MT) plates, the design of equipment to deliver samples and reagents into all assay wells on these plates in a single operation, and the development of computer-linked MT plate spectrophotometers capable of rapidly reading chromogenic substrate-based enzyme assays. In 1981, we quickly exploited these new tools in our development of a rapid, high-throughput, miniaturized liquid BIA for use in our natural products screening program for antitumor compounds.

Simple yet important modifications were introduced into the liquid BIA to establish an MT version of the assay that could be employed in screening. First, the reagent volumes had to be reduced to accommodate the maximum 270-µl capacity of an MT well. Second, it was recognized that the precise quantitation of enzyme-specific activity called for in the original procedure would have to be replaced with a semiquantitative enzyme determination to provide a simpler, less labor-intensive screening tool. The protocol for the MT screen (10) is outlined in Figure 4. Since timing of reagent addition was critical, and a large number of assay plates was being processed in screening, the Bellco Minispense II dispenser proved to be indispensable to accomplish these operations. The A_{405} of the MT wells was determined using an Artek plate-reading device. This instrument

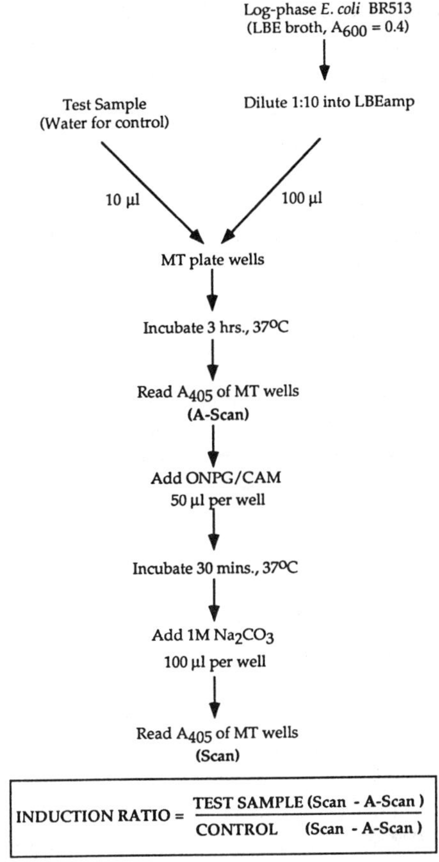

Figure 4 The MT-BIA protocol. LBE and the log-phase *E. coli* BR513 culture used as the assay inoculum were prepared as described in Ref. 8. LBEamp consisted of LBE supplemented with 10 µg/ml of ampicillin. ONPG/CAM contained *o*-nitrophenyl-β-D-galactopyranoside (ONPG), 2 mg/ml, and chloramphenicol (CAM), 50 µg/ml. ONPG yields the yellow-colored product *o*-nitrophenol upon hydrolysis by β-galactosidase. Reagents were added simultaneously to all wells of an MT plate using a Bellco Minispense II dispenser. The A_{405} of the assay wells was determined by an automated MT plate-reading device from Artek Systems Corp.

could read all wells of an MT plate in approximately 1.5 minutes, and the data were stored in a computer (an early model Apple II) that was an integral part of the unit, a feature not available on comparable readers at the time.

The expedient use of this system in screening was dependent upon the design by Artek of a software package, customized to our specifications, which processed our data to permit a rapid selection of actives. We had decided to conduct an initial A_{405} reading of each assay plate after the induction period (the A-Scan). After the half-hour enzyme assay, a second reading of each plate was completed (the Scan). The software then subtracted the A-Scan from the Scan value such that each well was blanked against itself. This computation was extremely important for screening microbial fermentation broths, which can contribute colored medium ingredients, pigments, and cellular material that could interfere with a spectrophotometric enzyme assay. To further simplify the process of locating actives, an additional routine was written, which computed the ratio of each test sample value to that of an uninduced control. In screening, any sample yielding a ratio of ≥3.0 was selected as an active prioritized for further study. Ratios of >0.8 to 1.2 were considered to be inactive and of >1.2 to <3.0 marginally active. In order to avoid missing cultures producing high-potency DNA-damaging activity, which yielded a toxic response in the assay (potentially false negatives), all samples with a ratio of ≤0.8 were titrated in a second test. Very few of the toxic samples were found to be true BIA actives.

The original data from the screening experiment in which the calicheamicins were first discovered are presented in Figure 5. All of the values utilized in the data-processing scheme are clearly depicted in this report. Well number 3-G with a ratio of 8.718 represents our first detection of a culture producing this new family of DNA-damaging antibiotics. It is estimated that the active fermentation sample contained approximately 100 pg/ml of the calicheamicins. Other cultures from subsequent screening experiments were found to produce these compounds as well. In a comparison in the MT-BIA, calicheamicin γ_1^I was found to be roughly four to five orders of magnitude more active than bleomycin (Fig. 6).

In this MT-BIA screening campaign, 256 cultures out of a total of 21,500 tested (1.2%) were detected with reproducible activity. All prioritized cultures were refermented, and those confirming the original activity in the MT-BIA were chemically evaluated for preliminary identification of potentially novel leads.

III. BIOACTIVITY-GUIDED LEAD DEVELOPMENT: THE AGAR PLATE BIA

Although the MT-BIA was employed for primary screening of microbial fermentation samples, the agar plate BIA was still found to be unparalleled in its versatility to support fermentation studies and chemical isolation, purification, and identification efforts. The resistance of this version of the assay to interferences by solvents was a major attribute contributing to its utility for bioautography- and bioactivity-guided fractionation of antibiotic components using various techniques (Fig. 7A). In addition, yield increases could be monitored using the agar plate version of the assay by titrating fermentation broths to an induction endpoint (Fig. 7B).

ARTEK V-BEAM READER

		1	2	3	4	5	6	7	8	9	10	11	12
A-		1- A	2- A	3- A	4- A	5- A	6- A	7- A	8- A	9- A	10-A	11-A	12-A
	SCAN	+0.000	+0.325	+0.350	+0.300	+0.306	+0.312	+0.319	+0.349	+0.350	+0.280	+0.306	+0.359
	A-SCAN	+0.050	+0.214	+0.179	+0.184	+0.184	+0.170	+0.178	+0.176	+0.176	+0.266	+0.167	+0.200
	RATIO	+0.000	+1.144	+1.232	+1.056	+1.077	+1.099	+1.123	+1.229	+1.232	+0.986	+1.077	+1.264
B-		1- B	2- B	3- B	4- B	5- B	6- B	7- B	8- B	9- B	10-B	11-B	12-B
	SCAN	+0.284	+0.298	+0.305	+0.074	+0.331	+0.268	+0.306	+0.320	+0.317	+0.329	+0.324	+0.330
	A-SCAN	+0.155	+0.161	+0.184	+0.253	+0.169	+0.160	+0.168	+0.166	+0.164	+0.165	+0.157	+0.152
	RATIO	+1.000	+1.049	+1.074	+0.261	+1.165	+0.944	+1.077	+1.127	+1.116	+1.158	+1.141	+1.162
C-		1- C	2- C	3- C	4- C	5- C	6- C	7- C	8- C	9- C	10-C	11-C	12-C
	SCAN	+0.297	+0.131	+0.300	+0.327	+0.356	+0.302	+0.331	+0.304	+0.310	+0.365	+0.310	+0.330
	A-SCAN	+0.160	+0.273	+0.170	+0.180	+0.177	+0.222	+0.178	+0.173	+0.179	+0.178	+0.153	+0.173
	RATIO	+1.046	+0.461	+1.056	+1.151	+1.254	+1.063	+1.165	+1.070	+1.092	+1.285	+1.092	+1.162
D-		1- D	2- D	3- D	4- D	5- D	6- D	7- D	8- D	9- D	10-D	11-D	12-D
	SCAN	+0.344	+0.314	+0.305	+0.330	+0.334	+0.327	+0.347	+0.134	+0.196	+0.341	+0.307	+0.311
	A-SCAN	+0.163	+0.175	+0.181	+0.207	+0.177	+0.183	+0.306	+0.261	+0.188	+0.183	+0.167	+0.156
	RATIO	+1.211	+1.106	+1.074	+1.162	+1.176	+1.151	+1.222	+0.472	+0.690	+1.201	+1.081	+1.095
E-		1- E	2- E	3- E	4- E	5- E	6- E	7- E	8- E	9- E	10-E	11-E	12-E
	SCAN	+0.909	+0.333	+0.097	+0.205	+0.310	+0.318	+0.328	+0.346	+0.150	+0.321	+0.322	+0.400
	A-SCAN	+0.175	+0.187	+0.251	+0.210	+0.195	+0.176	+0.255	+0.379	+0.272	+0.174	+0.170	+0.245
	RATIO	+3.201	+1.173	+0.342	+0.722	+1.092	+1.120	+1.155	+1.218	+0.528	+1.130	+1.134	+1.408
F-		1- F	2- F	3- F	4- F	5- F	6- F	7- F	8- F	9- F	10-F	11-F	12-F
	SCAN	+2.258	+0.361	+0.105	+0.344	+0.330	+0.337	+0.322	+0.254	+0.320	+0.320	+0.352	+0.288
	A-SCAN	+0.168	+0.190	+0.256	+0.195	+0.202	+0.208	+0.204	+0.164	+0.179	+0.180	+0.180	+0.171
	RATIO	+7.951	+1.271	+0.370	+1.211	+1.162	+1.187	+1.134	+0.894	+1.127	+1.127	+1.239	+1.014
G-		1- G	2- G	3- G	4- G	5- G	6- G	7- G	8- G	9- G	10-G	11-G	12-G
	SCAN	+2.484	+0.427	+2.476	+2.229	+0.285	+0.285	+0.285	+0.293	+0.286	+0.283	+0.292	-0.287
	A-SCAN	+0.176	+0.302	+0.184	+0.197	+0.166	+0.163	+0.166	+0.158	+0.152	+0.152	+0.151	+0.151
	RATIO	+8.746	+1.504	+8.718	+7.849	+1.004	+1.004	+1.004	+1.032	+1.007	+0.996	+1.028	+1.011
H-		1- H	2- H	3- H	4- H	5- H	6- H	7- H	8- H	9- H	10-H	11-H	12-H
	SCAN	+1.235	+0.312	+0.324	+0.296	+0.283	+0.276	+0.290	+0.288	+0.295	+0.281	+0.277	+0.269
	A-SCAN	+0.177	+0.164	+0.168	+0.165	+0.168	+0.159	+0.162	+0.159	+0.159	+0.157	+0.152	+0.152
	RATIO	+4.349	+1.099	+1.141	+1.042	+0.996	+0.972	+1.021	+1.014	+1.039	+0.989	+0.975	+0.947

```
FILTER   -> 405 NM
BLANK    -> A-SCANNED PLATE
LOT #    -> 000-000
RATIO WELL 1-B = 0.294
```

Figure 5 First detection of the calicheamicins using the MT-BIA. The underscored well contained a sample from our culture that was ultimately found to produce the calicheamicins. In column A on all screening plates, the uninduced control was placed in well 1-B, and the known BIA-active antibiotic bleomycin was included as a positive control in concentrations of 0.5, 1.0, 2.5, 5.0, 10.0, and 25.0 μg/ml in wells 1-C through 1-H, respectively.

CALICHEAMICIN   BLEOMYCIN

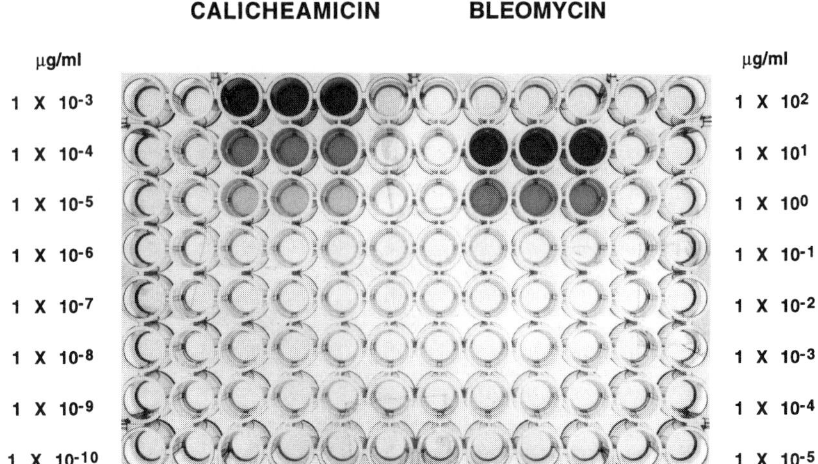

Figure 6 A comparison of calicheamicin γ_1^I and bleomycin activities in the MT-BIA. Serial 10-fold dilutions of the antibiotics were prepared in 50% DMSO, and 10-μl samples of these solutions were dispensed into the wells of an MT plate to yield the indicated final drug concentrations in the MT-BIA.

The protocol employed for the agar plate BIA (11) is presented in Figure 8. The major modification introduced in our procedure involved the bulk preparation of *E. coli* BR513 cell pellets that were resuspended in buffer, held at 4°C, and used to prepare numerous assay plates over a 4-day period during each week. Since it is critical in the BIA that the cells are maintained in log phase, this bulk process had to be conducted with extraordinary care to assure that the cultures were kept at 4°C from the time an A_{600} of 0.4 had been attained until the preparation of the cell pellet suspensions had been completed. This development permitted us to avoid the daily preparation of log-phase cells, which would have delayed the availability of assay plates to our scientists until much later in the workday.

On a routine basis, BIA plates were supplied by a centralized assay laboratory at a rate of 50–75 plates per day to support the studies being conducted on our various screening leads. Plates were prepared early in the morning for distribution to the various fermentation microbiologists and natural products chemists, who applied their samples for testing. Plates were returned at the end of the day for addition of the agar overlay containing the chromogenic β-galactosidase substrate. Each scientist was then able to read his or her results immediately so that studies could quickly progress the next day. The successful use of the agar plate BIA in the development of the calicheamicins was a tribute to the carefully

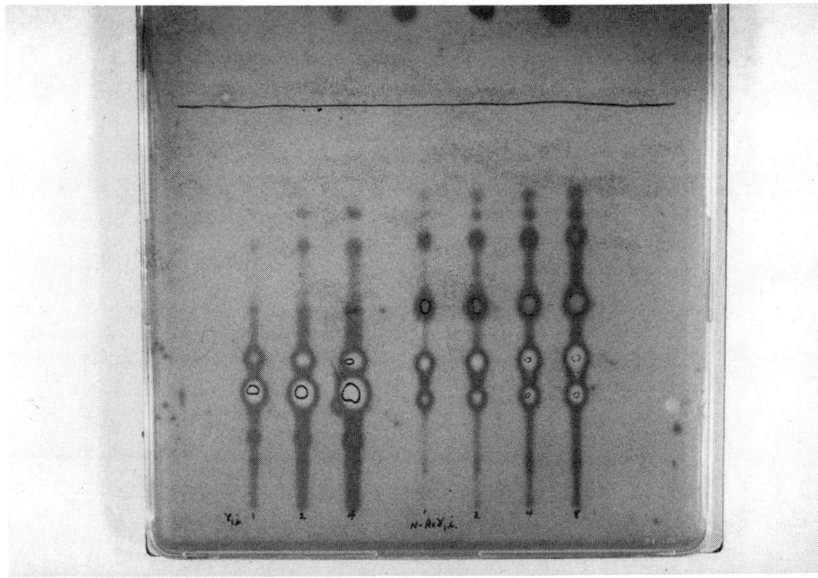

(A)

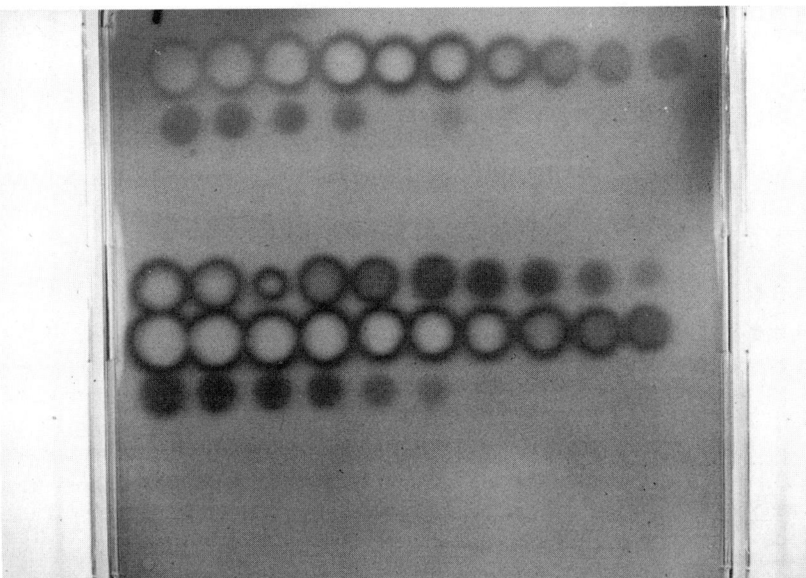

(B)

Figure 7 Applications of the agar plate BIA to fermentation extract analysis. (A) Component profiling by bioautography. (B) Screening for enhanced bioactivity by titration.

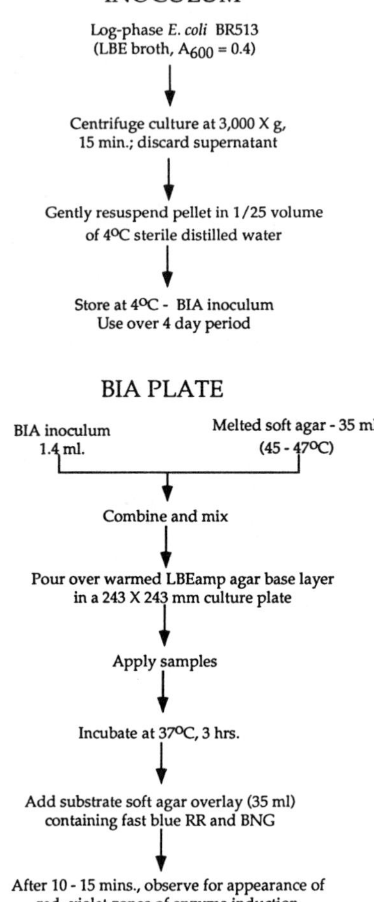

Figure 8 The agar plate BIA protocol. LBE agar and the log-phase *E. coli* BR513 culture used as the assay inoculum were prepared as described in Ref. 8. LBEamp agar consisted of LBE agar supplemented with 10 µg/ml of ampicillin. The substrate soft agar overlay contained 84 mg of fast blue RR and 14 mg of 6-bromo-2-naphthyl-β-D-galactopyranoside (BNG). Upon hydrolysis by β-galactosidase, the BNG enzyme substrate yielded a product that interacted with fast blue RR to produce the red-violet color. As a positive control, bleomycin was spotted on all plates (10 µl) at concentrations of 0.5, 1.0, 2.5, and 5.0 µg/ml.

controlled, reproducible protocol designed by the assay laboratory staff and the spirit of cooperation they established with all other scientists in the program.

IV. CONCLUDING REMARKS

The BIA represents a revolutionary, early application of reporter gene fusion technology in the development of a microbial assay to detect compounds interacting with a specific cellular target. Drs. Elespuru and Yarmolinsky are to be credited with their insight and imaginative use of advanced microbial genetics in providing this useful tool to the scientific community. Since that time, the techniques of molecular biology have made the use of reporter genes a routinely applicable, quickly accomplished process in the development of screens for new drug discovery. New natural products as exciting as the calicheamicins will continue to be found as a result.

REFERENCES

1. A. Lwoff, *Bacteriol. Rev., 17,* 269 (1953).
2. J. S. Gots, T. J. Bird, and S. Mudd, *Biochim. Biophys. Acta, 17,* 449 (1955).
3. N. Otsuji, M. Sekiguchi, T. Iijima, and Y. Takagi, *Nature, 184,* 1079 (1959).
4. J. Lein, B. Heinemann, and A. Gourevitch, *Nature, 196,* 783 (1962).
5. H. Endo, M. Ishizawa, T. Kamiya, and S. Sonoda, *Nature, 198,* 258 (1963).
6. B. Heinemann and A. J. Howard, *Appl. Microbiol., 12,* 234 (1964).
7. K. E. Price, R. E. Buck, and J. Lein, *Appl. Microbiol., 12,* 428 (1964).
8. R. K. Elespuru and M. B. Yarmolinsky, *Environ. Mutagen., 1,* 65 (1979).
9. R. K. Elespuru and R. J. White, *Cancer Res., 43,* 2819 (1983).
10. M. Greenstein, T. Monji, R. Yeung, W. M. Maiese, and R. J. White, *Antimicrob. Agents Chemotherap., 29*(5), 861 (1986).
11. R. J. White, W. M. Maiese, and M. Greenstein, in *Manual of Industrial Microbiology and Biotechnology* (A. L. Demain and N. A. Solomon, eds.), American Society for Microbiology, Washington, DC, 1986, pp. 24–31.
12. R. K. Elespuru, in *Topics in Environmental Physiology and Medicine, Short-Term Tests for Chemical Carcinogens* (H. Stich and R. H. C. San, eds.), Springer-Verlag, New York, 1981, pp. 1–11.

3

Taxonomy, Fermentation, and Yield Improvement

Amedeo A. Fantini* and Raymond T. Testa
Lederle Laboratories, American Cyanamid Company, Pearl River, New York

I. INTRODUCTION

In the early 1980s, a screening program aimed at the discovery of antitumor agents produced by microorganisms was initiated. This program was based on testing of fermentation beers in a modified biochemical prophage-induction assay (BIA), which specifically detects compounds binding or interfering with DNA synthesis (1,2). Active compounds induce the production of β-galactosidase, which is readily detected in an agar assay by a characteristic reddish-purple pigmentation (see Chapter 2).

The discovery of potential antitumor agents by the BIA, while not completely effective in detecting all such compounds, proved to be a useful approach in this program, particularly as it dealt with complex fermentation mixtures. One of the cultures obtained was LL-E33288. The culture was isolated from a chalky (caliche) soil sample collected in Texas, utilizing a medium emended with novobiocin, which is effective for selecting members of the genus *Micromonospora* (3).

II. TAXONOMY

Actinomycetes are generally classified on the basis of their morphology, physiology, cell wall chemistry, and whole cell composition (4,5).

**Present affiliation*: Fermentation Consulting Services, New City, New York.

Colonies of LL-E33288, particularly on dextrin-containing media, are usually yellow to orange and eventually turn dark brown to black as spores mature. This, in conjunction with microscopic examination, which revealed absence of aerial mycelium and presence of single spores on the substrate mycelium, suggested that LL-E33288 was a member of the genus *Micromonospora*.

Lechevalier et al. (6) established that the composition of actinomycete cell walls is particularly useful in determining the generic status of a culture. While nine cell wall types were reported, the most common (I–IV) show the presence of peptidoglycans that contain diaminopimelic acid (DAP). The latter occurs in three isomeric forms, with the *meso* and the L-forms of diagnostic significance. Cell wall types II–IV can frequently be further characterized by the detection of specific sugars found in whole-cell hydrolysates.

Cell wall analysis of culture LL-E33288 showed the presence of the *meso* isomer of DAP, together with major amounts of the 3-OH derivative of the latter. Further, xylose and traces of arabinose were found in whole-cell sugar hydrolysates. The above studies assign culture LL-E33288 to cell wall type II and to type D sugar pattern, which are diagnostic characteristics for the genus *Micromonospora*. Genera other than *Micromonospora* (*Actinoplanes, Amorphosporangium, Ampullariella, Dactylosporangium*) have a type II cell wall, but *Micromonospora* is distinguished by single spores on the substrate mycelium and the absence of aerial mycelium (7).

Parallel morphological studies of various *Micromonospora* species suggested similarities between culture LL-E33288 and *Micromonospora echinospora* ssp. *pallida*, NRRL-2996 (Tables 1 and 2). Comparison studies of carbohydrate utilization patterns and physiological reactions of the two cultures are shown in Tables 3 and 4. In these studies cultures LL-E33288 and *Micromonospora echinospora* ssp. *pallida* were shown to differ sufficiently in spore and substrate mycelial pigmentation, growth on salicylate and at 45°C, and decarboxylation of mucate to be considered distinctive subspecies of *M. echinospora*. Culture LL-E33288 was thus designated *M. echinospora* ssp. *calichensis,* from the caliche clay soil sample from which it was isolated.

M. echinospora ssp. *calichensis* (LL-E33288) was deposited with the Culture Collection Laboratory, Northern Regional Research Center, USDA, Peoria, IL, under accession number NRRL-15839.

III. FERMENTATION STUDIES

Micromonospora echinospora ssp. *calichensis* (LL-E33288) produces a family of compounds with extremely potent activity against bacteria, fungi, and in vivo against experimental tumor systems (8–10). These compounds have been collectively labeled calicheamicins, and the several components produced were assigned letters of the Greek alphabet based on their HPLC retention times (11). The first

Table 1 Comparison of Macromorphology of Culture LL-E33288 and
Micromonospora echinospora ssp. *pallida* NRRL-2996

ISP agar medium	Spores	Vegetative mycelium[a]	Soluble pigments
		LL-E33288	
Yeast-malt (ISP 2)	None	Dark orange-yellow (72)	None
Oatmeal (ISP 3)	None	Colorless—pale orange-yellow (73)	None
Inorganic salts-starch (ISP 4)	Slight border of black spores	Dark orange-yellow (72) to light yellow-brown (76)	Light brownish
Glycerol-asparagine (ISP 5)	None	Pale orange-yellow (73) colorless	None
		NRRL-2996	
Yeast-malt	None	Beige-medium yellow (87m light)	None
Oatmeal	None	Gray-yellow (90, light)	None
Inorganic salts-starch	None	Gray-yellow (90)	None
Glycerol-asparagine	None	Colorless	None

ISP, International Streptomyces Project.

[a] ISCC, National Bureau of Standard Centroid Color Charts, Publication 440, Washington, DC, 1976.

two components isolated and characterized were β^{Br} and γ^{Br}. The Br superscript indicates the presence of bromine in the calicheamicin structure.

Yields from early fermentations of culture LL-E33288 proved to be very low, in the range of ≤ 1 ng/ml, and below the detection limits of the then-current HPLC system. More suitable fermentation conditions and the induction of mutants with improved biosynthetic potential had to be developed to obtain sufficient material for biological testing and structure determination.

The original BIA activity expressed by culture LL-E33288 was detected in fermentations of medium A (Table 5). Slight yield improvements were obtained with various modifications, such as those in media B and C. Since culture LL-E33288 produced only slight growth in these media, an effort was made to increase cell mass in fermentations. Substitution of dextrin as a carbon source resulted in sub-

Table 2 Comparison of Macromorphology of Culture LL-E33288 and *Micromonospora echinospora* ssp. *pallida* NRRL-2996

Agar medium	LL-E33288	NRRL-2996
Pablum	V: Beige	Beige
	S: Slight black	Slight black
	P: None	None
Yeast–Czapek	V: Beige	Beige
	S: None	None
	P: None	Slight soluble brownish
Czapek	V: Beige	Orange
	S: Slight black	Slight black
	P: None	Slight brown
Yeast–dextrose	V: Tan	Tan
	S: Moderate Black	Slight black
	P: Slight dark	Slight brown
Nutrient	V: Colorless to tan	Colorless
	S: Slight black	Slight black
	P: None	None
Nutrient–glycerol	V: Colorless to light beige	Colorless
	S: None	Slight black
	P: None	None
Bennett's dextrin	V: Colorless to beige	Colorless to beige
	S: Slight black	Slight black
	P: None	None
Glucose–asparagine	V: Colorless to light orange-beige	Colorless to light orange beige
	S: None	Slight black
	P: None	None

V, Growth of vegetative mycelium; S, spores; P, soluble pigment.

Table 3 Physiological Reactions of Culture LL-E33288 and *Micromonospora echinospora* ssp. *pallida* NRRL-2996

	LL-E33288	NRRL-2996
Hydrolysis of		
Casein	+	+
Xanthine	−	−
Hypoxanthine	−	−
Tyrosine	+	+
Adenine	−	−
Gelatin	+	+
Potato starch	+	+
Esculin	+	+
Production of		
Nitrate reductase	+	+
Phosphatase	W	W
Urease	−	−

Table 3 Continued

	LL-E33288	NRRL-2996
Growth on		
Salicin	−	+
5% NaCl	−	−
Lysozyme broth	−	−
Decarboxylation of		
Acetate	+	+
Benzoate	−	−
Citrate	−	−
Lactate	+	+
Malate	−	V
Mucate	−	+
Oxalate	−	−
Propionate	+	+
Pyruvate	+	+
Succinate	−	−
Tartrate	−	−
Acid from		
Adonitol	−	−
Arabinose	+	+
Cellobiose	+	+
Dextrin	+	+
Dulcitol	−	−
Erythritol	−	−
Fructose	+	+
Galactose	V	−
Glucose	−	−
Glycerol	−	−
Inositol	−	−
Lactose	−	−
Maltose	+	+
Mannitol	−	−
Mannose	+	+
Methyl α-D-glucoside	−	−
Melibiose	−	−
Raffinose	+	+
Rhamnose	+	+
Salicin	+	+
Sorbitol	−	−
Sucrose	+	+
Trehalose	+	+
Xylose	+	+
Methyl β-D-xyloside	−	−
Growth at		
10°C	−	−
42°C	+	+
45°C	+	−

+, Positive; −, negative; V, variable; W, weak.

Table 4 Carbohydrate Utilization of Culture LL-E33288 and *Micromonospora echinospora* ssp. *pallida* NRRL-2996

	LL-E33288	NRRL-2996
Arabinose	+	+
Cellulose	−	−
Fructose	+	+
Glucose	+	+
Inositol	−	−
Mannitol	−	−
Raffinose	±	−
Rhamnose	+	+
Sucrose	+	+
Xylose	+	+

[a] +, Utilized; ±, weakly utilized; −, not utilized.

stantially enhanced vegetative growth; however, antibiotic yields were further reduced to almost zero.

Other modifications of the media, carbon and nitrogen sources, pH, fermentation temperature, aeration, and harvest times generated few significant changes in yield. The problem of marginal yields was further aggravated by the absence

Table 5 Media Employed in Early Stages of This Study

A. *Seed medium S*

Yeast extract	0.5 g
Beef extract	0.3 g
Tryptose	0.5 g
Dextrin	2.4 g
Dextrose	0.5 g
CaCO$_3$	0.4 g
H$_2$O-TAP	100 ml

B. *Fermentation medium*

	A	B	C
Bacto peptone	0.5 g	—	—
Dextrose	1.0 g	0.5 g	0.5 g
Molasses	2.0 g	2.0 g	2.0 g
CaCO$_3$	0.1 g	—	—
Soya peptone	—	0.5 g	—
Peptone/Marcor	—	—	0.5 g
H$_2$O-Tap	100 ml	100 ml	100 ml

of a simple, rapid quantitation procedure to monitor fermentation beers. Prior to the development of a satisfactory HPLC system, fermentations were monitored as follows:

1. BIA dilution in microtiter plates (see Chapter 2)
2. Agar diffusion assay against *Escherichia coli* and *Bacillus subtilis*
3. Thin layer chromatography (TLC) on silica gel plates (Brinkman) developed in a solvent system of ethyl acetate:isopropyl alcohol (97:3) saturated with KH_2PO_4 (0.1 M), with visualization via bioautography on BIA plates

None of the above were particularly quantitative, but in toto they gave sufficient information to guide the progress being made. TLC followed by bioautography eventually proved to be a very informative qualitative tool as yields were improved (Fig. 1). Using this procedure the effects of media and mutants on the changes of the component ratios of the LL-E33288 complex could be monitored. For example, strain UV 784 was selected for further study as a producer of major components, and strain UV 1523 was selected as producer of the faster-moving minor components.

Since most of the activity produced in fermentations of culture LL-E33288 appeared to be associated with the mycelium, samples were routinely prepared for TLC and HPLC in a uniform manner. Fermentation beers (10 ml) were extracted with an equal volume of ethyl acetate by vigorous mixing in a GLAS-COL vortexer for 3 minutes. The samples were centrifuged, and 5-ml aliquots of the organic phase were pipetted off for HPLC analyses. Similarly, 1-ml aliquots of the same organic phase were transferred to a vial, evaporated to dryness, and redissolved in 50 μl of ethyl acetate just prior to spotting on TLC plates.

IV. DEVELOPMENT OF MUTANTS

Concurrently with efforts to optimize the fermentation media, studies were initiated to develop mutants with improved biosynthetic potential. A spore suspension of parent culture LL-E33288 (NRRL-15839) was plated, and 50 randomly selected single colonies were isolated (labeled NS1 to NS50). Fermentation of these isolates showed a pattern in which those with moderate sporulation were generally better producers of the LL-E33288 complex. Isolate NS6 was selected as representative of this group. Isolate NS12, a heavily sporulating isolate, was selected as typical of the poor producers.

Using isolate NS6 as the starting culture, spore suspensions were again prepared and exposed to *N*-methyl-*N*-nitroso-guanidine (NTG) or ultraviolet (UV) irradiation. The NTG procedure was essentially as described by Delic et al. (12) with a mutagen concentration of 1.0 mg/ml and exposure periods of 2–3 hours. For the UV procedure, spore suspensions were exposed to shortwave UV for various time periods, followed by dilution and plating as described by Fantini (13).

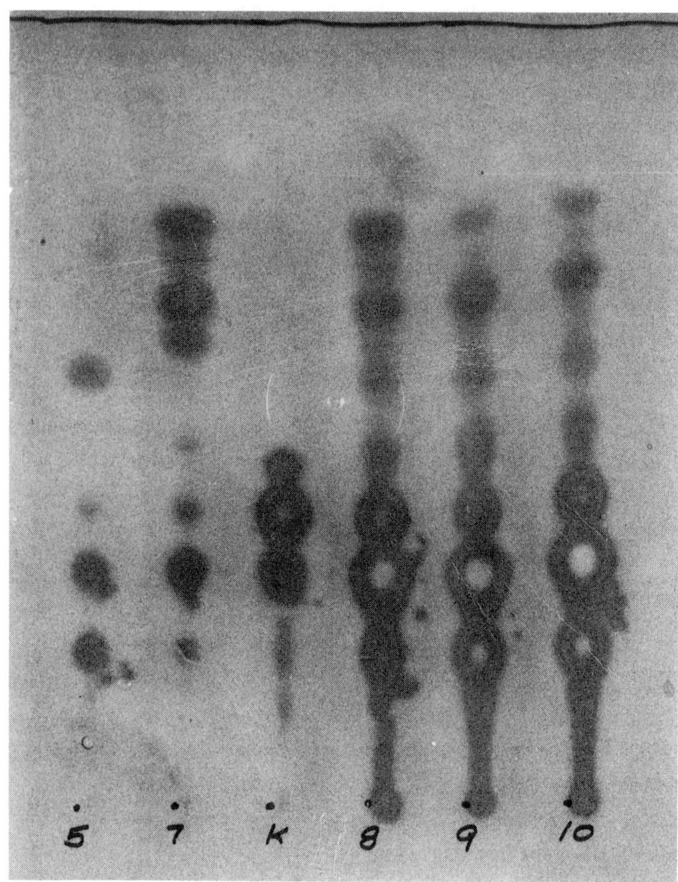

Figure 1   Thin layer chromatography followed by bioautography of extracts of various isolates after exposure to UV light. Lane 5, UV1122; lane 7, UV1523; lane k, control; lane 8, UV784; lane 9, UV959 and lane 10, UV1010.

The energy emitted by the UV source employed was 300 $\mu W/cm^2$, with exposure periods ranging from 45 seconds to 20 minutes. The sequence in the development of the more significant mutants of culture LL-E33288 is given schematically in Figure 2; the number of isolated survivors following mutagenic treatment is shown in parentheses, while key isolates are shown in brackets.

No significantly improved isolates were generated from UV irradiation until exposure times were increased to 20 minutes. One of the isolates obtained from this rather drastic treatment was UV610, which produced yields of about

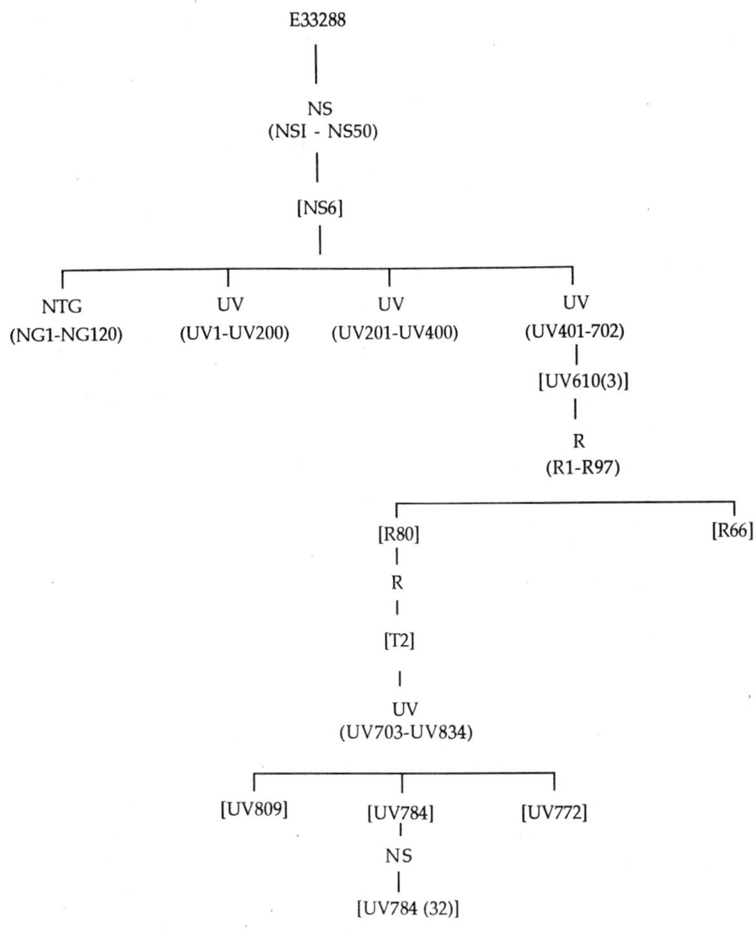

Figure 2 Derivation of key isolates of culture LL-E33288.

0.4 µg/ml. This yield, while still inadequate, represented a 40-fold improvement over that of the parent culture when fermented in the best media then available. Isolate UV610 was then streaked on agar, and subisolate UV610(3) was selected for further mutation studies.

In view of the highly potent antibacterial and antineoplastic nature of the LL-E33288 complex, it was inferred that once a limited concentration of the antibiotic was biosynthesized, it could become toxic or inhibitory to the producing culture, thus limiting further synthesis. An effort was made to obtain isolates resistant to the LL-E33288 antibiotic complex. This type of deregulated mutant has been reported by Unowsky and Hoppe (14) to have enhanced biosynthetic potential.

Vegetative growth of isolate UV610(3) was inoculated to 50 ml of medium #C (Table 5) supplemented with 8.0 μg/ml of LL-E33288β^{Br}. This concentration was severalfold higher than any achieved by fermentation at that time. The flask was incubated at 28°C on a rotary shaker, and aliquots were removed and plated on a daily basis. A resistant population was observed after day 7, and the experiment was continued for 17 days. A total of 97 colonies was isolated (R1 to R97), and isolates R66 and R80 were selected as improved producers of the LL-E33288 complex (~ 4 μg/ml) (Fig. 2).

Mutant LL-E33288-R66 was deposited with the Culture Collection Laboratory, USDA, Peoria, IL, under accession number NRRL-15975.

V. EFFECT OF HALIDES ON FERMENTATION

While fermentation and mutation studies were continuing, isolation of the first major components of the LL-E33288 complex was accomplished. Initial mass spectral analysis indicated the presence of both bromine and sulfur in the chemical structure, and these members of the LL-E33288 family were designated β^{Br} and γ^{Br}, respectively (11).

The discovery of bromine in these antibiotics suggested that this halogen, not a common component of fermentation media except possibly in trace amounts, could be a limiting factor in biosynthesis. Various bromides were then added to fermentation media, but little effect on the yield was obtained. Composition of the best medium incorporating NaBr (medium D) is shown in Table 6.

It was then decided to supplement a fermentation medium with potassium iodide. The most immediate consequence of iodide supplementation was a strong suggestion of improved yields, based on increase in the zones of inhibition in agar diffusion assays against *B. subtilis* and *E. coli,* and the enhanced response detected in the TLC with BIA bioautography. When these same fermentation extracts were submitted for HPLC analysis, however, yields of β^{Br} and γ^{Br} showed little change, but two new peaks chromatographing slightly slower than β^{Br} and γ^{Br} were detected. These new peaks proved to be iodinated analogs β^{I} and γ^{I}. This interesting event eventually led to the discovery of a whole family of iodinated analogs of the LL-E33288 complex (15,16).

Iodides other than KI were added to fermentation media, but none proved superior in producing enhanced yields. Various concentrations of crystalline iodine were also added to media and also resulted in production of iodinated compounds. The composition of two representative iodine-containing media (media E and F) is shown in Table 6.

The supplementation of fermentation media with halides, particularly iodide, resulted in a number of interesting and dramatic effects, several of which are depicted in Figure 3 with strain R66 grown in medium E (Table 6):

1. Fermentation media supplemented with exogenous bromides, and those media not thus supplemented, result in the exclusive biosynthesis of brominated members of the LL-E33288 complex.
2. The major component produced under condition 1. above is β^{Br}.
3. Fermentation media supplemented with iodides produce primarily iodinated members of the complex.
4. The major component produced under condition 3. above is γ^I and not β^I as expected.
5. Fermentation media containing iodides produce enhanced yields of iodinated compounds when compared to brominated homologs in bromide containing media.
6. Fermentation media supplemented with both bromide and iodide salts produce both brominated and iodinated components, but the iodinated members predominate.
7. Preliminary studies based on HPLC retention times suggest that fluoride may also be incorporated when the latter is added to fermentation media as sodium fluoride.

Table 6 Optimized Media for Calicheamicin Production

	Medium		
	D	E	F
Sucrose	2.0 g	0.5 g	1.0 g
$FeSO_4 \cdot 7H_2O$	0.01 g	0.01 g	0.01 g
$MgSO_4 \cdot 7H_2O$	0.02 g	0.02 g	0.02 g
$CaCO_3$	0.25 g	0.25 g	0.1 g
Peptone/Marcor	0.2 g	0.4 g	—
Molasses	0.5 g	0.25 g	0.25 g
NaBr	0.05 g	—	—
KI	—	0.01 g	0.05 g
Casamino acids	—	—	0.04 g
H_2O-Tap	100 ml	100 ml	100 ml

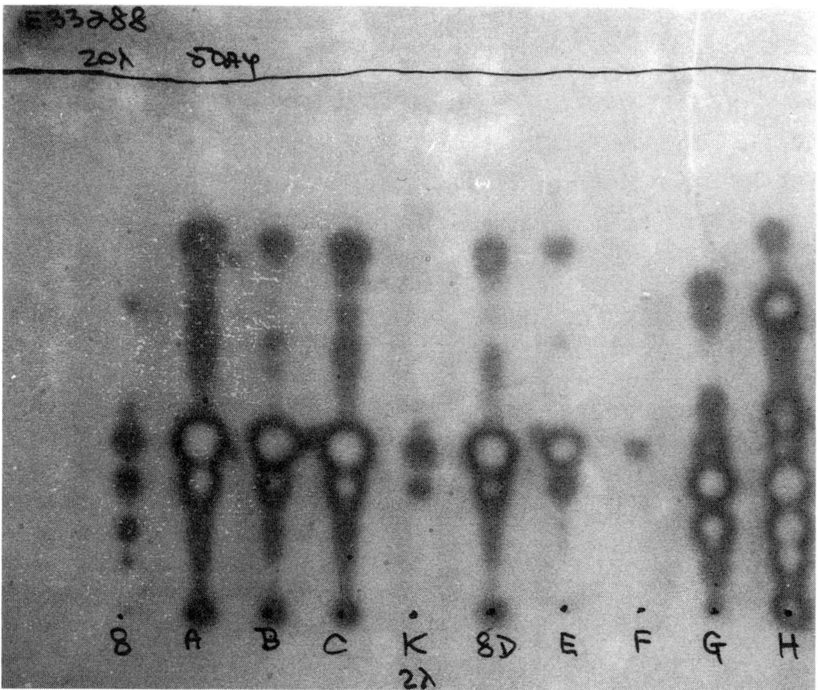

Figure 3 Thin layer chromatography followed by bioautography of strain R66 grown in medium E (Table 6) with the following additions: lane 8, NaBr (0.05); lane A, KI (0.05%); lane B, KI (0.1%); lane C, KI (0.2%); K-control, no addition; lane 8D, KI and NaBr (0.05% each); lane E, KF (0.05%); lane F, Na F$_2$ acetate (0.05%); lane G, NaBr + primagen; lane H, KI + primagen.

VI. DERIVATION OF MUTANT UV784

While improved yields ($\sim$4 μg/ml) of the γ^I were obtained from fermentations of mutant R66 in a KI-containing medium, efforts in the strain development program continued in order to obtain sufficient material for chemical and biological studies. Isolate R80, essentially similar to R66 in its biosynthetic potential, was used as the starting culture. The procedure employed was as previously described and consisted of exposing a vegetative population of R80 to a relatively higher concentration (12 μg/ml) of LL-E33288 β^{Br}.

A spore suspension from one such survivor, labeled T2, was then further exposed to another round of UV irradiation for 20 minutes. From the 131 colonies isolated (labeled UV703–UV834) and fermented, mutant UV784 was selected as an improved producer (Fig. 2). A number of subisolates of UV784 were also fermented and UV784(32), when grown under optimized fermentation conditions, produced yields of 10–11 µg/ml in flasks.

Isolate UV784 was deposited with the Culture Collection Laboratory, USDA, under accession number NRRL-18149.

VII. EFFECTS OF HALIDES ON SPECIFIC PRODUCTIVITY OF CALICHEAMICIN AND ESPERAMICIN

A. Calicheamicin

When the structural relationships between the calicheamicins and the esperamicins became known (17) (Figs. 4,5), a fermentation study was undertaken to evaluate the stimulation by halide supplementation of the specific productivity of the producing cultures (18). This proved of particular interest in view of the lack of a halide constituent in the esperamicins.

While the calicheamicins are produced by a member of the genus *Micromonospora,* the esperamicins are produced by *Actinomadura verrucosospora,* ATCC 39334. The *A. verrucosospora* utilized in our studies was ATCC 27299, Nonomura and Ohara, which is the type strain (1971). The *A. verrucosospora* ATCC 39334 culture was not available at the time of this study.

The effect of halides on production of calicheamicins is shown quantitatively in Table 7. Bromide supplementation gave an increase in brominated γ and β with no effect on growth (packed cell volume), such that a parallel increase in specific productivity is observed. With iodide supplementation, two new iodinated compounds are produced, γ and β, with yields substantially exceeding those observed for the brominated members of the complex. Again, growth is not affected, so

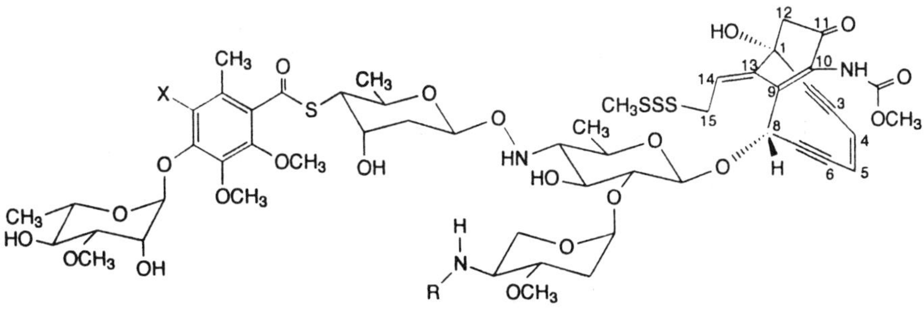

β_1^{Br} R = (CH₃)₂CH   X = Br

γ_1^{I} R = CH₃CH₂   X = I

Figure 4 Chemical structures of calicheamicins β_1^{Br} and γ_1^{I}.

Table 7 Effect of Halides on Production of Calicheamicins by *M. echinospora* ssp. *calichensis* NRRL-18149

Halide added (%)	Components (µg/ml)				PCV (ml)	Specific productivity (µg/ml ÷ PCV)			
	γ^{Br}	β^{Br}	γ^{I}	β^{I}		γ^{Br}	β^{Br}	γ^{I}	β^{I}
None	0	0.001	0	0	1.4	0	0.0007	0	0
BR$^-$ (0.05)	0.7	0.05	0	0	1.4	0.5	0.036	0	0
I$^-$ (0.01)	0	0	9.8	2.6	1.4	0	0	7.0	1.86

PCV, packed cell volume.

that a parallel increase in specific productivity of the iodinated components is seen. These results suggest that in addition to stimulating the biosynthetic enzymes involved in the halogenation of these antibiotics, iodine is utilized as a preferred substrate.

B. Esperamicin

In a parallel study, the effect of halide supplementation on antibiotic production by *A. verrucosospora* was determined using the medium shown in Table 8. Both

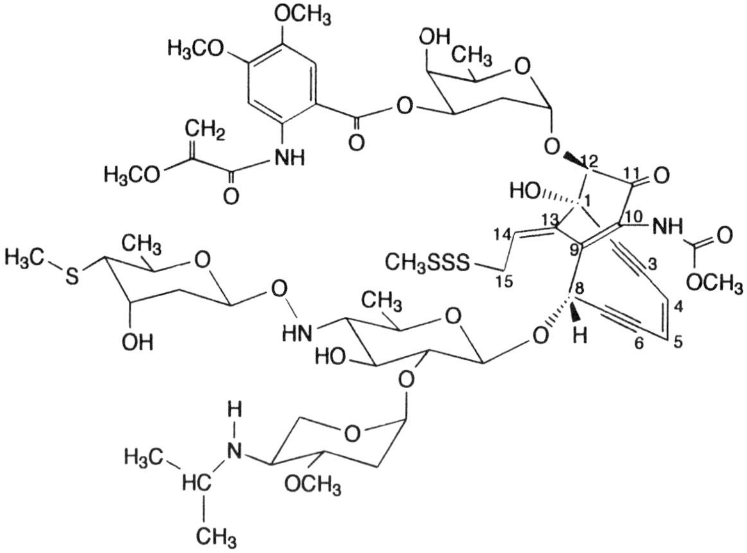

Figure 5 Chemical structure of esperamicin A$_1$.

Table 8　Fermentation Medium (Medium H) for Esperamicin Production by *Actinomadura verrucosospora* ATCC 27299

Dextrose	0.5 g
Molasses	1.5 g
CaCO$_3$	0.1 g
NaNO$_3$	0.2 g
KI or NaBr	0.01 g
Cottonseed flour	1.0 g
H$_2$O-Tap	100 ml

Table 9　Effect of Halides on Antibiotic Production by *A. verrucosospora* ATCC 27299

Halide added (%)	Antibiotic[a] (μg/ml)	PCV (ml)	Specific productivity (μg/ml ÷ PCV)
None	0.1	2.75	0.036
I$^-$ (0.01)	4.1	2.75	1.49
Br$^-$ (0.01)	>5.7	2.75	2.07

[a] Major component.
PCV, Packed cell volume.

iodide and bromide supplementation induce an increase in antibiotic production, no effect on growth, and a parallel increase in specific productivity (Table 9).

Thus, even though a halogen is not a component of the esperamicin molecule, there is a pronounced stimulation in antibiotic biosynthesis. Further, bromide appears to produce a greater stimulation in esperamicin yields, whereas iodide stimulation is greater for calicheamicin production.

VIII.　OPTIMIZATION OF FERMENTATION CONDITIONS

Improved isolates were routinely preserved in cryotubes as vegetative growth at –70°C. Inoculum for fermentations was prepared in two stages: stage I consisted of 50 ml of medium #S (Table 5) in a 250-ml Erlenmeyer flask incubated for 4 days on a rotary shaker (200 rpm) at 28°C, after inoculation with 1.5 ml of the frozen preserved culture. For stage II, a 3.0-ml volume of stage I was transferred to 50 ml of the same medium in a 250-ml "baffled" flask (BELLCO: 2540-00250), which was incubated for 2 days on a rotary shaker (250 rpm) at 28°C.

Stage II inoculum (2.5 ml) was used to inoculate 50 ml of fermentation medium in the 250-ml "baffled" flasks. Fermentations were carried out on a rotary shaker (250 rpm) at 28°C for 6 days. When larger fermentation volumes were desired, the same inoculum/medium ratio was maintained in larger "baffled" flasks (BELLCO: 2540-00500). The use of baffled flasks, both for inoculum preparation and fermentations, in conjunction with increased shaker rpm resulted in increased production of the calicheamicins.

IX. PRODUCTION OF MINOR MEMBERS OF THE LL-E33288 COMPLEX

Other members of the LL-E33288 complex are normally coproduced by fermentation and significant quantities were isolated by Lee et al. (19). Yields of some components were also selectively enhanced by changes in media or by the mutants obtained. For example, greater amounts of the α components were produced by increasing the concentration of peptone or other complex nitrogenous sources in the fermentation medium.

Frequently, mutants of LL-E33288 have shown different responses to changes in fermentation conditions. Normally, isolates R66, R80, and T2 in medium #E (Table 6) produce very similar TLC patterns. However, when fermented in a medium containing fish meal (Fig. 6) mutant T2 displayed a very different biosynthetic potential (lanes 32, 33, and 34). Further, in a fermentation medium with peptone and an increased sucrose concentration, T2 produced substantially altered component ratios (lanes 37 and 38 as compared to 35 and 36).

Mutants UV784(32) and UV772 in media #E and #F produced essentially comparable yields of β^I, γ^I, and δ^I (Table 10). When fermented in medium #G (Table 11), mutant UV772 produced much improved yields of δ^I ($\sim 7.8\ \mu g/ml$), while UV784(32) gave generally poor results. Thus mutant UV772 in medium #G became the combination of choice for the selective biosynthesis of the δ^I component. The composition of media #E and #F is shown in Table 6.

Table 10 Biosynthetic Potential of Mutants UV784(32) and UV772 in Different Media

		Components ($\mu g/ml$)		
Mutant	Medium	β^I	γ^I	δ^I
UV784(32)	E	2.4	8.4	1.0
UV772	E	1.9	8.6	1.9
UV784 (32)	F	8.8	7.5	ND
UV772	F	5.8	6.2	ND
UV784(32)	G	0.7	1.1	0.9
UV772	G	1.7	4.1	7.8

ND, Not determined.

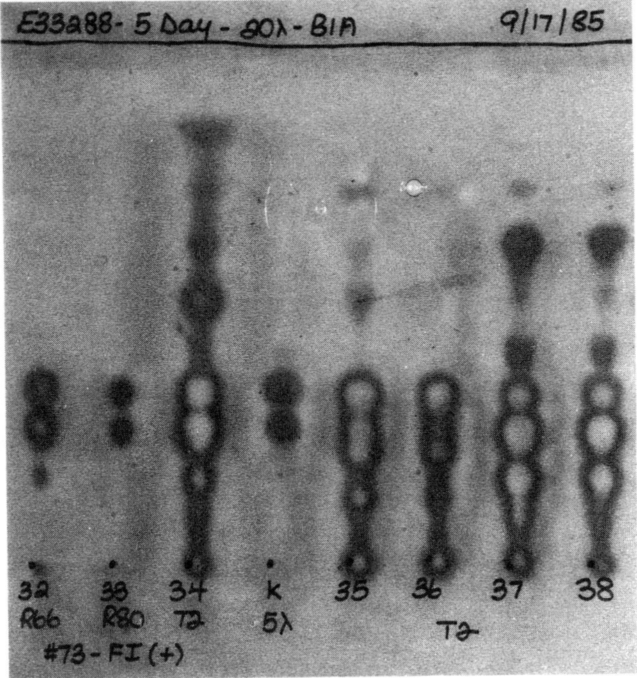

Figure 6 Thin layer chromatography of extracts from mutants fermented in different media. Detection by bioautography.

X. SUMMARY

Culture LL-E33288, identified as *Micromonospora echinospora* spp. *calichensis,* produces a complex of antibiotics designated the calicheamicins with β and γ as the major components. These novel compounds have shown unusually potent activity in vivo against a panel of tumors and in vitro against both gram-positive and gram-negative bacteria and fungi.

Yields from early fermentations were in the range of ≤1 ng/ml necessitating a medium and strain improvement program to obtain sufficient material for further study. Mutagen-induced isolates and the development of deregulated mutants selected for increased resistance to the toxic effects of the antibiotic produced were the major methods used to obtain higher antibiotic yields. The mutants obtained, in conjunction with the development and formulation of an iodine containing medium, resulted in not only significantly improved yields but also the biosynthesis of a whole new family of iodinated members of the LL-E33288 complex, distinct from the originally discovered brominated series.

Table 11 Medium G for
Enhanced Production of δ
Component by Mutant
UV772

Dextrose	0.5 g
Molasses	3.0 g
$CaCO_3$	0.1 g
$NaNO_3$	0.2 g
KI	0.01 g
Meat peptone	1.0 g
H_2O-Tap	100 ml

Table 12 Key Stages in LL-E33288 Fermentation Yield Improvement

LL-E33288	Yield	Comments
Parent	~1 ng/ml	
Parent	~10 ng/ml	Improved medium
NS6	~0.01–0.1 μg/ml	
UV610	~0.4 μg/ml	
R66	~3.3 μg/ml	KI medium
UV784	~5.8 μg/ml	KI medium
UV784(32)	~10.0 μg/ml	KI medium plus increased aeration

The key stages in yield improvement for culture LL-E33288 are summarized in Table 12. Assuming a starting yield of 1 or 0.1 ng/ml, the yields obtained when the laboratory phase of this study was terminated represent a 10,000- to 100,000-fold improvement for the major components of the complex. Additionally, substantial contributions were made in the biosynthesis and induction of several minor components not originally observed.

REFERENCES

1. R. K. Elespuru and M. B. Yarmolinsky, *Environ. Mutagen., 1,* 55 (1979).
2. R. K. Elespuru and R. J. White, *Cancer Res., 43,* 2819 (1983).
3. T. Cross and R. W. Attwell, in *Spore Research* (A. N. Barker, G. W. Gould, and J. Wolf, eds.), Academic Press, London, 1973, p. 11.
4. E. B. Shirling and D. Gottlieb, *Int. J. Syst. Bacteriol., 16,* 313 (1966).
5. M. P. Lechevalier and H. A. Lechevalier, in *Actinomycete Taxonomy,* No. 6 (A. Dietz and D. W. Thayer, eds.), Society for Ind. Micro., Arlington, VA, 1980, p. 227.
6. H. A. Lechevalier, M. P. Lechevalier, and N. N. Gerber, *Adv. Appl. Microbiol., 47,* 47 (1971).

7. G. M. Luedemann, in *Bergey's Manual of Determinative Bacteriology* (R. E. Buchanan and N. E. Gibbons, eds.), Williams and Wilkins, Baltimore, MD, 1974, p. 846.
8. A. A. Fantini, J. D. Korshalla, F. Pinho, N. A. Kuck, M. J. Mroczenski-Wildey, M. Greenstein, W. M. Maiese, and R. T. Testa, Abstracts of the 26th Interscience Conference on Antimicrobial Agents and Chemotherapy, New Orleans, LA, 1986, p. 137.
9. J. P. Thomas, S. G. Garvajal, H. L. Lindsay, R. V. Citarella, R. E. Wallace, M. D. Lee, and F. E. Durr, Abstracts of the 26th Interscience Conference on Antimicrobial Agents and Chemotherapy, New Orleans, LA, 1986, p. 138.
10. W. M. Maiese, M. P. Lechevalier, H. A. Lechevalier, J. D. Korshalla, N. Kuck, A. A. Fantini, M. J. Mroczenski-Wildey, J. Thomas, and M. Greenstein, *J. Antibiot., 42,* 558 (1989).
11. M. D. Lee, G. O. Morton, T. S. Dunn, D. R. Williams, J. K. Manning, M. Siegel, C. C. Chang, and D. B. Borders, Abstracts of the 26th Interscience Conference on Antimicrobial Agents and Chemotherapy, New Orleans, LA, 1986, p. 137.
12. V. Delic, D. A. Hopwood, and E. J. Friend, *Mutat. Res., 9,* 167 (1970).
13. A. A. Fantini, in *Antibiotics, Methods in Enzymology* (J. H. Hash, ed.), Academic Press, New York, 1975, p. 24.
14. J. Unowsky and D. C. Hoppe, *J. Antibiot., 31,* 662 (1978).
15. M. D. Lee, T. S. Dunne, M. M. Siegel, C. C. Chang, G. O. Morton, and D. B. Borders, *J. Am. Chem. Soc., 109,* 3464 (1987).
16. M. D. Lee, T. S. Dunne, C. C. Chang, G. A. Ellestad, M. M. Siegel, G. O. Morton, W. J. McGahren, and D. B. Borders, *J. Am. Chem. Soc., 109,* 3466 (1987).
17. J. Golic, J. Clardy, G. Dubay, G. Groeneworld, H. Kawaguchi, M. Konishi, B. Krishinan, H. Ohkuma, K. Saitoh, and T. W. Doyle, *J. Am. Chem. Soc., 109,* 3469 (1987).
18. A. A. Fantini, W. M. Maiese, and M. Greenstein, Abstracts of the 27th Interscience Conference on Antimicrobial Agents and Chemotherapy, New York, 1987, p. 150.
19. M. D. Lee, J. K. Manning, D. R. Williams, N. A. Kuck, R. T. Testa, and D. B. Borders, *J. Antibiot., 42,* 1070 (1989).

4

Identification, Isolation, and Structure Determination

May D. Lee
Microcide Pharmaceuticals, Inc., Mountain View, California

I. INTRODUCTION

The calicheamicins were discovered in the mid-1980s through the use of the biochemical induction assay (BIA) (see Chapter 1). At least 15 distinct calicheamicin components were produced by the fermentations of different strains of *Micromonospora echinospira* spp. *calichensis*. Only seven of these were isolated in large enough quantity to be fully characterized; their chemical structures are shown in Figure 1. Details of the isolation and structure elucidation of these compounds have been reported (1–3). This chapter will focus on aspects of identification and discovery that have not been published before and the interesting chemistry discovered during the structure elucidation.

II. IDENTIFICATION OF THE CALICHEAMICINS AS NEW ENTITIES OF INTEREST

The screening approach that led to the discovery of the calicheamicins at the Medical Research Division of American Cyanamid is summarized in Figure 2. Key to the approach was the use of the BIA as the primary assay and P388 and B16 tumor-bearing animal models as the confirmatory test. Only those cultures that yielded preparations with T/C > 150 for P388 and T/C > 125 for B16 progressed beyond the screening stage. During the 2-year period, the fermentation

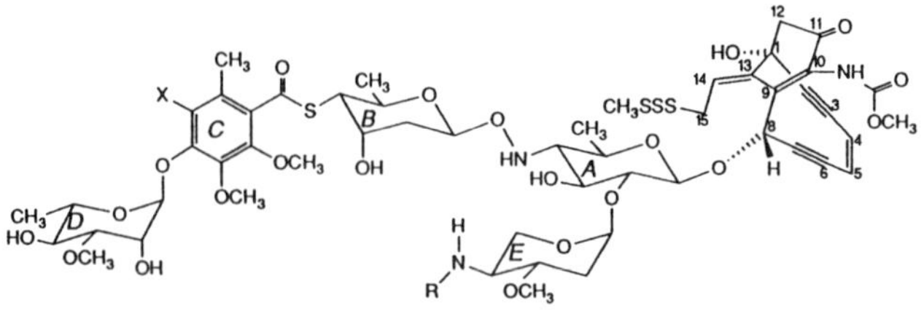

Calicheamicin β_1^{Br} (1)	R = $(CH_3)_2CH$	X = Br
Calicheamicin γ_1^{Br} (2)	R = CH_3CH_2	X = Br
Calicheamicin β_1^{I} (3)	R = $(CH_3)_2CH$	X = I
Calicheamicin γ_1^{I} (4)	R = CH_3CH_2	X = I
Calicheamicin δ_1^{I} (5)	R = CH_3	X = I

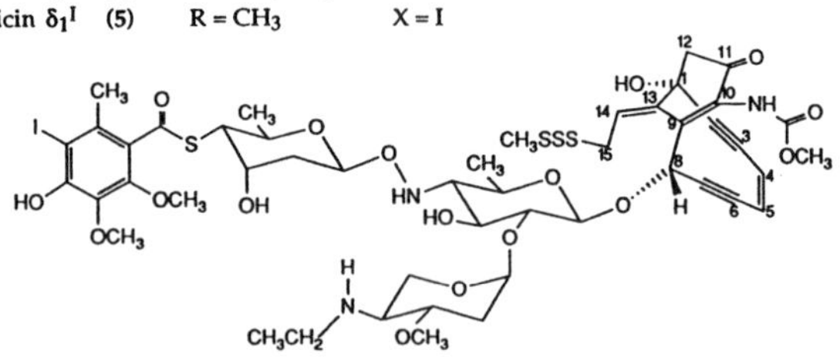

Calicheamicin α_2^{I} (6)

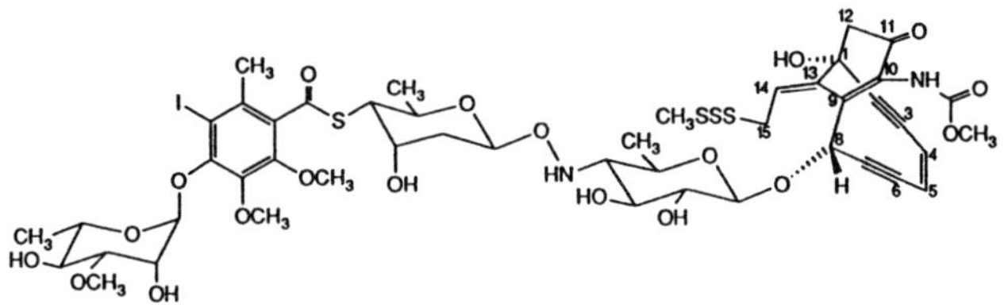

Calicheamicin α_3^{I} (7)

Figure 1 Chemical structures of calicheamicins β_1^{Br}, γ_1^{Br}, β_1^{I}, γ_1^{I}, δ_1^{I}, α_2^{I}, and α_3^{I}.

broths of approximately 22,000 cultures were screened. Cultures (3–5%) yielding BIA-positive fermentation broths were refermented and reassayed, and the broths with confirmed activity in the BIA (25–40%) progressed into the dereplication stage.

The goal of our program was to discover BIA-positive antitumor agents of novel chemical structures. We were not interested in new agents of known structure classes or agents of macromolecular nature. A dereplication scheme was set up using whole fermentation extracts which had been partially purified by Sep-Pak C_{18} cartridges. These samples were analyzed by three HPLC systems to identify the presence of members of the anthracycline, the mitomycin, the streptonigrin, the kidamycin, and the bleomycin families of known BIA-positive antitumor agents. The macromolecular BIA-active agents in general did not absorb on C_{18}-bonded silica and did not pass through 10,000 MW cut-off

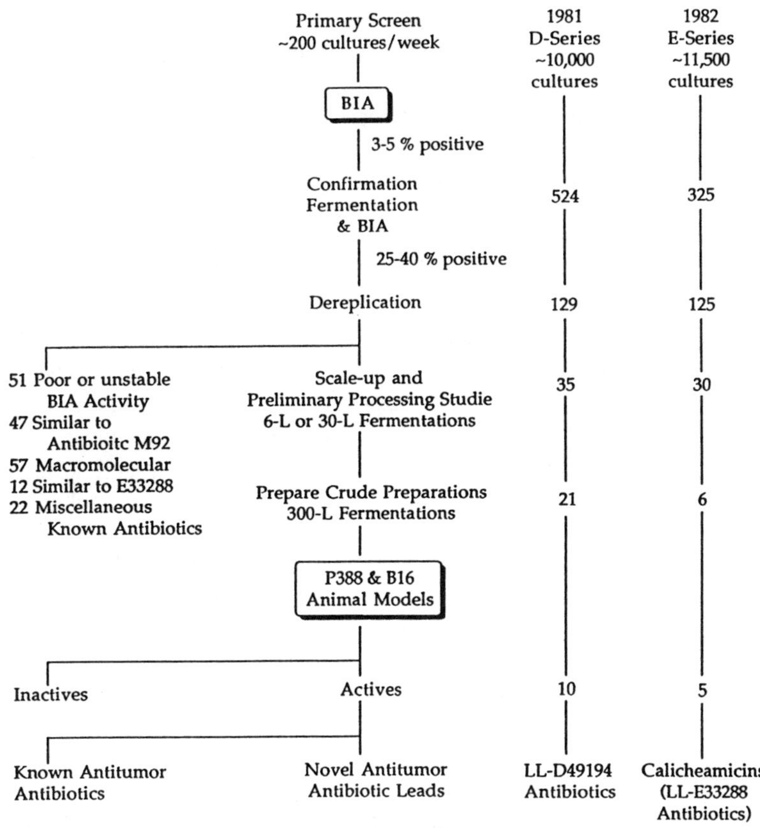

Figure 2 The screening approach used for the discovery of the calicheamicins.

ultrafilitration membranes. The biological activities of the unidentified samples were then evaluated by BIA and antibacterial assay against sensitive gram-negative and gram-positive bacteria. Attempts were then made to prioritize and to group these cultures producing potentially novel BIA-positive agents in order to eliminate duplicates based on all of the information collected and the morphology of the producing organisms. Cultures passed the scrutiny were scaled up in 30-liter fermenters for preliminary processing studies and further chemical identification (the LL-D49194 antibiotics were identified new but related to the trioxacarcins at this stage) (4). Those scaled up successfully and remained unidentified were fermented in 300-liter fermenters to prepare enough material for evaluation in murine tumor models P388 and B16. The test results of a preparation derived from culture LL-E33288 were outstanding, showing potency and efficacy comparable to that of adriamycin. Since the preparation was estimated to contain less than 1% of the compounds responsible for the BIA activity, and the BIA activity could be distinguished from other antitumor antibiotics in the literature, we knew we had an extremely potent novel antitumor agent in our hand, and the isolation and characterization of these new antibiotics, the calicheamicins, became the top priority of our program.

III. ISOLATION OF THE BROMINATED CALICHEAMICINS

Large-scale (300-, 1500-, 3000-liter) production of the calicheamicins by the parent culture LL-E33288 (NRRL 15839) were not reproducible. The fermentation titers ranged from approximately 0.001 to 0.1 μg/ml. Most of the calicheamicins (monitored by the BIA in our initial isolation studies) found in the fermentation broths were associated with the mycelium and were recovered by extracting the whole fermentation mash with ethyl acetate. Alternatively, an organic solvent such as acetone or acetonitrile was added to the fermentation broth to solubilize the antibiotics; the antibiotics in the solution were then adsorbed onto a polymeric resin such as Diaion HP20 for further processing. In any event, the crude extracts were further purified by selective solubilization and precipitation to enrich the antibiotic content to at least 0.1% (by weight) before further purification by column chromatography.

Thin layer chromatography (TLC)–bioautography studies of the calicheamicin complex before chromatographic purification showed the presence of three BIA-positive components, named α, β, and γ according to their elution order. As the purity of the complex improved through chromatographic purification, more components could be observed, and the designations α_1, α_2, α_3, α_4, β_1, β_2, γ_1, and δ_1 were assigned. The β_1 [1] component, the major component produced by the fermentation of strain NRRL 15839, was the first member of the complex to be isolated and characterized. An 18-mg sample was isolated through repeated column chromatography using silica gel, Sephadex LH-20, and C_{18}-bonded silica, starting with a 26-g sample (containing $\sim$0.3% of β_1) derived from a 1500-liter fermentation containing $\sim$0.1 μg/ml of the antibiotic (5). The γ_1 [2] component was isolated from a later fermentation after we perfected the solation technique.

IV. RECOGNITION OF A NEW STRUCTURAL CLASS

Evaluation of calicheamicin β_1 revealed that it was active in the BIA and against gram-positive bacteria at concentrations of <1 ng/ml and was approximately 4000-fold more active than adriamycin when evaluated in p388 and B16 animal models. The presence of bromine in calicheamicin β_1 was first suggested by low mass fragment ions (EIMS) exhibiting typical bromine isotope pattern and was confirmed by electron spectroscopy for chemical analysis (ESCA), which, in addition, revealed the presence of sulfur and nitrogen. The extreme potency and the presence of both sulfur and bromine placed calicheamicin β_1 outside of any known chemical structure class. It, in fact, was exactly what our screening program was searching for. The NMR data of the β_1 component was complex and suggested a molecular weight of > 1000 as well as the presence of a number of glycosides. All the observations indicated that it would be a real challenge to determine its chemical structure and that gram quantities of material would be required.

V. DISCOVERY OF THE IODINATED CALICHEAMICINS

A strain and fermentation-improvement program was initiated with the goal of improving the fermentation titer of the new antibiotics of interest, hopefully to > 100 μg/ml, in order to provide material for structure elucidation and further antitumor evaluation. Extracts of fermentations with increased antibacterial and BIA activity were analyzed by TLC-bioautography and by HPLC. In order to detect the β_1 component in the fermentation broth at concentrations as low as 0.1 μg/ ml, each sample of the whole fermentation mash was partially purified as shown in Figure 3A prior to HPLC analysis. The HPLC trace of a sample prepared from a fermentation whole mash (strain NS6) containing 0.3 μg/ml of the β_1 component is shown in Figure 3B.

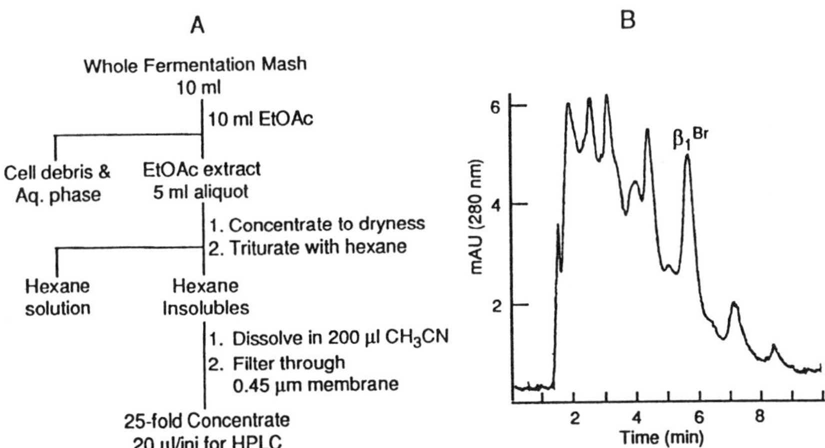

Figure 3 HPLC quantitation of calicheamicin β_1^{Br} in the fermentation broth. (A) Prechromatographic sample concentration procedure. (B) HPLC trace: Sepralyte C_{18}, 5 μm, 4.6 mm $\times$ 25 cm (Analytichem); CH_3CN – 0.2 M NH_4OAc, pH 7.0 (60:40), 1.5 ml/min; UV detection at 280 nm. The concentration of calicheamicin β_1^{Br} in this fermentation was calculated to be 0.3 μg/ml.

A major discrepancy was observed between the TLC-bioautography and the HPLC assay results of fermentations conducted in media supplemented with iodine or iodide salts. The TLC-bioautography results of these fermentation extracts indicated a dramatic increase of the fermentation titers of both the β_1 and the γ_1 components, while HPLC analysis did not show improved yields of either components. Instead, a new peak chromatographing a little slower than β_1 was observed. Could the iodide/iodine-supplemented fermentations be producing an analog of calicheamicin β_1, which could not be separated by TLC but could be separated by HPLC from β_1? More provocatively, could the new component be the iodine analog of calicheamicin β_1? How could we be sure of any of these without actually isolating and characterizing the new component? What we needed was a calicheamicin-specific detector for HPLC—a detection method more specific than the BIA.

During a bioassay development study it was discovered, by serendipity, that the antibacterial activity of calicheamicin β_1 disappeared completely when dithiothreitol (DTT) was added to the assay medium. Is the bioactivity of calicheamicin β_1 antagonized by DTT, or is calicheamicin β_1 unstable in the presence of DTT? If calicheamicin β_1 is decomposed by DTT, HPLC analysis of the above fermentation extracts before and after treatment with DTT would allow us to confirm whether the new peak observed in the iodine/iodide-supplemented fermentations was an analog of calicheamicin β_1. To answer these questions, the stability of acetonitrile solutions of calicheamicin β_1 in the presence of various concentrations of DTT was investigated using HPLC as the analytical tool. The studies revealed that a 1000-fold molar excess of DTT decomposed calicheamicin β_1 completely in 10 minutes; a 10-fold molar excess of DTT decomposed 20, 60, and 85% of calicheamicin β_1 after 2, 20, and 60 minutes, respectively. Consequently, a 50- to 100-fold excess of DTT and a minimum reaction time of one hour was selected for treating the fermentation extracts before HPLC analysis. The HPLC traces of such an experiment using samples prepared from the fermentations of strain R66 (NRRL 15975) using media supplemented with NaBr and with NaI are shown in Figure 4. Results such as shown in Figure 4 convinced us that the new component in the iodide-supplemented fermentation of strain R66 (as well as a number of other strains derived during the strain improvement work) was an analog of calicheamicin β_1 and intensified our interest in its isolation and characterization. The new series of compounds were designated as calicheamicins α_1^I, α_2^I, α_3^I, β_1^I, β_2^I, γ_1^I, and δ_1^I to distinguish them from the original calicheamicin components, and a Br superscript was added to the designation of the original calicheamicin components. When strain R66 was fermented in pilot plant scales, calicheamicin γ_1^I instead of β_1^I was produced as the major component of the complex (Fig. 5). Further laboratory fermentation studies revealed that the ratio of γ_1^I to β_1^I can be changed by varying the amounts and types of nitrogen source used for the fermentation.

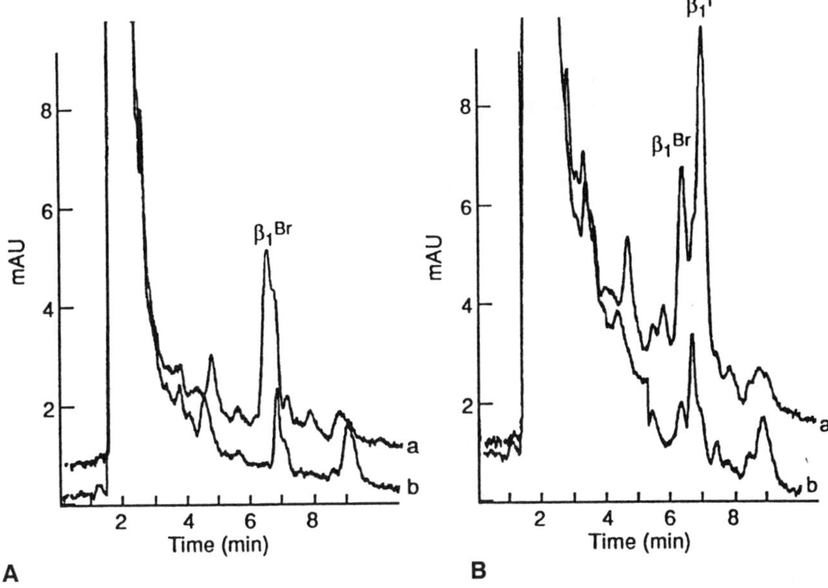

Figure 4 HPLC analyses of fermentation extracts before (trace a) and after (trace b) treatment with DTT. (A) From a NaBr-supplemented fermentation of strain R66; (B) from a NaI-supplemented fermentation of strain R66. HPLC conditions: Sepralyte C_{18}, 5 μm, 4.6 mm × 25 cm (Analytichem); CH_3CN – 0.2 M NH_4OAc, pH 7.0 (55:45), 1.5 ml/ min; UV detection at 280 nm.

VI. ISOLATION OF THE IODINATED CALICHEAMICINS

The iodinated calicheamicins were first isolated from isolate R66. Further strain improvement work resulted in the isolation of strain UV785 (NRRL 18149), which produced ~ 10 μg/ml of calicheamicin γ_1^I. The bulk of the calicheamicins used for chemical, biochemical, and biological studies described in this book were isolated from the fermentations of strain UV785 (which also produced substantial amounts of calicheamicin δ_1^I) as described below and in Figure 6.

The calicheamicin complex was recovered by extracting the whole fermentation mash with one equal volume of EtOAc. The EtOAc solution containing the calicheamicins was concentrated and selectively precipitated to give the crude calicheamicin complex (6.4% γ_1^I, 3.7 δ_1^I, and small amounts of α_1^I, α_3^I, and β_1^I). The individual components were separated by reversed phase column chromatography and further purified by silica gel normal phase or Sephadex LH-20 partition column chromatography. The amount of calicheamicin α_2^I present in the crude calicheamicin complex was approximately the same as that of calicheamicin α_3^I.

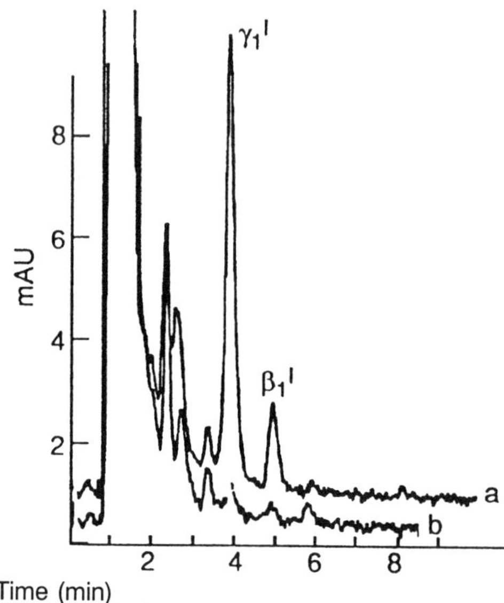

Figure 5   HPLC analysis of a fermentation extract prepared from the broth of a fermentation of strain R66 in a 3000-liter fermenter before (trace a) and after (trace b) addition of DTT. HPLC conditions: NOVA-PACK C_{18} Radial Pack, 4 μm, 5 mm × 10 cm cartridge (Waters); CH_3CN – 0.2 M NH_4OAc, pH 7.0 (50:50), 1.2 ml/min; UV detection at 280 nm. The concentration of calicheamicin γ_1^I in this fermentation was estimated to be 2.0 μg/ml.

However, due to the much higher retention of the α_2^I component in the reversed phase system used to separate the individual components, it was not recovered after the Sepralyte C_{18} column chromatography. In the course of degradation studies, it was found that calicheamicin α_2^I could be prepared from calicheamicin γ_1^I by mild acid hydrolysis.

VII. CHROMATOGRAPHIC CHARACTERIZATION OF THE CALICHEAMICINS

The TLC systems used routinely to analyzed the calicheamicin samples are shown below and the R_f values for the individual components are listed in Table 1.

Adsorbent: Silica gel 60 F254 precoated aluminum sheets (E. Merck)
Solvent system I: 3% 2-propanol in EtOAc saturated with 0.1 M KH_2PO_4 (aqueous)
Solvent system II: EtOAc–MeOH (95:5)

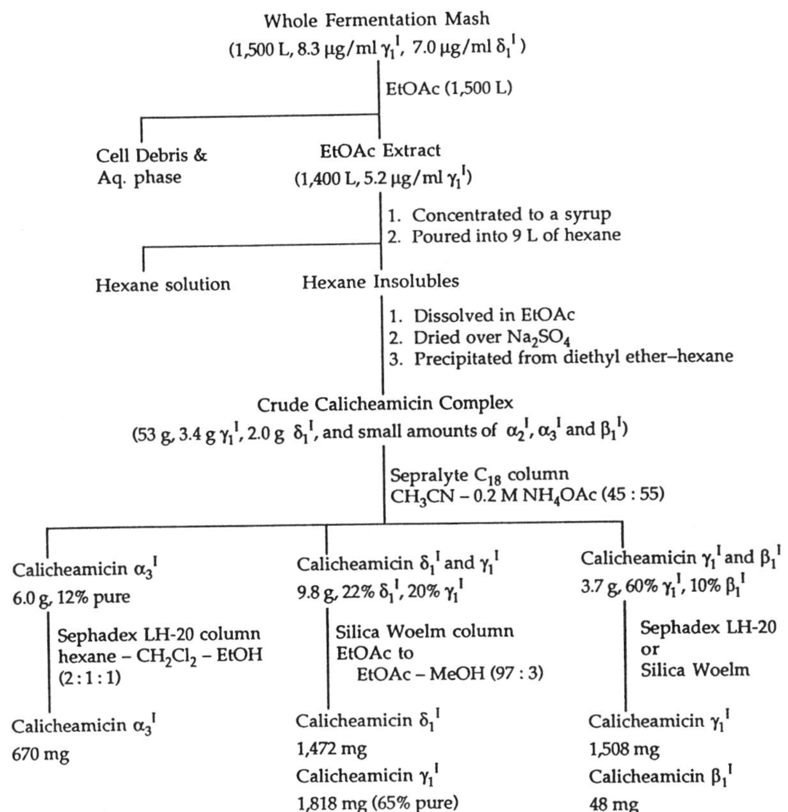

Figure 6 Process for the isolation of the iodinated calicheamicins from the fermentation of strain UV785.

Table 1 TLC Characterization of the Calicheamicin Components

	Rf value	
Calicheamicin components	Solvent system I	Solvent system II
$\alpha_1^{Br}\ \alpha_1^I$	0.80	0.79
$\alpha_2^{Br}\ \alpha_2^I$	0.75	0.73
$\alpha_3^{Br}\ \alpha_3^I$	0.69	0.61
α_4^{Br}	0.64	0.54
$\beta_2^{Br}\ \beta_2^I$	0.41	0.45
$\beta_1^{Br}\ \beta_1^I$	0.35	0.36
$\gamma_1^{Br}\ \gamma_1^I$	0.28	0.27
δ_1^I	0.19	

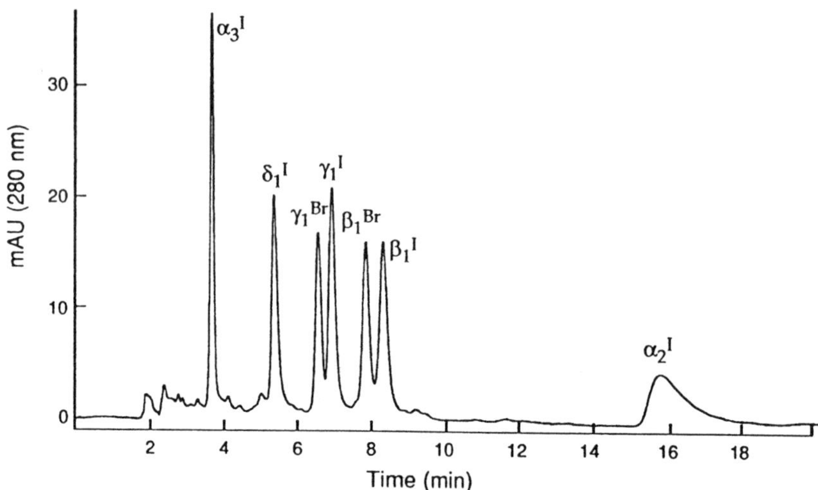

Figure 7   HPLC separation of a mixture containing 0.1 mg/ml of calicheamicin α_2^I and 0.05 mg/ml of each of the other component using the following conditions: Ultrasphere-ODS, 5 μm, 4.6 mm × 25 cm, CH_3CN – 0.2 M NH_4OAc, pH 6.0 (55:45), 1.0 ml/min, 5 μl/inj, UV detection at 280 nm.

The corresponding components of the brominated and the iodinated series cannot be separated by TLC, however, they can be separated by HPLC as shown in Figure 7. In general, it was not practical to separate the brominated components from the corresponding iodinated analogs in preparative scales. Fortunately, the fermentation condition that gave the best yield of the iodinated calicheamicins produced negligible amounts of the brominated components, and when the fermentations were not supplemented with iodides no iodinated components were produced.

VIII. STRUCTURAL DIFFERENCES BETWEEN THE CALICHEAMICIN COMPONENTS

Extensive degradation, nuclear magnetic resonance (NMR), and mass spectroscopic studies were carried out on calicheamicin γ_1^I, the most abundant component of the complex. No chemical degradation was carried out with the other components; instead their chemical structures were assigned by comparing their spectroscopic data with those of calicheamicin γ_1^I. Early in our structure work before we knew the chemical structure of calicheamicin γ_1^I, it was quite evident that (1) the difference between the brominated and the iodinated series was the replacement of a Br atom for an I atom on an aromatic ring (ring C), (2) the difference between the β_1, γ_1, and δ_1 components was the presence of an $NHCH(CH_3)_2$, $NHCH_2CH_3$, or $NHCH_3$ moiety, respectively, on a glycoside (ring E), (3) the same gycoside (ring E) was missing in the α_3 component, and (4) the α_2 component is the γ_1 component without the substituted rhamnose unit (ring D). Some of these structural differences could be readily observed when the ^1H and ^{13}C NMR data of the different calicheamicins were compared side by side (see Table 2 and Fig. 8).

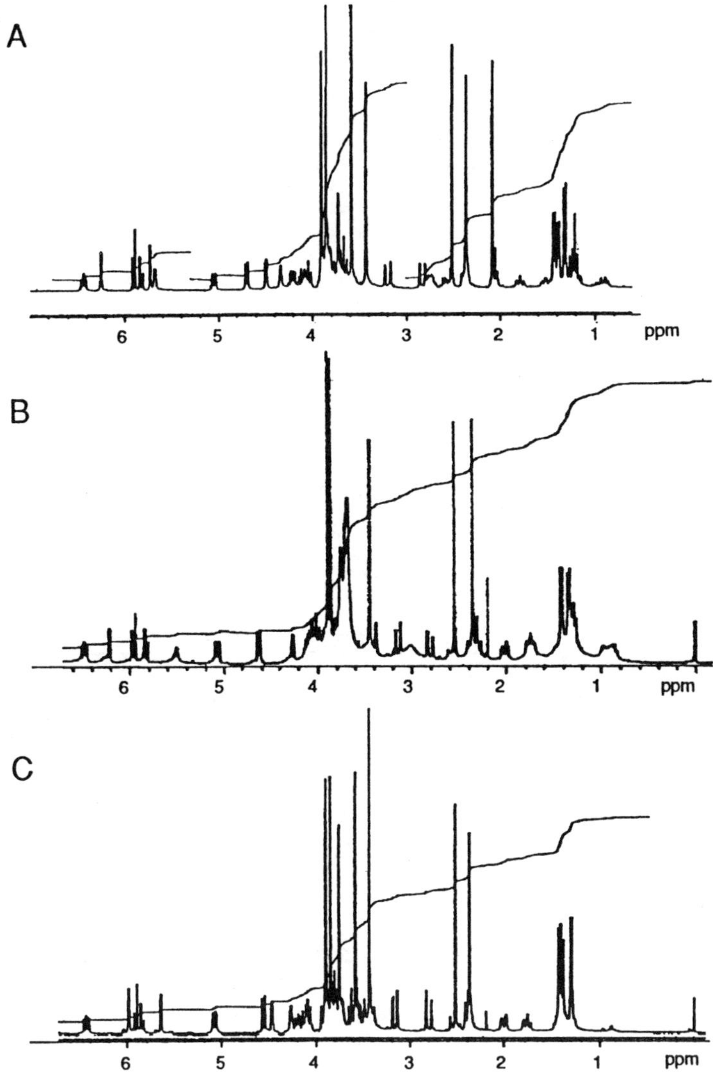

Figure 8 ^1H NMR (300 M Hz) spectra of (A) calicheamicin γ_1^I **[4]** NH_4OAc salt in $CDCl_3$); (B) calicheamicin α_2^I **[6]** $CDCl_3 - CD_3OC$), and (C) calicheaminic α_3^I **[7]** ($CDCl_3 - CD_3OD$).

Table 2 ^{13}C NMR Correlations of Some Calicheamicins

Atom no.	$\beta_1^{Br}[\mathbf{1}]^a$	$\beta_1^{I}[\mathbf{3}]^a$	$\gamma_1^{Br}[\mathbf{2}]^b$	$\gamma_1^{I}[\mathbf{4}]^c$	$\alpha_2^{I}[\mathbf{6}]^b$	$\alpha_3^{I}[\mathbf{7}]^b$	$\delta_1^{I}[\mathbf{5}]^d$
1	72.1 (s)	72.2	71.1	72.2 (s)	71.8	72.1 (s)	71.9
2^e	100.8 (s)	100.8	101.3	101.0 (s)	100.8	101.0 (s)	101.0
3^e	88.2 (s)	88.1	88.4	88.1 (s)	87.4	87.6 (s)	88.1
4	123.4 (d)	123.4	123.0	123.4 (d)	122.7	123.4 (d)	123.3
5	124.4 (d)	124.4	124.9	124.4 (d)	125.1	124.7 (d)	124.7
6^e	83.3 (s)	83.3	82.9	83.0 (s)	82.6	83.1 (s)	82.8
7^e	100.1 (s)^f	100.1^f	98.8^f	100.3 (s)^f	100.4^f	98.6 (s)	99.0^f
8	71.1 (d)	71.1	71.1	71.2 (d)	71.0	70.9 (d)	70.9
9	131.2 (s)^f	131.2^f	131.1	131.0 (s)	131.3^f	130.7 (s)	131.2^f
10	138.8 (s)^f		138.0	139.1 (s)	137.0	136.8 (s)	139.2^f
11	191.7 (s)	192.3	192.5	191.9 (s)	192.8	192.4 (s)	192.5
12	54.6 (t)	54.8	51.1	54.7 (t)	53.8	53.7 (t)	54.5^f
13	145.7^f		146.5^f	145.1 (s)	145.8^f	142.3 (s)^f	146.0^f
14	126.5 (d)	126.4	126.9	126.3 (d)	126.3	127.3 (d)	126.3
15	39.2 (t)	39.2	39.5	39.4 (t)	39.6	39.2 (t)	39.2
15-SSSCH$_3$	22.8 (q)	22.8	22.8	22.8 (q)	22.7	22.7 (q)	22.8
10-NHCOOCH$_3$	154.8		155.6	154.5 (s)	155.5	154.7 (s)	155.0^f
10-NHCOOCH$_3$	52.7 (q)	52.8	52.7	52.7 (q)	53.3	53.3 (q)	52.9
1A	99.7 (d)	99.6	100.0	99.6 (d)	98.2	103.4 (d)	99.6
2A	76.1 (d)	76.2	76.1	76.0 (d)		74.5 (d)	76.1
3A	69.7 (d)	69.6	70.1	69.8 (d)	70.3	70.1 (d)	69.9
4A	66.9 (d)	68.4	67.2	67.2 (d)	67.7	67.1 (d)	67.0
5A	68.4 (d)	68.4	68.23	68.5 (d)	69.6	70.0 (d)	68.2
6A	17.64 (q)	17.6	17.9	17.7 (q)	17.7	18.0 (q)	17.8
1B	99.7 (d)	99.6	100.2	99.7 (d)	100.1	100.1 (d)	99.9
2B	36.9 (t)	36.9	37.6	37.0 (t)	37.4	37.4 (t)	37.2
3B	68.4 (d)	68.4	68.18	68.4 (d)	67.9	68.0 (d)	68.1
4B	51.7 (d)	51.6	51.6	51.8 (d)	51.3	51.5 (d)	51.4
5B	69.1 (d)	69.1	69.7	69.2 (d)	69.7	69.5 (d)	69.4
6B	18.9 (q)	18.9	19.0	19.0 (q)	18.8	19.0 (q)	18.9

1C	130.2 (s)	130.1	130.4	130.3 (s)	127.1	130.4 (s)	130.3
2C	149.3 (s)	150.9	149.5	150.7 (s)	149.2	150.5 (s)	150.6
3C	144.6 (s)		144.7	143.1 (s)	137.1	143.1 (s)	143.1
4C	149.5 (s)	151.8	149.6	151.6 (s)	151.6	151.6 (s)	151.6
5C	115.1 (s)	93.6	115.3	93.5 (s)	85.4	93.7 (s)	93.7
6C	130.8 (s)	133.4	131.8	133.4 (s)	133.1	133.5 (s)	133.5
1C-CO-	192.4 (s)	192.6	192.9	192.4 (s)	193.2	192.6 (s)	192.9
6C-CH$_3$	19.7 (q)	25.4	19.7	25.4 (q)	24.7	25.3 (q)	25.4
2C-OCH$_3$	61.7 (q)	62.2	61.9	61.7 (q)	61.4	61.8 (q)	61.8
3C-OCH$_3$	61.0 (q)	60.9	61.1	60.9 (q)	60.7	61.0 (q)	61.0
1D	102.5 (d)	102.6	103.0	102.7 (d)		103.1 (d)	102.9
2D	68.0 (d)	67.0	69.4	67.2 (d)		67.3 (d)	67.0
3D	81.0 (d)	80.8	81.0	81.0 (d)		80.8 (d)	80.8
4D	71.9 (d)	71.8	71.8	72.0 (d)		71.3 (d)	71.4
5D	70.2 (d)	70.4	70.8	70.5 (d)		70.8 (d)	70.7
6D	17.60 (q)	17.6	17.6	17.6 (q)		17.5 (q)	17.6
3D-OCH$_3$	57.2 (q)	57.2	57.3	57.3 (q)		57.3 (q)	57.3
1E	97.4 (d)	97.4	97.8	97.4 (d)	98.0		97.5
2E	34.3 (t)	34.3	34.0	34.1 (t)	33.1[f]		33.9
3E				75.8 (d)		76.6	
4E	57.8 (d)	57.9	59.3	60.2 (d)	60.7		60.8
5E	62.4 (t)	61.6	61.8	61.3 (t)	61.2		61.3[f]
3E-OCH$_3$	56.3 (q)	56.3	56.3	56.3 (q)	56.3		56.4
4E-NE-$\underline{C}$H$_2$CH$_3$			42.1	42.2 (t)	41.4		
4E-NE-CH$_2\underline{C}$H$_3$			14.4	14.4 (q)	12.0		
4E-NH-CH($\underline{C}$H$_3$)$_2$	47.8 (d)	47.9					
4E-NH-CH($\underline{C}$H$_3$)$_2$	22.4 (q)	22.4					
4E-NH-CH($\underline{C}$H$_3$)$_2$	23.5 (q)	23.4					
4E-NH-CH$_3$							33.3

[a] 75.5 MHz, CDCl$_3$.
[b] 75.5 MHz, CDCl$_3$/CD$_3$OD.
[c] 75.5 MHz, CDCL$_3$, a 1:1 acetate salt of **6** was used.
[d] 126 MHz, CDCL$_3$/CD$_3$OD.
[e] Assignments for these carbons could be reversed.
[f] Low-intensity signals.

IX. MOLECULAR FORMULA OF CALICHEAMICIN γ_1^I

The molecular weight of calicheamicin γ_1^I [4], 1367, was first suggested by a $M+H$ ion in fast atom bombardment mass spectroscopy (FABMS), although the ion current was weak and the accuracy of the high-resolution data was questionable. A molecular formula of $C_{54\text{-}56}H_{73\text{-}77}IN_3O_{20\text{-}22}S_4$, however, could be inferred based on other analytical and spectroscopic data such as ^{1}H NMR, ^{13}C NMR, ESCA, and elemental analysis. N-acetylcalicheamicin γ_1^I [8] afforded an intense $M+H$ ion and its exact mass was determined to be 1410.2954 corresponding to $C_{57}H_{77}IN_3O_{22}S_4$ (Δ 0.26 mmu) and a molecular formula of $C_{57}H_{76}IN_3O_{22}S_4$ for N-acetylcalicheamicin γ_1^I. The molecular formula for calicheamicin γ_1^I was calculated to be $C_{55}H_{74}IN_3O_{21}S_4$ and confirmed, much later, by a second high-resolution FABMS measurement ($M+H$, m/z 1368.2878 Δ 5.7 mmu) using the sulfolane matrix.

X. CHEMICAL STRUCTURE OF THE GLYCOSIDIC SIDE CHAIN OF CALICHEAMICIN γ_1^I

The NMR data of N-acetylcalicheamicin γ_1^I and calicheamicin γ_1^I revealed the presence of four glycosidic units, however, the identity of glycosides could not be determined readily due to considerable NMR signal overlap. Hydrochloric acid–catalyzed methanolysis of N-acetylcalicheamicin γ_1^I (Scheme I) resulted in the isolation and characterization of compounds **9** to **14** and resolved the structures of rings C, D, and E of the intact antibiotic. The isolation of compound **11** was a mystery at the time. None of the above degradation products were BIA positive.

It was of great interest at this juncture to isolate methanolysis products of higher molecular weight and especially those with the portion of the molecule responsible for the BIA activity remaining intact. A number of reaction conditions were investigated, and the study culminated in the procedure shown in Scheme II. A concentrated methanolic solution of calicheamicin γ_1^I was loaded onto a strong cation exchange (Dowex 50W-X8, H+ form) column that had been preequilibrated with methanol. The antibiotic was adsorbed on the resin through ionic interaction with the ethylamino group of ring E. The column was then eluted with large volumes of methanol to affect methanolysis catalyzed by the sulfonic acid residues on the resin. Methanolysis occurred at all possible sites as indicated by the arrows (Scheme II). As the methanol eluted from the column, it carried the methanolysis products with it, effectively removing the extremely acid-labile calicheamicin pseudoaglycon [17] and other reaction products (**9** and its β-anomer and **15, 16** and their α-anomers) from the acidic environment.

The isolation and characterization of compounds **15** and **16** allowed us to solve the structure of the third glycoside in calicheamicin γ_1^I and assign the portion of

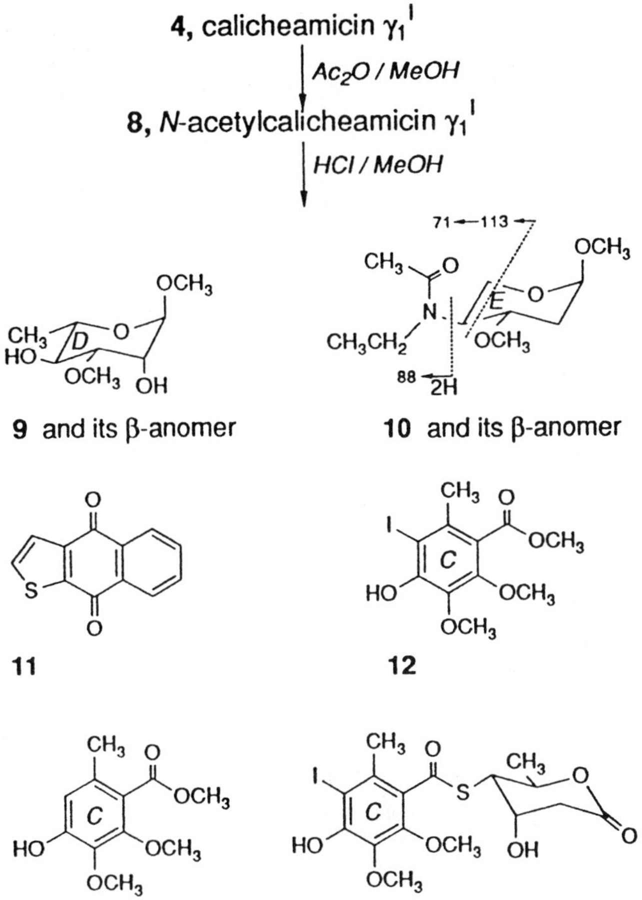

4, calicheamicin γ_1^I

$\big\downarrow$ *Ac$_2$O / MeOH*

8, *N*-acetylcalicheamicin γ_1^I

$\big\downarrow$ *HCl / MeOH*

9 and its β-anomer

10 and its β-anomer

11

12

13

14

Scheme I

the structure containing rings B, C, and D. The NMR data of calicheamicin pseudoaglycon clearly showed that it contained rings B and C as well as another glycoside (ring A) and the aglycon. Careful analysis of the COSY data and the coupling constances of the ring protons allowed us to assign the chemical structure of ring A, the fourth glycoside present in calicheamicin γ_1^I. The attachment of ring E to ring A was first suggested by mass spectral fragmentation patterns and was eventually confirmed by comparison of the A-ring proton chemical shifts of peracetylated pseudoaglycon [17] and the hexaacetate of the glycosidic chain.

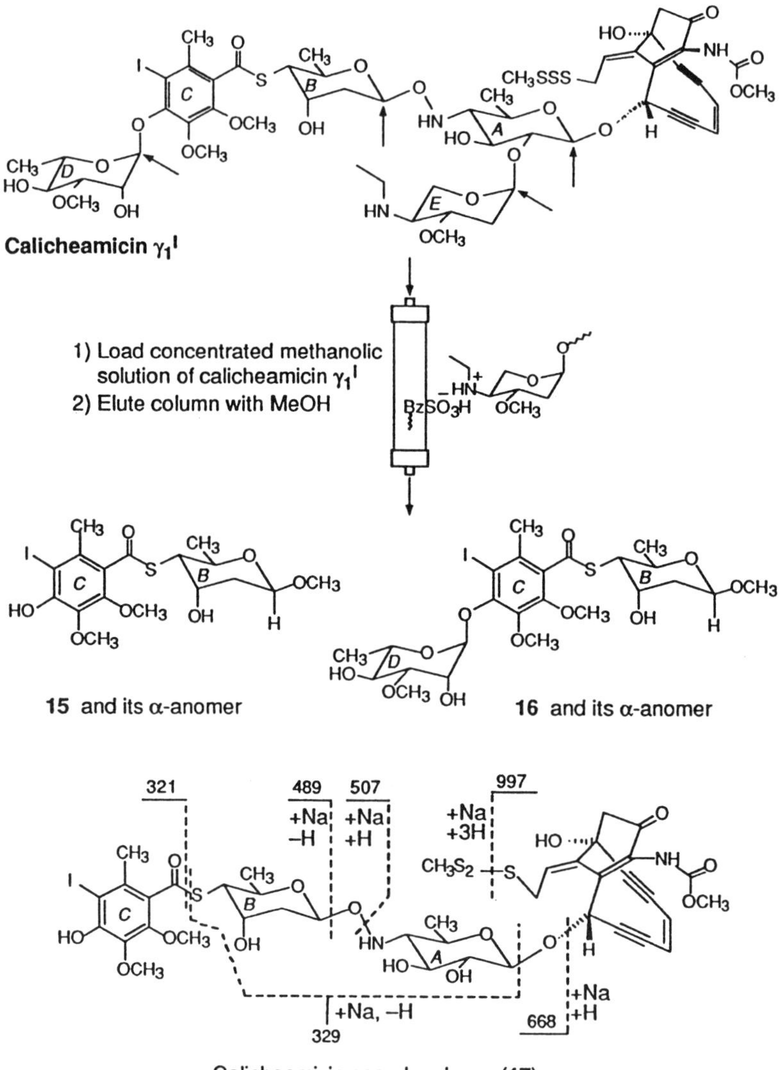

Calicheamicin pseudoaglycon (17)

Scheme II

XI. CHEMICAL STRUCTURE OF THE CALICHEAMICIN AGLYCON

A. NMR Data of the Calicheamicin Aglycon

After assigning the chemical structures of rings A–E, the remaining signals in the NMR spectra of calicheamicin γ_1^I [4] and the calicheamicin pseudoaglycon [17] were attributed to the aglycon (Table 3). Unfortunately, there was very little connectivity information for working out its chemical structure.

B. Reaction of the Calicheamicin Aglycon with NaBH₄/CH₃I

In order to provide one more proton for NMR connectivity studies, compound **17** was reduced with NaBH$_4$ using a solvent mixture of EtOH and CH$_3$I to afford dihydrocalicheamicin pseudoaglycon [18] (Scheme III). Initially, CH$_3$I was used as a cosolvent in order to scavenge any free thiol group that might be generated as a side reaction from the reduction of the thioester linkage between rings B and C. Ultimately, however, it served as a buffer for the reaction. When CH$_3$I was not included, the reaction mixture became too basic for either the starting material [17] or the reaction product [18] to survive. A comparison (Scheme III) of the NMR data of the aglycon portion of [17] and [18] allowed us to identify the following structural units in the calicheamicin aglycon:

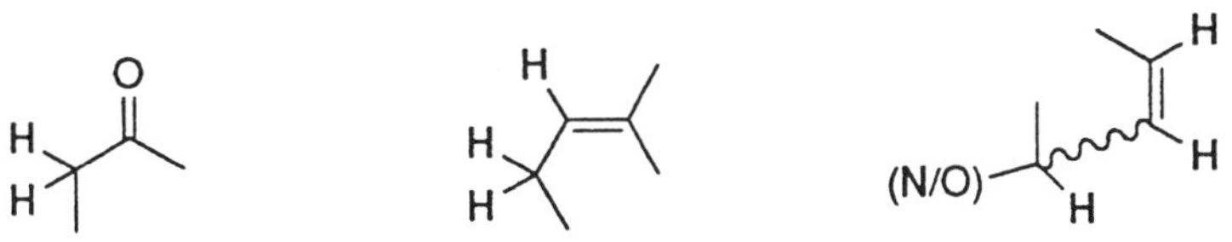

C. Reaction of the Calicheamicin Aglycon with Triphenylphospine

The sulfur chemistry of the calicheamicin aglycon was investigated in order to isolate a major degradation product where the aglycon was transformed or partially degraded. Among many other reactions, calicheamicin pseudoaglycon [17] was allowed to react with triphenylphosphine, and the cycloaromatized calicheamicin pseudoaglycon [19] was isolated. Based on NMR data it was quite clear that the glycosidic portion of the molecule remained intact in the product but drastic changes took place in the aglycon. One intriguing bit of information stood out: the FABMS data indicated that the molecular formula of the product is CS$_2$ less than the starting material, while the NMR data revealed that a methyl group was missing in the product. During the reaction process, three protons from the environment/solvents must have been incorporated into the final prod-

Table 3 ^{1}H NMR (300 MHz, CDCl$_3$) and ^{13}C NMR data of Calicheamicin Pseudoaglycon [17]

Atom no.	^{13}C (mult)	^{1}H (mult, J, intgrtn)	^{1}H-^{1}H COSY	Atom no.	^{13}C (mult)	^{1}H (mult, J, intgrtn)	^{1}H-^{1}H COSY
1	72.5 (s)			1A	103.5 (d)	4.60 (d, 7.7, 1H)	3.64
2[a]	100.4 (s)			2A	74.5 (d)	3.64 (bt, 8.2)	4.60, 3.98
3[a]	87.5 (s)			3A	70.1 (d)	3.98 (bt, 10.0)	3.64, 2.44
4	124.1 (d)	5.89 (s, 1H)	5.93	4A	67.2 (d)	2.44 (t, 9.8)	3.98, 3.79
5	124.2 (d)	5.89 (s, 1H)		5A	69.6 (d)	3.79 (m)	2.44, 1.39
6[a]	83.9 (s)			6A	17.8 (q)	1.39 (d, 6.1, 3H)	3.79
7[a]				1B	99.7 (d)	5.06 (bd, 10, 1H)	1.78, 2.04
8	71.3 (d)	5.99 (s, 1H)	5.89	2B	36.8 (t)	1.78 (bdd, 13, 10, 1H)	5.06, 4.32, 2.04
9	130.6 (s)					2.04 (md, 13, 1H)	5.06, 4.32, 1.78
10	136.3 (s)			3B	68.2 (d)	4.32 (m, 1H)	1.78, 2.04, 3.72
11	191.8 (s)			4B	51.6 (d)	3.72 (dd, 11, 2.3)	4.32, 4.07
12	53.3 (5)	2.84 (d, 16.8, 1H)	3.22	5B	69.1 (d)	4.07 (m)	3.72, 1.43
		3.22 (d, 168.8 1H)	2.84	6B	19.1 (q)	1.43 (d, 6.2, 3H)	4.07
13	140.7 (s)[b]			1C	126.8 (s)		
14	127.5 (d)	6.45 (dd, 9.8, 5.3, 1H)	3.87, 4.12	2C	148.8 (s)		
15	39.1 (t)	3.87 (m)	6.45, 4.12	3C	136.4 (s)		
		4.12 (m)	6.45, 3.87	4C	150.9 (s)		
10-NH<u>C</u>OOCH$_3$	154.3 (s)			5C	84.4 (s)		
10-NHCOO<u>C</u>H$_3$	53.6 (q)	3.77 (s, 3H)		6C	133.2 (s)		
15-SSSCH$_3$	22.8 (q)	2.52 (s, 3H)		1C-CO-	192.0 (s)		
				2C-OCH$_3$	61.5 (q)	3.91 (s, 3H)	
				3C-OCH$_3$	61.0 (q)	3.88 (s, 3H)	
				6C-CH$_3$	24.7 (q)	2.34 (s, 3H)	

[a] The assignments for these carbons could be reversed.
[b] Very low-intensity signal.

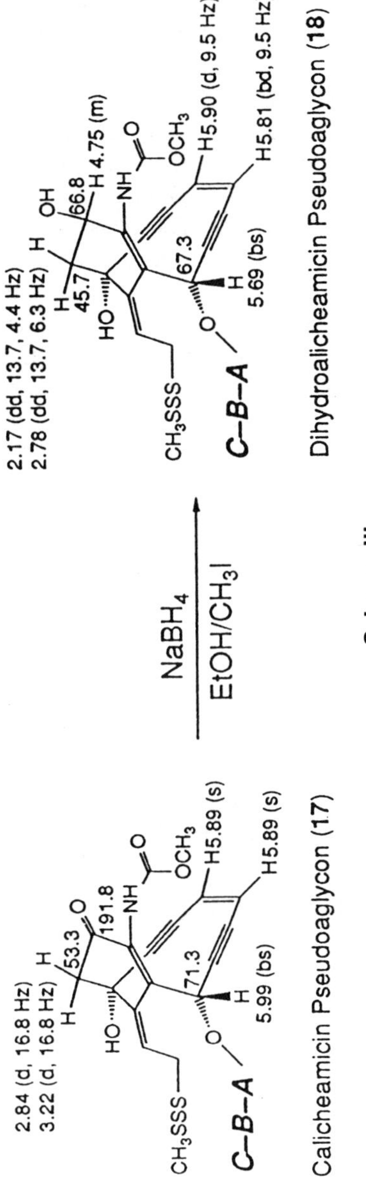

2.17 (dd, 13.7, 4.4 Hz)
2.78 (dd, 13.7, 6.3 Hz)
H
OH
66.8
H 4.75 (m)
45.7
H
HO
NH
O
OCH3
H5.90 (d, 9.5 Hz)
67.3
H5.81 (bd, 9.5 Hz)
CH3SSS
C–B–A
H 5.69 (bs)
Dihydroalicheamicin Pseudoaglycon (18)
NaBH4
EtOH/CH3I
Scheme III
2.84 (d, 16.8 Hz)
3.22 (d, 16.8 Hz)
H
53.3
191.8
O
NH
O
OCH3
H5.89 (s)
HO
71.3
H5.89 (s)
CH3SSS
C–B–A
H 5.99 (bs)
Calicheamicin Pseudoaglycon (17)

uct. In order to locate these newly acquired protons, we studied the cyclo-aromatization reaction using deuterium-labeled solvents. A mixture of CH_2Cl_2 and CH_3OH was used initially due to the solubility of the reaction components. The ^1H NMR spectra of compound **19** isolated from the reaction using CH_2Cl_2/CD_3OD as solvent was identical to that isolated from the initial reaction. The aromatic portion of the ^1H NMR spectrum of the reaction conducted in CD_2Cl_2/CD_3OD showed clearly, however, that two of the four consecutive aromatic protons in the newly formed aromatic ring were deuterated and that the two remaining protons were *ortho* to each other (Fig. 9). Careful NMR analysis in a number of different solvents allowed us to conclude unambiguously that the deuterium incorporation was in the *para* positions of the new aromatic ring. The source of the deuterium indicated a free radical reaction mechanism and suggested the existence of a benzene-1,4-diyl reaction intermediate for the conversion of compound **17** to **19**. When the chemical structure of the calicheamicin aglycon was determined, the cycloaromatization reaction mechanism (see Scheme V) was proposed to accommodate this experimental observation.

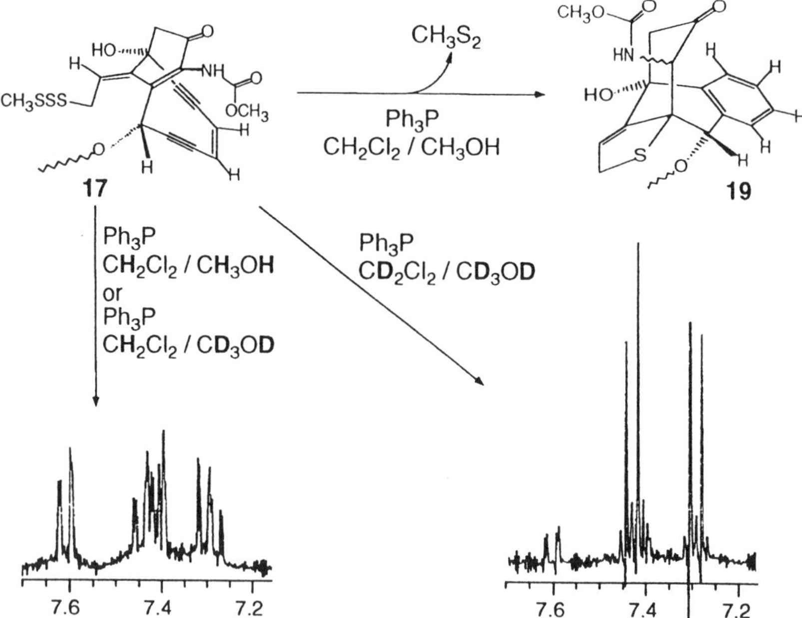

Figure 9 The cycloaromatization of the calicheamicin pseudoaglycon **[17]** in the presence of deuterated solvents. ^1H NMR spectra of the aromatic region of the cycloaromatized pseudoglycon **[19]** clearly demonstrated the 1,4-incorporation of deuterium (see Scheme V) and the source of deuterium.

Extensive NMR studies were conducted on compound **19** and allowed us to assign the structural units shown below to the cycloaromatized calicheamicin aglycon. It was not possible, however, to connect these units unambiguously to form a single structure for the cycloaromatized aglycon.

D. Retro-Aldol Cleavage of the Cyclized Calicheamicin Pseudoaglycon

Since NMR data did not provide sufficient information to assign the structure of the cycloaromatized aglycon, further degradation studies were initiated. Treatment of compound **19** with a saturated solution of K_2CO_3 in methanol at room temperature for 30 minutes afforded compound **11** as the only isolatable product (Scheme IV). In order to isolate the intermediate of the above conversion, the reaction was terminated at 5 minutes by the addition of excess acetic anhydride while the mixture was cooled in a icewater bath, and compounds **22** and **23** were isolated. Compound **22** crystallized out in the NMR tube and suitable crystals were prepared for x-ray analysis. The x-ray structure of compound **22** (Scheme IV) (1) revealed the hydroxyamino sugar linkage between rings A and B, (2) determined glycosides A and B to be in the D-configuration, and (3) provided the basic framework for the structure of the cycloaromatized aglycon. The chemical structure of the cycloaromatized calicheamicin pseudoaglycon [19] was assigned based on the structure of compound **22** and the structural information derived from the NMR studies.

E. Characterization of a Modified Dihydrocalicheamicin Aglycon

Concurrent with the studies described above, attempts were made to prepare dihydrocalicheamicin pseudoaglycon [18] via the Dowex 50W-X8 (H^+)–catalyzed methanolysis of dihydrocalicheamicin γ_1^I. Instead of the expected product [18], des-SS-methyl-dihydrocalicheamicin aglycon [24] was isolated (Fig. 10). The IR spectrum of compound **24** showed a weak absorption at 2190 cm^{-1} for the almost

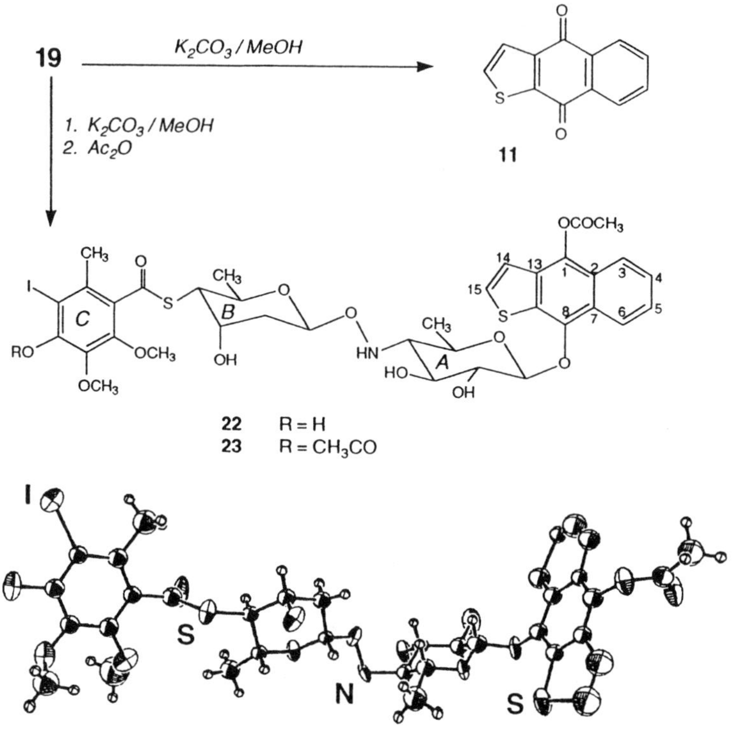

Scheme IV

symmetrical enediyne system—the first and the only time this band was observed during the structural work. The chemical structure of compound **24** was determined based on (1) the careful comparison of its NMR data (including COSY, ^{1}H-^{13}C direct and multiple bond correlations) with that of the aglycon portion of dihydrocalicheamicin pseudoaglycon [**18**], (2) the chemical structure of the cycloaromatized calicheamicin pseudoaglycon [**19**], and (3) the presence of a conjugated symmetrical acetylenic system supported by the IR band described above and the carbons with no attached proton resonating at 86.1, 87.6, 97.7, and 102.0 ppm. The structure of the calicheamicin aglycon was then proposed based on the structure of compound **24** and rationally accounted for the loss of a S_2CH_3 unit during the formation of the cycloaromatized pseudoaglycon (**19**).

A more recent CD measurement of calicheamicin γ_1^I confirmed the characteristic negative Cotton effect (311 nm, $\Delta\varepsilon$ –55; 272 nm, $\Delta\varepsilon$ +63), centered around the dienone chromophore and the absolute configuration of the calicheamicin aglycon to be as drawn in this report.

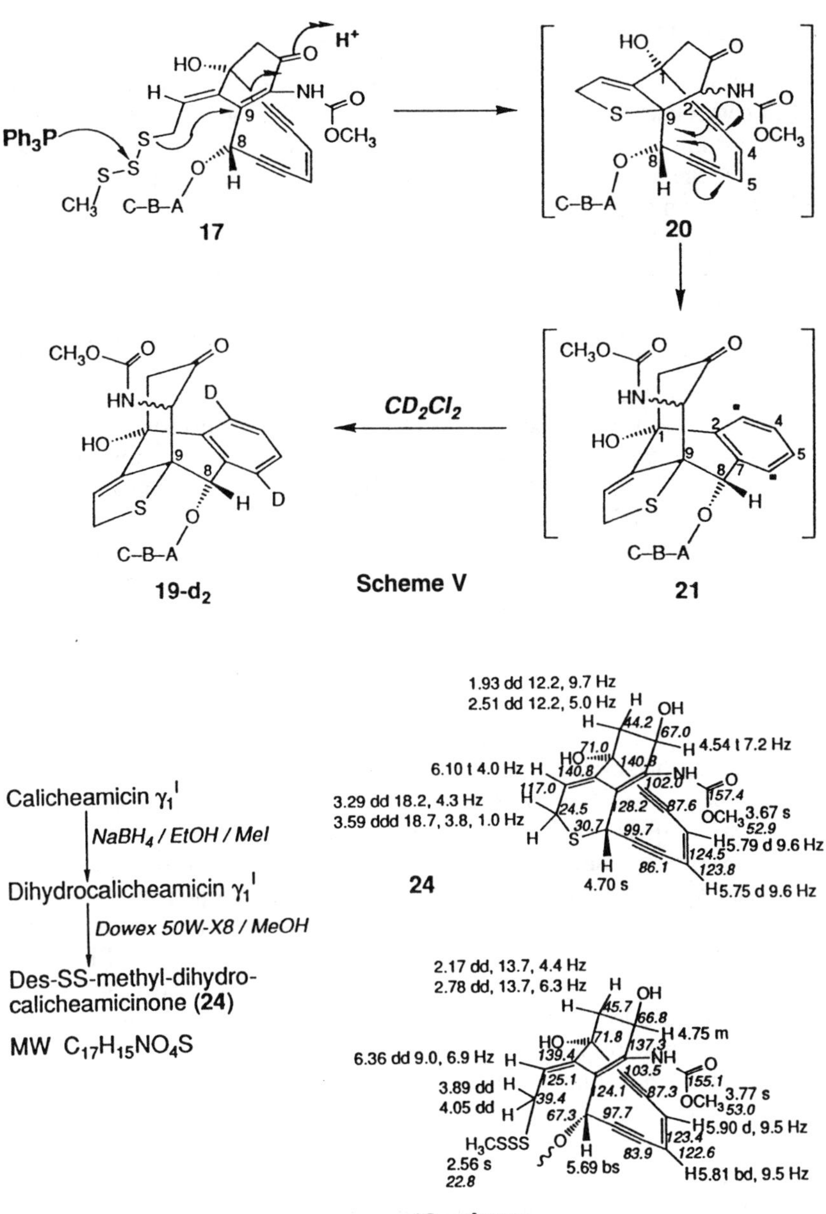

Figure 10 Conversion of dihydrocalicheamicin γ₁ᴵ to des-SS-methyl-dihydrocalichea micinone [24]. ¹H and ¹³C NMR data of 24 revealed that it was the dihydrocalicheamicin aglycon without the SSCH₃ group.

XII. THE CYCLOAROMATIZATION REACTION

As described in Section IX.C., the transformation of calicheamicin pseudoaglycon [17] to compound **19** occurred via a benzene-1,4-diyl intermediate. In order to account for this experimental observation, the following sequence of events was proposed (Scheme V): (1) triphenylphosphine attack at the allylic trisulfide, (2) Michael reaction of the resulting thiolate or thiol with the α,β-unsaturated ketone, (3) tautomerization of the resulting enol to the corresponding keto [20], (4) cyclization of compound **20** to generate the 1,4-diyl (**21**), (5) deuterium atom abstraction from solvent CD_2Cl_2 to give the isolated reaction product **19**-d_2. During the Dowex 50W treatment of dihydrocalicheamicin γ_1^I, in the absence of a driving force for the β-addition at C-9, the thiol displaced the glycoside at C-8 instead, and resulted in the formation of compound **24**.

When Scheme V was proposed initially, it was the best explanation we could offer for our experimental data concerning the chemistry and the structure of the calicheamicin aglycon. The β-addition step was in accordance with the observation that the conversion of compound **17** to **19** was much slower in the absence of methanol. The cyclization of the enediyne system via a 1,4-diyl was supported by Bergman's work on 1,4-dehydrobenzene (6–8). Examination of models suggested that the enediyne system in compound **20** was considerably more flexible than that in compound **17**, increasing the probability for C-2 and C-7 to be at close enough proximity for cyclization to occur. It was not possible to build a cyclized model with both bridge-head double bonds present, providing an explanation for the calicheamicins' existence. According to this model, neither calicheamicin ε (the cycloaromatized calicheamicin γ_1^I), which was prepared from calicheamicin γ_1^I as well as isolated from the fermentation broth (9), nor esperamicin X (10,11) were natural products; rather, they were degradation products of the corresponding natural products. The calicheamicins β_1^{Br}, γ_1^{Br}, α_2^I, α_3^I, β_1^I, γ_1^I, and δ_1^I, N-acetylcalicheamicin γ_1^I, the calicheamicin pseudoaglycon [17], the dihydrocalicheamicin pseudoaglycon [18], and dihydrocalicheamicin γ_1^I were potent DNA-damaging agents as demonstrated by their activity in the BIA. Compound **19** and calicheamicin ε, however, were completely inactive in the BIA. These observations led us to propose that the cyclo-aromatization process shown in Scheme V was responsible for the potent DNA-damaging effects of the calicheamicins and that the 1,4-diyl [21] is the actual active species in the DNA-cleavage process (12–15). Theoretical aspects of the cycloaromatization process as well as the mechanistic aspects of the DNA cleavage process by calicheamicin γ_1^I and other endiyne antibiotics have been studied in great detail. These studies will be reviewed in other chapters of this book.

REFERENCES

1. M. D. Lee, T. S. Dunne, M. M. Siegel, C. C. Chang, G. O. Morton, and D. B. Borders, *J. Am. Chem. Soc., 109,* 3464 (1987).

2. M. D. Lee, T. S. Dunne, C. C. Chang, G. A. Ellestad, M. M. Siegel, G. O. Morton, W. J. McGahren, and D. B. Borders, *J. Am. Chem. Soc., 109,* 3466 (1987).

3. M. D. Lee, T. S. Dunne, C. C. Chang, M. M. Siegel, G. O. Morton, G. A. Ellestad, W. J. McGahren, and D. B. Borders, *J. Am. Chem. Soc., 114,* 985 (1992).

4. W. M. Maiese, D. P. Labeda, J. Korshalla, N. Kuck, A. A. Fantini, M. J. Wildey, J. Thomas, and M. Greenstein, *J. Antibiot., 43,* 253 (1990).

5. M. D. Lee, J. K. Manning, D. R. Williams, N. A. Kuck, R. T. Testa, and D. B. Borders, *J. Antibiot., 42,* 1070 (1989).

6. T. P. Lockhart, P. B. Comita, and R. G. Bergman, *J. Am. Chem. Soc., 103,* 4082 (1981).

7. T. P. Lockhart and R. G. Bergman, *J. Am. Chem. Soc., 103,* 4091 (1981).

8. H. N. C. Wong and F. Sondheimer, *Tetrahedron Lett., 21,* 217 (1980).

9. G. A. Ellestead, P. R. Hamann, N. Zein, G. O. Morten, M. M. Siegel, M. Pastel, D. B. Borders, and W. J. McGahren, *Tetrahedron Lett., 30*(23), 3033 (19??).

10. J. Golik, J. Clardy, G. Dubay, G. Groenewold, H. Kawaguchi, M. Konishi, B. Krishnan, H. Ohkuma, K. Saitoh, and T. W. Doyle, *J. Am. Chem. Soc., 109,* 3461 (1987).

11. J. Golik, J. Clardy, G. Dubay, G. Groenewold, H. Kawaguchi, M. Konishi, B. Krishnan, H. Ohkuma, K. Saitoh, and T. W. Doyle, *J. Am. Chem. Soc., 109,* 3462 (1987).

12. N. Zein, A. M. Sinha, W. J. McGahren, and G. A. Ellestead, *Science, 240,* 1198 (1988).

13. N. Zein, W. J. McGahren, G. O. Morton, J. Ashcroft, and G. A. Ellestad, *J. Am. Chem. Soc., 111,* 6888 (1989).

14. N. Zein, M. Poncin, R. Nilakantan, and G. A. Ellestad, *Science, 244,* 697 (1989).

15. C. A. Townsend, J. J. DeVoss, W. Ding, G. O. Morton, G. A. Ellestad, N. Zein, A. B. Tabor, and S. L. Schreiber, *J. Am. Chem. Soc., 112,* 9669 (1990).

5

Disulfide Calicheamicins and the Chemistry of the Allylic Trisulfide Group

William J. McGahren, * **Wei-Dong Ding, and George A. Ellestad**
*Lederle Laboratories, American Cyanamid Company, Pearl River,
New York*

I. INTRODUCTION

In a recent review on enediyne anticancer antibiotics, it was remarked that natural products chemistry continues to uncover invaluable leads for new scientific ventures (1). This reflects a previous observation in the β-lactam area that, with few exceptions, products from microorganisms have been the inspiration for the design of new β-lactams in clinical use (2). The discovery of calicheamicin has shown that, once again, the isolation and study of natural products has led to the design of potentially useful drugs. This chapter discusses calicheamicin γ_1^I disulfide exchange chemistry, which permitted the preparation of linkers for use in the attachment of monoclonal antibodies (mAbs). The immunoconjugate derivatives of calicheamicin may be of therapeutic value as antitumor agents even though the parent calicheamicin γ_1^I was considered too toxic for clinical consideration. In addition, the isolation and structures of some calicheamicin disulfide analogs obtained, along with the corresponding trisulfides, are presented.

From sodium iodide–supplemented fermentations of *Micromonospora echinospora* spp. *calichensis,* five iodinated metabolites were obtained, namely, calicheamicins α_2^I, α_3^I, β_1^I, γ_1^I, and δ_1^I (Fig. 1). All of these natural products contain (1) an enediyne warhead, (2) a carbohydrate DNA targeting portion, and (3) an allylic trisulfide-triggering device (3). This kind of imagery is normally associated with modern warfare. Since the U.S. government declared war on cancer

---

*Retired

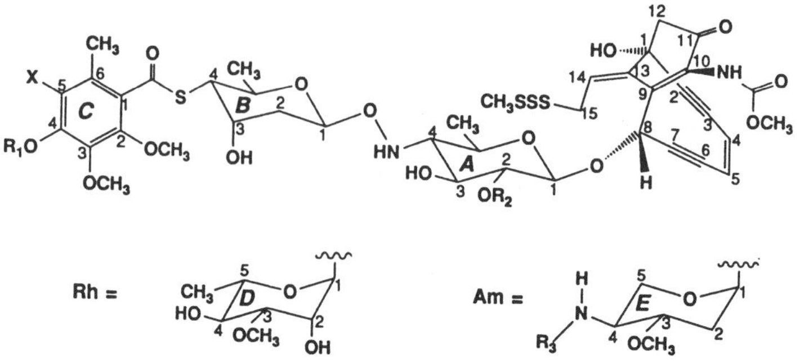

Figure 1 Structures of naturally occurring calicheamicins.

CALICHEAMICIN	R_1	R_2	R
α_2^I	H	AM	Et
α_3^I	Rha	H	--
β_1^I	Rha	AM	CH[CH$_3$]$_2$
γ_1^I	Rha	AM	Et
δ_1^I	Rha	AM	CH$_3$

in the early 1970s it is not unexpected that such nomenclature would be used in connection with powerful new anticarcinogens. Once intuitive concepts regarding the structure of γ_1^I began taking shape, and with the knowledge of its extraordinary antitumor activity in hand, these terms crept into common usage among chemists referring to this metabolite.

When calicheamicin γ_1^I is put into solution with double-stranded DNA under appropriate conditions, it can wreak havoc on the genetic material (4,5). The mechanism of its action involves the priming by bioreductive cleavage of the allylic trisulfide to a thiolate anion, which initiates Michael addition at C_9 of the α,β-unsaturated ketone entity, leading to a Bergman cyclization of the enediyne to a p-phenylene diradical. The diradical is the armed warhead, and because of the carbohydrate-targeting portion, it is already strategically positioned in the minor groove of the DNA to abstract hydrogen atoms from the proximal hydrogens of the deoxyribose sugars on both strands. As a result of these hydrogen atom abstractions, oxidative strand lesions occur, resulting in serious genetic damage (Scheme I).

Of particular interest in this chapter is the chemistry of the allylic trisulfide, which includes a number of intriguing facets. These include its role in activating the enediyne warhead, exchange chemistry with nonreducing thiols to prepare linkers for conjugating monoclonal antibodies, and the isolation from fermenta-

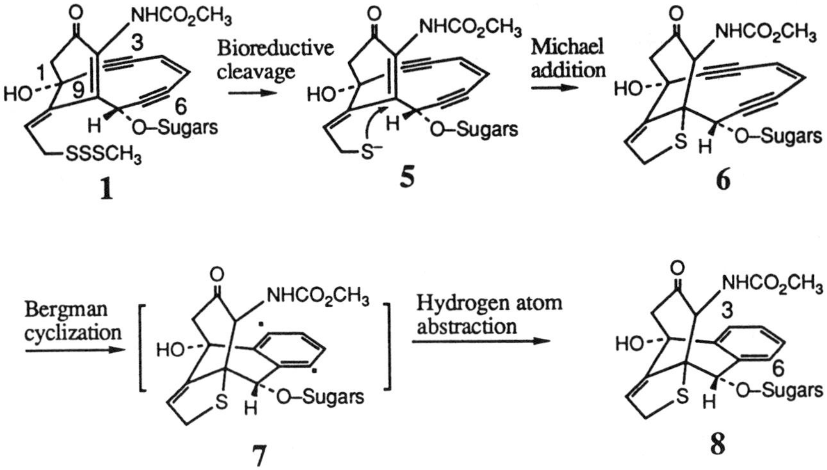

Scheme I Bioactivation of calicheamicins.

tion broths of several variants of this structural entity. Clearly, the most obvious and important feature of this chemistry was the observation that in vitro, in the presence of reducing thiols, extremely low concentrations of γ_1^I produce double-stranded cuts in supercoiled, covalently closed DNA. The reducing thiol cleaves the allylic sulfur-sulfur bond to generate a thiolate anion (**5**), which initiates the chemical cascade of events shown in Scheme I. However, in the absence of thiols, a 10-fold or greater increase in the γ_1^I concentration results in essentially the same cutting results. It is not obvious what the priming mechanism is under such conditions. But it is clear that the drug concentration is a controlling factor. In their review, Nicolaou and Dai asked how the producing organism protects itself against such a dangerous molecule (1). One possible answer is that calicheamicin biosynthesis is tightly controlled. When extruded into the aqueous environment, the metabolites are essentially insoluble due to their extreme lipophilic character. This concentration control by the *Micromonospora* is evidenced by the extreme difficulty of increasing the concentration of the γ_1^I metabolite in the broth to above 50 mg/liter.

II. ISOLATION OF CALICHEAMICIN-RELATED TRACE COMPONENTS

Iodine-supplemented fermentations of *Micromonospora echinospora* yielded γ_1^I at between 0.5 and 5 mg/liter as the major metabolite, while the most abundant minor component, δ_1^I, was produced at between 10 and 20% of the concentration of the major metabolite (3). The δ_1^I preparations from a few fermentations, while appearing to be pure by HPLC, did not respond in normal fashion to the biochemical induction assay (BIA). In this test a genetically altered *Escherichia coli* along with a chemical dye on an agar plate are used to detect DNA-damaging compounds (6). Pure preparations of calicheamicins are positive in the BIA test, but after treatment with excess dithiothreitol (DTT) they are negative. The γ_1^I preparations in question remained positive after DTT treatment. By adjusting the pH of the acetate buffer used in the HPLC system from 6.4 to 4.5, the apparently pure δ_1^I peak could be resolved into two barely separated peaks.

By adding a slight excess of DTT to a solution of the impure δ_1^I preparation in acetonitrile, the δ_1^I component was rapidly degraded, and the DDT unreactive material (at least under these conditions) accounting for the remaining peak was readily isolated in pure form. Fast atom bombardment mass spectroscopy (FABMS) indicated that the new material had a molecular weight of 1335, or 32 mass units less than γ_1^I. A proton NMR spectrum appeared to be identical with a spectrum of γ_1^I except that the SCH_3 signal, normally observed at $\delta2.52$, shifted to $\delta2.36$ (7). Together with the mass spectral data this was compelling evidence that the new material was a disulfide version of γ_1^I (8). Consequently, the new metabolite was dubbed γ_2^I. The question immediately arose as to whether the allylic disulfide was an effective triggering device in view of its stability to DTT. When tested in vitro, in DNA cutting experiments, it was found that γ_2^I behaved similarly to γ_1^I except that it was 4–6 times less potent. This result led to an intensive effort to uncover other, potentially useful, disulfide calicheamicins (see below).

It is appropriate at this stage to discuss the discovery of two other trace components in fermentation broths of the *Micromonospora* organism, which has a bearing on the versatility of the allylic trisulfide entity. The two components in question were found in early, iodine-rich fermentations but for the most part are barely detectable in more recent, higher γ_1^I-producing broths. The first of these components to be isolated was ε, and the determination of the structure of this material enabled the understanding of the mechanism presented in Scheme 1 (3,9). All of the ε preparations isolated from broth contained between 5 and 10% of a less polar peak. When a solution of one of these preparations in acetonitrile was treated with $(Et_2N)_3P$, the minor peak disappeared with concomitant increase in the area of the major peak. This reagent is known to excise sulfur from a disulfide to yield the corresponding monosulfide (10). Patient, HPLC peak-shaving procedures yielded about 35 mg of the minor component labeled ζ. FABMS data indicated that ζ had a molecular weight of 1323. The proton spectrum of ζ in $CDCl_3$ was very similar to that of ε with a few notable exceptions. The geminal hydrogens at C-12 in the ^1H NMR spectrum of ε appear as doublets [J = 16.6 Hz) at $\delta2.80$ and $\delta3.20$. In the spectrum of ζ they are shifted to $\delta2.60$ and $\delta2.85$, respectively, with a coupling constant of 12.6 Hz. In addition, the olefinic proton of the dihydrothiophene ring (a broad signal at $\delta6.30$ in ε) appears as a doublet of doublets at $\delta7.10$ in ζ. These shifts and changes in coupling constants are

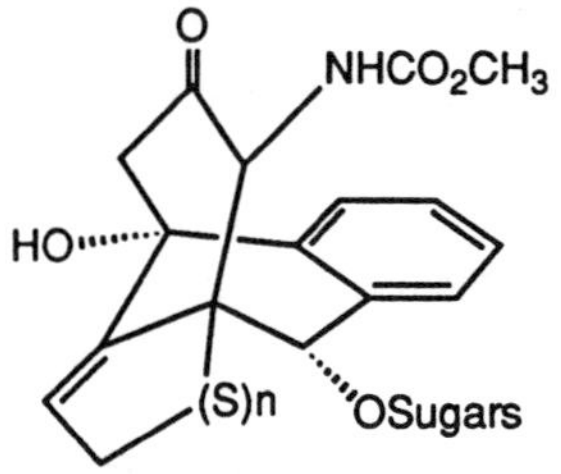

Figure 2 Calicheamicin γ_1^I degradation products.

consistent with the change from a 5-membered thiophene to a 6-membered dithiene ring.

Within a month after the isolation of the first ε preparation from fermentation broth it was discovered that pure ε could be prepared by reacting γ_1^I with Ph$_3$P in methylene chloride. However, examination of the reaction mixture under a variety of conditions never showed any evidence of ζ formation. The structures of ε and ζ are shown in Figure 2.

III. CHEMISTRY OF THE PH$_3$P-γ_1^I REACTION

The origin of ε and ζ in the fermentation broth is not certain. Degradation of γ_1^I due to the presence of certain enzymes and/or thiols is a distinct possibility. In later fermentations in which the levels of γ_1^I have been enhanced, very little evidence of these compounds has been detected. When the strong thiophile Ph$_3$P is allowed to react with γ_1^I in CH$_2$Cl$_2$, a solid precipitate appears. Recovery and purification of this solid shows it to be the dimer CAL-SSS-CAL (8,11). The dimer is relatively insoluble in CH$_2$Cl$_2$, hence it precipitates and is protected from further attack by Ph$_3$P. When the reaction is carried out in methanol, a solvent in which the dimer is soluble, ε is the only calicheamicin product observed. The two byproducts Ph$_3$PO and Ph$_3$PS were also isolated from this reaction in approximately equal amounts. In addition, CH$_3$SSCH$_3$ and CH$_3$SH were identified in the reaction solution by GC-MS. Most of the products mentioned can be accounted for by Scheme II, many of the individual steps of which have precedent in the literature (12).

$$CAL\text{--}SSSCH_3 \; + \; PPh_3 \; \rightleftharpoons \; CAL\text{--}S^- \; + \; Ph_3PSSCH_3^+$$

$$CAL\text{--}S^- \longrightarrow \; \longrightarrow \; \longrightarrow \; \varepsilon$$

$$CAL\text{--}SSSCH_3 \; + \; PPh_3 \; \rightleftharpoons \; CAL\text{--}SS^- \; + \; Ph_3PSCH_3^+$$

$$CAL\text{--}SSSCH_3 \; + \; PPh_3 \; \rightleftharpoons \; CAL\text{--}SSPPh_3^+ \; + \; CH_3S^-$$

$$CAL\text{--}SS^- \; + \; CAL\text{--}SSPPh_3^+ \longrightarrow \; CAL\text{--}SSS\text{--}CAL \; + \; Ph_3PS$$

Scheme II Explanation of Products ε, CAL-SSS-CAL, and Ph$_3$PS.

However, Scheme 2 does not explain the presence of Ph_3PO, nor does it account for the absence of ζ. Treatment of ε with Ph_3P gave no sign of the oxide, whereas in a reaction of diallyl trisulfide with Ph_3P the sulfide was formed but no Ph_3PO was detected. Hence, the cleavage of the allylic trisulfide itself is not responsible for the Ph_3PO formation. The oxygen uptake in the γ_1^I reaction is immediate and is easily determined by monitoring oxygen uptake using an oxygen electrode.

That the oxygen in Ph_3PO does indeed originate from molecular oxygen derives from the fact that no oxide is formed when the reaction is carried out in the absence of oxygen. Also, the use of an $^{18}O_2$ atmosphere resulted in the isolation of $Ph_3P^{18}O$. This is likely a result of the formation of superoxide by univalent reduction of molecular oxygen by thiyl radicals, arising from the *p*-phenylene diradical intermediate formed on the path to ε (13). The total absence of ζ is unexpected in those reactions since there is little doubt that something like the conversion to CalSS$^-$ to ζ definitely does occur in fermentations.

IV. CONVERSION OF γ_1^I TO DISULFIDE CALICHEAMICINS

Attempts to form di- or monosulfide analogs of γ_1^I using $(Et_2N)_3P$ were unsuccessful. The first indication that the allylic trisulfide-triggering device could be altered, while at the same time leaving the enediyne portion intact, came from the reaction of γ_1^I in ethanol with $NaBH_4$ in the presence of excess methyl iodide. Two products were isolated from this reaction, namely, the expected dihydro γ_1^I (3) and a slightly more polar material. FABMS showed that this new compound had a molecular weight of 1337, which seemed to indicate the loss of sulfur from dihydro γ_1^I. NMR data confirmed this conclusion since the spectra of both materials were virtually identical except for the position of the SCH_3 signal at $\delta 2.38$ in the more polar product labeled dihydro γ_2^I. Figure 3 depicts these dihydro compounds. Both compounds were BIA active, and in vitro DNA-cutting experiments showed that dihydro γ_1^I was about as effective as γ_1^I. The mechanism of Scheme I cannot apply in this instance, since the α,β-unsaturated ketone is gone, thus

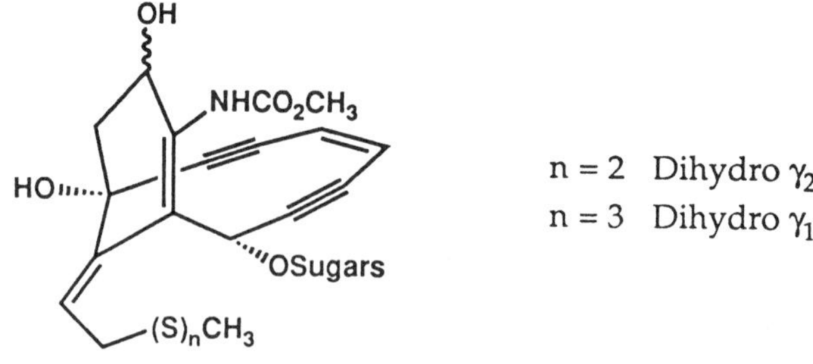

Figure 3   Dihydro-calicheamicins.

eliminating the possibility of Michael addition. Treatment of a solution containing both these dihydro compounds with DTT left the dihydro γ_2^I unaffected, but the dihydro γ_1^I was presumably converted to dihydro ε, since the converted product appeared to co-chromatograph with the $NaBH_4$ reduction product of ε. This brings up the question of whether a thiyl radical is involved. Under aerobic conditions thiyl radicals as well as hydroperoxy radicals might be formed from thiol and oxygen (14,15). Thiyl addition to the double bond of the allylic alcohol, therefore, would not be dependent on the electron-withdrawing properties of an eneone for removal of the bridgehead double bond by a Michael reaction.

It has already been mentioned that when γ_1^I was reacted with thiols such as β-mercaptoethanol or DTT in alcoholic solvents, the only isolable product was ε. Later it was decided to look at the effect of volatile, nonreducing thiols on γ_1^I under a variety of conditions. When propyl mercaptan and γ_1^I were dissolved in methylene chloride at room temperature, no reaction occurred. When the reaction was carried out in acetonitrile, HPLC monitoring showed the smooth, virtually quantitative conversion of γ_1^I to a slightly less polar, single product. The reaction was complete in about 2 hours and indeed, using stoichiometric amounts of both reactants, it went to completion overnight at $-20°C$.

The isolated product, I, was shown by FBMS to have a molecular weight of 1363 or 4 mass units less than γ_1^I. In the ^1H NMR spectrum of product I, the SCH_3 signal at $\delta2.52$ was replaced by a methylene multiplet at $\delta2.58$. Two new signals were observed: a terminal methyl at $\delta0.92$ and another methylene at $\delta1.59$. The data indicated that a methyl dithiolate had been replaced by a propyl thiolate, which neatly explained the loss of 4 mass units.

When the same reaction was run using ethyl mercaptan as the volatile thiol, the initial HPLC profile was quite disconcerting since it seemed to indicate that no reaction had occurred. Despite appearances, the reaction was processed to yield a product, II, which had a molecular weight of 1349. The proton spectrum of product II showed a mercaptomethylene signal at $\delta2.64$ and a terminal methyl at $\delta1.18$. The consternation mentioned above was due solely to the coincidence that γ_1^I and product II co-chromatographed in the HPLC system used.

Reaction of γ_1^I with a slight excess of the stenchy, gaseous methyl mercaptan yielded material that was identical with the natural product γ_2^I. Close HPLC monitoring of this reaction revealed that the dimer CAL-SSS-CAL is formed in significant amounts early in the reaction. The concentration was found to rise until roughly equivalent to the remaining γ_1^I, at which point the concentrations of these two species fell off, in parallel, until only the disulfide calicheamicin remains. These results are shown in Scheme III.

$$CAL\text{-}SSSCH_3 + CH_3SH \rightarrow CAL\text{-}SSCH_3 + CH_3\,SS^-$$
$$CAL\text{-}SSSCH_3 + CH_3SS^- \rightarrow CAL\text{-}SS + CH_3\text{-}SSSCH_3$$
$$CAL\text{-}SSSCH_3 + CALSS^- \rightarrow CAL\text{-}SSS\text{-}CAL + CH_3\,SS^-$$

Scheme III   Dimer Formation in the Conversion of γ_1 to Disulfide Calicheamicins.

Not only is this reaction solvent dependent, but it appears to be internally base catalyzed. In the case of γ_1^I general base catalysis is provided by the basic nitrogen of the amino sugar E. The *N*-acetyl derivative fails to react until triethylamine is added, in which case reaction occurs in the normal, smooth fashion. Based on the kinetic studies of Overman and O'Connor on the effect of proximal amino groupings on the reductive cleavage of disulfides with Ph_3P in aqueous dioxane, it is unlikely that the ethylamino sugar in the protonated or free base form participates directly in the calicheamicin allylic trisulfide cleavage (16).

When pure calicheamicin γ_1^I was reacted with methyl mercaptan, a virtual quantitative yield of calicheamicin γ_2^I was realized. The molecular weight was shown to be 1321, and the proton spectrum showed the expected upfield shift of the $-SCH_3$ signal. Biological evaluation of the disulfide calicheamicins mentioned so far in mice infected with P388 leukemia cells indicated that they were between 5- and 10-fold less effective than γ_1^I. This means that these materials are still potent antitumor agents. However, the therapeutic indices of all of them were still unacceptable low. In other words, such drugs cannot be injected into the blood stream at the concentrations needed to destroy tumors. The best hope of their being used clinically depends on targeting. To complete the modern warfare analogy, delivery systems would have to be provided. For that purpose tumor-selective monoclonal antibodies these quantities are now available would seem to be the answer.

Because the conversion of γ_1^I to the various disulfide derivatives was so gentle and smooth, the notion developed that these procedures could be used to attach linkers to γ_1^I, converting it into a variety of γ_2^Is without serious loss of antitumor effectiveness. The free ends of the linkers could consist of acidic, basic, or active ester groups, which could be used to bind covalently with the mAbs. Such conjugates would have one other powerful advantage. Enzymes capable of hydrolyzing disulfide linkages are indigenous in humans, and hence, at the target sites, the huge protein carriers could be cleaved off, allowing the primed warheads to cause essentially selective damage on the genetic material of the cancerous cells.

A question remained as to whether thiols with carbonyl or amino polar groups would undergo the smooth replacement reactions observed with alkyl thiols. When 3-mercaptoproprionic acid was reacted with γ_1^I in acetonitrile at $-20°C$, the reaction went to completion over a slightly longer period of time. The product, III, was considerably more difficult to purify because of the free carboxyl group. The molecular weight turned out to be 1393 as expected, and the proton spectrum showed the mercapto methylene at $\delta 2.70$ and the carboxylic methylene at $\delta 2.94$. Upon reaction of dimethylaminoethanethiol hydrochloride with γ_1^I the product, IV, was readily isolated and by FABMS had a molecular ion at an m/e of 1393 mass units. The proton spectrum, in deuterated aqueous solution, showed an intense dimethylamino peak at $\delta 2.90$, which is where this signal appeared in the spectrum of the starting thiol. Since product IV was isolated as the hydrochloride salt it was water soluble, and because of that one might have expected some difference in bioactivity. However, no improvement was noted in acute toxicity tests in mice, while the antitumor activity against murine P388 leukemia was perhaps a little lower than those of other disulfide calicheamicins.

To prepare a disulfide derivative with the active p-nitrophenyl ester on the free end of a linker, it was necessary to prepare the thiol reagent. Initially, 3-mercaptoproprionic acid was doubly butylated in methylene chloride using isobutylene in the presence of a drop of concentrated sulfuric acid catalyst. The product was converted by acid reflux to the free acid, which was readily esterified using p-nitrophenol and a carbodimide. The mercapto group was then unmasked using mercuric acetate in trifluoroacetic acid, and the mercury was precipitated using hydrogen sulfide in dimethylformamide (17). The desired product was purified by silica gel chromatography and reacted with γ_1^I in acetonitrile to a virtual quantitative yield of product V. By FABMS the molecular weight was determined to be 1514 and the proton spectrum had all the expected signals including doublets [J $\sim$ 9Hz] at $\delta 8.30$ and $\delta 7.30$ for the protons of the nitrophenyl ring.

The γ_1^I to γ_2^I displacement reaction was studied for a number of other thiols such as 1-methyl-1-propanethiol, 2-methyl-2-propanethiol, and the doubly protected cysteine, t-BOC-Cys-t-Bu. These reactions were run at a concentration of 200 μg/ml in acetonitrile. Conversions appeared to be quantitative by HPLC, but the products were not isolated. Table 1 contains a list of the early disulfide calicheamicins that were prepared and analyzed.

Later studies using the sulfur exchange reaction described here led to the selection of the linker 3-mercaptopropionyl hydrazide. This linker has been attached

Table 1 Disulfide Calicheamicins

Compound	X	Mol. wt.	Formula
Derivatives of the general formula CAL-SS-X			
γ_2^I	CH_3	1335	$C_{55}H_{74}IN_3O_{21}S_3$
I	$CH_2CH_2CH_3$	1363	$C_{57}H_{78}IN_3O_{21}S_3$
II	CH_2CH_3	1349	$C_{56}H_{76}IN_3O_{21}S_3$
III	CH_2CH_2COOH	1393	$C_{57}H_{76}IN_3O_{21}S_3$
IV	$CH_2CH_2N[CH_3]_2 \cdot HCl$	1428.5	$C_{58}H_{82}ClIN_4O_{21}S_3$
V	$CH_2CH_2CO_2PhNO_2$	1514	$C_{63}H_{81}IN_4O_{25}S_3$
Derivatives of the formula CAL^1-SS-X where CAL^1 = CAL $-$ CH$_2$			
δ_2	CH_3	1321	$C_{54}H_{72}IN_3O_{21}S_3$
Dihydro δ_2	CH_3	1323	$C_{54}H_{74}IN_4O_{21}S_3$
Derivatives of the formula CAL^2-SS-X where CAL^2 = CAL $+$ 2H			
Dihydro γ_2	CH_3	1337	$C_{55}H_{76}IN_3O_{21}S_3$

Table 2 In Vitro Antibacterial Activities of Calicheamicins Expressed as Minimal Inhibitory Concentrations (μg/ml)

Organism	Calicheamicin γ_2	Product IV	Calicheamicin γ_1
Escherichia coli CMC 84-11	0.25	0.5	0.06
Escherichia coli #311	0.25	0.5	0.06
Escherichia coli ATCC 25922	0.12	0.5	0.06
Klebsiella pneumoniae CMC 84-5	0.25	1.0	0.12
Klebsiella pneumoniae AD mp.	0.12	0.25	0.03
Enterobacter cloacae CMC 84-4	0.5	2.0	0.12
Enterobacter aerogenes lo 83-44	0.5	1.0	0.12
Serratia marcescens CMC 83-27	0.25	1.0	0.03
Serratia marcescens F35 mp.	0.25	1.0	0.03
Morganella morganii lo 83-18	0.5	2.0	0.12
Proteus stutzer CMC 83-82	1.0	2.0	0.12
Citrobacter diversus K-82-24	0.5	1.0	0.12
Citrobacter freundii lo 83-13	0.5	0.5	0.03
Acinetobacter CMC 83-19	0.25	0.5	0.015
Acinetobacter lo 83-49	0.25	1.0	0.015
Pseudomonas aeruginosa 12-4-4 mp.	0.25	1.0	0.12
Pseudomonas aeruginosa ATCC 27853	0.12	0.5	0.06
Staphylococcus aureus Smith mp.	0.001	0.002	0.00012
Staphylococcus aureus SSC 82-21	0.0005	0.004	0.00012
Staphylococcus aureus ATCC 25923	0.0005	0.004	0.00012
Staphylococcus aureus ATCC 29213	0.001	0.004	0.00025
Staphylococcus aureus SSC 82-23	0.001	0.002	0.00012
Staphylococcus aureus VGH 84-21	0.001	0.002	0.00012
Staphylococcus aureus VGH 84-47	0.001	0.004	0.00025
Staphylococcus epidermidis CMC 83-133	0.001	0.002	0.00025
Staphylococcus ATCC 12228	0.001	0.004	0.00025
Streptococcus faecalis ATCC 29212	0.002	0.004	0.00025
Streptococcus faecalis UGH 84-65	0.004	0.004	0.00025
Streptococcus faecalis CMC 83-53	0.004	0.004	0.0005
Streptococcus faecalis UCl 85-20	0.002	0.004	0.0005
Streptococcus faecalis lo 83-28	0.004	0.004	0.00025

Agar dilution method using a Mueller-Hinton II medium.

to N-acetyl γ_1^I, and the resultant disulfide calicheamicin was covalently bonded to an mAb (7F11C7) specific for human, fat globule, membrane antigen present on a variety of tumors (18). This mAb conjugate caused tumor regression of the MX-1 and Lung-78, non–small-cell lung carcinoma xenographs and resulted in long-term, tumor-free survivors in both murine models (19,20). Studies of similar conjugates in humans are planned.

V. ANTIBIOTIC ACTIVITY OF CALICHEAMICINS

In addition to antitumor effectiveness, calicheamicins exhibit powerful antibiotic activity in vitro, particularly against gram-positive organisms. Because of their acute and long-term toxicities, they are never likely to be used as antiinfectives. Table 2 illustrates the antibiotic power of γ_1^I and also that the disulfide calicheamicins, γ_2^I and product IV, are about an order of magnitude less effective than γ_1. This loss in activity mirrors the loss in antitumor activity and would seem to indicate that the mode of action is still by attack on the bacterial genetic material. The two or more orders of magnitude of greater activity against gram positives is simply a reflection of the difficulties molecules of this size have in penetrating the outer membrane of the gram negatives.

At the outset of this chapter it was noted how natural products discovery frequently anticipates subsequent, significant drug developments in antiinfective chemotherapy. The isolation and study of γ_1^I and γ_2^I led eventually to the mAb conjugate work, which may produce a drug of use in antitumor chemotherapy.

REFERENCES

1. K. C. Nicolaou and W.-M. Dai, *Angew. Chem., 30,* 1387 (1991).
2. A. G. Brown, *Pure Appl. Chem., 59,* 475 (1987).
3. M. D. Lee, T. S. Dunne, C. C. Chang, M. M. Siegel, G. O. Morton, G. A. Ellestad, W. J. McGahren, and D. B. Borders, *J. Am. Chem. Soc., 114,* 985 (1992).
4. N. Zein, A. M. Sinha, W. J. McGahren, and G. A. Ellestad, *Science, 240,* 1198 (1988).
5. N. Zein, M. Poncin, R. Nilikantan, and G. A. Ellestad, *Science, 244,* 697 (1989).
6. R. K. Elespura and R. J. White, *Cancer Res., 43,* 2819 (1983).
7. E. Block, in *Reactions of Organosulfur Compounds,* Academic Press, New York, 1978, p. 287.
8. G. A. Ellestead, P. R. Hamann, N. Zein, G. O. Morton, M. M. Siegel, M. Pascal, D. B. Borders, and W. J. McGahren, *Tetrahedron. Lett., 30,* 3033 (1989).
9. N. Zein, W. J. McGahren, G. O. Morton, J. Ashcroft, and G. A. Ellestad, *J. Am. Chem. Soc., 111,* 6888 (1989).
10. D. N. Harpp and J. G. Gleason, *J. Am. Chem. Soc., 93,* 2437 (1971).
11. P. Magnus, R. T. Lewis, and F. Bennett, *J. Chem. Soc., Chem. Comm.,* 916 (1989).
12. D. N. Harpp and R. A. Smith, *J. Am. Chem. Soc., 104,* 6045 (1982).
13. D.-H. Chin and I. H. Goldberg, *Biochemistry, 25,* 1009 (1986).
14. K. Fujiwara, A. Kurisaki, and M. Hirama, *Tetrahedron Lett., 31,* 4329 (1990).
15. G. Fava, G. Reichenbach, and U. Peron, *J. Am. Chem. Soc., 89,* 6696 (1967).
16. L. E. Overman and E. M. O'Connor, *J. Am. Chem. Soc., 98,* 771 (1976).
17. O. Nishimura, C. Kitada, and M. Fujino, *Chem. Pharm. Bull., 26,* 1576 (1978).
18. P. R. Hamann, L. M. Hinman, and J. Upeslacis, *Abstr. 5th Int. Conf. Monoclonal Antibody Immunoconjugates For Cancer, 99,* 63 (1990).

19. L. M. Hinman, R. E. Wallace, P. R. Hamann, F. E. Durr, and J. Upeslacis, *Abstr. 5th Int. Conf. Monoclonal Antibody Immunoconjugates For Cancer, 84*, 59 (1990).
20. A. T. Menendez, L. M. Hinman, P. R. Hamann, J. Upeslacis, and F. E. Durr, *Abstr. 5th Int. Conf. Monoclonal Antibody Immunoconjugates For Cancer, 100*, 63 (1990).

6

Preparation of Conjugates to Monoclonal Antibodies

Lois M. Hinman, Philip R. Hamann, and Janis Upeslacis
Lederle Laboratories, American Cyanamid Company, Pearl River,
New York

I. CURRENT APPROACHES TO ANTIBODY-BASED CANCER THERAPIES

In the 1950s and 1960s, many efforts to make "magic bullets" for targeted therapy were undertaken. While some small therapeutic advantage could be seen from targeting in early animal studies, the first true breakthrough in the targeting field did not occur until the mid-1970s, with the development of the hybridoma technology that allowed for the production of large quantities of homogeneous monoclonal antibodies (mAbs) (1). The ability to prepare mAbs selective for well-defined antigens on human cells has generated a great deal of excitement in many areas of biomedical research (see Refs. 2 and 3 for recent reviews). In the field of cancer, the proof of principle that mAbs can be targetted to specific antigens, abundant or overexpressed on tumor cells, has been shown many times, and the first mAb-imaging agent has recently been approved for diagnosis of colorectal and ovarian carcinoma (4). Other mAb-based products have been approved for reversal of tissue rejection in renal transplant patients and for imaging of myocardial tissue (5). However, no mAb-targeted cancer therapy has as yet been approved for human use (6).

Many obstacles have been encountered in the development of mAb-based therapies as described in detail elsewhere (7,8). One problem that has been a major limiting factor results from the fact that, although the mAbs generated by the hybridoma technology bind to human antigens, they are murine proteins, which can be highly immunogenic in humans. Most patients injected with murine mAbs develop HAMA (human antimouse antibodies) in response to the foreign protein, and this limits the therapeutic potential of mAb-based treatments by limiting multiple dosing regimens (9). Recently, new technologies to produce humanized or human mAbs that are much less likely to be immunogenic in patients have been developed. The use of humanized mAbs to target therapeutic agents is becoming the state-of-the-art in the field, and several mAb-based therapies using humanized mAbs are beginning clinical evaluations (10,11).

The active agents that have been attached to mAbs and tested clinically to date fall into three general categories: isotopes, phytotoxins (protein toxins of plant or bacterial origin), and standard anticancer drugs. Isotope conjugates are by far the most advanced clinically, and even in studies using murine mAbs, some therapeutic effects have been seen in the clinic with radioimmunotherapy (RIT). New directions in RIT include the use of fragments for more rapid blood clearance to minimize the myelosuppressive effects of the radiotherapy and the use of humanized mAbs as the targeting agents (12). Immunotoxins (IT), which are mAb constructs that deliver one of the protein synthesis–inhibiting bacterial or plant phytotoxins, such as ricin or *Pseudomonas* exotoxin, show impressive antitumor effects in vitro or in vivo in animal models for a wide range of tumors. IT therapy at first appeared highly exciting, but in clinical trials immunogenicity is dose limiting in all except the most highly immunosuppressed patients (13). The challenge with IT therapy at this time is to overcome the inherent immunogenicity of the constructs (14,15).

In contrast with RIT and IT therapy, however, little clinical promise has been seen with mAb-based targeting of any standard chemotherapeutic agents (7,16). In addition to the problems of HAMA, the major limitation seen in all efforts to target standard chemotherapeutic agents is their relatively low potency, which is often reduced by the modifications required for linking them to mAbs. To address the issue of potency, one new strategy that has recently emerged is to target drugs that have potency near to that of the protein toxins without their inherent immunogenicity. Recent reports have been made on the targeting of several such antibiotics including the antimitotic maytansinoid derivatives (17) and the protein synthesis–inhibiting tricothecenes (18). We have also reported from our laboratories on the targeting of the DNA-active calicheamicins (19,20). As we intend to develop conjugates of the calicheamicins attached to humanized mAbs for human use, considerations of linker design, analog selection, and characteristics of an effective mAb for selective delivery to a tumor are all being addressed. We have recently published preclinical data on the structure-activity profile of calicheamicin conjugates with the internalizing antipolymorphic epithelial mucin (anti-PEM) mAb, CT-M-01, which binds to the PEM antigen abundant on a number of solid tumors including breast, ovarian, and non–small-cell lung (19,21).

Our studies to date show that some analogs of the calicheamicins are highly promising agents for targeted therapy, and the structural features of the drug that appear to be important for conjugate activity will be summarized in this review. The disulfide exchange chemistry that has allowed for the attachment of linkers onto the calicheamicins for conjugation is described in detail elsewhere in this volume.

Most of the preclinical and clinical studies to date in the field of mAb-based drug targeting have used mAbs of the IgG class, as shown in Figure 1. Whole IgG molecules (150 kD) consist of four disulfide cross-linked chains, referred to as the heavy and light chains. In some cases fragments, (Fab')$_2$ or Fabs, which are prepared from whole antibodies by removal of the Fc fragment through enzymatic digestion or directly through genetic engineering techniques, have been used as targeting agents (see Figure 1). In humanized mAbs most of the residues in the amino acid framework of the murine mAb are replaced with those characteristic of a human IgG, with care being given in the engineering process to minimizing changes in the structure or conformation of the antigen-binding site (9,10).

Many of the functionalized side chains of amino acid residues in the framework of a 150 kD IgG molecule or its fragments (whether murine or humanized) can be used for attachment of small molecules (22). The specific problem that arises in conjugating small molecules to mAbs is that the addition of the ligand to the antibody molecule can interfere with the binding of the mAb to its target antigen, either by modifying a residue in the hypervariable regions or by significantly altering the conformation of the antigen-recognition sites.

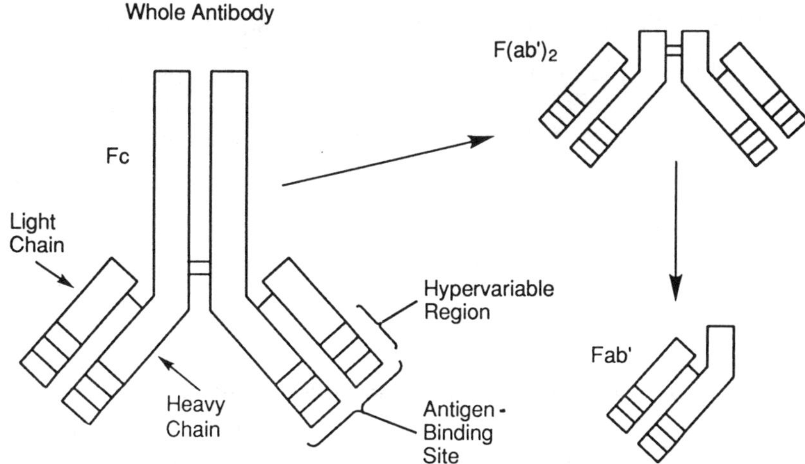

Figure 1   A schematic representation of an IgG molecule and commonly prepared fragments used in conjugation reactions.

Investigators have used a number of different strategies in preparing drug–mAb conjugates (23–25). The amino acid residues most commonly modified in the preparation of conjugation are lysines and cysteines, the latter being frequently employed in the construction of ITs with F(ab')$_2$ fragments. Because of their hydrophilicity, which generally makes them solvent available, and their susceptibility to chemical modification, the ε-amino groups of lysines have been most commonly used for drug attachment. However, as lysines tend to be abundant throughout the structure of the mAb, modifying too many lysines is likely to result in modification of a residue in the hypervariable region of the mAb and interfere with binding of the mAb to its target antigen. The possibility of this happening can only be assessed experimentally and differs from mAb to mAb and drug to drug.

Another approach to modifying whole IgG molecules is to use the carbohydrate residues present on the Fc region (26). Oxidation of the 1,2-diols in the carbohydrate chain with periodic acid allows for the attachment of drugs containing various nucleophiles such as a hydrazide. This approach has been taken with a number of drugs and for the delivery of chelated metals as well.

The preparation of a carbohydrate-linked drug–mAb conjugate is a three-step process involving modification of the drug to contain a hydrazide functionality, oxidation of the carbohydrates of the mAb with periodic acid to produce aldehydes for reaction with the hydrazides, and conjugation of the modified protein with the drug hydrazide to form a Schiff-base linkage, followed by subsequent purification and characterization of the resulting conjugate. Detailed descriptions of the synthesis of intermediates and the preparation of carbohydrate-based calicheamicin conjugates with whole IgGs are given below.

II. MODIFICATION OF THE CALICHEAMICINS FOR LINKING

Prior to conjugation, the calicheamicins must be modified to contain a linker that can be used as a site of attachment. As mentioned above, the disulfide exchange reaction provides a convenient way to incorporate a linking site into the drug structure. To modify calicheamicins for linking, two steps are required: first, an appropriate thiol hydrazide to use in the disulfide exchange reaction must be prepared and, second, it must be attached to the drug. The reaction of calicheamicin γ_1^I [1] (γ_1^I can be written as γ_1^I-SSSCH$_3$ to emphasize the presence of the trisulfide trigger) with a thiol hydrazide, in this case 3-mercaptopropionyl hydrazide [2], is shown schematically in Figure 2. Once the hydrazide disulfide [3] is purified, it can be reacted with the oxidized carbohydrates of a mAb as described below. The preparation of a variety of thiol hydrazides used in our studies, as well as the corresponding hydrazide-containing calicheamicin disulfides, are described in detail in Section VI.

Carbohydrate-linked conjugates of five different calicheamicin analogs, which vary in the integrity of the rhamnose and amino sugars, have been synthesized.

Calicheamicin γ_1^{I}-SSSCH$_3$ [**1**] +

2

$\xrightarrow{\text{16 hrs, -15°C, MeCN}}$

3

Calicheamicin γ_1^{I}-SS

Figure 2   The preparation of a thiol hydrazide derivative of γ_1^I.

These five analogs are shown in Figure 3. All of these analogs contain the bicyclic "warhead," which is responsible for causing double-stranded breaks in DNA, as well as the methyl trisulfide, which is a bioreducable trigger for the drug. The structure of most potent "parent" compound, calicheamicin γ_1^I [**1**], contains both the rhamnose and the amino sugar. The α_2^I analog [**4**] is missing the rhamnose, while

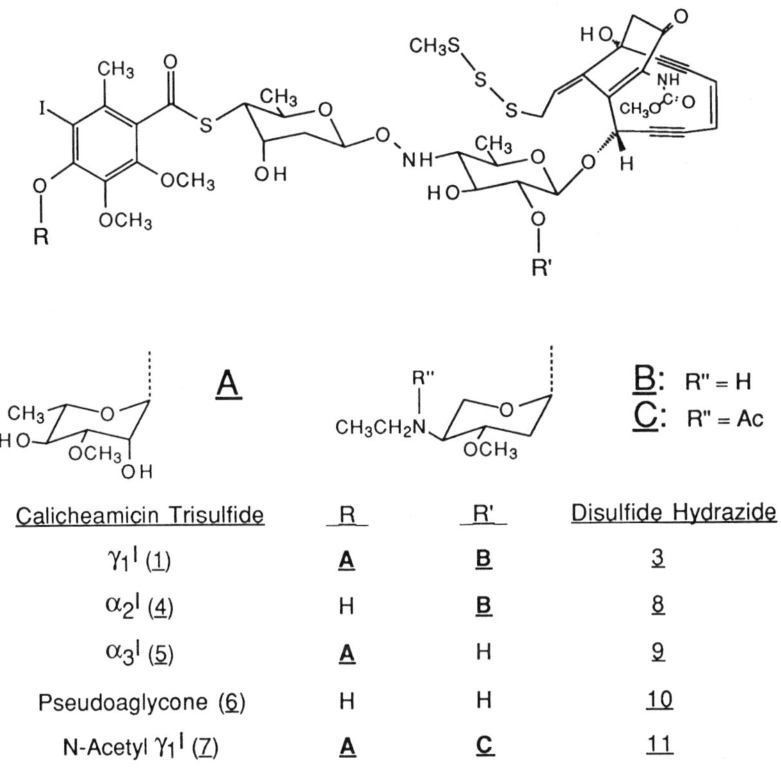

Calicheamicin Trisulfide	R	R'	Disulfide Hydrazide
γ_1^I (**1**)	**A**	**B**	**3**
α_2^I (**4**)	H	**B**	**8**
α_3^I (**5**)	**A**	H	**9**
Pseudoaglycone (**6**)	H	H	**10**
N-Acetyl γ_1^I (**7**)	**A**	**C**	**11**

Figure 3   Structural analogs of the calicheamicins used in these studies.

α_3^I [5] is missing the amino sugar and the pseudoaglycone (PSAG) [6] lacks both the rhamnose and amino sugars. *N*-Acetyl γ_1^I [7] can be made by acylating γ_1^I in methanol with an excess of acetic anhydride. For each of these five analogs, a disulfide hydrazide has been prepared by reaction with compound **2** in analogy with the formation of compound **3**.

The antitumor effects of the five trisulfide calicheamicin derivatives along with their respective hydrazides were studied in vivo in the P388 leukemia model (Table 1), as reported previously (19,20). In each experiment, the test drug was administered IP to normal mice carrying P388 leukemia as well as to a comparable group of nontumored animals. The lethality of the drugs in the nontumored animals was used to determine maximum tolerated dose (MTD). In Table 1, the increase in survival of treated animals is reported as the percent increase in lifespan (%ILS) for each analog and its hydrazide, respectively, at two doses: the optimal dose (OD) that gives the greatest %ILS in the P388 animals, and the MTD, determined in the nontumored animals.

Several conclusions can be made from these data. For all five trisulfide calicheamicins, the MTD was less than the OD. For example, the greatest increase in lifespan resulting from treatment with any of these derivatives was 150% for the α_2^I calicheamicin, at a dose eightfold higher than the MTD. The potency of the hydrazides was two- to eight-fold less than that of the corresponding parent compounds for all analogs. These data confirm the previous observation that although the calicheamicins are highly potent, toxicity limits their therapeutic efficacy as single agents (20). However, their impressive potency makes them viable candidates for targeting, particularly if targeting can improve the therapeutic potential of the drugs by reducing toxicity at effective doses. The hydrazide de-

Table 1 Comparison of Antitumor Effects and Lethality of Calicheamicin Analogs and Corresponding Disulfide Hydrazides

Calicheamicin		Trisulfide			Hydrazide	
		OD (μg/kg)	MTD (μg/kg)		OD (μg/kg)	MTD (μg/kg)
γ_1^I	**1**	5	1.25	**3**	5	2.5
		(123%)[a]	(86%)		(83%)	(75%)
α_2^I	**4**	10	1.25	**8**	10	5
		(150%)	(75%)		(130%)	(83%)
α_3^I	**5**	40	10	**9**	80	80
		(109%)	(73%)		(73%)	(73%)
PSAG	**6**	160	40	**10**	not tested	
N-Acetyl γ_1^I	**7**	40	20	**11**	160	160
		(123%)	(79%)		(63%)	(63%)

[a] Numbers of parentheses refer to % increase in lifespan compared with a nontumored control.
Source: Ref. 19.

rivatives for each of these calicheamicins (referred to as "simple" hydrazides, compared with those discussed in Sec. V) have therefore been conjugated to mAbs and evaluated for potency and specificity as described below.

III. PREPARATION OF CARBOHYDRATE-LINKED CONJUGATES OF CALICHEAMICIN γ_1^I

A procedure for the preparation of hydrazide-linked conjugates of calicheamicin γ_1^I is outlined schematically in Figure 4 and described in detail below. The oxidation of the mAb and the conjugation reaction are both conveniently done in pH 5.5 acetate buffer. The preparation of conjugates of the other four analogs [4–7] follows the same general procedure, using the appropriate "simple" disulfide hydrazides [8–11] indicated in Figure 3, the syntheses of which are described in Section VI. These hydrazone conjugates had drug loadings of two to three molecules of calicheamicin per molecule of mAb and retained greater than 85% of the immunoaffinity of the unmodified mAb.

mAb at a concentration of ~10 mg/ml in 50 mM sodium acetate buffer, pH 5.5, containing 0.1 M sodium chloride was oxidized with ~15 mM periodic acid added to 0.2 M sodium acetate. The oxidation was allowed to proceed in the dark with stirring at 4°C for 45 minutes, at which time the oxidized mAb was desalted on a Sephadex G-25 column. The degree of oxidation of the antibody was assessed by reaction with *p*-nitrophenylhydrazine (NPH) as described previously (19). The oxidized mAb was reacted with an excess of drug hydrazide at 0.5–1.0 mg/ml. The hydrazides were dissolved in dimethylformamide (DMF) and added to the aqueous solution of mAb. The concentration of the drug stock in DMF was adjusted so that the final concentration of DMF in the reaction was 15%.

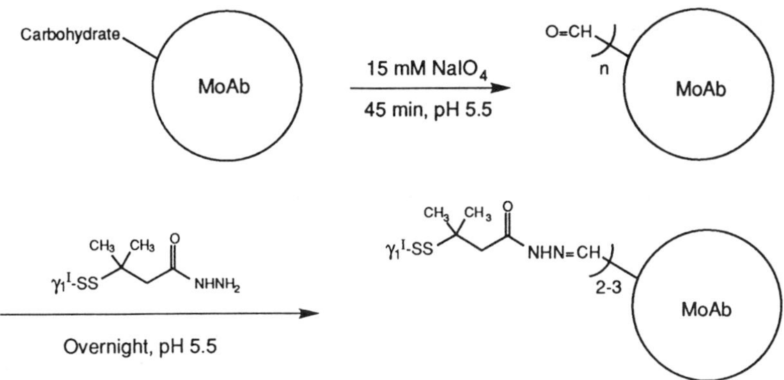

Figure 4 A schematic for the preparation of a carbohydrate-linked conjugate of calicheamicin γ_1^I.

Reaction was allowed to proceed overnight at room temperature with gentle shaking. A 10% volume of 0.1 M acethydrazide was added, and shaking was continued for one hour. The conjugate was desalted on a Sephadex G-25 column using 50 mM phosphate buffer at a pH of 7.4 with 100 mM NaCl, filtered, and purified on S-200 gel exclusion chromatography to remove aggregates. The final pooled and concentrated monomer was analyzed for aggregate by gel exclusion HPLC (Zorbax GF 250) and for free drug by reverse-phase HPLC (C-18 with a 50 mM ammonium phosphate/acetonitrile gradient). Drug loading was determined spectroscopically using the extinction coefficients of both the antibody ($\varepsilon_{280\,nm}$ = 1.43 ml/mg) and the drug ($\varepsilon_{333\,nm}$ = 2.85 ml/mg). A correction for the contribution of the drug to protein absorbance was made using ($A_{280\,corr}$ = A_{280} − (3 × A_{333}), as described previously (19). Drug loadings of 2–3 M/M are normal. (Cyanoborohydride, 0.5 M overnight, was added at the end of the reaction in early studies in an attempt to reduce the hydrazones. However, as this step has not proven to be beneficial with respect to the biological profile for any conjugates, nor can the reduction be confirmed, it has been excluded in recent work. The acethydrazide used at the end of the conjugation is important to add to block any unreacted aldehydes and thus minimize aggregate formation.) After conjugation, the products are neutralized to pH 7.4 to minimize hydrazone hydrolysis during purification and storage. The final conjugates release some free hydrazide in storage over time, but the in vitro and in vivo activity profiles remain unchanged even after extended storage (months). Conjugates can be lyophilized if long-term storage is desired.

IV. BIOLOGICAL ACTIVITY OF CONJUGATES OF VARIOUS CALICHEAMICIN ANALOGS

A. Activity and Specificity of Calicheamicin γ_1^I Hydrazone Conjugates

Calicheamicin γ_1^I was conjugated with the anti-PEM mAb, CT-M-01, according to the procedure described above and tested for activity and specificity in vitro. In a typical study, calicheamicin γ_1^I [1] and two conjugates: a CT-M-01–γ_1^I hydrazone conjugate that binds to the breast carcinoma line, MX-1, and a γ_1^I hydrazone conjugate prepared with Lym-2, a mAb specific for human B lymphocytes that does not bind to any solid tumors, were studied. In Figure 5, the cytotoxic effects of calicheamicin γ_1^I and the two γ_1^I conjugates are compared on the MX-1 breast carcinoma cells, which binds and internalizes CT-M-01, but not Lym-2, and rat sarcoma XC cells, which do not bind either antibody. These data show that the CT-M-01 conjugate was specifically cytotoxic toward the MX-1 cells and not active on the nontarget line. From dose titration data, the nonbinding Lym-2 conjugate was at least 10-fold less active than the CT-M-01 conjugate or γ_1^I on the MX-1 line, although this Lym-2 conjugate was highly active against

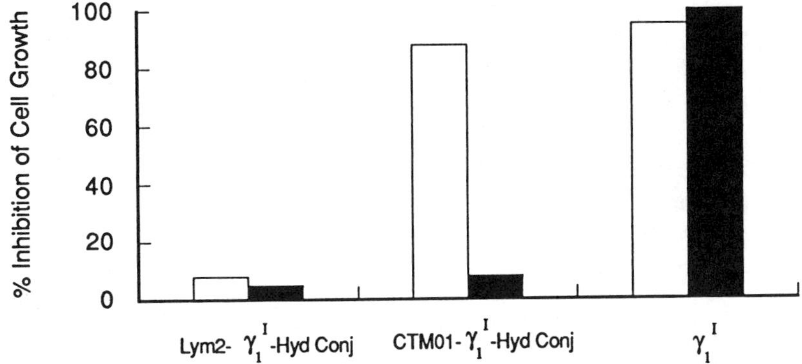

Figure 5 A comparison of the in vitro cytotoxicity of γ_1^I and conjugates of γ_1^I-hydrazide with CT-M-01 and Lym-2 on the MX-1 and XC-RM cells. 10^6 cells were incubated for 30 minutes with 20-ng equivalents of γ_1^I or antibody conjugates loaded with 20-ng equivalents of γ_1^I. After 3 days of growth, the cells were pulsed with ^{3}H thymidine and the inhibition of cell growth resulting from the treatment was calculated relative to the growth of the untreated control cells. □, Target cells (MX-1); ■, nontarget cells (RC-XM).

its own antigen-positive target line, HS Sultan, under similar experimental conditions (data not shown). Data such as these show the selectivity of the calicheamicin conjugates in vitro.

Antitumor effects of the CT-M-01–γ_1^I hydrazide conjugate were also seen in vivo against the MX-1 human breast carcinoma implanted subcutaneously in nude mice. The conjugate was administered at three dose levels (as three doses given 4 days apart). The top dose (25 µg/kg × 3) was lethal to all animals treated by day 21, while at lower doses the conjugates produced a dose-related inhibition of tumor growth. As indicated in Table 2, for the CT-M-01–γ_1^I hydrazone con-

Table 2 Comparison of Efficacy of Calicheamicin–CT-M-01 Hydrazide Conjugates: Effects on Growth of the MX-1 Tumor in Athymic Mice

Conjugate	MED[a] (µg/kg × 3)	MTD[a] (µg/kg × 3)	TR (MTD/MED)	Tumor size[a] (% of control)	Tumor-free survivors at day 100
γ_1^I-Hyd [3]	12.5	12.5	1	13.6	0/6
α_2^I-Hyd [8]	50.0	30.0	< 1	43.6	0/6
α_3^I-Hyd [9]	< 25.0	> 100.0	> 4	0.0	6/6
PSAG-Hyd [10]	> 350.0	> 350.0	< 1	78.7	0/6
N-Acetyl γ_1^I-Hyd [11]	< 25.0	> 100.0	> 4	0.0	6/6

[a] Measured at 35 days post–tumor implantation, $n = 6$ per test group, $n = 10$ in the control group.
Source: Ref. 19.

jugate, one dose of the conjugate, 12.5 μg/kg × 3, was effective and minimally toxic, producing an average of 87% reduction in the size of the tumor at 35 days post–tumor implantation in the four out of six surviving animals. In this study, calicheamicin γ_1^I itself was lethal at one-fifth this dose (MTD for γ_1^I < 2.5 μg/ kg × 3), and the drug hydrazide and a noncovalent mixture of the drug hydrazide and mAb (prepared to simulate the concentrations of both drug and mAb in the conjugates) were both lethal and noneffective at a dose of 6.3 μg/kg × 3. CT-M-01 itself did not inhibit the growth of the tumor at doses up to 0.5 mg/dose × 3 doses (>10 times the dose administered in this test as a conjugate).

From these results it was clear that conjugation of calicheamicin γ_1^I to CT-M-01 decreased the toxicity of calicheamicin γ_1^I more than five-fold and, more importantly, allowed the delivery of a therapeutically effective dose of drug to the tumor. However, treatment with the CT-M-01–γ_1^I hydrazone conjugates did not produce any complete regressions of the MX-1 tumor or result in any long-term survivors. As the MTD and the MED (minimum effective dose) for this conjugate against the MX-1 tumor in vivo were both approximately 12.5 μg/kg × 3, a therapeutic ratio (TR = MTD/MED) or ~1 could be estimated for CT-M-01–γ_1^I hydrazone conjugates. While this compares favorably with the fractional TRs of the drug derivatives or drug–mAb mixtures, an effort to further increase the TR for these conjugates by looking at the properties of conjugates of other calicheamicin derivatives was pursued.

B. In Vivo Activity of CT-M-01 Conjugates of Calicheamicin Variants

The in vivo activity against the MX-1 tumor of the "simple" hydrazide derivatives of the four other calicheamicin analogs described earlier conjugated to CT-M-01 is also summarized in Table 2. These data show that structural variations in the drug had a profound effect on the TR of their conjugates, which did not necessarily correspond with the activity of the drugs as single agents (see Table 1). For example, the CT-M-01 conjugate of α_2^I, the analog missing the rhamnose from the putative DNA-binding region of the drug and next in potency to γ_1^I against P388, had a TR < 1 and showed no antitumor effects at nonlethal doses. In contrast, conjugates of α_3^I and N-acetyl-γ_1^I, analogs that contain the rhamnose but are modified at the amino sugar (see Fig. 3), were highly efficacious over a fourfold dose range, showing an improved therapeutic window (TR > 4) compared with γ_1^I (see Table 2). Both of these conjugates exhibited dramatic antitumor activity, inhibiting the growth of the MX-1 tumor at nonlethal doses and producing long-term tumor-free survivors (>100 days) at the 100 μg/kg dose. The parent drug trisulfides [**5** and **7**] included in the tests as controls were inactive at nonlethal doses. One possible explanation for the superiority of the conjugates of the two calicheamicin derivatives lacking the basic amino sugar (α_3^I and

N-acetyl γ_1^I) over those of γ_1^I is a role for the basic sugar in the triggering of the disulfide. This has been examined by others (27) and shown not to play a role in the solution chemistry of the methyl trisulfides. The biological role of the amino sugar has not been established. One possibility is that the basic amino sugar plays a role in the ability of the compounds to penetrate intracellular membranes or in other ways to efficiently relocate to the nucleus, although this needs to be established.

The fifth variant of calicheamicin conjugated to CT-M-01 was the PSAG [6], which is missing both the rhamnose and the amino sugar. The PSAG is significantly less potent than the other derivatives against P388 leukemia. As shown in Table 2, this conjugate was ineffective and nonlethal even at doses 28-fold higher than the MTD for the γ_1^I conjugate. This is interesting in that it indicates that a conjugate of a derivative that contains the "warhead" of calicheamicin, but not the terminal sugars, could not perform effectively, even when delivered into the cell on an internalizing mAb. Due to this low potency, PSAG conjugates were not studied further.

V. HYDRAZIDE LINKER VARIATIONS: EFFECTS ON BIOLOGICAL STABILITY OF HYDRAZONES AND CONJUGATES

There is significant precedent in the literature, particularly in the study of ricin–mAb conjugates, to suggest that bulky groups near the disulfide of the linker can significantly affect both conjugate stability and potency. The triggering of a calicheamicin requires reduction of the thiol bond (trisulfide in the parent drug or disulfide for the drug derivatives or conjugates). It was therefore of interest to see how structural variation of the simple hydrazide linker would affect the ease of reduction of the disulfide bond in the hydrazide derivatives, that is, how easily the warhead is triggered. In a biological system, the most likely reducing agent to accomplish this cleavage is glutathione. To address the question of the relative stability of various calicheamicin disulfides to reduction with glutathione, the four hydrazides of calicheamicin γ_1^I, shown in Figure 6, were studied. These γ_1^I hydrazides were all prepared from the corresponding thiol hydrazides: 3-mercaptopropionyl hydrazide [2] for the synthesis of the γ_1^I "simple" hydrazide [3], p-mercaptodihydrocinnamyl hydrazide [12] for the synthesis of the γ_1^I aryl hydrazide [13], 3-mercaptobutyryl hydrazide [14] for the synthesis of the γ_1^I monomethyl hydrazide [15], and 3-mercaptoisovaleryl hydrazide [16] for the synthesis of γ_1^I dimethyl hydrazide [17]. The synthesis of these compounds are given in Section VI of this chapter.

To compare the rates of decomposition of these compounds in the presence of glutathione, the following procedure was followed. Stock solutions of each of the hydrazides of γ_1^I (simple [3], aryl [13], monomethyl [15], and dimethyl [17])

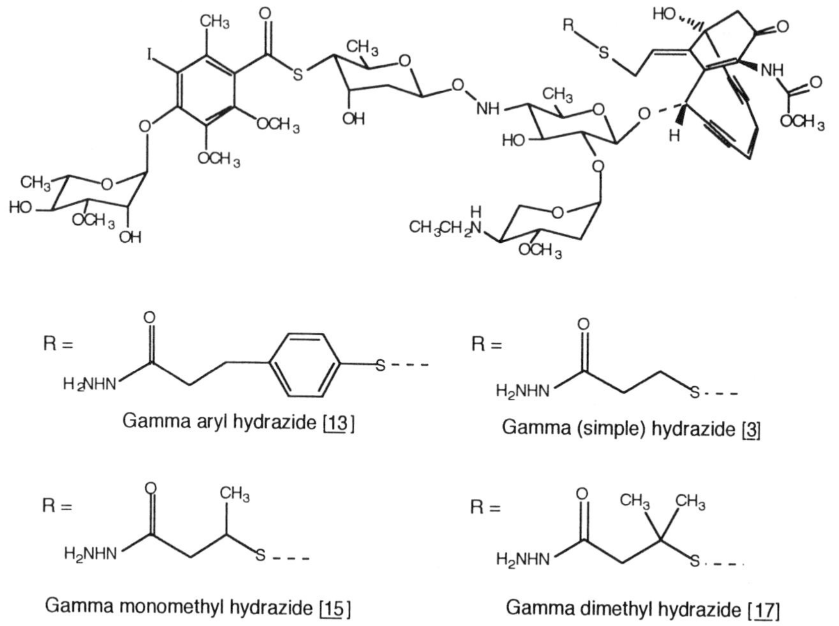

Figure 6 Variations in the structure of the hydrazide linkers of calicheamicin γ_1^I derivatives.

were prepared in ethanol at a concentration of 200 µg/ml. A 100-µl aliquot of each of these was added separately to 900-µl aliquots of 1 mM glutathione in pH 7.0 phosphate (50 mM with 100 mM NaCl). The disappearance of each particular γ_1^I hydrazide was monitored over time by reverse-phase HPLC (C-18 as described above). The concentration of glutathione was assayed before and after this experiment with Ellman's reagent (28). The results of these studies are presented in Table 3, which shows the time course for the decomposition of each of the hydrazides as a result of glutathione reduction.

As these data show, the order of stability of these hydrazides is aryl < simple < monomethyl < dimethyl. For comparative purposes, it should be noted that the aryl disulfide [13] is roughly as stable as γ_1^I [1] itself (data not shown). The disulfide hydrazide formed with a primary thiol [3] is ~1.5 times more stable than either the aryl hydrazide or γ_1^I itself. The more hindered disulfides formed from secondary [15] or tertiary [17] thiols are somewhat more stable at all time points measured. It is interesting to note that hindered disulfides of ITs are 100–1000 times more stable than their nonhindered counterparts (see Refs. 29 and 30). Although the differences in stability from glutathione may appear modest, the effect is reflected in the biological profile of these conjugates. In Figure 7,

Table 3 % Loss of Starting Hydrazide

Hydrazide of γ_1^I	Loss (%) at:		
	30 min	2 hr	6 hr
Aryl [13]	85	100	nd
Simple [1]	55	92	100
Monomethyl [15]	19	52	90
Dimethyl [17]	12	30	nd

the antitumor effects of the aryl [13], the "simple" [3], and the dimethyl [17] hydrazide-linked conjugates of γ_1^I with CT-M-01 are compared on the MX-1 xenograft tumor. As in the studies described above, the conjugates were administered as three intraperitoneal injections (to groups of six mice per treatment group) on days 4, 7, and 11 post–tumor implantation, and the size of the tumor was measured every 7 days post–tumor implantation. As these data indicate, the simple hydrazide conjugate produced a significant reduction in the size of the tumor at the nonlethal dose of 12.5 µg/kg × 3 doses, in agreement with the results de-

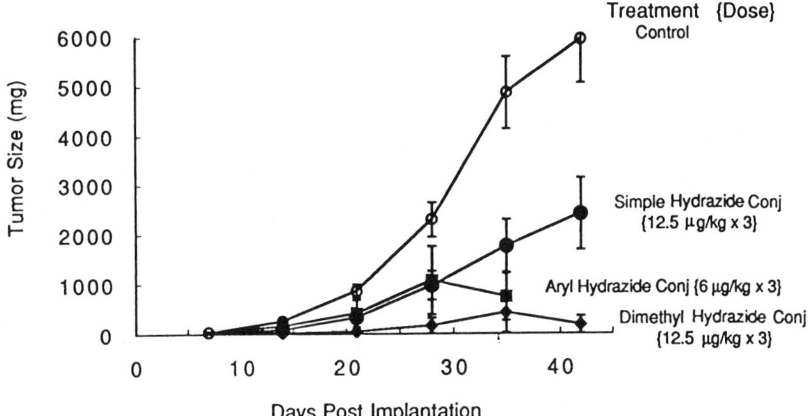

Figure 7 Antitumor effects of CT-M-01 conjugates of γ_1^I prepared with the "simple" [3], the aryl [13], and the dimethyl [17] hydrazide linkers on the MX-1 xenograft tumor. Athymic mice implanted with the subcutaneous MX-1 breast carcinoma were treated s4d × 3, IP, with the conjugate and controls. All animals treated with the aryl conjugate died by day 35, and the animals in the other groups were all alive at day 42. In all test groups $n = 6$, and in the control group $n = 10$; error bars represent ±SEM for each data point.

scribed in Table 2. The less stable aryl-linked conjugate was more toxic than the simple hydrazide and ineffective at lower nontoxic doses, and the more stable dimethyl hydrazide conjugate was more effective than the simple hydrazide conjugate at its optimal dose of 12.5 μg/kg × 3. The monomethyl hydrazide conjugate was comparable to the dimethyl conjugate in activity and toxicity in this study (data not shown). Similar results were seen when the hindered hydrazide linkers were used to compare the activity of conjugates of N-acetyl γ_1^I as previously reported in studies on the MX-2 breast carcinoma (19). Our data suggest that conjugates prepared with hindered hydrazide linkers have a better therapeutic profile than the "simple" hydrazides, which are themselves clearly more effacious than the less stable aryl hydrazides.

Based on these results, conjugates were prepared with the hindered dimethyl linkers using the two calicheamicin derivatives that had already shown superior therapeutic ratios, N-acetyl γ_1^I and α_3^I, as indicated in Table 2. The strong antitumor effects of CT-M-01 conjugates of α_3^I dimethyl hydrazide [18] and N-acetyl γ_1^I dimethyl hydrazide [19] on a non–small-cell lung carcinoma xenograft, Lu78, are shown in Figure 8.

In this study, the α_3^I dimethyl hydrazone–CT-M-01 conjugate was tested over a fourfold dose range, and at day 28, 23 of the 24 treated animals were alive and tumor-free. There was one death in the 265 μg/kg dose group. The N-acetyl γ_1^I dimethyl hydrazone conjugate was tested at two doses, 125 and 165 μg/kg, and 11 of the 12 treated animals were tumor-free at day 28. Using the formula for TR described previously, a TR > 4 was seen with the conjugates in this study. Neither the α_3^I [5], N-acetyl γ_1^I [7], α_3^I dimethyl hydrazide [18] nor N-acetyl γ_1^I dimethyl hydrazide [19] produced significant tumor inhibition at any dose against the Lu78 model.

Our studies defining the activity profile of calicheamicin derivatives conjugated through different linkers incorporated into the drug through disulfide exchange are continuing with a variety of internalizing mAbs specific for both leukemias and solid tumors.

VI. SYNTHETIC DETAILS OF THE PREPARATION OF INTERMEDIATES FOR CALICHEAMICIN CONJUGATION

A. Preparation of Thiol Hydrazides

1. *3-Mercaptopropionyl Hydrazide [2]*

To 5.4 ml (3 eq) of anhydrous hydrazide in 100 ml of refluxing tetrahydrofuran under argon was added dropwise 9.2 ml (83 mmol) of methyl 3-mercaptopropionate in 50 ml tetrahydrofuran over 2 hours. The solution was refluxed an additional 2 hours, evaporated, and then diluted and evaporated twice with 300 ml of toluene. The product was applied to a plug of silica gel with 5%

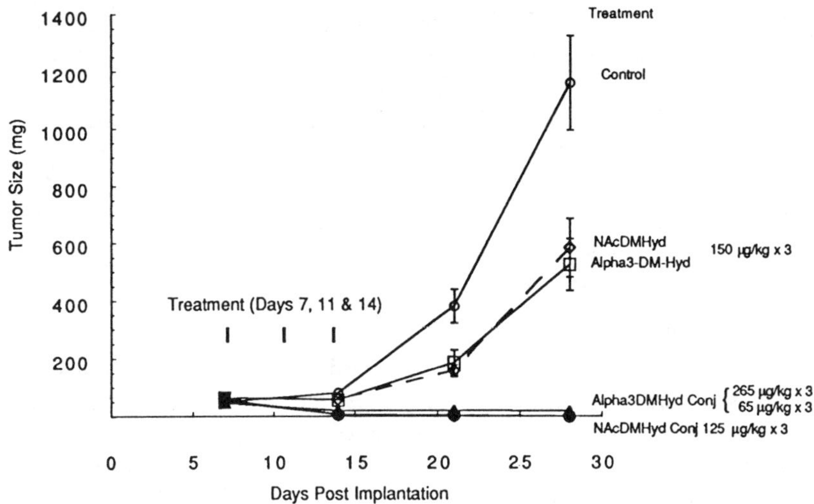

Figure 8 A comparison of the antitumor effects of CT-M-01 conjugate of N-acetyl γ_1^I dimethyl (NAcDM) hydrazide and α_3^I dimethyl (Alpha3DM) and drug hydrazide controls on the Lu78 xenograft tumor. Athymic mice implanted with the subcutaneous Lu 78 non–small-cell lung carcinoma were treated q4d $\times$ 3, IP. The N-acetyl γ_1^I hydrazide and α_3-DM hydrazide were not effective at nonlethal doses. There were four out of six survivors in the α_3^I dimethyl hydrazide conjugate-treated group at the higher dose and six of six tumor-free survivors at lower doses, with significant tumor regressions in all conjugate treatment groups. In all test groups $n = 6$, and in the control group $n = 10$; error bars represent $\pm$SEM for each data point.

ethyl acetate/chloroform and eluted from the plug with 20% methanol/chloroform. The resultant 3-mercapto-propionyl hydrazide was a slightly pink oil that solidified when cooled but melted at room temperature.

NMR(CDCl$_3$): δ 6.87 (br s, 1H, NH), 3.94 (br s, 2H, NH$_2$), 3.45 (m, 2H, CH$_2$), 2.48 (m, 2H, CH$_2$), 1.80 (m, 1H, SH); CI-MS: 121 (MH$^+$), 138 (M-NH$_4^+$); IR: 3303, 3066 (NH), 2554 (SH), 1669, 1634 (NC=O) cm^{-1}; Anal. Calcd for C$_3$H$_8$N$_2$OS: C, 29.99; H, 6.71; N, 23.31; S, 26.68. Found: C, 30.14; H, 6.75; N, 23.12; S, 26.32.

2. p-*Mercaptodihydrocinnamyl Hydrazide* [*12*]

To 500 mg (2.75 mmol) of p-mercaptodihydrocinnamic acid was added 15 ml methanol containing one drop of concentrated sulfuric acid. This reaction was refluxed for 5 hours and then cooled to ambient temperature. Hydrazine (1.5 ml) was added and the resultant mixture was refluxed for 2 hours under argon and then stirred for 10 hours at ambient temperature. A 200-mg portion of dithiothreitol was added to reduce any disulfides present, and the reaction mixture was cooled to –15°C. The resultant crystals were filtered, washed with a mixture of ether and methanol, and then dried in a vacuum oven (50°/5 μm/10 hr) to give *p*-mercaptodihydrocinnamyl hydrazide.

NMR(d6-DMSO): δ 8.95 (s, IH, SH), 7.41 (d, J = 8.2 Hz, 2H, ArH), 7.21 (d, J = 8.2 Hz, 1H, ArH), 4.15 (br s, 1H, NH), 3.34 (br s, 2H, NH$_2$), 2.79 (t, J = 7.7 Hz, 2H, CH$_2$), 2.29 (t, J = 7.7 Hz, 2H, CH$_2$); CI-MS: 197 (MH$^+$), 214 (M-NH4$^+$); IR: 3320, 3208 (NH), 2554 (SH), 1631 (NC=O) cm^{-1}; Anal. Calcd for C$_4$H$_{10}$N$_2$OS: C, 55.08; H, 6.16; N, 14.27; S, 16.33. Found: C, 54.05; H, 6.10; N, 14.70; S, 16.29.

3. *3-Mercaptobutyryl Hydrazide* [*14*]

To 17.2 g (0.2 moles) of crotonic acid was added 18 ml (0.26 moles) of thioacetic acid. This mixture was heated at reflux under argon for 6 hours. The excess thioacetic acid was removed under aspirator vacuum, and the resultant oil was dissolved in 100 ml absolute ethanol containing 200 μl of concentrated sulfuric acid. This reaction was refluxed for 10 hours and then reduced in volume under aspirator vacuum. Hexanes were added, and the resultant solution was washed successively with two portions of saturated sodium bicarbonate and one portion of water. This solution was then dried with magnesium sulfate, filtered, and reduced in volume to an oil. This crude product was dissolved in 250 ml of methanol containing 12 ml of hydrazine, and the resultant mixture was refluxed for 10 hours under argon. The reaction mixture was reduced in volume and then distilled rapidly by Kugelrohr and crystallized from a mixture of chloroform–hexane to give 3-mercaptobutyryl hydrazide.

NMR(CDCl$_3$): δ 6.87 (br s, 1H, NH), 3.94 (br s, 2H, NH$_2$), 3.45 (mult, 1H, CH), 2.48 (dd, J = 5.6 & 14.6 Hz, 1H, CH$_2$) & 2.33 (dd, J = 8.9, 14.6 Hz, 1H, CH$_2$), 1.80 (d, J = 6.5 Hz, 1H, SH), 1.39 (d, J = 6.9 Hz, 3H, CH$_3$); CI-MS: 135.2 (MH$^+$), 152.2 (M-NH$_4^+$); IR: 3303, 3066 (NH), 2254 (SH), 1669, 1634 (NC=O) cm^{-1}; Anal. Calcd for C$_4$N$_{10}$N$_2$OS: C, 35.80; H, 7.51; N, 20,88; S, 23.89. Found: C, 35.91; H, 7.48; N, 20.63; S, 24.02.

4. *3-Mercaptoisovaleryl Hydrazide* [*16*]

To 10 g (0.1 moles) of 3,3-dimethyl acrylic acid was added 9 ml (0.13 moles) of thioacetic acid. This mixture was heated at reflux under argon for 6 hours. The excess thioacetic acid was removed under aspirator vacuum, and the resultant oil was dissolved in 100 ml absolute ethanol containing 200 μl of concentrated sulfuric acid. This reaction was refluxed for 34 hours before addition of 16 ml of hydrazine. The resultant mixture was refluxed for 24 hours under argon. The reaction mixture was reduced in volume and then dissolved in a mixture of brine and saturated sodium bicarbonate. The product was extracted with several volumes of chloroform. The combined chloroform layers were dried with magnesium sulfate, filtered, and reduced in volume to an oil. This oil was purified by flash chromatography with a methanol–chloroform gradient and then crystallized from chloroform-hexanes to give 3-mercaptoisovaleryl hydrazide.

NMR (CDCl$_3$): δ 7.27 (br s, 1H, NH), 3.93 (br s, 2H, NH$_2$), 2.47 (s, 2H, CH$_2$), 2.22 (s, 1H, SH), 1.51 (s, 1H, CH$_3$); Cl-MS: 149.2 (MH$^+$), 166.2 (M-NH$_4^+$); IR: 3291, 3219, 3117 (NH), 2549 (SH), 1652, 1625 (NC=O) cm^{-1}; Anal. Calcd for C$_5$H$_{12}$N$_2$OS: C, 40.52; H, 8.16; N, 18.90; S, 21.63. Found: C, 40.41; H, 8.08; N, 18.94; S, 21.68.

B. Preparation of Calicheamicin Disulfides

A general procedure for the preparation of all of the calicheamicin hydrazide disulfides used in these studies is presented below, and selected chemical properties for each compound are included in Table 4. To a 1–5 mg/ml solution of the appropriate calicheamicin trisulfide in acetonitrile at –15°C is added 3 equivalents of the appropriate thiol-hydrazide in a minimum amount of acetonitrile and one equivalent of triethylamine. The reaction is stirred at –15°C, monitoring the completion of the reaction using reverse-phase (C-18) HPLC. The solvent is then evap-

Table 4 Specific Chemical Properties of Calicheamicin Disulfide Hydrazides

Calicheamicin	#	Retention time (min) % MeCN[a]	RT of SM (min) % MeCN[a]	FAB-MS m/z
γ_1^I simple hydrazide	10	5.0 (41%)[b]	5.5 (56%)[b]	1408 (M+H$^+$)
α_2^I simple hydrazide	11	2.6 (58%)	7.5 (58%)	1248 (M+H$^+$)
α_3^I simple hydrazide	12	2.1 (45%)[b]	5.7 (45%)[b]	1251 (M+H$^+$)
PSAG simple hydrazide	13	2.8 (50%)	7.9 (50%)	1091 (M+H$^+$)
N-Ac-γ_1^I simple hydrazide	14	2.5 (50%)	6.6 (50%)	1450 (M+H$^+$)
γ_1^I aryl hydrazide	15	5.4 (43%)	13.4 (43%)	1484 (M+H$^+$)
γ_1^I methyl hydrazide	16	3.5 (43%)	13.4 (43%)	1422 (M+H$^+$)
γ_1^I dimethyl hydrazide	17	3.9 (43%)	13.4 (43%)	1436 (M+H$^+$)
α_3^I dimethyl hydrazide	18	3.4 (Grad)[c]	5.0 (Grad)[c]	1279 (M+H$^+$)
N-Acetyl γ_1^I dimethyl hydrazide	19	2.5 (50%)	6.6 (50%)	1478 (M+H$^+$)

[a] Isocratic analytical C18-HPLC with acetonitrile/50 mM NH$_4$H$_2$PO$_4$.

[b] Isocratic analytical C18-HPLC with acetonitrile/100 mM NH$_4$O$_2$CCH$_3$.

[c] Gradient analytical C18-HPLC with 35–65% acetonitrile/50 mM NH$_4$H$_2$PO$_4$ (Waters' gradient #5).

All of the above compounds gave NMR spectra similar to the corresponding starting material except for the absence of the absorbence for the -SSMe group and the presence of absorbances expected for the new linker portion.

orated and the residue is chromatographed on silica gel with a 5–15% methanol-in-chloroform gradient to yield the desired product in 50–90% yield.

VII. FUTURE DIRECTIONS FOR ANTIBODY-TARGETED THERAPIES

While the proof of principle that any targeted cytotoxic agent can be effective clinically has yet to be established, impressive preclinical data, such as seen in the studies reported here with the targeted calicheamicins linked to an internalizing mAb, look most promising, and the first clinical evaluations of calicheamicin derivatives conjugated with humanized antibodies are expected within the next two years. The targeting of a potent agent such as a calicheamicin may provide an effective new approach to cancer therapy, yet it is just one of a variety of new approaches to the development of targeted cancer therapeutics. In addition to using mAbs as "magic bullets" to deliver potent cytotoxic drugs, radioisotopes, and protein toxins, researchers are currently looking at mAbs as agents to sensitize cells to chemotherapeutic drugs, modify cellular effector functions, or block cellular receptors.

Regardless of the approach, however, clinical success with mAbs will require the generation of human/humanized mAbs with low immunogenicity that can be used in multiple dosing regimens. Using a combination of a human or humanized antibody and a potent low molecular weight cytotoxic drug, such as calicheamicin, it should be possible to optimize therapeutic benefit with limited side effects. Further research into ways to improve tumor penetration and overcome the problems related to the heterogeneity of antigen expression should lead to additional improvements in mAb-based therapies in the near future.

REFERENCES

1. G. Kohler and C. Milstein, *Nature, 256,* 495 (1975).
2. S. J. Russell, M. B. Llewelyn, and R. E. Hawkins, *Br. Med. J., 305,* 1424 (1992).
3. G. A. Pietersz and I. F. C. McKensie, *Immunol. Rev., 129,* 57 (1992).
4. S. Clark, *Curr. Opin. Invest. Drugs, 2,* 164 (1992).
5. G. A. Heaver, *Ann. Rep. Med. Chem., 27,* 179 (1992).
6. L. J. Sannes, *Spectrum Biotech. Applications, 26,* 1 (1992).
7. D. A. Goldenberg, *Am. J. Med., 94,* 297 (1993).
8. H. Thomas, *Drugs Today, 28,* 311 (1992).
9. P. W. H. I. Parren, *Hum. Antibod. Hybridomas, 3,* 137 (1992).
10. J. S. Sandhu, *Crit. Rev. Biotech., 12,* 437 (1992).
11. L. M. Hinman and G. Yarranton, *Annu. Reports Med. Chem., 28,* (1993), in press.
12. D. J. Buchsbaum and T. S. Lawrence, *Antibody, Immunoconj. Radiopharm., 4,* 245 (1991).

13. E. S. Vitetta, M. Stone, P. Amlot, J. Fay, R., May, M. Till, J. Newman, P. Clark, D. Cunningham, V. Ghetie, J. W. Uhr, and P. E. Thorpe, *Cancer Res., 51,* 4052 (1991).
14. J. Mendelson, *J. Clin. Oncol., 9,* 2088 (1991).
15. P. W. Cobb and C. F. Lemaistre, *Semin. Hematol., 29,* 6 (1992).
16. R. A. Reisfeld and M. Schrappe, in *Therapeutic Monoclonal Antibodies* (C. Borrebaeck and J. Larrick, eds.), Stockton Press, New York, 1990, p. 57.
17. R. V. Chari, B. A. Martell, J. L. Gross, S. B. Cook, S. A. Shah, W. A. Blattler, S. J. McKenzie, and V. S. Goldmacher, *Cancer Res., 52,* 127 (1992).
18. A. C. Morgan, F. T. Comezoglu, R. Manger, B. Jarvis, P. G. Abrams, and G. Sivam, in *Therapeutic Monoclonal Antibodies* (C. Borrebaeck and J. Larrick, eds.), Stockton Press, New York, 1990, p. 143.
19. L. M. Hinman, P. R. Hamann, R. Wallace, A. T. Menendez, F. E. Durr, and J. Upeslacis, *Cancer Res., 53,* 1 (1993).
20. M. Lee, F. Durr, L. Hinman, P. Hamman, and G. Ellestad, in *Advances in Medical Chemistry,* Vol. 2 (B. E. Maryanoff and C. A. Maryanoff, eds.), JAI Press, Greenwich, CT. 1993, p. 31.
21. L. M. Hinman, P. R. Hamann, C. F. Beyer, R. Wallace, J. Upeslacis, J. Adair, T. Baker, and A. Mountain, *Proc. Am. Assoc. Cancer Res., 34,* 479 (1993).
22. M. Brinkley, *Bioconjugate Chem., 3,* 2 (1992).
23. G. A. Koppel, *Bioconjugate Chem., 1,* 13 (1990).
24. J. Upeslacis and L. M. Hinman, *Ann. Rev. Med. Chem., 23,* 151 (1988).
25. J. Upeslacis, *Am. J. Pharm. Ed., 56,* 464 (1992).
26. J. D. Rodwell and T. J. McKearn, U.S. Patent No. 4,671,958, June 9, 1987.
27. K. D. Cramer and C. A. Townsend, *Tetrahedron Lett., 32,* 4635 (1991).
28. H. Deakin, M. G. Ord, and L. A. Stocken, *Biochem. J., 89,* 296 (1963).
29. D. A. Goff and S. A. Carroll, *Bioconjugate Chem., 1,* 381 (1990).
30. L. Greenfield, W. Bloch, and M. Moreland, *Bioconjugate Chem., 1,* 400 (1990).

7

Genetic Analysis of Calicheamicin Biosynthesis

David M. Rothstein
Myco Pharmaceuticals, Inc., Cambridge, Massachusetts

I. INTRODUCTION

The genetic analysis of calicheamicin biosynthesis involved several approaches, including the mutagenesis of *Micromonospora echinospora*, the isolation and characterization of mutants blocked in calicheamicin biosynthesis, the analysis and their defective or partial calicheamicin products, the construction of libraries of *Micromonospora echinospora* DNA, and the identification of calicheamicin biosynthetic genes.

Mutagenesis of antibiotic-producing organisms has proved to be an effective means of generating high-producing variants (2,25,26) and of isolating blocked mutants that aid in the dissection of biosynthetic pathways (2,22,24,25). Using blocked mutant strains, it is also possible to generate novel products by biological conversion of modified intermediates (2,24,25). In order to identify mutants that fail to produce calicheamicin, the biological induction assay (BIA) (8), a quick and reliable plate assay that can detect pg quantities of calicheamicin, was crucial. It was also necessary to mutagenize the producing organism, since the frequency of spontaneous mutants that failed to produce calicheamicin was too low. This chapter will describe protocols that were effective in mutagenizing the calicheamicin producer *Micromonospora echinospora* leading to the isolation and characterization of mutants blocked specifically in the calicheamicin biosynthetic pathway (27).

Blocked mutants often make partial products or intermediates, which can provide information about the biosynthetic pathway. For example, if a pathway requires enzymes A, B, and C, in that order, to make the final product, a mutant that lacks enzyme C activity may still make an intermediate that is secreted into the growth medium as a result of catalysis by enzymes A and B. Furthermore, the intermediate may be taken up and converted to the final product by a second mutant that lacks enzyme A activity but retains enzyme C function, which catalyzes the final step in the pathway. This cross-feeding mechanism, whereby two blocked mutants together make the final product, is called co-synthesis. In a linear biosynthetic pathway, the secreting strain is defective in a later biosynthetic step (e.g., defective enzyme C) and the converting strain in an earlier step in the biosynthetic pathway (lacking enzyme A). In the elegant experiments of Dr. J. McCormick's group at Lederle Laboratories, a collection of mutants blocked in the chlortetracycline biosynthetic pathway was analyzed. The polyketide was found to be produced first, followed by ordered modifications of the pretetramid (22). Other antibiotic pathways have also been analyzed by this approach (2,24).

Micromonospora echinospora normally produces several active forms of calicheamicin, which have in common the aglycon moiety, containing the enediyne (15), which cleaves DNA by a free radical mechanism (31), and an oligosaccharide moiety, which is variable, especially in the amino sugar E (Fig. 1). Characterization of calicheamicin intermediates produced by blocked mutants indicates a branched pathway and suggests that intermediates can derive from either calicheamicin moiety (Sec. III). In addition mutants are described that are defective in producing specific forms of calicheamicin (Sec. III).

Although co-synthesis of final product suggests that nonproducing mutants contain lesions in biosynthetic genes, it is still possible that other explanations could account for the loss of antibiotic formation. Many secondary metabolites, including calicheamicin, are produced after the growing phase (4,19), and their appearance is often dependent on normal development during the stationary phase. The loss of any function that blocks development during the stationary phase could therefore interfere with calicheamicin production. There are examples among actinomycetes of small molecule effectors that are secreted into the growth medium and that are essential for normal development during stationary phase, such as A factor of *Streptomyces griseus* (5). A mutation affecting a nutritional function could also lead indirectly to loss of antibiotic function. Several approaches can provide stronger evidence that genetic lesions are in biosynthetic genes. First, there is strength in numbers. One shouldn't rely on just two co-synthesizing mutants. Second, if a mutant appears to grow poorly or contains an auxotropic defect resulting in a nutritional requirement, the strain should be regarded with suspicion. When in doubt, throw it out. Third, it is preferable to obtain independent evidence that mutants contain a defect specifically in the biosynthetic pathway. One example

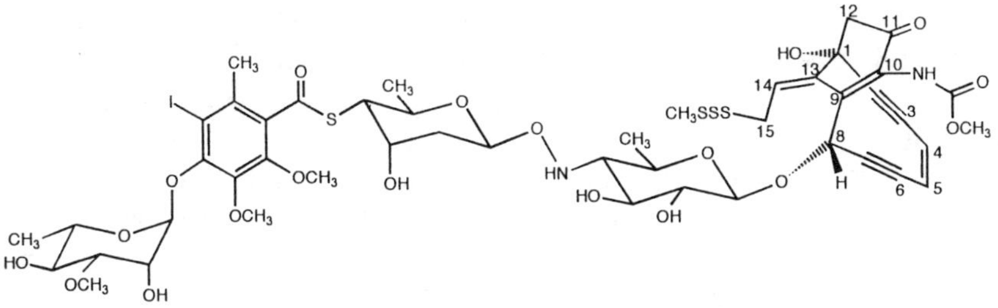

Calicheamicin α_3^I

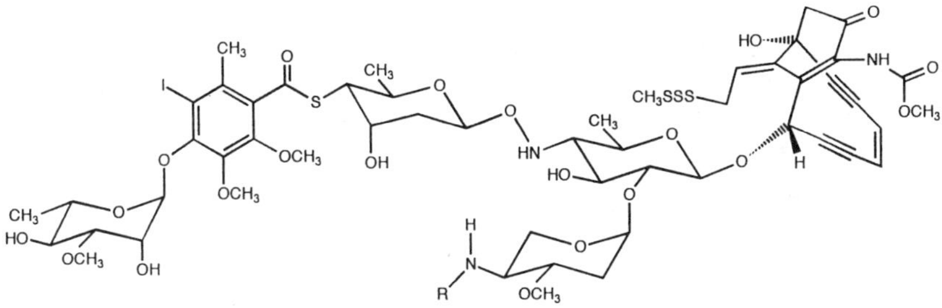

Calicheamicin β_1^I R = (CH$_3$)$_2$CH
Calicheamicin γ_1^I R = CH$_3$CH$_2$
Calicheamicin δ_1^I R = CH$_3$

Figure 1 Chemical structures of calicheamicins α_3^I, β_1^I, γ_1^I, and δ_1^I. Calicheamicin forms have the common core structure shown. The α form lacks the amino sugar E. The β, γ, and δ forms differ in the amino substituent of sugar E. Psuedoaglycon, a fragment of calicheamicin derived by methanolysis, lacks both the D and E sugars.

for *M. echinospora* mutants is the conversion of the pseudoaglycon fragment to calicheamicin (Sec. III).

Blocked mutants also provide an opportunity to clone antibiotic biosynthetic genes by genetic complementation (9,12,29). The characterization of such genes provides the possibility to study the gene products that catalyze the biosynthetic reactions, and thus can provide complementary information about calicheamicin biosynthesis. In order to clone *M. echinospora* genes, libraries containing random DNA fragments from *M. echinospora* were cloned into vectors that could replicate in *Escherichia coli* or *Streptomyces lividans,* two bacteria that have useful and well-studied genetic systems (Sec. IV). However, genetic complementation also requires the ability to transform cloned DNA into blocked mutant strains. Our limited success in transforming *M. echinospora* is summarized in Section V. The development of an efficient transformation system for *M. echinospora* would lead to the rapid cloning of most or all of the calicheamicin biosynthetic genes. Other methods of cloning these biosynthetic genes are described in Section V.

There are several advances that could be achieved if biosynthetic genes were cloned. DNA sequences of biosynthetic genes could suggest functions for gene products involved in this very interesting biosynthetic pathway by comparing the deduced protein sequences to those of known enzyme functions. One method to facilitate the study of a particular enzyme is to overexpress its gene after subcloning into a host such as *E. coli*. Then the isolation of biosynthetic enzymes might be facilitated. Furthermore, the cloning of biosynthetic genes ultimately can result in increased yields of product by cloning and expressing the biosynthetic gene encoding the rate-limiting enzyme back into the producing organism. It could also be possible to generate novel products by cloning biosynthetic genes into strains that make related compounds, such as the esperamicin producer. Such genes could endow the host organism with the ability to carry out new reactions on the enediyne nucleus, a process called *mutasynthesis* (11,13,28).

II. MUTAGENESIS PROTOCOLS FOR *Micromonospora echinospora*

A. Mutagenesis of a Multicellular Microorganism

Because *M. echinospora* grows as a multicellular mycelia, it is difficult to isolate a mutant that fails to produce calicheamicin if it is growing within a mass of producing cells. One method of reducing the number of cells within mycelia is to fracture them by sonication (1). A second approach is to allow the mycelia to differentiate into spores, which are single cells (7,10). Theoretically, growth (growing out) for several generations after mutagenesis can maximize expression of recessive mutations even among unicellular organisms. Just after mutagenesis an individual cell contains one mutagenized DNA strand and a wild-type DNA strand. Thus the cell has the capacity to generate a mixture of mutant and wild-type progeny following cell division. Previously described mutagenic protocols, however, were effective when fractionation or sporulation was used before mutagenesis (1,7,10), perhaps because the mutagenic agent kills at a high enough frequency so that only one daughter cell survived the treatment.

B. Mutagenesis with NTG

N-Nitro-*N*-methyl-*N*-nitroso-guanidine (NTG) works most effectively on the DNA replication fork of growing cells (23). Therefore a protocol was designed for growing cells with the expectation of high mutational frequencies. A well-aerated culture of mycelia growing at 30°C in mid-log phase was exposed to 1 mg/ml of NTG in buffered GER medium (pH 7.6) (27). After 35 minutes, culture aliquots were centrifuged and washed three times with GER medium.

Mutagenized cells were grown out on GER plates for 4 days at 28°C, so that a mutant cell would grow into a localized cluster of cells within the mycelial mass. Mycelia were resuspended in 10% sucrose and fragmented by sonication. Two criteria were utilized to titer fragmentation. Colony-forming units were measured as a function of sonication time, and cells were examined by microscopy. Colony forming units were maximal after 7 seconds of sonication. Mycelia were sonicated longer, for 20 seconds, to assure that only small fragments containing few cells remained (MSE Soniprep 150 sonicator, amplitude 16 μm). Microscopic examination revealed that most mycelial clusters were reduced in size to two to three cell lengths. Such small clusters of cells were likely to be genetically uniform and were diluted and inoculated onto GER plates to obtain discrete colonies or stored at –70°C in 20% glycerol.

Alternatively, mutagenized cells were grown out on slants containing yeast dextrose medium. After incubation at 30°C for 4 weeks, a spore preparation was made by filtration as described (27). Spores were diluted and inoculated on GER plates to obtain discrete colonies.

C. Mutagenesis with Ultraviolet Light

Cells were grown in GER medium to mid-log phase, and 5×10^9 cells were harvested by centrifugation, washed, and sonicated in order to fragment mycelia, as described above. It was important to sonicate prior to UV treatment to prevent shading of interior cells within a mycelial mass (protection from UV light). It was also important to resuspend fractionated mycelia in a clear solution with a large surface area (20% glycerol in a Petri dish) to permit maximum penetration of UV light (27). After exposure for 120 seconds (2.4 j/m^2/sec of UV light at 256 nm), cells were either removed and inoculated onto GER plates for outgrowth or stored at –70°C. Outgrown mycelia were fragmented and treated as described above.

D. Screening for Blocked Mutants

Mutants defective in calicheamicin production were identified by inoculating colonies in wells of 24-well plates (Corning) containing 73-3I medium (27) and one glass bead. After vigorous aeration for one week at 28°C (ample time for the wild type to produce calicheamicin), fermentations were spotted on the BIA plate to identify mutants that failed to produce calicheamicin.

A nonproducing culture was discarded if it exhibited a phenotype suggesting that it carried an extraneous mutation that could prevent calicheamicin production. Examples included mutants that appeared to grow poorly or that were found to have a nutritional requirement. Mutants were also discarded if they failed to produce orange pigment during stationary phase, which was an indication that cells were not developing normally during the stationary phase, when calicheamicin is produced (4,19). (Pigmentless mutants, however, could produce normal amounts of calicheamicin, demonstrating that blocked mutants would not be lost by using pigment formation as a criteria of normal development.)

Fifteen nonproducing mutants of 480 survivors were derived following NTG treatment. Of the fifteen, 9 of 240 tested were isolated after fragmenting the mycelia and 6 were isolated following sporulation. One mutant of 480 tested was derived from UV mutagenesis. NTG mutagenesis, then, was the more effective method of obtaining mutants. The high frequency of calicheamicin nonproducers (over 3% of the NTG-mutagenized cells) is not so extraordinary if one considers the complexity of calicheamicin (Fig. 1) and the number of gene products that must be involved in its biosynthesis. The calicheamicin pathway is therefore likely to be a large genetic target.

Other useful mutants were identified that had acquired nutritional requirements. They could grow on GER agar medium but not on minimal agar medium supplemented as described (6). In all, six classes of auxotrophs were selected using NTG mutagenesis: requirers of (1) aromatic amino acids, the predominant class, (2) tryptophan, (3) uracil + arginine (probably mutated in the carbamoyl phosphate synthetase gene), (4) adenine, (5) lysine, and (6) histidine. From the UV mutagenesis, requirers of (1) organic sulfur, the predominant class, (2) threonine, and (3) histidine were isolated. Most auxotrophs contained a single, defined nutritional requirement, consistent with a mutation at a single genetic locus, rather than multiple mutations. The auxotrophs obtained may prove to be useful genetic markers (18). The organic sulfur requirers may also be useful in labeling calicheamicin with radioactive cysteine or methionine.

III. ANALYSIS OF BLOCKED MUTANTS

A. Conversion of the Pseudoaglycon to Calicheamicin by Blocked Mutants

The pseudoaglycon of calicheamicin lacks two sugar substituents (15) (Fig. 2) and is formed by methanolysis. If the addition of a pure chemical, a fragment of the calicheamicin molecule, is sufficient to overcome the genetic defect of a particular mutant, then the mutant must be defective in manufacturing this fraction of the calicheamicin molecule. Stationary phase cultures of three putative blocked mutant strains, DR43, DR46, and DR1316, were supplemented with the pseudoaglycon. Because the pseudoaglycon retains diminished but detectable BIA activity, extracts of cultures were subjected to thin layer chromatography to sep-

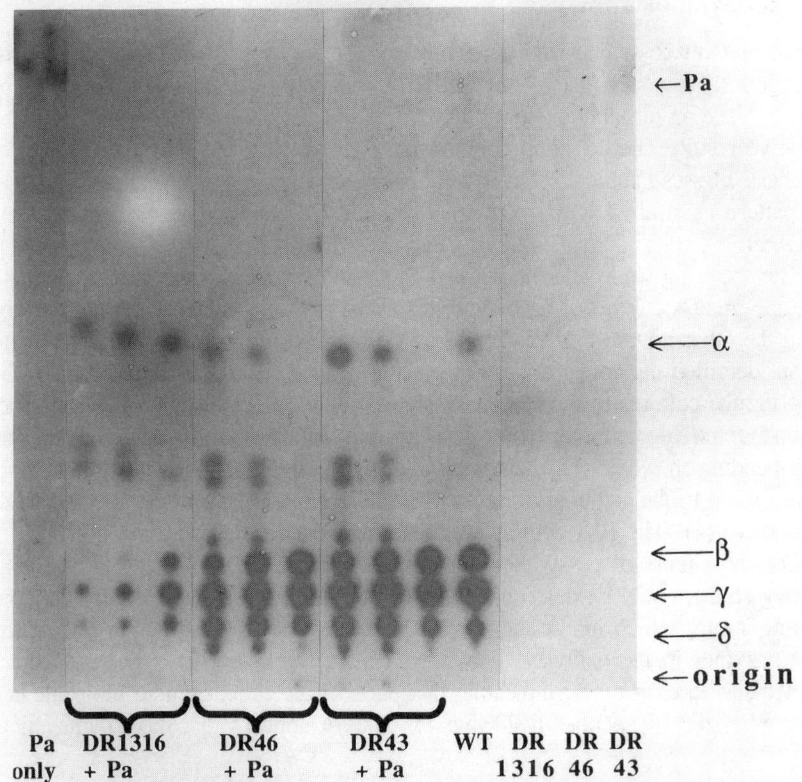

Figure 2 Conversion of pseudoaglycon (Pa) to calicheamicins by blocked mutant strains DR43, DR46, and DR1316. Cultures of the indicated strains were grown to stationary phase in 24-well trays. Then 0.2, 1, or 5 μg of pseudoaglycon (Pa) was added and cultures continued to incubate overnight. Calicheamicins were extracted with acetone/ethyl acetate, subjected to thin layer chromatography, and applied to a BIA plate to detect calicheamicins as described. Samples from cultures without added Pa, as well as those with 0.2, 1, and 5 μg of Pa (from right to left) are indicated. The origin of the TLC plate, pseudoaglycon, and of α, β, γ, and δ calicheamicin forms are indicated. (From Ref. 27.)

arate calicheamicin from the added pseudoaglycon, and then the thin layer plate was tested for BIA activity (27). Figure 2 indicates that the pseudoaglycon was converted to calicheamicins by all three mutant strains. Thus, these mutants are unable to synthesize a chemical bond or substituent found within the pseudoaglycon.

B. Co-Synthesis Studies

If two mutants co-synthesize calicheamicin, then they must contain lesions in distinct genes. However, if two mutants fail to co-synthesize, no conclusion can be drawn, since an unstable or nondiffusable intermediate may be responsible for the negative result. The 15 nonproducing mutants were sorted into 10 distinct co-synthesis classes (Table 1). One additional mutant exhibited the same co-synthesis pattern as strain DR210, and four additional mutants were similar to strain DR1014.

The secreting strain and the converting strain were determined by supplementing one mutant culture of a co-synthesizing pair with a cell-free extract derived from the other mutant culture. Production of calicheamicin following supplementation identified the converting and secreting cultures. Extracts were prepared by growing the cultures to the stationary phase, adding an equal volume of acetone, mixing, removing cell debris by centrifugation, drying down the supernatant, and resuspending in water. Extracts were added to cultures of blocked mutants that were grown to the stationary phase, when calicheamicin is produced in the wild-type strain (4). The BIA activity was determined the following day.

For most pairs of co-synthesizing mutants (Table 1), the secreting and converting strains could be determined (Table 2). Strain DR43 was usually the converting strain, which might suggest that it contains a lesion affecting one of the first enzymes in the pathway. However, strains DR43 and DR123 secreted intermediates to each other, indicating that parts of the calicheamicin molecule can be synthesized independently (Table 1). Thus it appears that the calicheamicin

Table 1 Co-Synthesis Pattern of Blocked Mutants

	DR 210	DR 118	DR 1014	DR 91	DR 123	DR 58	DR 1712	DR 1316	DR 46	DR 43
DR210	−	+	−	−	−	−	−	−	−	+
DR118	+	−	+	−	−	+	−	+	+	+
DR1014	−	+	−	−	−	+	+	+	+	+
DR91	−	+	−	−	+	+	+	+	+	+
DR124	−	+	−	+	−	+	+	+	+	+
DR58	−	−	+	+	+	−	+	+	+	+
DR1712	−	−	+	+	+	+	−	+	+	+
DR1316	−	−	+	+	+	+	+	−	+	+
DR46	−	+	+	+	+	+	+	+	−	+
DR43	+	+	+	+	+	+	+	+	+	−

+, Calicheamicin was detected when the indicated mutant strains (e.g., DR210 and DR118) were grown together; −, no calicheamicin was detected when the indicated strains were grown together.
Source: Ref. 27.

Table 2 Secreter-Converter Relationships Among Blocked Mutants

Extract	Converting strain	Amount detected[a]	Phase partitioning (solvent/water)
DR46	DR43	100	Water
DR1712	DR43	100	Water
DR1316	DR43	10	Water
DR118	DR43	1	nd
DR210	DR43	1	nd
DR123	DR43	1	nd
DR43	DR123	30	Ethyl acetate
DR1316	DR46	3	Ethyl acetate
DR118	DR46	1	nd
DR46	DR123	1	nd
DR210	DR118	15	nd
DR118	DR123	1	nd

[a] Amount determined as %, compared to the conversion by strain DR43 of the intermediate produced by strain DR46.

nd, Not determined.

pathway is branched (see also below). It is therefore possible that particularly stable and/or diffusable intermediates produced by each of the other blocked mutants may complement the defect of strain DR43.

C. Characterization of Calicheamicin Intermediates

One ultimate goal of blocked mutant studies is the identification of intermediates of the calicheamicin pathway. Although this goal has not yet been achieved, some information about the nature of intermediates comes from solvent extraction experiments, and other interesting features from detailed analysis of co-synthesis products.

Solvent-extractable and aqueous fractions were prepared by mixing up equal volumes of ethyl acetate to cultures and collecting the solvent phase. The aqueous phase was saved after cell debris was removed by centrifugation. All samples were lyophilized to dryness, the solvent-extractable material was resuspended in a small volume of ethanol, and the aqueous phase was resuspended in water. The material from up to five volumes of secreting culture was added back to a stationary phase culture of the converting strain, and BIA activity was assessed the next day.

Strain DR43 produced an intermediate that was water insoluble and very hydrophobic. The intermediate, converted by strain DR123, was extracted into ethyl acetate or even into hexane. The aglycone moiety is extremely hydrophobic, so the favored hypothesis is that the intermediate produced by strain DR43 derives from the aglycone moiety. DR43, according to this hypothesis, is capable of making the aglycone moiety but is deficient in making a substituent of the oligosaccharide moiety. In keeping with the hypothesis, intermediates converted by strain DR43 were water soluble. Since the oligosaccharide moiety is the more polar region of the calicheamicin molecule, it is likely that such water-soluble intermediates are derived from that moiety. Furthermore, strains DR43 and DR46 co-synthesized the beta form, but not the gamma form, of calicheamicin, whereas the wild-type strain produced both the beta and gamma forms as major products (Fig. 3). The simplest explanation is that the soluble intermediate produced

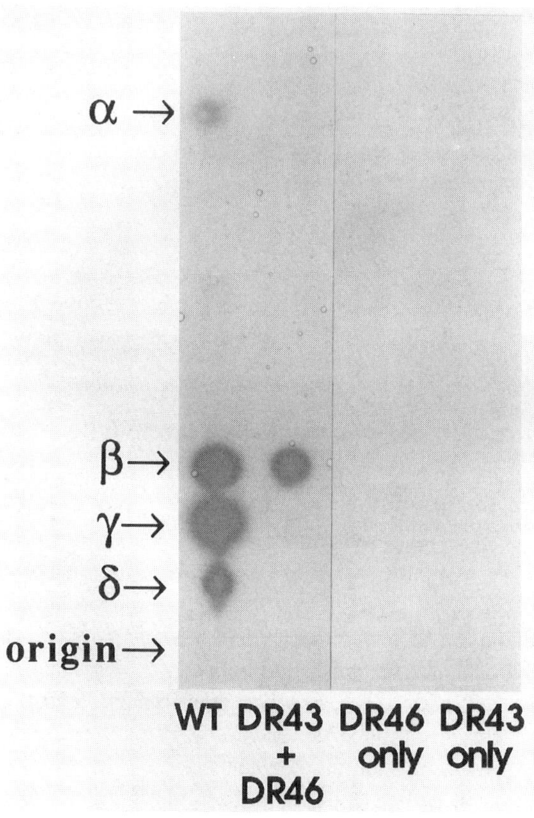

Figure 3 Blocked mutant strains DR43 and DR46 co-synthesized the β, but not the γ calicheamicin form. Cultures of the wild type (WT), strain DR43, and strain DR46, were grown separately, and strain D43 and DR46 were grown together. Calicheamicins were extracted with ethyl acetate, separated by thin layer chromatography, and applied to a BIA agar plate as described. The origin of the TLC plate and of calicheamicins α, β, γ, and δ, are indicated. (From Ref. 27.)

by strain DR46 contains the isopropyl amino sugar E (Fig. 1), predetermining that the beta form is made in the co-synthesis. Again the evidence suggests that strain DR43 requires a chemical bond or entity found within the thiobenzoate-carbohydrate tail, provided either by pseudoaglycon or by water-soluble intermediates produced by strains DR46, DR1316, or DR1712.

The analysis of intermediates also reinforces the notion that the calicheamicin biosynthetic pathway, unlike the tetracycline pathway, is branched. As discussed previously, strains DR43 and DR123 secreted intermediates to each other, indicating a branched pathway (Table 2). It is also noteworthy that strain DR1316 produced two intermediates with distinct chemical properties: a water-soluble intermediate converted by strain DR43, and an ethyl acetate-extractable intermediate converted by strain DR46. Thus, distinct intermediates of the calicheamicin pathway can be synthesized within one blocked mutant, indicating that parts of the calicheamicin molecule can be synthesized independently (Table 2).

The purification of intermediates requires a reliable assay to track the intermediate. The water-soluble intermediate produced by strain DR46 was assayed by adding back to strain DR43 cultures that had been grown to stationary phase. The following day the BIA assay revealed the presence of the intermediate. The intermediate of strain DR46 was processed on a large scale by passing supernatant through a column containing XAD2 beads and eluting with methanol. Recovery was estimated to approach 100%. After drying and resuspending in water, the material was further purified by reverse-phase column chromatography with C18 or by partition chromatography on Sephadex LH-20. Either 1, 10, or 180 μl from each fraction tested was assayed for the intermediate by adding back to 0.8 ml of the converting culture that had grown into stationary phase, and the BIA activity was determined the following day (Fig. 4). The amount of intermediate in fractions, relative to the starting material, indicated that most of the intermediate was recovered. The intermediate appears stable when stored as a partially purified solution at –20°C.

The hydrophobic intermediate produced by strain DR43 was tracked by adding back to the converting culture, strain DR123. This intermediate could be separated by concentrating the cells by centrifugation or filtration and extracting with acetone. After the cell debris was removed by centrifugation, the extracted material was dried, resuspended in water, and the intermediate was found to partition into the organic phase when an equal volume of methylene chloride was added.

D. Mutants Defective in Producing Specific Calicheamicin Intermediates

To screen for mutants exhibiting an altered profile of calicheamicin components, fermentations were extracted by adding 325 μl of organic solvents (8/5 acetone/ethyl acetate V/V) to 0.8 ml of culture broth. Samples were vortexed, centrifuged,

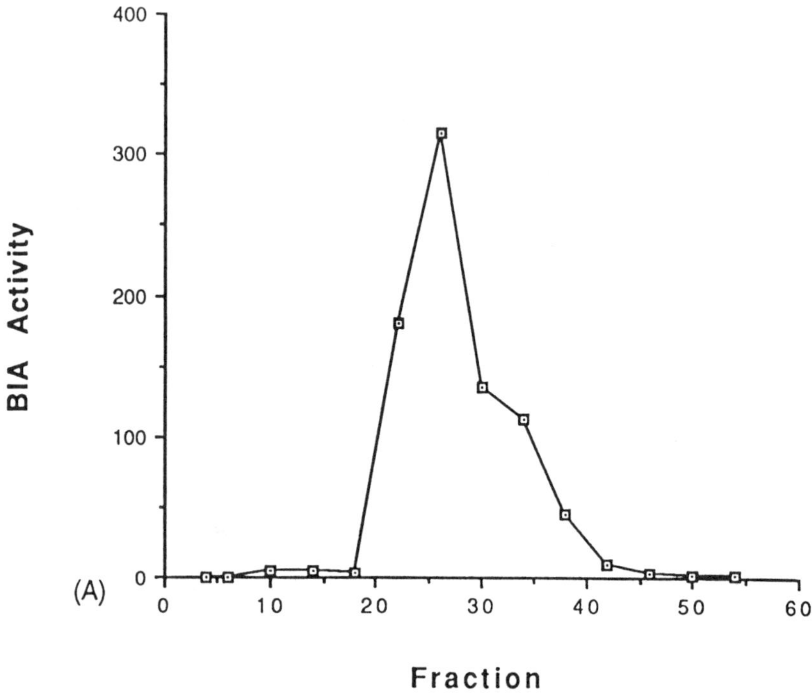

Fraction

Figure 4 Chromatography of the intermediate secreted by strain DR46. The intermediate was concentrated by passing supernatant of a stationary culture of strain DR46 over XAD2 beads and eluting with methanol. After drying and resuspending, the eluate was subjected to C18 reversed-phase column chromatography (A), or LH20 chromatography (B). Fractions were eluted with methanol/H_2O, dried, and resuspended in their original volume with water. 1, 10, or 180 μl of each fraction was added to 0.8 ml of the converting culture, strain DR43, grown to the stationary phase. The following day the BIA activity of fractions and of original sample was determined. The BIA activity, in arbitrary units (the amount of intermediate found in the mg of crude preparation/fraction for (A), or relative to ml of supernatant/fraction for (B)) is indicated.

and 10 μl of the top phase was applied to a thin layer chromatography plate (27). The predominant calicheamicin forms of wild-type cultures were beta and gamma, which differ in substituents on the amino sugar (Fig. 1). Figure 5 shows profiles of two mutant strains that were detected by screening NTG-treated cells using thin layer chromatography. Strain DR414 produced only the delta form, and strain DR1122 produced delta and gamma forms.

These mutants were apparently blocked in a biosynthetic step(s) essential for producing the other calicheamicin component(s). The existence of such mutants

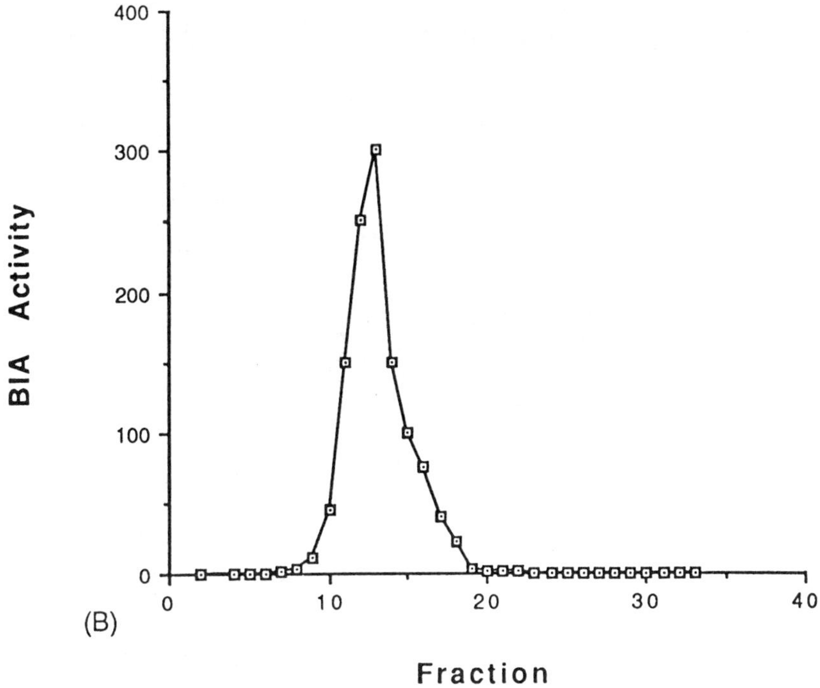

suggest that the conversion of delta, beta, and gamma forms may involve the sequential addition of methyl groups onto the nitrogen of amino sugar E (Fig. 1). We do not as yet know, however, whether each mutant strain contains a genetic defect resulting in the loss of a single enzyme function.

IV. MOLECULAR BIOLOGY OF *Micromonospora echinospora*

A. Constructing Libraries of *M. echinospora* DNA

To construct DNA libraries, the *Micromonospora* chromosome was partially digested with Sau3A1 restriction enzyme, and large fragments were isolated following agarose gel electrophoresis or following sucrose gradient centrifugation as described (20). The fragments were cloned into derivatives of plasmid pBR322, and *E. coli* was transformed. Alternatively, large fragments of *M. echinospora* DNA were cloned into a cosmid shuttle vector constructed by Mike Ryan and Jason Lotvin, to be described in a future publication (personal communication). This vector has the advantage that large fragments of approximately 25 kb of *M. echinospora* DNA (encoding 25 average-sized structural genes) were ligated to

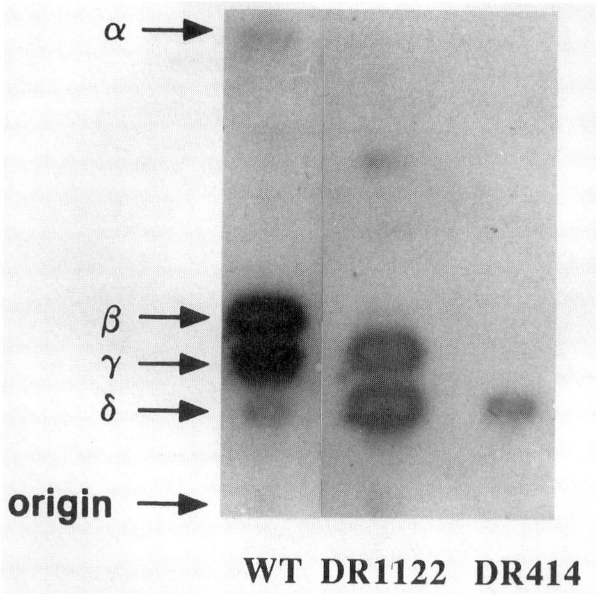

Figure 5 Mutants with altered profiles of calicheamicin forms. Cultures of the indicated strains were extracted with acetone/ethyl acetate, subjected to thin layer chromatography, and applied to a BIA agar plate to detect calicheamicins as described. The origin and the α, β, γ, and δ calicheamicin forms are indicated. (From Ref. 27.)

two other DNA fragments. These vector fragments, or arms, contain the *cos* site essential for λ packaging, origins of plasmid replication, and selectable markers, enabling the ligated DNA to be packaged into bacterial virus particles or, subsequently, to exist as a plasmid in either *E. coli* or in *S. lividans*. The ligation with the cosmid arms was packaged as described to form lambda virus particles (20), which infected *E. coli*. The plasmic form of the cosmid was prepared and was used to transform *S. lividans,* selecting for thiostrepton resistance.

B. Strategies to Identify Calicheamicin Biosynthetic Genes

Biosynthetic genes for other antibiotics have been cloned using a variety of strategies (9,29). The following approaches to clone calicheamicin biosynthetic genes were considered:

1. Clone into *Micromonospora* strains blocked specifically in the calicheamicin pathway (27), and screen for genetic complementation.
2. Identify clones that hybridize with the *actI* gene, a polyketide synthetase gene of actinohodin biosynthesis (12).

3. Select for clones that confer calicheamicin resistance, since in some organisms resistance genes are linked to antibiotic biosynthetic genes.
4. Clone the entire pathway into a naive host, *S. lividans*.
5. Screen clones for the ability to make a calicheamicin intermediate by co-synthesis with a *Micromonospora* blocked mutant strain.
6. Identify and isolate a biosynthetic enzyme, sequence part of the protein, and make a probe to identify the DNA encoding the protein.
7. Clone into *Micromonospora;* screen for increased antibiotic production.

Cloning by genetic complementation of blocked mutants is an excellent way to clone biosynthetic genes, because it assumes nothing about the number of required genes, the linkage of genes, or the expression of genes in foreign hosts. It is the most direct method to clone biosynthetic genes. Mutants blocked specifically in the calicheamicin biosynthetic pathway were described in Sections II and III. However, obstacles to cloning genes into *M. echinospora* are serious impediments to large-scale (shotgun) cloning into *M. echinospora* (see below).

It is likely that part of the calicheamicin molecule (Fig. 1)—either the aglycone backbone and/or the multi-substituted phenyl ring—is synthesized by a polyketide mechanism. The proposed polyketide synthetase may be encoded by a gene that is homologous to *actI* of *S. coelicolor* (12). By performing a colony hybridization with the *E. coli* libraries containing *Micromonospora* DNA, the *actI* homolog of *Micromonospora* was identified. It would be interesting to assess whether inactivation of this gene in the *Micromonospora* chromosome results in a mutant blocked in calicheamicin biosynthesis. Such an experiment would require overcoming obstacles in transferring DNA into *M. echinospora,* which are discussed below.

Bacteria generally have mechanisms to protect against drugs that they produce. Often genes that encode resistance are linked to biosynthetic genes (9,29). To select for calicheamicin resistance among *S. lividans* transformants carrying *Micromonospora* DNA, transformants were incubated on agar medium with extracts containing calicheamicin. Several independently isolated clones that survived exposure to calicheamicin contained plasmid with a similar restriction pattern, indicating that the *Micromonospora* DNA within the plasmids contained common sequences that protected against calicheamicin.

There is little possibility of cloning the entire calicheamicin biosynthetic pathway. This approach is predicated on the notion that all of the biosynthetic genes are genetically linked in one region of the chromosome, as is the case for some biosynthetic pathways. Furthermore, all of the genes for the pathway would have to be located within 25 kb of DNA, which is the size of *Micromonospora* inserts within each cosmid. However, it is probable that more than 25 Kb of DNA (enough information for approximately 25 genes) is essential for encoding all the enzymes to carry out the many steps involved in making such a complicated molecule. It was therefore not surprising that none of 3000 cosmid transformants of *S. lividans* tested produced calicheamicin, which was assessed by utilizing the BIA (8).

The fifth approach, to clone part of the biosynthetic pathway, is a more realistic possibility. In this strategy, *Micromonospora*-blocked mutants that co-synthesize calicheamicin, described earlier in the chapter, are utilized. A pair of blocked mutants, grown together, can make calicheamicin by a cross-feeding mechanism (co-synthesis), whereas neither mutant alone can make the entire molecule. The secreting strain makes an intermediate that is taken up by the converting strain, which incorporates it into the final product. In this strategy, a transformant of *S. lividans* is the potential screening strain; the 25 kb of cloned *Micromonospora* DNA must contain the information to synthesize the intermediate for this method to succeed. Two *Micromonospora* blocked mutant strains, DR43 and DR123, were utilized as converter strains in these experiments. Again 3000 clones were co-grown with either the blocked mutant strain DR43 or DR123 by mixing together 0.6 ml of *S. lividans* transformants with 0.6 ml of the converting culture. No BIA activity was detected after 5 days' growth. Control experiments showed that co-synthesis was not inhibited by the presence of faster-growing *Streptomyces* cells in the culture. For cloning any one particular gene function, 3000 transformants represents a fivefold redundancy of the *M. echinospora* chromosome, meaning that the chances that a particular gene is not once represented among the 3000 transformants are vanishingly small. It is possible that genes required to make an intermediate are not linked and/or that the amount of information to encode for making an intermediate exceeds 25 kb. It is always possible that the required genes for making an intermediate were cloned into *S. lividans* but were not expressed.

The sixth approach, reverse genetics, requires a purified biosynthetic enzyme from *Micromonospora,* which is not yet available. The seventh approach, cloning the rate-limiting enzyme in calicheamicin biosynthesis, thereby improving calicheamicin production, requires improvements in the methods for cloning in *Micromonospora* (see below).

C. Transformation of Plasmid DNA into *M. echinospora*

The transformation of *M. echinospora* with plasmid DNA required overcoming four obstacles: (1) protoplasting of the organism to allow the entry of DNA, (2) regenerating the protoplasts, (3) selecting transformants with an effective marker (e.g., a drug-resistance determinant), and (4) identifying a plasmid that replicates efficiently in *M. echinospora*. A summary of these findings follows; more details are described elsewhere (18).

The important features enhancing the formation of protoplasts, that is, cells devoid of the cell wall, were the age of the culture (48–60 hours of growth in

GER medium at 28°C), and the addition of glycine to 0.15% in the growth medium, which results in smaller mycelial fragments that break up more easily following lysozyme treatment. Regeneration required 0.15 M sucrose as osmotic stabilizer (other osmotic stabilizers were not effective) and a growth rate–limiting nitrogen source (e.g., RM medium). Curiously, in medium containing a good nitrogen source, mucoid colonies resulted that required the continued propagation of osmotically stabilized medium. Because sucrose is a favored carbon source, there was no possibility of testing the effect of alternative carbon sources.

Most *Streptomyces* plasmids rely on the thiostrepton resistance determinant as the selectable marker. Unfortunately, *M. echinospora* is partially resistant to thiostrepton, preventing its use in selecting for transformants. To maximize the possibility that the kanamycin resistance marker would be expressed in *M. echinospora* transformants, DNA fragments containing *M. echinospora* promoters were inserted in plasmid pIJ486 (30). The combination of a *M. echinospora* promoter region followed by the kanamycin resistance gene was inserted within each plasmid that was tested for transformation of *M. echinospora*.

The major obstacle in developing a cloning system in *M. echinospora* is identifying a plasmid that is well maintained. The natural source of plasmids is actinomycetes, since in general, plasmids from outside the actinomycete group do not replicate in these organisms. Transformation was detected using a derivative of plasmid pIJ486 described above, which conferred kanamycin resistance. Using this derivative, transformants were detected when kanamycin was added 5 days after incubation of regenerating protoplasts, albeit at a frequency that was too inefficient to consider shotgun cloning into *M. echinospora*. This plasmid has a replicating mechanism (replicon) that works well in *Streptomyces* spp. (9,29) and in some *Micromonospora* strains (14,21). However, in *M. echinospora* transformants, plasmid could only be detected by Southern analysis, using ^{32}P-labeled probe, and not by ethidium bromide staining (18). Thus the plasmid was not well replicated and/or well maintained in *M. echinospora*. Transformation with a number of other plasmids (9,29), which were modified to contain a kanamycin resistance determinant as the selectable marker, were not successful.

D. Expressing Biosynthetic Genes During the Stationary Phase

Calicheamicin is produced by *M. echinospora* during the stationary phase (4,19). Thus, if biosynthetic genes were cloned, then it would be desirable, and maybe even essential, to express these genes during the stationary phase. An expression system was developed for expressing cloned genes during the stationary phase in *M. echinospora*. It relies on a subclone of the 0.4 kb fragment from *M. echinospora,* containing only the P1 promoters and not the P2 promoter (3,4). The mechanism of regulation of the P1 promoters is at the level of transcription. There is a form of RNA polymerase that is only found in *M. echinospora* during the stationary phase (16,17). This form of RNA polymerase recognizes the P1 promoters. Thus, if calicheamicin biosynthetic genes were cloned, they could be expressed at the time that calicheamicin is produced by ligating such structural genes, and their translational start signals, after the P1 promoter signals. Then transcription of cloned genes would be dependent on the RNA polymerase enzyme that was only present in *M. echinospora* during stationary phase.

V. SUMMARY

The isolation of mutant strains of *Micromonospora echinospora* blocked in the production of calicheamicin provides a means for elucidation of the calicheamicin biosynthetic pathway. These mutants probably contain lesions in genes of this pathway for the following reasons. Each of the 16 mutants co-synthesized calicheamicin with at least two other mutants (Table 1). All three mutants tested were able to make calicheamicin when supplemented with the pseudoaglycon fragment (Fig. 2). Furthermore, strain DR46 secreted an intermediate that strain DR43 converted to the beta, but not the gamma calicheamicin component (Fig. 3), suggesting that the intermediate contained the isopropylamino sugar E (Fig. 1).

These studies indicate that calicheamicin is produced by a branched, rather than a linear pathway. A reasonable working hypothesis is that the aglycon and oligosaccharide moieties are synthesized independently. One intriguing possibility is that strain DR43 can synthesize the aglycon domain of the molecule, which accounts for its production of the hydrophobic intermediate. Strain DR43 appears to require a chemical bond or entity found within the thiobenzoate-carbohydrate tail, provided either by pseudoaglycon or by water-soluble intermediates produced by strains DR46, DR1316, or DR1712.

Additional mutants were isolated that produced an altered profile of calicheamicin components (Fig. 5). These mutants suggest the possibility that methyl groups are added to the amino sugar sequentially, resulting in the conversion of the methyl amino sugar to the ethyl amino sugar, which would subsequently be converted to the isopropyl amino sugar.

The cloning of some calicheamicin biosynthetic genes may have been accomplished by the identification of the *actI* homolog from *Micromonospora* and the cloning of a resistance gene(s) conferring some protection against extracts containing calicheamicin. However, cloning for the capacity to make calicheamicin intermediates was unsuccessful. The cloning of biosynthetic genes by genetic complementation of blocked mutant strains, which has proved to be a powerful approach for other biosynthetic systems, awaits improvements in the frequency of plasmid transformation. In particular, an alternative vector is required that replicates more efficiently and/or is better maintained in *Micromonospora echinospora*.

The analysis of blocked mutant strains and the cloning of calicheamicin biosynthetic genes are two complementary approaches to learning about the biosynthetic pathway of the calicheamicins and the gene products catalyzing the biosynthetic reactions. Both approaches provide possibilities of generating novel calicheamicin derivatives.

ACKNOWLEDGMENTS

I thank Ellen Baum, Ling-Shen Lin, and Susan Love for carrying out many of the experiments described in this chapter, Bill Maiese for his support, May Lee for helpful discussions and for providing pseudoaglycon, Cindy McElroy and Joann Manning for technical assistance, and Marcia Osburne and Valerie Bernan for valuable discussions.

REFERENCES

1. R. H. Baltz, in *Manual of Industrial Microbiology and Biotechnology* (A. L. Demain and N. A. Solomon, eds.), American Society for Microbiology, Washington, DC), 1986, pp. 184–190.
2. R. H. Baltz and E. T. Seno, *Ann. Rev. Microbiol., 42,* 547 (1988).
3. E. Z. Baum, M. J. Buttner, L.-S. Lin, and D. M. Rothstein, *J. Bacteriol., 171,* 6503 (1989).
4. E. Z. Baum, S. F. Love, and D. M. Rothstein, *J. Bacteriol., 170,* 71 (1988).
5. T. Beppu and S. Horinouchi, *Planta Med., 57,* S44 (1991).
6. R. W. Davis, D. Botstein, and J. R. Roth, *Advanced Bacterial Genetics,* Cold Spring Harbor Laboratory, Cold Spring Harbor, NY, 1980.
7. V. Delic, D. A. Hopwood, and E. J. Friend, *Mutat. Res., 9,* 167 (1970).
8. R. K. Elespuru and R. J. White, *Cancer Res., 43,* 2819 (1983).
9. D. A. Hopwood, M. J. Bibb, K. F. Chater, and T. Kieser, *Methods Enzymol., 143,* 106 (1987).
10. D. A. Hopwood, M. J. Bibb, K. F. Chater, T. Kieser, C. J. Bruton, H. M. Kieser, D. J. Lydiate, C. P. Smith, J. M. Ward, and H. Schrempf, *Genetic Manipulation of* Streptomyces; *A Laboratory Manual,* The John Innes Foundation, Norwich, U.K., 1985.
11. D. A. Hopwood, F. Malpartide, H. M. Kieser, H. Ikeda, J. Duncan, I. Fujii, B. A. M. Rudd, H. G. Floss, and S. Omura, *Nature, 314,* 642 (1985).
12. D. A. Hopwood and D. H. Sherman, *Ann. Rev. Genetics, 24,* 37 (1990).
13. C. R. Hutchinson, C. W. Borell, M. J. Donovan, F. Kato, H. Motamedi, H. Nakayama, S. L. Otten, R. L. Rubin, S. L. Streicher, and K. J. Stutzman-Engwall, *Ann. NY Acad. Sci., 646,* 78 (1991).
14. G. H. Kelemen, I. Financsek, and M. Jarai, *J. Antibiot., 42,* 325 (1989).
15. M. D. Lee, J. K. Manning, D. R. Williams, N. A. Kuck, R. T. Testa, and D. B. Borders, *J. Antibiotic., 42,* 1070 (1989).

16. L.-S. Lin and D. M. Rothstein, *J. Bacteriol.*, *174*, 3111 (1992).

17. L.-S. Lin and D. M. Rothstein, *J. Gen. Microbiol.*, *138*, 1881 (1992).

18. S. F. Love, W. M. Maiese, and D. M. Rothstein, *Appl. Environ. Microbiol.*, *58*, 1376 (1992).

19. W. M. Maiese, M. P. Lechevalier, H. A. Lechevalier, J. Korshalla, N. Kuck, A. Fantini, M. J. Wildey, J. Thomas, and M. Greenstein, *J. Antibiotics*, *42*, 558 (1989).

20. T. Maniatis, E. F. Fritsch, and J. Sambrook, *Molecular Cloning: A Laboratory Manual,* Cold Spring Harbor Laboratory, Cold Spring Harbor, NY, 1982.

21. Matsushima, P. and R. H. Baltz, *J. Antibiot.*, *41*, 583 (1988).

22. J. R. D. McCormick, U. Hirsch, N. D., Schollander, and A. P. Doerschuk, *J. Am. Chem. Soc.*, *82*, 5006 (1960).

23. J. H. Miller, *Experiments in Molecular Genetics,* Cold Spring Harbor Laboratory, Cold Spring Harbor, NY, 1972.

24. S. Omura and Y. Tanaka, in *Macrolide Antibiotics: Chemistry, Biology, and Practice* (S. Omura, ed.), Academic Press, Inc. New York, 1984, pp. 199–229.

25. S. W. Queener, *Ann. Rev. Microbiol.*, *32*, 593 (1978).

26. S. W. Queener and D. H. Lively, in *Manual of Industrial Microbiology and Biotechnology* (A. L. Demain and N. A. Solomon, eds.), American Society for Microbiology, Washington, DC, 1986, pp. 155–169.

27. D. M. Rothstein and S. F. Love, *J. Bacteriol.*, *173*, 7716 (1991).

28. W. R. Strohl and N. C. Connors, *Mol. Microbiol.*, *6*, 147 (1992).

29. P. K. Tomich, *Antimicrob. Agents Chemother.*, *32*, 1465 (1988).

30. J. M. Ward, G. R. Janssen, T. Kieser, M. J. Bibb, M. J. Buttner, and M. J. Bibb, *Mol. Gen. Genet.*, *203*, 468 (1986).

31. N. Zein, A. M. Sinha, W. J. McGahren, and G. A. Ellestad, *Science, 240,* 1198 (1988).

8

Biological Activities of Calicheamicin

Frederick E. Durr, Roslyn E. Wallace, Raymond T. Testa, and Nydia A. Kuck
Lederle Laboratories, American Cyanamid Company, Pearl River, New York

I. ANTITUMOR ACTIVITY OF CALICHEAMICIN

A. In Vivo Antitumor Activity

The biological activity of the calicheamicin complex of antibiotics was first detected in a modified biochemical prophage induction assay (1) used in the laboratory to screen fermentation broths for DNA-damaging agents. The in vivo studies initially carried out with the earliest antibiotic preparations showed these antibiotics to have significant antitumor activity at extremely low treatment doses against a number of experimental murine tumors. For example, the β_1 component was highly effective against the P388 leukemia in mice when given intraperitoneally (IP) on a day 1, 5, and 9 treatment schedule, producing an overall 95% increase in life span (%ILS) with 2 of 30 mice surviving 30 days at the optimal dose of 1.25–2.5 μg/kg. Similar doses given on the same schedule produced a 40% ILS with three of six long-term (60 days) survivors when β_1 was tested against B16 melanoma and a 59% ILS when tested against colon 26. This degree of activity was equal to or greater than the DN2 activity criteria established by the NCl for these tumors (2). The degree of activity against P388 leukemia and the solid tumor B16 melanoma was especially exciting. Other members of the calicheamicin complex proved to be equally potent and effective in these three tumor models. The efficacy of the γ_1^I component, which eventually was chosen as the lead candidate for development, against a panel of intraperitoneally implanted murine tumors is shown in Table 1. In other studies (not shown) it was determined that γ_1^I was more effective against B16 melanoma on the q4d $\times$ 3 schedule than when administered as a single dose or on a qd $\times$ 9 schedule. In these studies the γ_1^I derivative given at 1.2 μg/kg produced a survival pattern similar to that of doxorubicin administered at 800 μg/kg on its optimal schedule of qd $\times$ 9 (3).

As new preparations of calicheamicin γ_1^I were evaluated for activity over time, it was observed that the optimal IP dose of the antibiotics against P388 leukemia on the q4d $\times$ 3 schedule varied between 0.6 and 5.0 μg/kg with a median dose of 2.5 μg/kg, which produced an average of 20% survivors at 30 days. Significant antitumor activity (ILS $\geq$ 25%) was also demonstrable at doses as low as 0.15 μg/kg. Dose-scheduling studies carried out against P388 leukemia provided no evidence for schedule dependency, but the IP q4d $\times$ 3 schedule has become our standard treatment regimen on the basis of the performance of the calicheamicin derivatives against B16 melanoma and other solid tumors when given on that schedule.

Limited studies on the effect of route of administration of calicheamicin against IP-implanted P388 leukemia have indicated that the antibiotic was effective by the IP route but was ineffective when given subcutaneously (SC) or orally (3). Intravenous (IV) administration was effective against IV-injected P388 leukemia, and when given IP or IV, calicheamicin γ_1^I was shown effective against SC-implanted human tumor xenografts, such as human breast (MX-1) and ovarian carcinoma (H207).

Although the γ_1^I derivative was not extensively tested against human tumor xenografts, the *N*-acetyl γ_1^I calicheamicin derivative was tested against a wide spec-

Table 1 Activity of Calicheamicin γ_1^I Against Murine Tumors[a]

Treatment, IP q4d $\times$ 3 (μg/kg)[c]	%ILS[b]			
	P388	L-1210	B-16	Colon 26
10.0	—	−41	−40	−41
5.0	64	56	−15	38
2.5	105	22	68	46
1.25	68	17	176 (33[d])	22
0.6	45	11	74	27

[a] All tumors were propagated and used for testing in general accordance with the protocols described by the NCI.
[b] Median survival time of treated (T) divided by control (C) mice in days, reported as percent increase in life span (%ILS). An ILS of $\geq$25% is considered necessary to demonstrate activity.
[c] Three doses administered at 4-day intervals.
[d] Percent of survivors among the treated mice.

trum of tumors as a result of its inclusion in comparative efficacy trials carried out with monoclonal antibody conjugates made with this derivative (see below). Although 10- to 20-fold less potent than the γ_1^I derivative, N-acetyl γ_1^I, given IP on an q4d $\times$ 3 schedule (typically started on day 5–7) produced significant inhibitory effects (>58% inhibition of tumor growth) against 2 of 4 breast carcinomas, 3 of 3 lung carcinomas, 2 of 3 ovarian carcinomas, and 1 of 1 epidermoid carcinomas. No activity was demonstrated against 7 of 7 colon carcinomas or against representatives of pancreatic, melanoma, osteosarcoma, B-cell lymphoma, myeloma, or myeloid tumors (R. E. Wallace and D. Lindh, unpublished results). The human tumor spectrum is shown in Table 2.

Table 2 N-Acetyl Calicheamicin γ_1^I: Antitumor Activity Spectrum Against Human Tumor Xenografts

Tumor type	Response
Breast carcinoma	
MX1	+
MX2	+
MCF7	0
Lung carcinoma	
LX1, SCLC	+
LU-8, NSCLC	+
A549, NSCLC	+
Ovarian carcinoma	
H207	+
A2780	+ +
OVCAR-3	0
Colon carcinoma	
LS174T	0
CO77	0
CX1	0
SW620	0
HCT15	0
SW948	0
COLO205	0
Miscellaneous tumors	
Pancreas, lymphoma, myeloma, melanoma, osteosarcoma	0
Epidermoid carcinoma, KB	±

0, <58% tumor inhibition; ±, 58–64% tumor inhibition; +, reproduced 65–85% tumor inhibition; + +, 86–100% tumor inhibition-regression.

B. Preliminary Toxicity Studies

Being cognizant of literature reports of delayed toxicity associated with another highly potent antitumor antibiotic, CC1065 (4), we injected various calicheamicin derivatives (β_1, β_2, γ_1^I) into normal mice and held them for possible mortality over a period of 3–8 months. All the derivatives tested displayed delayed toxicity, which became pronounced only after 60 days and occurred at doses below the optimally effective doses of the derivatives (vs. P388 leukemia). As indicated in Table 3, calicheamicin γ_1^I displays acute toxicity at doses above the optimally effective dose of 2.5 µg/kg but produces delayed lethality at a dose below the optimal dose (1.25 µg/kg). With most derivatives of calicheamicin it is very likely that their delayed toxicity would have escaped detection in our standard antitumor tests because tumored unresponsive mice would have died earlier than 60 days or the apparently "cured" mice would normally have been sacrificed by 60 days or earlier (S. G. Carvajal and J. P. Thomas, unpublished results).

It has also been demonstrated that γ_1^I calicheamicin is most toxic when given by the IP route and least toxic by the oral route, not surprisingly matching the most and least efficacious treatment routes. The maximum tolerated (nonlethal) doses of γ_1^I given on an q4d × 3 schedule by the oral, SC, IV, and IP routes were 20, 5, 1.2, and 0.6 µg/kg, respectively. It is perhaps of some importance to point out that the lower tumor inhibitory doses (0.3–0.6 µg/kg) either were not or were only minimally associated with lethal toxicity and that the clinically relevant IV route of administration was slightly less toxic than the IP route.

Similar delayed lethality has been observed in treated rats, but there were no serum chemistry abnormalities (BUN, SGOT, SGPT, bilirubin) on days 10–53 among rats that eventually died of treatment with calicheamicin. The cause of death in mice and rats is not yet known, but hepatocellular pleomorphism is the most common finding at necropsies performed 4–8 months after administration of calicheamicin (J. Tiner, unpublished results). Although other tissue changes have been observed, none appear to explain the delayed lethal toxicity; but as described

Table 3 Lethal Toxicity of Calicheamicin γ_1^I in Normal Mice

Treatment, IP q4d × 3 (µg/kg)	Dead/Total	Range (day of death up to 320 days)
10	23/24	12–74
5	35/36	15–54
2.5	23/36	15 ⩾ 320
1.25	6/30	87 ⩾ 320
0.6	0/30	None dead
0.3	0/6	None dead

earlier, greatly reduced levels of ATP and NAD+ could perhaps account for the more acute aspects of cell death.

Chemical modification of the calicheamicin molecule has not yet led to derivatives with a reduced propensity to induce delayed toxicity. While derivatives have tended to be considerably less potent, they have retained their delayed lethality characteristics at doses below their optimally effective antitumor doses as determined against P388 leukemia. For example, the MTD for N-acetyl γ_1^I calicheamicin is 10 µg/kg and the optimally effective IP dose is 40 µg/kg when given on an q4d × 3 schedule. Also, calicheamicin α_3 shows an MTD of 5 µg/kg and its optimally effective dose level is 40 µg/kg on the same treatment schedule (Table 4). Although the overall therapeutic index of these derivatives has not much changed as a result of chemical modification, they have been shown to possess certain superior qualities, including reduced lethal toxicity when conjugated to monoclonal antibodies, as is described in a later section. The overall antitumor spectrum of calicheamicin γ_1^I and the N-acetyl γ_1^I is summarized in Table 5.

C. Cell Culture Studies with Calicheamicin

The discovery of calicheamicin in a biochemical prophage induction assay that detected DNA-damaging agents led to an early test of its cytogenetic effects on

Table 4 Activity and Toxicity Profiles of Calicheamicin Antibiotics

	Activity (P388 leukemia)		Lethal toxicity	
Dose (µg/kg)		%ILS	Dead/Total	Range (days)
Calicheamicin γ_1^I N-acetyl				
80		29	18/18	10–44
40[a]		123	28/30	14≥237
20		79	13/30	47≥271
10[b]		54	0/30	>280
5		57	0/12	>280
2.5		41	0/12	>280
Calicheamicin α_3				
80		89	12/12	12–17
40[a]		93	12/12	26–35
20		71	11/12	36≥300
10		66	1/12	143≥300
5[b]		45	0/6	>300
2.5		45	0/6	>300

[a] Optimally effective IP dose, q4d × 3 against P388 leukemia. Pooled data from 2–5 tests.
[b] Maximum nonlethal IP dose, q4d × 3 in normal mice.

Table 5 Calicheamicin Antitumor Spectrum[a]

Activity demonstrated:	
Murine leukemias	P-388, L-1210
Murine solid tumors	B-16 melanoma
	Colon 26
	M 5076
Human tumor xenografts	Breast, MX-1, MX-2
	NSCLC, A549
	NSCLC, Lu-78
	SCLC, LX-1
	Ovarian, H207
	Ovarian, A2780
	Cervical, ME-180 (marginally active)
	Epidermoid, KB
No activity demonstrated:	
Murine solid tumor	Lewis Lung carcinoma
Human tumor xenografts	Ovarian, OVCAR 3
	Pancreatic, P-105
	Osteosarcoma, KHOS
	Melonoma, LOX; Colo-38
	Melanoma, SK-MEL-28
	Lymphoma, RAJI
	Myeloma, SULTAN
	Colon, LS 174T; SW620; SW948
	Colon, CO77; CX-1; HCT-15; COLO205

[a] Results achieved with calicheamicin γ_1^I or *N*-acetyl calicheamicin γ_1^I administered IP on a q4d $\times$ 3 schedule.

mammalian cells in culture. Because one of the earliest fully characterized components of the calicheamicin family of antibiotics was the β_1^{Br} derivative (5), the availability of that derivative led to its being used in initial studies. The β_1^{Br} component was subsequently found to be essentially equipotent and equiactive to the γ_1^I component that was to become the primary focus of attention.

In the cytogenetic assessment, human fetal lung (diploid) fibroblasts were exposed to the β_1 derivative for 22 hours at 37°C, the cells treated by standard procedures and Giemsa-stained metaphases scored for chromosome aberrations (R. E. Wallace and D. Lindh, unpublished results). The antibiotic's potency and DNA-damaging attributes were confirmed by the finding that $\geq$50% of the treated cells displayed significant numbers of aberrations including chromosome and chromatid breaks and accentric fragments when exposed to 10 pg/ml of the β_1 derivative. It is perhaps interesting to note that the cleavage of supercoiled plasmid DNA (by γ_1^I) in a cell-free environment requires at least 10 ng/ml to effect a significant frequency of single and double strand breaks.

In more standard cytotoxicity assays the β_1^{Br} component was "sterilizing" to the human colon carcinoma cell line, WiDr, as determined in a clonogenic assay, when cells were treated with ca 20 pg/ml of the antibiotic for 2 hours. The IC_{50} for the β_1^{Br} component in several tests ranged from 4 to 8 pg/ml. When this derivative was tested for effects on cycling and noncycling WiDr cells, it was found that cycling cells were about 15- to 20-fold more sensitive to the antibiotic than the plateau phase cells (R. E. Wallace and D. Lindh, unpublished results). Calicheamicin β_1^{Br} was also examined for its potential to affect tubulin and thereby cause proliferating cells to collect in the metaphase stage of the cell cycle. Human fetal lung diploid fibroblasts were treated with concentrations of β_1^{Br} ranging from 0.6 to 750 pg/ml, colchicine was added after an 18-hour incubation, and the cells evaluated at 22 hours postexposure to drug. Whereas the known tubulin binder, vincristine, increased the frequency of cells in metaphase from background levels of 8.5% to levels of 23–35%, calicheamicin β_1^{Br} produced a dose-related inhibition in the occurrence of mitotic figures. Although direct tubulin-binding experiments were not carried out, it is concluded that the mechanism of action of calicheamicin does not include significant effects on tubulin (R. E. Wallace and D. Lindh, unpublished results).

Another natural component of the calicheamicin family, the γ_1^I derivative, was shown to be quite comparable in potency to the β_1^{Br} component. γ_1^I showed an IC_{50} of around 3 pg/ml in clonogenic assays carried out with the human T-cell lines Molt-4 and T-8402, but the melanoma cell line SK-Mel-28 was less sensitive, showing an IC_{50} of 20 pg/ml. In pulse-exposure experiments in which cells were treated with drug for 5–30 minutes followed by 4 days' growth, the IC_{50} for γ_1^I calicheamicin determined by uptake of ^3H-thymidine ranged from 0.18 to 0.75 ng/ml against a number of human tumor cell lines. In contrast, the chemically modified N-acetyl calicheamicin γ_1^I derivative showed IC_{50}s up to 10-fold higher (0.3–7.6 ng/ml) depending on the tumor cell lines. This difference was similar to the relationship determined for these two derivatives in in vivo studies. Experiments in which cells were exposed to the drug continuously for up to 4 days generally showed IC_{50}s 16- to 30-fold lower compared with pulse exposure experiments.

D. *p*-Glycoprotein (MDR)–Mediated Resistance to Calicheamicin

As natural products, the calicheamicins could be anticipated to share certain characteristics with other natural products, such as the ability to induce multiple drug resistance (MDR) operating via a p-glycoprotein efflux pump (i.e., p170). Indeed, it was demonstrated that the N-acetyl γ_1^I derivative was >50-fold less potent

Table 6 Sensitivity of Human Tumor Cell Lines with and Without the MDR Phenotype to Calicheamicin[a]

Cell line	IC$_{50}$ (ng/ml)	
	N-acetyl γ_1^I	γ_1^I
OVCAR-3/S	0.73	0.002
OVCAR-3/R[b]	>100	0.11
KB/S	0.87	0.02
KB/R[c] (8-5)	11.8	0.04
SW620	0.25	0.001
SW620/R[d]	18.8	0.03
MCF-7/S	0.58	0.006
MCF-7/R[e]	>100	0.1

[a] Proliferation assay—incorporation of ^{3}H-TdR after 3 days' exposure to drug.
[b] Ovarian, OVCAR 3 cell line made resistant to bisantrene (6).
[c] Epidermoid carcinoma line resistant to colchicine.
[d] Colon carcinoma cell line, SW620, resistant to doxorubicin.
[e] Breast carcinoma cell line, MCF-7, resistant to doxorubicin.

against breast MCF-7 cells resistant to doxorubicin and >135-fold less potent against a bisantrene-resistant subline of OVCAR 3 than against the parental cell lines of each (A. T. Menendez, unpublished results). Both of the above resistant cell lines have been shown to display the typical MDR phenotype (6). The resistance patterns of calicheamicin γ_1^I and the N-acetyl derivative against four human cell lines are summarized in Table 6. Of some interest is the observation that MDR human tumor cell lines resistant to N-acetyl calicheamicin γ_1^I are 2- to 10-fold more sensitive to the parent, natural γ_1^I derivative.

As with other natural products, calicheamicin is capable of inducing the typical MDR phenotype in human breast tumor cells exposed to increase concentrations of drug in vitro. These cells display gp170, and their resistance can be overcome by adding drug in the presence of verapamil and other known MDR-reversal agents (7).

II. ANTIBACTERIAL ACTIVITY OF CALICHEAMICIN

The calicheamicin's exhibited highly potent in vitro antibacterial activity. In vitro activity was determined by a standard agar dilution method. Calicheamicin components were dissolved in DMSO or MeOH, then diluted with distilled water to bring the solvent content to 10% before further dilution in Mueller-Hinton medium. The Steers inocula replicator was used to apply 10^5 CFU of each test organism to agar plates containing twofold serial dilutions of the agents. The minimum inhibitory concentration (MIC) was determined as the lowest concentration that inhibited growth of the organism after 20 hours of incubation. The exceptionally high potency of the agents made it necessary for certain precautions to avoid skips in the MIC readings. Pipettes were changed for each twofold dilution step. Wells and inoculation prongs of the Steers apparatus were changed for each agent to avoid carry over into the next series.

The antimicrobial activity of the calicheamicins against a spectrum of gram-positive and gram-negative bacteria is shown in Table 7. The individual components of the calicheamicins exhibited very potent activity against gram-positive bacteria with most MIC values in the pg/ml range. The MIC values for gram-negative bacteria were significantly higher (0.06–0.5 μg/ml). The β and γ components were similar in potency, and only minor differences were noted for the bromine- vs. iodine-containing antibiotics.

The in vivo activity of calicheamicin β_1 was tested in mice against acute lethal infections produced by IP injection of *Staphylococcus aureus* Smith or *Streptococcus pyogenes* C203. A single dose of 64 μg/kg administered SC or IV was tolerated by normal mice with no untoward toxic signs for the test period of 7 days. No protection was observed for either of the infections where doses of 64–0.25 μg/kg were administered SC or IV 30 minutes after the IP injection of the infecting organisms. Administered IP, normal mice tolerated ≤4 μg/kg. Protection against the *S. aureus* Smith injection was observed when doses of 4 or 1 μg/kg of β_1 were administered IP after infection. Apparently absorption and distribution of the SC and IV doses of the agent was not rapid enough to protect the mice from the acute lethal peritoneal infection. With IP treatment, the agent produced its potent antibacterial effect at the site of the infecting organism.

Table 7 In Vitro Antimicrobial Activity of the Calicheamicins

Organisms (strains tested)	MIC (μg/ml) range[a]			
	β_1^{Br}	β_1^{I}	γ_1^{Br}	γ_1^{I}
Escherichia coli (3)	0.12 ~ 0.25	0.25 ~ 0.5	0.25 ~ 0.5	0.25
Klebsiella pneumoniae (2)	0.12 ~ 0.25	0.5	0.5	0.25
Enterobacter sp. (2)	0.25 ~ 0.5	0.25 ~ 0.5	0.5	0.5
Serratia spp. (2)	0.12	0.25 ~ 0.5	0.25 ~ 0.5	0.12 ~ 0.25
Citrobacter spp. (2)	0.12	0.25 ~ 0.5	0.12 ~ 0.25	0.12 ~ 0.25
Acinetobacter spp. (2)	0.06 ~ 0.12	0.25	0.25	.06 ~ 0.12
Pseudomonas aeruginosa (2)	0.25 ~ 0.5	0.25 ~ 0.5	0.5 ~ 1.0	.12 ~ 0.25
Staphylococcus aureus (7)	≤0.00025	≤0.000031		≤0.000031
Enterococcus sp. (1)	0.0038	0.031	0.062	0.0078
Bacillus subtilis (1)	≤0.00025	≤0.000031	≤0.000031	≤0.000031

[a] MIC values were determined by the standard agar dilution method in Mueller-Hinton medium.

Other antibiotics in the enediyne class have exhibited high antibacterial potency. Tunac et al. (8) reported MIC values of ≤0.00006 µg/ml for veractamycin A against several gram-positive organisms. In their evaluation of dynemicin A, Miyoshi-Saitoh et al. (9) observed MIC values of ≤0.00008 µg/ml for gram-positive bacteria and values of 0.01–0.001 µg/ml for gram-negative organisms. Konishi et al. (10) also reported high in vitro potency for dynemicin A and its triacetate with MICs in the pg range. They also reported that low intraperitoneal doses of dynemicin A protected mice against the *Staphylococcus aureus* Smith infection.

REFERENCES

1. R. K. Elespuru and M. B. Yarmolinsky, *Environ. Mutagen., 1,* 55 (1979).
2. R. I. Geran, N. R. Greenberg, M. M. Macdonald, A. M. Schumacher, B. J. Abbott, *Cancer Chemother., 3,* 1 (1972).
3. J. P. Thomas, S. G. Carvajal, H. L. Lindsay, R. V. Citarella, R. E. Wallace, M. D., Lee, and F. E. Durr, Program and Abstracts; 26th Interscience Conference on Antimicrobial Agents and Chemotherapy, New Orleans, LA, Sept. 1986, American Society for Microbiology, Washington, DC; Abstr 229.
4. J. P. McGovern, G. L. Clarke, E. A. Pratt, and T. F. DeKoning, *J. Antibiot., 37,* 63 (1984).
5. W. M. Maiese, M. P. Lechevalier, H. A. Lechevalier, J. Korshalla, N. Kuck, A. Fantini, M. J. Wildey, J. Thomas, and M. Greenstein, *J. Antibiot., 42,* 558 (1984).
6. V. Ruszala-Mallon, J. Silva, D., Raventos-Suarez, and F. E. Durr, *Proc. Am. Assoc. Can. Res., 31,* 356 (Abst. 2110) (1990).
7. R. E. Wallace, D. Lindh, L. Greenberg, C. Raventos-Suarez, and F. E. Durr, *Proc. Am. Assoc. Cancer Res., 32,* 364 (Abst. 2163) (1991).
8. J. B. Tunac, B. D. Graham, S. W. Mamber, W. E. Dobson, and M. D. Lenzini, *J. Antibiot., 38,* 1337 (1985).
9. M. Miyoshi-Saitoh, N. Morisaki, Y. Tokiwa, and S. Iwasaki, *J. Antibiot., 44,* 1037 (1991).
10. M. Konishi, H. Ohkuma, K. Matsumoto, T. Tsuno, H. Kamei, T. Miyaki, T. Oki, and H. Kawaguchi, *J. Antibiot., 42,* 1449 (1989).

DNA-Cleaving Properties of Calicheamicin γ_1^I

George A. Ellestad and Wei-Dong Ding
Lederle Laboratories, American Cyanamid Company, Pearl River, New York

Nada Zein
Bristol-Myers Squibb Pharmaceutical Research Institute, Princeton, New Jersey

Craig A. Townsend
Johns Hopkins University, Baltimore, Maryland

I. INTRODUCTION

Calicheamicin γ_1^I (CLM) [1] (1,2), esperamicin A_1 [2] (3,4), dynemicin [3] (5), and neocarzinostatin [4] (6) are remarkable DNA-damaging agents that mediate strand cleavage through transient diradical intermediates (7). Indeed, it would seem that nature has designed these microbial metabolites specifically for defense against predator organisms (8). Insofar as the DNA-cleavage properties of calicheamicin γ_1^I and esperamicin A_1 are concerned, the structures can be divided into three domains, the physical and chemical properties of which all play important roles in DNA binding and cleavage. The first is the carbohydrate portion, which serves as a delivery or DNA-binding vehicle. The second is the allylic methyltrisulfide, which plays the part of a control or triggering device. Upon bioreductive cleavage of the allylic trisulfide, the allylic thiolate anion is formed which then adds to the α,β-unsaturated ketone system. This removes the structural rigidity associated with the bridgehead double bond (Bredt's rule) in the DNA-reactive third domain, which undergoes a geometric change to permit a Bergman reaction to occur where the enediyne undergoes aromatization (see Refs. 9 and 10 for review). The transient p-phenylene-diradical intermediate formed during the aromatization process initiates oxidative strand scission when bound to DNA by the abstraction of proximal hydrogen atoms from the targeted deoxyribose sugars. These transformations are summarized in Scheme 1. This chapter describes the initial exploratory DNA-

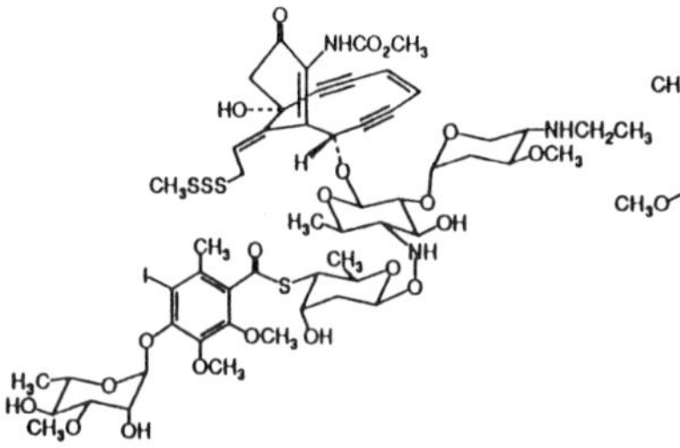

1 Calicheamicin γ_1^{I} 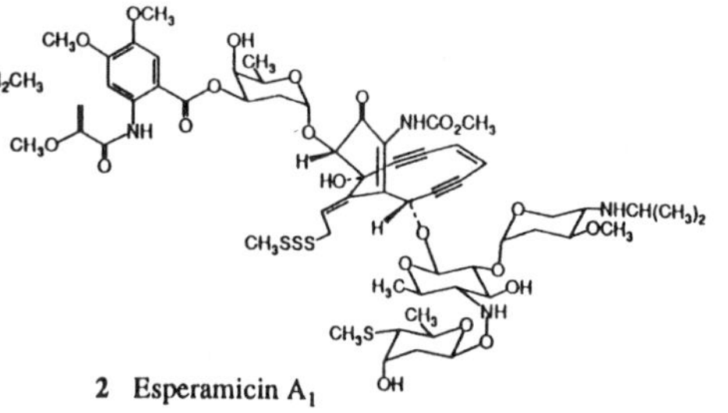   **2** Esperamicin A_1

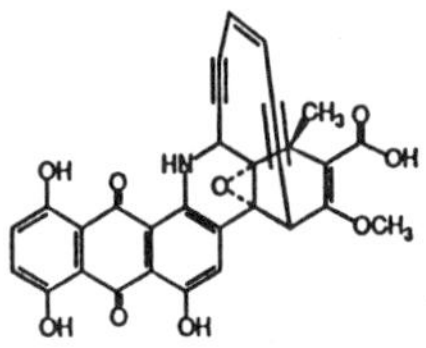

3 Dynemicin 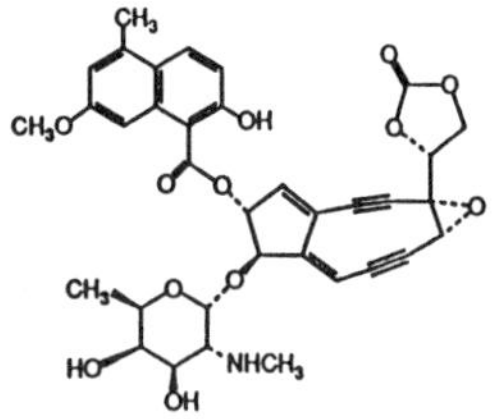   **4** Neocarzinostatin

binding/cleavage experiments with CLM carried out at American Cyanamid as well as more recent studies at several university laboratories. While these experiments support this general view of CLM–DNA interaction to a substantial extent, the molecular basis for the remarkable sequence discrimination of drug-induced cleavages of DNA remains to be determined.

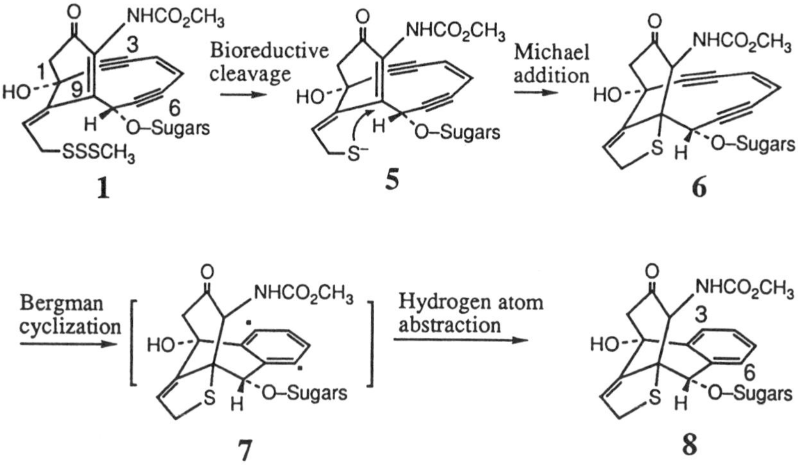

Scheme 1

II. CLEAVAGE OF PLASMID DNA

Early cleavage experiments carried out in the presence of reducing thiols with the replicative and nonreplicative forms of bacteriophage ΦX 174 and pBR322 indicated a clear preference for duplex DNA as analyzed by agarose gel electrophoresis (11). Single-stranded ΦX 174 was unaffected by CLM γ_1^I at concentrations up to 1.0 µg/ml compared with double-stranded ΦX 174 where large amounts of linear, form III DNA were formed with concentrations of drug as low as 0.01 µg/ml. More recently, Drak et al. at Yale examined the ratio of linear to nicked forms produced with double stranded ΦX 174 and observed values of 1:2 at a concentration of 1.5 nM (12). The statistics of forming double-stranded lesions directly from form I DNA at such low concentrations of drug is strongly suggestive that a single binding/cleavage event results in a double-stranded scission. These findings are consistent with strand cleavage mediated by a transient *p*-benzyne intermediate, which could conceivably abstract deoxyribose hydrogen atoms on opposite strands in a single cleavage event.

III. CLEAVAGE SPECIFICITY

These initial observations of double-strand DNA cleavage prompted more sophisticated experiments with 5′- and 3′–^{32}P end-labeled restriction fragments in conjunction with Maxam-Gilbert sequencing methodology to determine if the binding/cleavage of CLM γ_1^I exhibited any site discrimination (11). For the most part, these experiments were carried out with a 20 fold excess of DNA (in base pairs) over that of drug (0.36 mM). Conditions were identified that gave "one-hit kinetics." The first cleavage experiment with a restriction fragment derived from a *Streptomyces* promoter region provided evidence of surprising discrimination for a molecule of only 1367 daltons. Even under conditions where one-hit conditions did not obtain, nonpreferred sites were cleaved only weakly relative to the preferred sites. Although the exact nature of the sequences recognized and cleaved by the drug was not immediately apparent, it was clear that certain oligopyrimidine/oligopurine sites of four to six base pairs were principal targets, suggesting that the inherent asymmetry of these regions might be important for recognition by CLM. Subsequent cleavage experiments with a variety of ^{32}P end-labeled restriction fragments, primarily from *Streptomyces* promoter regions rich in GC-base pairs, led to the identification of two prominent binding/cleavage sites, 5′TCCT and 5′CTCT. However, other sites such as GCCT, TCCG, TCCC, TCTC, ACCT, TCCA provided similar cleavage patterns, the extent of which apparently depended upon the sequences themselves and the flanking sequences. Studies with a strand containing the 3′AGGA tetramer complementary to the 5′TCCT site indicated that the cleavage was staggered two nucleotides towards the 3′ side of the 3′NNAGGA sequence. This 3′ cleavage-offset suggested that CLM γ_1^I binds and cleaves in the minor groove of DNA.

This cleavage behavior was somewhat unexpected at the time because there was little obvious relationship to the more classical minor groove binders such as netropsin and distamycin, peptide antibiotics whose DNA binding is strongly biased towards A · T-rich tracts (13). Competition experiments with netropsin using a 5′ end–labeled SalI/BamHI fragments from pBR322 altered significantly the CLM binding/cleavage specificity. As seen in Figure 1, binding of netropsin in a preferred 5′ATTA tract prohibited CLM binding/cleavage at the adjacent 5′AGGA/TCCT tract (Lane 1), which is cleaved as expected in the absence of netropsin. Netropsin even prohibited cleavage at the bottom 5′TCCT tract, a site separated from the ATTA tract by three base pairs. It also suggested that the association constant for CLM/DNA binding was probably less than that of netropsin, which has been estimated to be as high as 10^9 M^{-1} for strong binding sites (14).

More recent studies have shown that CLM can bind and cleave certain A · T tracts in a pUC 19 restriction fragment, sometimes in preference to neighboring G · C-containing sequences cleaved by CLM γ_1^I in other contexts (Fig. 2) (15; S. Mah et al., unpublished results). These findings point strongly to some overlap in recognition sites between netropsin and CLM. Earlier cleavage studies with dodecamer 1 (Fig. 3), which contained a TCCT tract in the center flanked by an A · T pentamer on the 3′ side and a G · C trimer on the 5′ side, showed strong cleavage at the anticipated C in the 5′TCCT tract and little or no cleavage in the A · T-rich domain containing three sequential pyrimidines. These results indicate that in this dodecamer the TCCT site is preferred to that of the A · T region (16). The fact that CLM can bind and cleave both mixed G · C and A · T sites as well as some A · T-only sequences is unusual because of the differences in geometry between these sites due to the protruding of the 2-amino group of the G nucleotides into the minor groove (17,18).

No evidence for an intercalative association with DNA was obtained when CLM was incubated with plasmid DNA without reducing thiols. Agarose gel analysis (gel shift assay) of this mixture did not reveal any slower-moving bands (or any nicked or linear DNA forms) that would have suggested unwinding of the DNA, a property characteristic of intercalative agents (19).

IV. NATURE OF CALICHEAMICIN/DNA ASSOCIATION

Recent efforts to obtain information as to the strength of the association of CLM with DNA have led to estimates from 10^6 to $10^8 M^{-1}$. The Crothers and Danishefsky groups at Yale examined the CLM γ_1^I cleavage of a synthetic dodecamer 1 (Fig.3) containing a 5′TCCT site on sequencing gels and determined the drug concentration at half saturation/cleavage for this site (12). This gave Ka estimates of 3.3×10^7 to $1 \times 10^8 M^{-1}$ assuming equilibrium binding. In another study concerning the role of hydrophobic interactions between the drug and DNA,

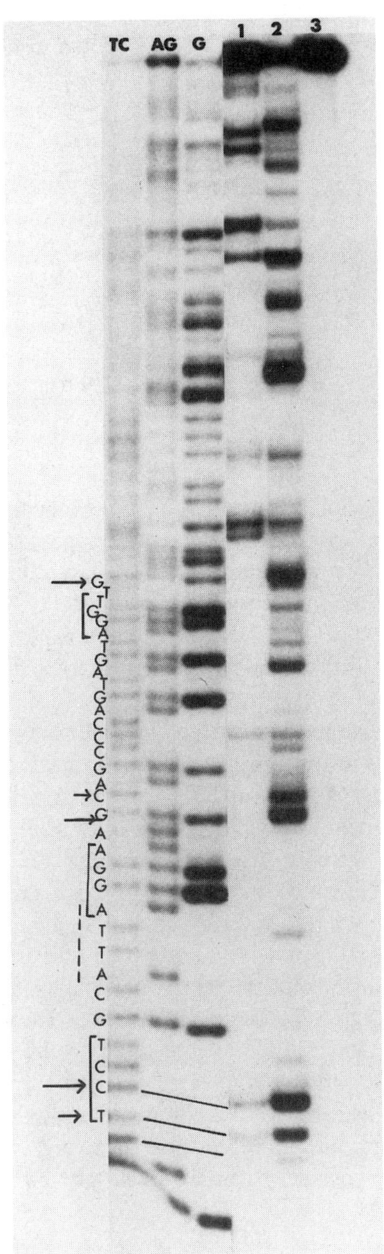

Figure 1 Autoradiogram of the reaction of calicheamicin γ_1^I with the 5′-end labeled fragment pBR322 SalI/BamHI. TC, AG, G are the Maxam Gilbert lanes. Lane 1, the DNA was treated with netropsin at 50 µg/ml in presence of β-mercaptoethanol for 15 mins at 37°C in 10:90 DMSO: 35mM tris-HCl, pH 7.5. The solution was then lyophilized, redissolved in buffer and treated with calicheamicin as described in lane 2. Lane 2, the DNA was treated with calicheamicin at 0.5 µg/ml in presence of β-mercaptoethanol at 37°C for 15 mins in 10:90 DMSO: 35mM tris-HCL, pH 7.5. The solution was then lyophilized, dissolved in loading buffer and analyzed on a 12% polacrylamide denaturing gel for 3 hours at 1200 volts. Lane 3, Control.

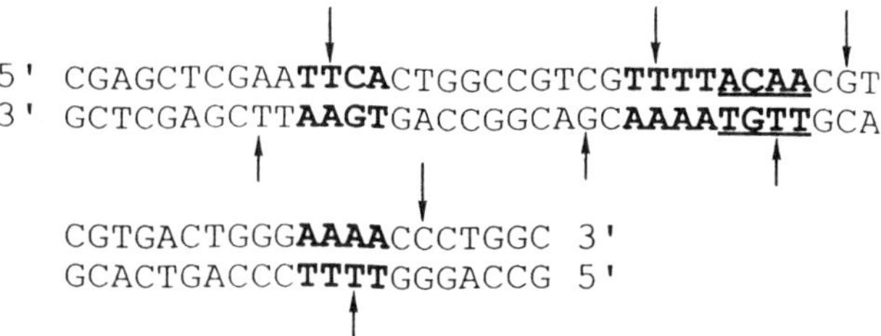

Figure 2 CLM γ_1^I cleavage pattern of a *Acc* 1-*Nde*1 fragment from pUC19. (From Ref. 15.)

binding constants of about 10^6 M^{-1} were estimated from Scatchard plots for TCCT, ACCT, and CTCT sequences based on the CLM γ_1^I–induced cleavage rates of pBR322 (20). These lower K_a values are an average of at least these three sequences rather than that derived from measuring the cleavage of a single TCCT site. Whatever the actual binding constant(s), the CLM/DNA association appears to be less than that for netropsin, consistent with the above-mentioned competition experiments.

The nature of the CLM/DNA association is not fully understood, although it appears that the ethylamino sugar is probably involved in general electrostatic attraction with the DNA and does not play a role in aqueous solution in deprotonation of the reducing thiol. This conclusion is based on kinetic studies in aqueous methanol on the bimolecular rate of trisulfide cleavage (21). Aminoethanethiol was chosen as the reducing agent because its pK_a of 8.3 is similar to that of reduced glutathione, the likely in vivo reducing thiol. The bimolecular rate constant for CLM γ_1^I was 2.8 $\pm$ 0.6 mM^{-1}s^{-1}, 1.7 $\pm$ 0.1 mM^{-1}s^{-1} for the *N*-acetyl derivative and 2.0 $\pm$ 0.4 mM^{-1}s^{-1} for the α_3 component, which lacks the ethylamino sugar. It had previously been proposed (16) that this sugar played an important role in the cleavage of the trisulfide moiety based on disulfide exchange reactions in acetonitrile (22). On the basis of these observations it was suggested that the amino sugar may act as a general base to deprotonate the attacking thiol or possibly stabilize an electrostatic transition-state involving the thiolate anion intermediate with a juxtaposed positively charged amino group. In

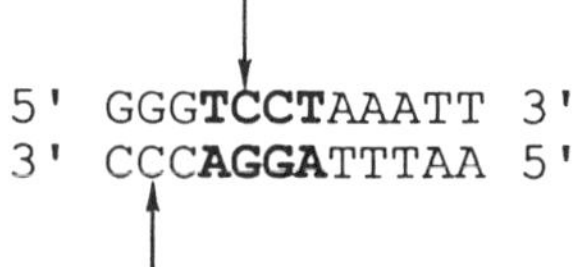

Figure 3 CLM γ_1^I cleavage pattern of dodecamer 1. (From Ref. 16.)

these disulfide exchange reactions, neutralization of the amine by acetylation or removal of this sugar resulted in essentially no disulfide exchange with nonreducing thiols. However, under the conditions of this reaction (anhydrous organic solvent), the amino sugar may simply provide a base for intermolecular thiol deprotonation and subsequent drug activation. In aqueous solution no kinetic advantage to the rate of thiol activation of CLM could be detected owing to the presence of the nearby amine.

These solution studies of CLM activation do not address the potential role of the DNA helix itself to organize and assist amino sugar–mediated thiol deprotonation and, hence, catalyze drug activation in the bound state. This appealing notion has been similarly raised in a related context examining the reactions of neocarzinostatin and thiol in an organic solvent mixture (23). To examine directly the possible role of DNA to enhance the rate of thiol-induced drug activation, the kinetics of CLM reaction with aminoethanethiol and glutathione were each examined in 30% aqueous methanol both in the presence and in the absence of calf thymus DNA (M. Chatterjee et al., unpublished results). An organic modifier was necessary to ensure drug solubility in the absence of DNA. Reaction with each of these thiols proceeded by comparatively rapid mixed disulfide formation with the added thiol, followed by slower decomposition to CLMε [8], the reduced form of the drug. The relative stability of the intermediate mixed disulfides had been previously observed allowing for their isolation and characterization (22). For neither reaction did the presence of DNA accelerate the rate over that observed in solution. In fact, in the presence of DNA the rates of both disulfide formation and its further reaction to CLMε were slightly *slower*. It would thus appear that attack of the CLM–DNA complex by thiolate is encumbered relative to drug free in solution presumably owing to steric effects and possibly electronic repulsion of thiolate approach to the negatively charged DNA polyanion.

The effect of the Hofmeister series of salts on the cleavage rate of CLM suggested that hydrophobic associations between the apolar surfaces of the very lipophilic drug and the reduced dielectric regions of the DNA minor groove could be important (20). For example, the poorly hydrated chaotropic salts such as $LiClO_4$ and LiCNS slowed down the DNA cleavage rate as measured on agarose gels with pBR322 as the substrate. This is believed to be due to the resultant increased solubility of CLM γ_1^I in water because of solvation of the apolar surfaces of the drug by these chaotropic salts. In contrast, the strongly hydrated and antichaotropic salt Na_2SO_4 increased the cleavage rate. It is believed that this is due to the salting-out property of this salt, which causes electrostriction of water molecules. This has been interpreted as indicating that the drug would rather remove itself from the aqueous environment and bind to the more hospitable minor groove, a finding not surprising for such a water-insoluble compound. Consistent with their middle position in the Hofmeister series, NaCl and LiCl had little effect on the cleavage rate, at least under the conditions of these experiments. This is a point that should be examined carefully with several concentrations of NaCl between 0 and 0.1 M.

A subsequent series of experiments corroborated the inferred hydrophobic effects from the above cleavage experiments with the Hofmeister series of salts. It has been pointed out that a characteristic feature of hydrophobic associations is the remarkable temperature dependence of binding between a very lipophilic ligand and its complementary hydrophobic binding site on a macromolecule. These interactions tend to increase between 4 and 25°C as the temperature is raised. This is in contrast to most other types of interactions in aqueous solutions, which tend to dissociate as the temperature is increased. However, around 25°C even hydrophobic complexes begin to dissociate. So the temperature dependence of binding of CLM to plasmid DNA (pBR322) was determined by measuring the rate of cleavage as a function of temperature between 10 and 40°C (20). Specifically, the amounts of DNA forms II and III produced in the cleavage reaction were quantitated by densitometry on agarose gels. The binding constants as determined from the above-mentioned Scatchard plots clearly show nonlinearity in this temperature range with increasing association up to about 27°C followed by a decrease as the temperature was further increased to 40°C. A plot of this relationship and the corresponding thermodynamic binding parameters is shown in Figure 4. These results suggest that binding between 10 and 27°C is entropy driven (negative heat capacity change, $\Delta C_p = -1.21$ kcal/T) consistent with binding-induced desolvation of CLM and DNA. It is also possible that binding-induced release of counterions makes a contribution to the favorable binding entropy observed in these experiments. In the event, it would seem that the net association of the drug with DNA is driven to a large extent by hydrophobic interactions occurring in the minor groove. However, the amino sugar also appears to play a role in this overall association process, presumably through nonspecific ionic interaction with the phosphate backbone. Based on structural information now available about the CLM · DNA complex (vide infra), such an interaction can be readily accommodated in model building. This proposed role for the amino sugar is supported by the observation that about 10^3 higher concentrations of CLM α_3, lacking the amino sugar, is required to achieve cleavage efficiencies equivalent to CLM γ_1^I itself (16).

Given that a hydrophobic driving force is significant in CLM/DNA binding, other factors such as hydrogen bonding from the deoxyribose sugars and nonbonded van der Waals contacts no doubt also play a role. However, the question remains as to how the CLM γ_1^I molecule recognizes a binding/cleavage site on DNA. Clearly, the finding that CLM can bind and cleave a variety of A · T-containing homopyrimidine tracts as well as those containing G · C sequences suggests that recognition of specific sequence cannot be correct and that inherent minor groove geometry alone may be too simplistic. G · C-only–containing regions are not recognized by the drug based on the initial cleavage studies. Spatially, the minor groove of G · C-containing tracts with the guanine amino groups protruding from the bottom of the groove is obviously different from that of tracts

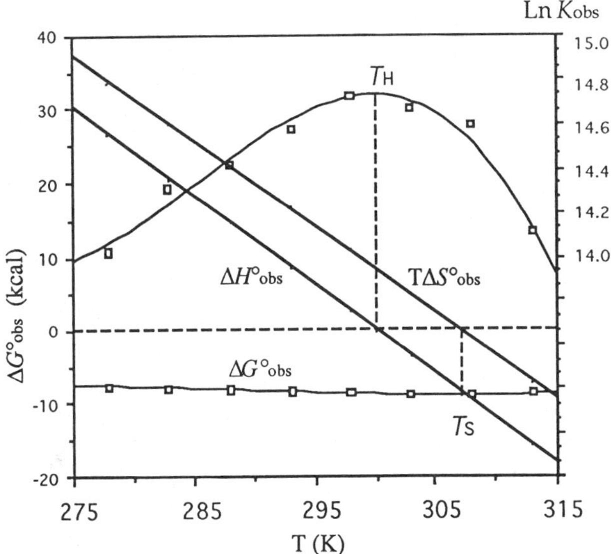

Figure 4 Thermodynamics for CLM/DNA binding, plotted as functions of T, ΔH° obs, TΔS obs, are calculated assuming ΔC_p is -1.21 kcal/T (From Ref. 20).

made up solely of A · T base pairs. But whether or not the width in these mixed A · T/G · C sites that CLM binds and cleaves is significantly different from the A · T-only sequences is questionable based on recent x-ray data (17). CLM may be recognizing and binding to sequences that are susceptible to drug-induced conformational changes (15,24,25), possibly related to sequence-dependent hydration (14,26–28).

In order to gain further insight into the nature of the TCCT/AGGA binding/ cleavage site, synthetic dodecamers **2–5** (Fig. 5) were prepared containing mis-

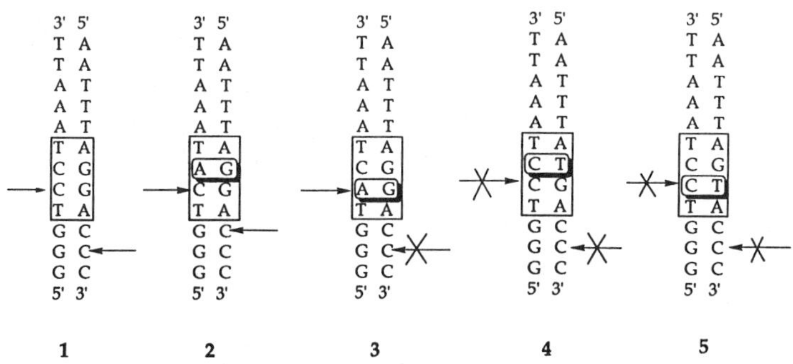

Figure 5 CLM γ_1^I cleavage of dodecamers **1–5**. (From Ref. 15.)

matches within the original TCCT tract (16). The creation of an A · G mismatch 5′TCAT/3′AGGA (dodecamer **2**) had no effect on the cleavage specificity of both strands. However, an A · G mismatch 5′TACT/3′AGGA (dodecamer **3**) prevented breakage on the AGGA strand but not on the TACT tetramer with cleavage at A. This result is not too surprising since it is known that an A · G mispair does not cause a significant deformation in the overall conformation of the DNA helix other than a local widening of the minor groove (29–31). Thus, an altered duplex geometry is better tolerated at the 3′ end of this tract than at the 5′ side. This is interesting in that the 5′ side of the site is where the aglycone is positioned with the carbohydrate tail positioned to the 3′ side (see discussion of the binding orientation below). This finding suggests that the tail portion of CLM γ_1^I is less discriminating than the enediyne part of the molecule. Such an interpretation is problematical, however, since it is difficult to attribute a specific binding role to one part of the molecule without considering the molecule as a whole (see below). In contrast to the dodecamers with A · G mispairs, neither of the two dodecamers containing T · C mismatches, 5′TCCT/3′AGTA and 5′TCCT3′ATGA (dodecamers **4** and **5**; Fig. 5), were susceptible to CLM γ_1^I binding/cleavage consistent with the fact that a T · C mismatch tends to result in more duplex instability than an A · G mispair (32).

While the overall rate-determining step in the activation of CLM γ_1^I for DNA cleavage (see Fig. 1) is the initial reductive cleavage of the allylic trisulfide (21), variable-temperature ^{1}H-NMR spectroscopic results showed that the dihydrothiophene intermediate **6** has a finite lifetime at physiological temperature (3–6 seconds) to be possibly the kinetically significant entity to recognize cleavage sites in the helix (33). Moreover, the movement of this reactive species along the DNA would be expected to be rapid. During the passage of the dihydrothiophene, it may encounter restricted steric environments that could be visualized, for example, to lower the activation barrier of Bergman rearrangement to diyl **7**. Thus, kinetic enhancements of DNA cleavage rates at certain sites might be observed to govern cleavage specificity. Circumstantial evidence to support this idea can be drawn from the cleavage behavior of structurally simpler co-metabolites of both CLM and esperamicin. In both families several metabolites are known having the same enediyne cleavage element but variously less elaborated carbohydrate side chains (1–4). The DNA-cleavage behavior observed generally among these compounds is site selectivity very similar or identical to that of the parent, but higher—often much higher—concentrations are required to achieve similar extents of DNA scission.

An interesting and important exception to this latter picture has emerged in the work of Walker et al., who have carried out cleavage experiments with a truncated version of CLM, CLMt (15). This derivative, which is missing the rhamnose, thiobenzoate, and thiosugar moieties, has been observed to cleave DNA essentially nonselectively. This finding suggests that cyclization kinetics do not significantly impact the sequence specificity of the intact drug as the effects of

Truncated calicheamicin

DNA interaction with the dihydrothiophene portions of both molecules presumably should be very similar. However, sequence specificity of cleavage is significantly diminished with CLMt, implying that cleavage specificity reflects binding affinity rather than kinetic effects imparted by interaction of the aglycone portion with the helix. Cleavage studies with racemic synthetic aglycone also showed no binding/cleavage sequence discrimination, but predominantly single-stranded breaks were found to occur (12). The observation that the truncated drug causes double-stranded lesions suggests that sugars A and B are sufficient to align the warhead in the minor groove for double-strand cutting. No groove specificity can be assigned from the cleavage experiments with the aglycone, but the observations with CLMt show that sugars A and B are sufficient to convert the aglycone to a double-strand cleaver similar to calicheamicin γ_1^I, but they are insufficient to afford the sequence specificity of strand scission observed for the intact drug containing the fully elaborated side chain.

Incisive experiments that demonstrate drug binding in the minor groove precede DNA cleavage and define the global structure of CLM–DNA complexes derive from hydroxyl radical footprinting studies with CLMε [8] (S. Mah et al., unpublished results). The spent form of the drug [8] is inert to DNA cleavage, but differs only by the absence of two hydrogen atoms from the structure of the 1,4-diyl [7] believed to be responsible for the initiation of DNA scission. Hydroxyl radical footprinting experiments of this material showed that CLMε bound where calicheamicin γ_1^I cleaved and that binding affinity largely paralleled cleavage efficiency. In particular, no sites of strong binding were observed in the footprinting experiments corresponding to weak or nonexistent cleavage. Similarly, no strong sites of cleavage were seen having only minimal footprints. Therefore, kinetic activation by the helix of dihydrothiophene closure appears to be of relatively little importance in determining the site selectivity of calicheamicin-induced cutting of DNA. Rather, thermodynamic effects brought about by the interaction of the activated drug with the DNA helix afford a variety of sites where both binding and subsequent observed cleavages are preferred.

The hydroxyl radical footprinting experiments additionally show that CLMε binding occurs in the minor groove in accord with observed cleavage data (see also atom transfer experiments below) and that the binding is asymmetric with respect to these cleavages, leading to the unified view that 5′-hydrogen abstraction occurs typically in a run of pyrimidines to direct the side chain to the 3′ side of this recognition sequence. This important generalization is in keeping with the chemical evidence from atom transfer experiments described below for a single 5′-TCCT site (34,35). That four to five bases are protected in these footprinting experiments and to roughly equal extents on both strands provides the clearest evidence to date locating the aryl-linked carbohydrate side chain in an extended conformation approximately equally disposed to both strands within the minor groove (S. Mah et al., unpublished results). This picture of the CLM–DNA complex is in accord with the proposed extended conformation of CLM in solution evidenced from NMR studies (36,37).

It has previously been proposed that the thiobenzoate moiety plays a dominant role in specificity (12,38), as opposed to a nonspecific one (16), through binding to the 2-amino group of a guanine nucleotide in 5′TCCT cleavage sites. The fact that certain A · T-only sites can be favorably recognized and cleaved (S. Mah et al., unpublished results, also ref. 15) argues against this hypothesis as the principal binding interaction conferring selectivity as does the lack of binding/cleavage at G · C-only sequences (11). The thiobenzoate apparently makes some contribution to specificity as shown by the lack of discrimination by the truncated drug CLMt that lacks this entity, although the role of the halogen substituent is not clear (38). It has been pointed out that the binding specificity of components measured in isolation can be misleading, since binding specificity and energetics rarely reflect just the sum of the individual components (15).

Recently reported footprinting experiments with synthetic aryltetrasaccharide prepared as the methyl glycoside of the corresponding domain in CLM have revealed binding in the general regions where CLM cleavage occurs and, indeed, affords protection to DNA from drug cleavage (39,40). Interestingly, with regard to the proposed role of the aryliodide in binding (38), Nicolaou has claimed that the desiodo aryltetrasaccharide does not footprint with DNase I as was seen for the synthetic iodo compound. Moreover, the regions of protection do not correspond exactly to presumed sites (11,16,34,35) of CLM binding, implying that the alygcone segment in combination with the aryltetrasaccharide portions of the drug both contribute to the binding and cleavage specificity in accord with arguments made earlier (15).

At this point it seems that the conformation of the glycosidic linkage between the aglycone and the sugars is critical in aligning the nucleolytic activity of the warhead in the minor groove so that optimal directionality is obtained with the targeted hydrogens on the deoxyribose sugars. ROESY experiments carried out by Kahne's group at Princeton on calicheamicin in both polar and nonpolar solvents, as well as low-temperature NMR experiments on synthetic model compounds, strongly suggest a significant degree of preorganization in the molecule. Furthermore, the studies with model compounds (37) showed that rotation around

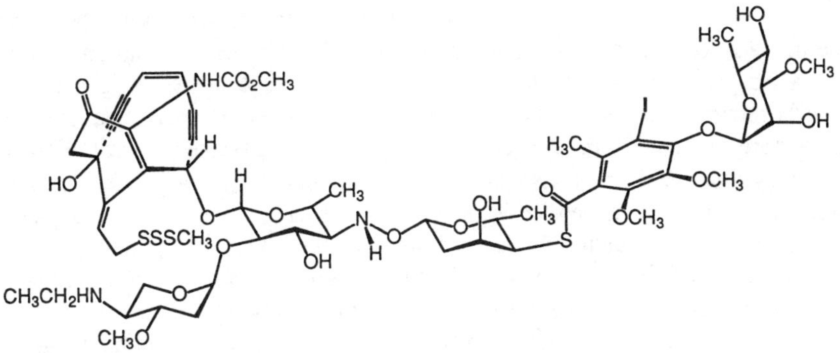

Figure 6 Preferred conformation of CLM γ_1^I based on interresidue NOE study. (From Ref. 36.)

the unusual N-O bond connecting sugars A to B is restricted as anticipated from earlier studies (36). Thus the N-O bond is a stereoelectronic feature key to enforcing a curvature to the molecule that is similarly isohelical with DNA (Fig. 6). Based on entropy arguments, some preorganization would seem necessary to obtain binding constants of 10^6–10^8 M^{-1}. In keeping with this view, an aryltetrasaccharide isomer containing the epimeric N-O linkage at C-4 of ring A was found to bind less efficiently to DNA than the natural configuration at this center (40).

CLM derivatives without the terminal rhamnose or the ethylamino sugar display the same cleavage specificity as the intact drug but require higher concentrations relative to that of the parent, indicating that these sugar appendages play little role in the sequence specificity but contribute largely to nonspecific binding (16).

V. CALICHEAMICIN-MEDIATED CLEAVAGE CHEMISTRY

Comparison of the electrophoretic mobilities of CLM-induced DNA-cleavage fragments with those obtained by Maxam-Gilbert sequencing reactions gave evidence as to the nature of the strand cleavage chemistry (11). With 5′-end–labeled restriction fragments as substrates, it was immediately clear that the drug-induced cleavage fragments co-migrated with the corresponding Maxam-Gilbert–produced fragments. This strongly suggested the formation of termini ending in 3′-phosphates. Evidence for the chemistry at the other side of the lesion was obtained with 3′-end–labeled fragments as substrates. In this case, the drug-induced cleavage fragments migrated as though they were two nucleotides longer than the corresponding chemically produced controls (11). Although an explanation of this phenomenon was not immediately apparent, Goldberg's findings with neocarzinostatin (41) suggested that treatment of the CLM γ_1^I reaction mixture with base might give fragments that co-migrated with the controls. This expectation was based on the neocarzinostatin cleavage chemistry in which 5′ hydrogen atom abstraction by this agent gives fragments ending in 3′ phosphates and 5′ aldehydes. Goldberg's studies showed conclusively that fragments ending with a 5′ aldehyde migrate as if they are two nucleotides longer than the chemically produced control oligonucleotides that end in phosphates. On treatment with base the terminal aldehyde–containing nucleoside is removed by a β-elimination reaction to give a fragment that now matches in electrophoretic mobility the corresponding control fragment. Therefore, treatment of the CLM γ_1^I–produced 3′-end–labeled oligonucleotide fragments with base gave oligonucleotides whose electrophoretic mobilities did indeed match the chemically produced controls, thus mimicking the neocarzinostatin cleavage chemistry. Therefore, CLM γ_1^I was inferred to abstract one of the C-5′ hydrogen atoms from the 5′ C of the 5′TCCT3′ tract.

On the complementary strand, it was not clear from these initial gel experiments which hydrogen(s) was(were) being abstracted. Oligonucleotide cleavage products derived from long restriction fragments labeled at the 5′ end appeared to migrate with the controls. However, with short synthetic dodecamers containing the TCCT site, the CLM-induced 3′ end–labeled cleavage fragment from the AGGA-containing strand migrated slightly faster than the control suggesting a 3′ terminus ending in a phosphoglycolate (16). This behavior is diagnostic of iron-bleomycin cleavage of DNA where 4′ hydrogen abstraction has been established (42).

The necessity of molecular oxygen for cleavage was clearly demonstrated in experiments in which oxygen in the reaction vessel was purged with argon (11). Under these mostly anaerobic conditions very little cleavage was seen by analysis of the reaction mixture on sequencing gels. Also, experiments were carried out in the presence of catalase and superoxide dismutase, but these enzymes had no obvious effect on the rate of cleavage or on the cleavage pattern. Therefore, based on these results and the specificity of the cleavage pattern, it was proposed that the nondiffusible, transient p-benzyne intermediate, formed during the CLM aromatization, abstracts hydrogen atoms from the C-5′ of the TCCT tract and C-4′ on the complementary strand. Dioxygen then reacts with these carbon-centered radicals and initiates strand scission most likely as summarized in Scheme 2. It must be remembered, however, that depending on the reaction conditions, there are two principal cleavage pathways for 4′ hydrogen abstraction based on the well-known studies of iron-bleomycin cleavage chemistry (42). The sensitivity of the relative proportions of 3′-phosphate or 3′-phosphoglyclate products to differing thiol concentrations has been observed in the reactions of calicheamicin with DNA to further support the proposed 4′-hydrogen abstraction (J. J. Hangeland and C. A. Townsend, unpublished results).

At this point an ^{1}H-NMR experiment was carried out (43) to prove chemically that CLM γ_1^I did indeed abstract hydrogen atoms from the deoxyribose sugars of DNA consistent with the inferences above from gel electrophoresis experiments

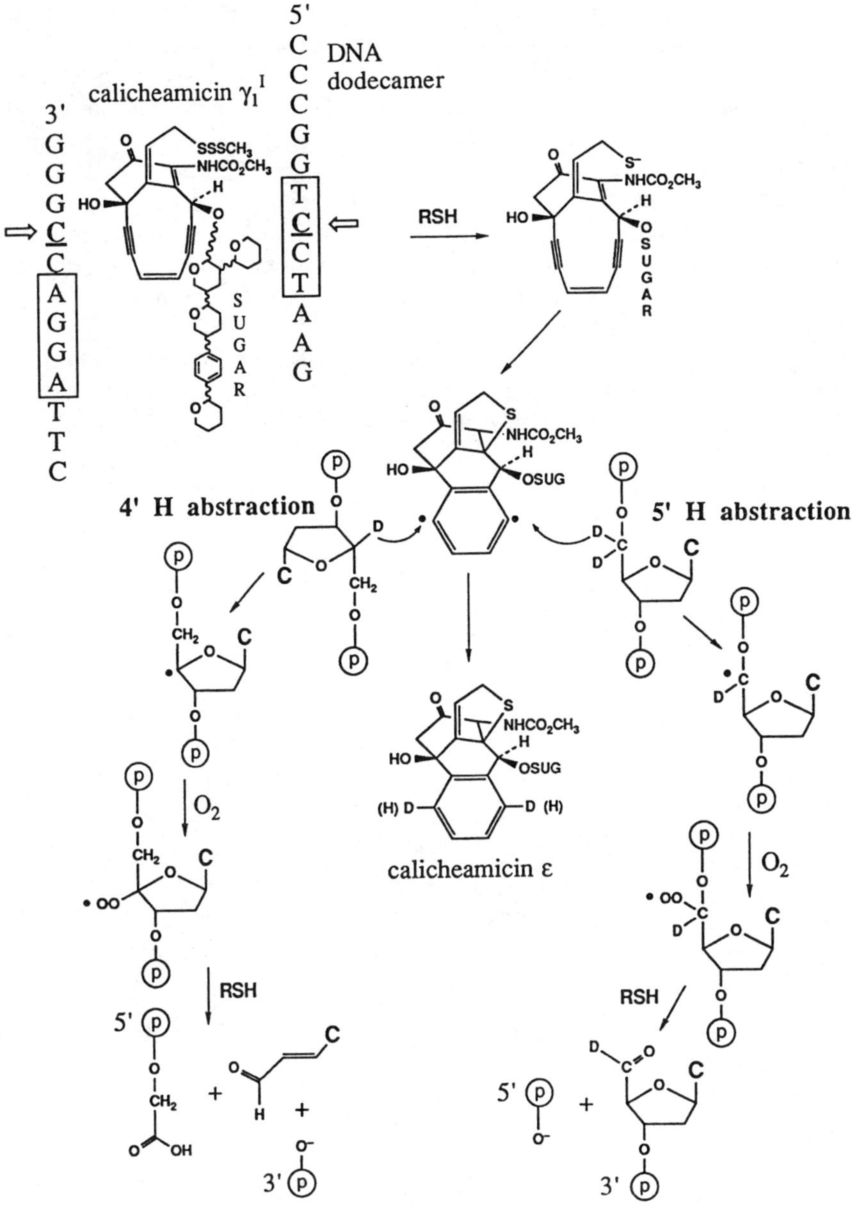
5'
C
C
C
G
G
T
C
C
T
A
A
G
DNA
dodecamer
calicheamicin γ_1^I
3'
G
G
G
C
C
A
G
G
A
T
T
C
SSSCH₃
NHCO₂CH₃
HO
H
O
SUGAR
RSH
S⁻
NHCO₂CH₃
H
OSUGAR
S
NHCO₂CH₃
H
HO
OSUG
4' H abstraction
5' H abstraction
D
C
CH₂
P
O₂
•OO
RSH
5'
CH₂
OH
H
3'
calicheamicin ε
(H) D
D (H)
5'
3'

Scheme 2

(11,16). Thus, sonicated calf thymus DNA was exchanged with D_2O as was the Tris buffer and methyl thioglycolate used as the reductant. Perdeuterated ethanol was used for solubilization of the drug. The reaction was scaled up (drug 0.36 μM and calf thymus ca. 3 μM in base pairs) so that the inactive aromatized end product, CLM ε [8], could be isolated by HPLC in quantities 0.75–1 mg) sufficient to determine the extent of deuterium transfer by ¹H-NMR. The ¹H-NMR spectrum of the isolated CLM ε showed conclusively that calicheamicin did in fact abstract nonexchangeable hydrogens only from the DNA. When the reaction was carried out without DNA, deuterium atoms (apparently from the deuteriothiol of methyl thioglycolate or possibly from the methylenes of perdeuterated ethanol) were transferred in better than 95% yield (Fig. 7).

In view of these results, samples of specifically labeled deoxycytidine dideuterated at C-5' were prepared for incorporation into the dodecamers **6** and **7** (Figure 8). Cleavage of these labeled substrates with CLM γ_1^I gave the deuterated ar-

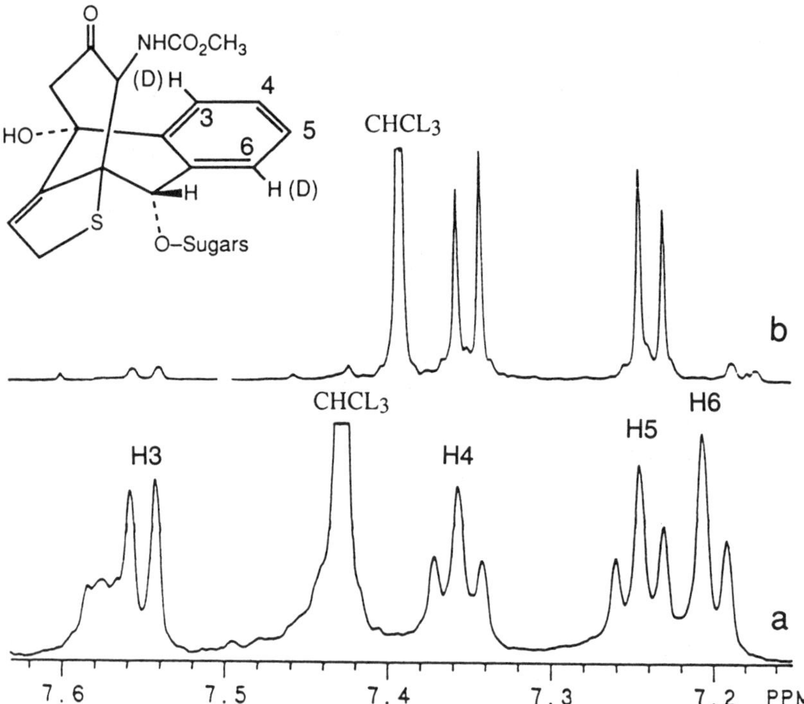

Figure 7   ¹H NMR of aromatic region of calicheamicin ε (8) isolated from the cleavage of calf-thymus DNA by calicheamicin γ_1^I. (a) Calicheamicin ε from a cleavage reaction carried out in a deuteriated medium and in the presence of deuterium exchanged calf-thymus DNA. (b) Calicheamicin ε from a cleavage reaction carried out in a deuteriated medium but without calf-thymus DNA (from ref. 43).

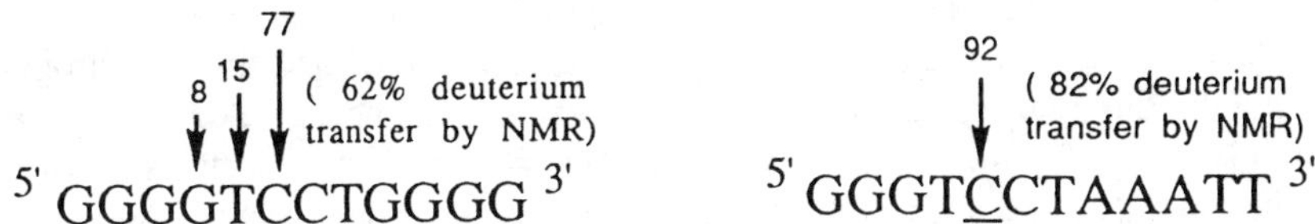

Figure 8 Summary of cleavage of dodecamers **6** (left) and **7** (right) as determined by high-resolution gel electrophoresis gel and NMR analysis of CLM ε. (From Ref. 34.)

omatized product whose ^{1}H-NMR spectrum showed deuterium incorporation at C-6 exclusively with transfer yields as indicated (34). This result not only confirmed the site of hydrogen atom abstraction, but also established the binding orientation of CLM γ_1^I with respect to the 5′TCCT/AGGA site such that the tail portion of the molecule was directed towards the 3′ side of the TCCT sequence as opposed to the 5′ side. Positioning of the tail portion towards the 5′ side of the TCCT sequence was suggested initially based on gel cleavage studies with the TCCT/AGGA sequence placed in the middle and at the 5′ and 3′ ends in synthetic dodecamers. These studies showed cleavage only at the two dodecamers with this tract at the middle and 3′ end, suggesting that the carbohydrate tail of the CLM molecule required duplex DNA at the 5′ side of the 5′TCCT site for binding (16).

Next, deoxycytidine deuterated at the 4′ position was prepared and incorporated into dodecamer **7** on the complementary AGGA-containing strand (35). Hydrogen atom abstraction from this labeled site occurred solely at C-3 of the drug to give CLM ε—but with only about 25% transfer efficiency. However, by moving the TCCT site two nucleotides towards the 3′ side and redesigning the dodecamer as **8** (Fig. 9), the transfer yield from the 4′ label of the deoxyribose to C-3 of CLM ε increased to 63% (35). An experiment with this dodecamer in the presence of deuterated solvent increased the atom transfer yield approximately 15%, indicative of the looseness of the abstraction process on this strand. The low transfer yield from abstraction at C-4′ in dodecamer **7** compared to that for **8** may be due to end effects on the labeled C-4′ as it is next to the terminal nucleotide in this strand. In any event, it is clear from these experiments that CLM

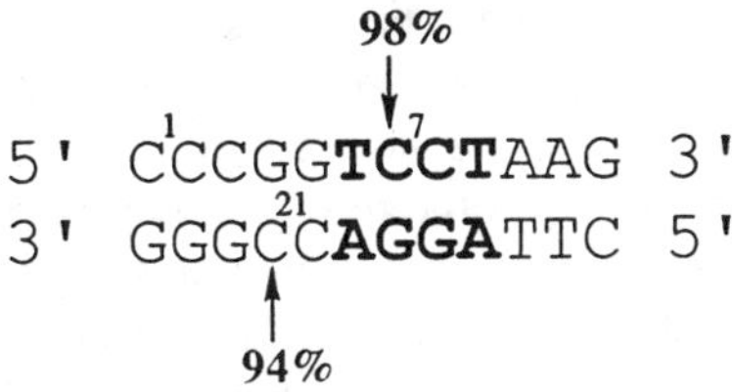

Figure 9 Dodecamer **8**. Percent of total cleavage at C^{21} was determined by high-resolution gel electrophoresis after piperidine treatment. (From Ref. 35.)

γ_1^I initiates oxidative strand scission with impressive accuracy by the abstraction of one of the 5′ hydrogens on the T<u>C</u>CT-containing strand and the 4′ hydrogen on the dC three nucleotides to the 3′ side of the complementary AGGA tract as summarized in Figure 9. No evidence for abstraction of the 1′ deuterium atom located in either strand in analogously labeled oligonucleotide **8** was observed.

It is readily apparent on examination of DNA models that it is the 5′*S*-hydrogen that points into the minor groove from each deoxynucleotide on either strand. The evidence from cleavage data gathered for CLM γ_1^I (35) and hydroxyl radical footprinting determinations (S. C. Mah et al., unpublished results) reinforce one another to point clearly toward minor groove binding. It would be predicted, therefore, that of the two diastereomic hydrogens at C-5′, the 5′*S* ligand should be removed to initiate scission in the TCCT recognition sequence. To this end 5′*S*- and 5′*R*-deuterated deoxycytidines were prepared by unambiguous methods from D-anhydroribose, activated for automated oligonucleotide synthesis and separately incorporated into dodecamer **8** (35). As anticipated for minor groove binding, transfer from the two forms of labeled DNA to CLM was highly selective, 89% from the 5′*S*-labeled oligonucleotide and <2% correspondingly from the 5′*R*-deuterated species.

In an effort to understand the nature of the strand cleavage (nicked vs. double-stranded) of esperamicin A_1, C, and CLM γ_1^I, Kishikawa et al. carried out a coupled kinetic analysis of the cleavage of these agents with closed circular plasmid DNA (PM2) using DNase I as a control for nicking (44). Analysis of the optical density data derived from agarose gel electrophoresis experiments showed that esperamicin A_1, like the enzyme, produces mainly single-stranded breaks. This behavior is in contrast to the cleavage data for esperamicin C (experamicin A_1 without the fucose-anthranilate moiety) and CLM γ_1^I, which fits a double-stranded kinetic model in which the rate constant for introducing the first break is followed by very fast cleavage on the complementary strand. This is consistent with a single activation event at the aglycone causing a double-stranded break. The single-stranded model for esperamicin A_1 suggests that one of the *p*-benzyne radicals is unproductive in that it reacts with solvent, the drug itself, or DNA but does not result in strand scission.

A high proportion of double-strand DNA damage is consistent with improved analytical methods developed for evaluation of the efficiencies of atom transfer determined from dodecamer **8**. In addition to using both ^{1}H-NMR and mass spectrometric methods to accurately establish the locations and efficiencies of deuterium transfer to generate CLMε, the occurrence of 4′-abstraction on the AGGA strand suggested the potential importance of abasic sites giving only partial scission on this strand when analyzed by electrophoresis. Thus, to evaluate the extent of true strand cleavage resulting from actual atom abstraction at the examined sites as a function of all cleavage on either strand, cleavage mixtures were treated with piperidine (35). The ^{32}P-labeled fragments were examined by phosphorimager after electrophoretic separation. The proportion of fragments generated by 5'-abstraction, that is, within the TCCT sequence, relative to uncut DNA was unchanged by base treatment. However, the AGGA strand resulted in the appearance of significantly larger proportions of cleavage fragments when examined analogously by gel electrophoresis and phosphorimager. Interestingly, the relative amount of cleavage at dC^{21} in **8** among all cleavage fragments from this strand remained remarkably constant despite extents of reaction of the intact dodecamer ranging from <10 to 90%. It is particularly notable that for the redesigned dodecamer **8** the selectivity of the cleavage at the indicated sites in Figure 9 on the TCCT strand was $98 \pm 1\%$ and $94 \pm 5\%$ on its complement. Therefore, atom transfer efficiencies of >80%, after correcting for solvent participation and small kinetic isotope effects (35), are indicative of very high extents of double-strand cleavage significantly in excess of the ratio 2:1 ss:ds reported by Drak et al. for averaged drug-cleavage behavior (12). Consideration of abasic sites arising from 4'-hydrogen abstraction was not evaluated in these experiments, and hence no base treatments of DNA were carried out to fully cleave the DNA. Accurate reflection of the true proportion of double-strand cleavage was probably not obtained in these experiments.

With regard to the drug-activation chemistry that takes place leading up to the formation of the phenylene diradical intermediate, low-temperature ^{1}H-NMR experiments using n-Bu$_3$P in methanol-d$_4$ showed that the dihydrothiophene has a significant half-life of 4.5 ± 1.5 sec at 37°C (33). The first-order rate constant determined over three half-lives is $5 \pm 2 \times 10^{-4}$ and gives a $\Delta G^{\neq}$ of 19.3 ± 0.2 kcal/mol, similar to that determined for the cyclization of neocarzinostatin (45). Indeed, the bimolecular thiol chemistry leading to this intermediate can be shown to be considerably slower than the rate of the Bergman aromatization. These are important observations with regard to the overall drug activation process for two reasons. The first is that while the initial reaction of calicheamicin γ_1^I with thiols is complex (33), it is overall rate-determining (21) consistent with the observed ability to isolate mixed disulfides with added thiols in high yield (22). This key finding has made possible the coupling of CLM to monoclonal antibodies to prepare immunoconjugates for selective drug delivery (see Chapter 8). Second, it was originally thought that once C-9 became sp^3 hybridized by allylic thiolate addition to the enone, aromatization would follow immediately. This is not the case, as formation of intermediate **6** is rate-limiting to an extent sufficient to quite possibly afford time to migrate to DNA in the cell and equilibrate along the helix to identify preferred binding/cleavage sites. This may help explain the question as to how CLM survives transport through the cell membrane without being triggered and inactivated before reaching the DNA target site.

VI. BIOCHEMICAL BASIS FOR CYTOTOXICITY

The potent DNA-cleavage properties of CLM γ_1^I strongly suggest that DNA is the principal cellular target. Whether the lipid membrane or other cellular entities are damaged by this agent and contribute to the overall cytotoxicity is uncertain. CLM γ_1^I caused significant chromosomal damage in human diploid fibroblast cells at pg/ml levels (11). A 50% inhibition of DNA synthesis (incorporation of [^{3}H]-thymidine) was observed in HeLa cells after treatment with 50 pg/ml of drug, whereas 15 ng/ml was necessary to cause a 50% inhibition of RNA synthesis (incorporation of [^{3}H]-uridine). Interestingly, an intermediate amount of CLM γ_1^I, 250 pg/ml, caused a 50% inhibition in protein synthesis (incorporation of [^{3}H]-leucine) (N. Zein et al., unpublished results). These findings strongly suggest that the inhibition of macromolecular synthesis is due to the binding and cleaving of duplex DNA by CLM γ_1^I.

Mitochondrial DNA damage in HeLa cells has been observed (T. Jones and N. Zein, unpublished results). Specific cleavage of mitochondrial DNA was suggested by the observation of discrete bands on agarose gels, and it will be interesting to see if the site of these lesions matches those observed in restriction fragments. The damage to mitochondrial DNA may explain the delayed lethality observed in non–tumor-bearing mice when injected with doses of CLM γ_1^I that prolonged the life of tumor-bearing mice. CC-1065 also causes delayed lethality in non–tumor-bearing mice and has been shown to damage mitochondrial DNA (46).

CLM γ_1^I has been found to cause a marked increase in poly(ADP-ribose)polymerase activity in promyelocytic HL-60 cells, apparently in response to extensive DNA damage. This resulted in a corresponding drop in NAD$^+$ levels, which paralleled cell death (47), suggesting that so much of the cell's energy is expended in trying to repair the CLM-induced DNA damage that energy levels are insufficient to maintain cellular viability.

In another study, fibroblasts from ataxia-telangiectasia (AT) patients were 40,000 times more sensitive to CLM γ_1^I than to bleomycin on a molar basis (48). It is well known that AT patients are extremely sensitive to ionizing radiation and are sensitive to DNA-damaging agents that cleave through the intermediacy of free radicals. This is suspected to be a result of defects in DNA repair in patients afflicted with this disease (49). CLM γ_1^I appeared to act in a similar manner to ionizing radiation in that it did not inhibit DNA synthesis in AT-derived cell lines.

A strong correlation between in vitro DNA damage and in vivo antitumor activity was observed with CLM derivatives. For example, *N*-acetyl CLM γ_1^I and the α_3 derivative, which lacks the basic ethylamino sugar, are less effective in prolonging the lifespan of mice challenged with experimental murine tumors and are also less effective in cleaving duplex DNA in vitro when compared with the parent drug (S. G. Caravajal and F. E. Durr, unpublished results). An explanation for this observation is not fully clear at this time but may point to an important role for the basic nitrogen in the ethylamino sugar moiety for uptake and/or DNA binding.

VII. SUMMARY

In conclusion, CLM γ_1^I is a potent DNA-damaging agent that binds and cleaves with sequence discrimination remarkable for such a small molecule. Strong chemical evidence has now been obtained that CLM γ_1^I binds and causes double-stranded cleavage at certain mixed G $\cdot$ C- and A $\cdot$ T-containing sequences in the minor groove with a notably strong preference towards homopyrimidine/homopurine tracts. Interestingly, it recognizes certain A $\cdot$ T-only sequences as well, suggesting that more than specific sequences or inherent groove geometry is involved in the binding/cleavage discrimination. Experiments with CLMt and particularly hydroxyl radical footprinting studies with CLMε show that cleavage specificity of the drug is largely determined by specificity of binding. Atom transfer experiments with DNA specifically labeled with deuterium reinforce and refine substantially earlier gel electrophoresis experiments indicating that 5'-hydrogen atom abstraction takes place on the targeted dC of a T<u>C</u>CT tract and 4'-abstraction occurs on the complementary strand two nucleotides to the 3' side of the 3'N<u>N</u>NAGGA tract. Furthermore, atom transfer takes place stereospecifically from the 5'S-hydrogen of the deoxyribose sugar to C-6 in the aromatized CLM ε and from the 4'-hydrogen of the sugar to C-3 of ε on the opposite strand providing unequivocal evidence for a single binding orientation with the tail portion oriented within the minor groove to the 3' side of TCCT site. Although a firm biochemical basis for the cytotoxicity of CLM γ_1^I is lacking, preliminary evidence strongly suggests that cellular DNA is a primary target of this potent antitumor agent.

ACKNOWLEDGMENTS

We wish to acknowledge helpful discussions with Professor T. D. Tullius (Johns Hopkins) during the course of this work. We also thank The National Institutes of Health (CA54421 to C.A.T.) for partial financial support.

Note Added in Proof Since the submission of this manuscript there have been a number of recent publications on the CLM association with DNA which either provide details of results mentioned in this chapter or describes completely new studies. Recent cleavage studies have shown that the major DNA cleavage event produced by CLM is a bistranded lesion which consists of a direct strand break resulting from 5' hydrogen abstraction on the TCCT-containing strand and an abasic site on the complementary <u>N</u>NAGGA strand resulting from C4' abstraction (50). Hydroxyl radical footprinting of CLMε shows that the carbohydrate-thiobenzoate tail portion lies in the minor groove in an extended conformation protecting approximately four nucleotides on each strand mainly to the 3' side of the C5' hydrogen abstraction on the TCCT- strand (51). This result is entirely consistent with the location of the enediyne established in earlier atom-transfer experiments but provides experimental evidence for the location of the aryl-linked carbohydrate side chain at a number of cleavage sites. Cleavage studies with long A-tracts and nucleosomal DNA suggest that CLM recognizes and cleaves sequences of DNA that have a narrow minor groove, and regions of DNA that may be susceptible to helix deformation (52). Evidence from circular dichroism studies suggests that the binding of CLM to DNA induces an optically detectable conformational change of B-form DNA (53). An NMR study of a CLM/DNA complex indicates a structural distortion of the CpC step of an ACCT sequence on CLM association (54). A very recent NMR study suggests the presence of two species in equilibrium which may explain the abstraction of two distant hydrogen atoms (55). The same group prepared the oligosaccharide potion of CLM with the iodo grouping replaced by bromo, chloro, fluoro, methyl and hydrogen which resulted in progressively weaker DNA binding (56). This pointed out again the importance of the iodo grouping for binding. However, it must not play a dominant role in binding specificity since CLM γ_1^I can bind and cleave AT only as well as GC-containing sequences. Full details of an analysis of hydroxylamine glycosidic linkages has appeared (57) as have results of a modeling study (58). Five of the six models predicted the correct DNA hydrogen abstraction pattern. Only one model, however, was consistent with all the available experimental data and which provided a clear rationale for the observed sequence specificity. DNA damage in HeLa nuclei and isolated nucleosome core particles has been examined for CLM, esperamicin A_1 (ESP A1), esperamicin C (ESP C) (A_1 without the deoxyfucose-anthranilate moiety) and neocarzinostatin (NCS). In nuclei, both NCS and ESP A_1 produced DNA damage limited to the linker region of the nucleosome, while CLM and ESP C damaged both the core and linker DNA (59). Recent studies investigated the complex early phase of CLM activation by thiols. Evidence is provided for the transient existence of intermediates leading to mixed disulfide formation and a minor process during initial encounter of thiolate with CLM to give directly dihydrothiophene [6] (60).

REFERENCES

1. M. D. Lee, J. K. Manning, D. R. Williams, N. A. Kuck, R. T. Testa, and D. B. Borders, *J. Antibiot., 42,* 1970 (1989).
2. M. D. Lee, T. S. Dunne, C. C. Chang, M. M. Siegel, G. O. Morton, G. A. Ellestad, W. J. McGahren, and D. B. Borders, *J. Am. Chem. Soc., 114,* 985 (1992).
3. J. Golik, J. Clardy, G. Dubay, G. Groenewold, H. Kawaguchi, M. Konishi, B. Krishnan, H. Ohkuma, K. Saitoh, and T. Doyle, *J. Am. Chem. Soc., 109,* 3461 (1987).
4. J. Golik, D. Dubay, G. Groenewold, H. Kawaguchi, M. Konishi, B. Krishnan, H. Ohkuma, K. Saitoh, and T. Doyle, *J. Am. Chem. Soc., 109,* 3462 (1987).

5. M. Konishi, H. Ohkuma, K. Matsumoto, T. Tsuno, H. Kamei, T. Miyaki, T. Oki, H. Kawaguchi, G. D. VanDuyne, and J. Clardy, *J. Antibiot,.* 42, 1449 (1989).

6. K. Edo, M. Mizugaki, Y. Koide, H. Seto, K. Furihata, N. Otake, and N. Ishida, *Tetrahedron Lett.,* 26, 331 (1985).

7. K. C. Nicolaou and W.-M. Dai, *Angew. Chem.,* 30, 1387 (1991).

8. R. A. Maplestone, M. J. Stone, and D. H. Williams, *Gene,* 115, 151 (1992).

9. R. G. Bergman, *Acc. Chem. Res.,* 6, 25 (1973).

10. T. P. Lockhart and R. G. Bergman, *J. Am. Chem. Soc.,* 103, 4091 (1981).

11. N. Zein, A. Sinha, W. J. McGahren, and G. A. Ellestad, *Science,* 240, 1198 (1988).

12. J. Drak, N. Iawasawa, S. Danishefsky, and D. Crothers, *Proc. Natl. Acad. Sci.,* 88, 7464 (1991).

13. C. Zimmer and U. Wähert, *Prog. Biophys. Molec. Biol.,* 47, 31 (1986).

14. L. A. Marky and K. J. Breslauer, *Proc. Natl. Acad. Sci.,* 84, 4359 (1987).

15. S. Walker, R. Landovitz, W.-D. Ding, G. A. Ellestad, and D. Kahne, *Proc. Natl. Acad. Sci.,* 89, 4608 (1992).

16. N. Zein, M. Poncin, R. Nilikantan, and G. A. Ellestad, *Science,* 244, 697 (1989).

17. K. Yanagi, G. G. Prive, and R. E. Dickerson, *J. Mol. Biol.,* 217, 201 (1991).

18. J. K. Sullivan and J. Lebowitz, *Biochemistry,* 30, 2664 (1991).

19. S. Satyanarayana, J. C. Dabarowiak, and J. B. Chaires, *Biochemistry,* 31, 9319 (1992).

20. W.-D. Ding and G. A. Ellestad, *J. Am. Chem. Soc.,* 113, 6617 (1991).

21. K. D. Cramer and C. A. Townsend, *Tetrahedron Lett.,* 32, 4635 (1991).

22. G. A. Ellestad, P. R. Hamann, N. Zein, G. O. Morton, M. M. Siegel, M. Pastel, D. B. Borders, and W. J. McGahren, *Tetrahedron Lett.,* 30, 3033 (1989).

23. A. G. Myers, P. M. Harrington, and B.-M. Kwon, *J. Am. Chem. Soc.,* 114, 1086 (1992).

24. D. L. Boger, H. Zarrinmayeh, S. A. Munk, P. A. Kitos, and O. Suntornwat, *Proc. Natl. Acad. Sci.,* 88, 1431 (1991).

25. D. Dasgupta, F. B. Howard, V. Sasisekharan, and H. T. Miles, *Biopolymers,* 30, 223 (1990).

26. V. P. Chuprina, U. Heinemann, A. A. Nurislamov, P., Zielenkiewicz, R. E. Dickerson, and W. Sanger, *Proc. Natl. Acad. Sci.,* 88, 593 (1991).

27. U. Heinemann and C. Alings, *J. Mol. Biol.,* 210, 369 (1989).

28. L. A. Marky and D. W. Kupke, *Biochemistry,* 28, 9982 (1989).

29. G. G. Prive, U. Heinemann, S. Chandrasegaran, L.-S. Kan, M. L. Kopka, and R. E. Dickerson, in *Structure and Expression* (M. H. Sarma and R. H. Sarma, eds.), Adenine, Schenectady, NY, 1988, Vol. 2, p. 27.

30. G. G. Prive, U. Heinemann, S. Chandrasegaran, L.-S. Kan, M. L. Kopka, and R. E. Dickerson, *Science,* 238, 498 (1987).

31. W. N. Hunter, T. Brown, N. N. Anand, and O. Kennard, *Nature,* 320, 552 (1986).

32. P. Modrich, *Annu. Rev. Biochem.,* 56, 435 (1987).

33. J. J. DeVoss, J. J. Hangeland, and C. A. Townsend, *J. Am. Chem. Soc.,* 112, 4554 (1990).

34. J. J. DeVoss, C. A. Townsend, W.-D. Ding, G. O. Morton, G. A. Ellestad, N. Zein, A. B. Tabor, and S. L. Schreiber, *J. Am. Chem. Soc.,* 112, 9669 (1990).

35. J. J. Hangeland, J. J. DeVoss, J. A. Heath, C. A. Townsend, W.-D. Ding, J. S. Ashcroft and G. A. Ellestad, *J. Am. Chem. Soc.*, *114*, 9200 (1992).

36. S. Walker, K. G. Valentine, and D. Kahne, *J. Am. Chem. Soc.*, *112*, 6428 (1990).

37. S. Walker, D. Yang, D. Kahne, and D. Gange, *J. Am. Chem. Soc.*, *113*, 4716 (1991).

38. R. C. Hawley, L. L. Kiessling, and S. L. Schreiber, *Proc. Natl. Acad. Sci.*, *86*, 1105 (1989).

39. J. Aiyar, S. J. Danishefsky, and D. M. Crothers, *J. Am. Chem. Soc.*, *114*, 7552 (1992).

40. K. C. Nicolaou, S.-C. Tsay, T. Suzuki, and G. F. Joyce, *J. Am. Chem. Soc.*, *114*, 7555 (1992).

41. I. H. Goldberg, *Acc. Chem. Res.*, *24*, 191 (1991).

42. G. H. McGall, L. E. Rabow, G. W. Ashley, S. H. Wu, J. W. Kozarich, and J. Stubbe, *J. Am. Chem. Soc.*, *114*, 4958 (1992)

43. N. Zein, W. J. McGahren, G. O. Morton, J. Ashcroft, and G. A. Ellestad, *J. Am. Chem. Soc.*, *111*, 6888 (1989).

44. H. Kishikawa, Y-P. Jiang, J. Goodisman, and J. Dabrowiak, *J. Am. Chem. Soc.*, *113*, 5434 (1991).

45. A. G. Myers and P. J. Proteau, *J. Am. Chem. Soc.*, *111*, 1146 (1989).

46. V. L. Reynolds, J. P. McGovren, and L. H. Hurley, *J. Antibiot.*, *39*, 319 (1986).

47. B. Zhao, S. Konno, J. M. Wu, and A. L. Oronsky, *Cancer Lett.*, *50*, 141 (1990).

48. N. Sullivan and L. Lyne, *Mutation Res.*, *245*, 171 (1990).

49. E. A. Hendrickson, X-Q. Qin, E. A. Bump, D. G. Schatz, M. O. Oettinger, and D. T. Weaver, *Proc. Natl. Acad. Sci.*, *88*, 4061 (1991).

50. P. C. Dedon, A. A. Salzberg, and J. Xu, *Biochemistry*, *32*, 3617 (1993).

51. S. C. Mah, C. A. Townsend, and T. D. Tullius, *Biochemistry*, *33*, 614 (1994).

52. S. C. Mah, M. A. Price, C. A. Townsend, and T. D. Tullius, *Tetrahedron*, *50*, 1361 (1994).

53. G. Krishnamurthy, W-d., Ding, L. O'Brien, and G. A. Ellestad, *Tetrahedron*, *50*, 1341 (1994).

54. S. Walker, J. Murnick, and D. Kahne, *J. Am. Chem. Soc.*, *115*, 7954 (1993). S. Walker, A. H. Andreotti, and D. Kahne, *Tetrahedron*, *50*, 1351 (1994).

55. L. G. Paloma, J. A. Smith, W. J. Chazin, and K. C. Nicolaou, *J. Am. Chem. Soc.*, *116*, 3697 (1994).

56. T. Li, Z. Zeng, V. A. Estevez, K. U. Baldenius, K. C. Nicolaou, and G. F. Joyce, *J. Am. Chem. Soc.*, *116*, 3709 (1994).

57. S. Walker, D. Gange, V. Gupta, and D. Kahne, *J. Am. Chem. Soc.*, *116*, 3197 (1994).

58. D. R. Langley, T. W. Doyle, and D. L. Beveridge, *Tetrahedron*, *50*, 1379 (1994).

59. L. Yu, I. H. Goldberg, and P. C. Dedon, *J. Biol. Chem.* *269*, 4144 (1994).

60. A. G. Myers, S. B. Cohen, and B. M. Kwon, *J. Am. Chem. Soc.*, *116*, 1255 (1994).

10

Fermentation and Isolation of Esperamicins

Kin Sing Lam and Salvatore Forenza
*Bristol-Myers Squibb Pharmaceutical Research Institute,
Wallingford, Connecticut*

I. INTRODUCTION

In our continuing search for microorganisms that produce novel antitumor
chemotypes, the supernatant from an actinomycete culture SA-24868 (strain ATCC
39334) showed extremely potent antitumor activity against P388 leukemia implanted in mice. At 160-fold dilution the culture supernatant still showed significant
antitumor activity. This actinomycete culture, identified as a new strain of
Actinomadura verrucosospora (1), was isolated from a soil sample collected at
Pto Esperanza, Misiones, Argentina. A family of extremely potent antitumor
antibiotics, with the trivial name esperamicins, was then isolated from this microorganism (2–7). The structures of esperamicins isolated from the fermentation
to date are shown in Figure 1. The esperamicins consist of a bicyclic core to
which are attached a trisaccharide and a substituted 2-deoxy-L-fucose. The bicyclic core contains a C-15 enediyne ring, an allylic trisulfide, and a bridgehead
enone.

At about the same time as the discovery of esperamicins, the isolation of
veractamycins (8–10), FR-900405 and FR-900406 (11,12), and calicheamicins
(13–16), enediyne antibiotics closely related to esperamicins, was also reported.
Veractamycin A and veractamycin B were later identified as esperamicin A_1 (esp
A_1) and esperamicin A_2 (esp A_2), respectively. FR-900405 and FR-900406 were

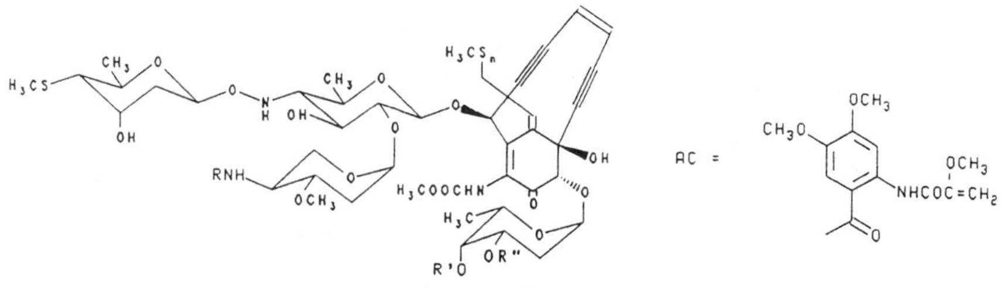

AC =

ESPERAMICIN	n	R	R'	R"
A_1	3	$CH(CH_3)_2$	H	AC
A_{1b}	3	CH_2CH_3	H	AC
A_{1c}	3	CH_3	H	AC
P	4	$CH(CH_3)_2$	H	AC
A_2	3	$CH(CH_3)_2$	AC	H
A_{2b}	3	CH_2CH_3	AC	H
A_{2c}	3	CH_3	AC	H

Figure 1   Structures of naturally occurring esperamicins.

identified as esperamicin A_{1b} (esp A_{1b}) and esperamicin A_{1c} (esp A_{1c}), respectively. Calicheamicins differ from esperamicins by the attachment of the aromatic chromophore to the trisaccharide moiety instead of to the enediyne ring. Also, esperamicins are nonhalogenated metabolites, while calicheamicins contain bromine or iodine. The extreme potency of these enediyne compounds against murine tumor models (17,18), their unique mode of action (19–27), their complex structures (3,4,13,15), and the low production of these agents in the bacterial cultures (1,8,14) generated a significant amount of excitement and challenges in the areas of microbial fermentation and chemistry.

In this review chapter, we describe the fermentation development of esp A_1, the most potent member of the esperamicin family, and the large-scale production and isolation of GMP grade esp A_1 for clinical evaluation. Through several years of extensive work in media development and strain improvement, we were able to improve the production of esp A_1 1000- to 2000-fold in the fermentation. Large-scale fermentation and isolation of esp A_1 was carried out at the National Cancer Institute (NCI)'s Frederick Cancer Research and Development Center (FCRDC) located in Frederick, Maryland. More than 40 grams of esp A_1 was isolated by FCRDC.

II. TAXONOMY OF THE PRODUCING ORGANISMS OF ESPERAMICINS

The producing strain of the esperamicin complex (ATCC 39334) has the following major taxonomic characteristics:

1. Aerial spore-chains: short, flexuous or hooked in shape
2. Spores: warty surface
3. Aerial mycelium: pinkish or bluish color
4. Substrate mycelium: pinkish in some media
5. Diffusible pigment: none
6. Mesophile
7. Cell-wall type III_B
8. Menaquinone system: MK-9(H_6) and MK-9(H_8)

These major characteristics indicate that strain ATCC 39334 belonged to the genus *Actinomadura*. As a result of comparison with the descriptions of 30 species including organisms disclosed in patents, strain ATCC 39334 appears most similar to *Actinomadura verrucosospora* (28,29). Strain ATCC 39334 was compared with the type strain *Actinomadura verrucosospora* KCC A-0147 and was found to be closely related to *Actinomadura verrucosospora* in its morphological, cultural, and physiological characteristics. Thus, strain ATCC 39334 was identified as a new strain of *Actinomadura verrucosospora*.

Veractamycins discovered at Parke-Davis and FR-900405 and FR-900406 discovered at Fujisawa are identical to the esperamicins produced by strain ATCC 39334 (Fig. 1). The producing culture of the veractamycins, strain ATCC 39363, was also identified as a new strain of *Actinomadura verrucosospora* (8). However, the growth characteristics of strain ATCC 39334 on the different carbon sources and some physiological characteristics are different from strain ATCC 39363 (Table 1). The producing culture of FR-900405 and FR-900406, strain ATCC 39100, was identified as a strain of *Actinomadura pulveracea* (11). Table 1 shows the difference in the carbohydrate utilization and physiological characteristics of strains ATCC 39334, ATCC 39363, and ATCC 39100. The differences in these characteristics demonstrated that strains ATCC 39334, ATCC 39363, and ATCC 39100 are novel strains of *Actinomadura* and may explain the differences in the metabolite production profiles in these strains.

III. ASSAY DEVELOPMENT

The original esperamicin-producing organism, strain ATCC 39334, produced extremely small amounts of esperamicin complex, estimated at about 0.1 µg/ml, in the initial fermentation medium. The major targeted compound, esp A_1, accounted for approximately 20–30% of the complex of 14–15 congeners. When

Table 1 Differences in the Carbohydrate Utilization and Physiological
Characteristics of *A. verrucosospora* ATCC 39334, *A. verrucosospora*
ATCC 39363, and *A. pulveracea* ATCC 39100

	Strain ATCC 39334	Strain ATCC 39363	Strain ATCC 39100
Utilization of carbon sources			
D-Fructose	+	+	−
D-Mannose	−	±	−
Lactose	−	+	−
D-Galactose	−	+	±
D-Trehalose	+	NT	−
Mannitol	+	+	−
Glycerol	+	+	±
Physiological characteristics			
Nitrate reduction	−	+	−
Milk peptonization	+	−	−

NT, Not tested.

an organism produces such a small amount of metabolite and the activities present
as a complex instead of a single active metabolite, it was extremely difficult to
isolate enough pure compound to serve as a standard for assay development.
Without a convenient and accurate assay, it was difficult to study and improve
the production of these antibiotics in the fermentation. In the early fermentation
and isolation study, in vitro biological activities such as cytotoxicity against tumor cell lines (30,31) and antimicrobial activity against *Bacillus subtilus* were used
to evaluate the samples. The media supporting improved production of the most
potent antibiotics in the complex can easily be detected using this biological activity guided evaluation of culture media even with only a slight increase in production. The production of esp A_1, the most potent member of the esperamicins,
was significantly increased in comparison to the other congeners during our media development study. The production of esp A_1 comprised about 75% of the
esperamicin complex in the fermentation using the improved production medium
(see below). Later a TLC system followed by bioautography with *B. subtilus*
provided some semiquantitative evaluation of the samples. Figure 2 shows the
protocol and the bioautogram of the TLC-bioautography of the extracts of strain
ATCC 39334. Four biologically active zones can be detected. The top biological active zone with Rf of 0.55 corresponded to esp A_1. In lane #4 of the
bioautogram, the sample did not contain any esperamicins. Once the authentic
standards were available, standard plots were constructed and the amount of

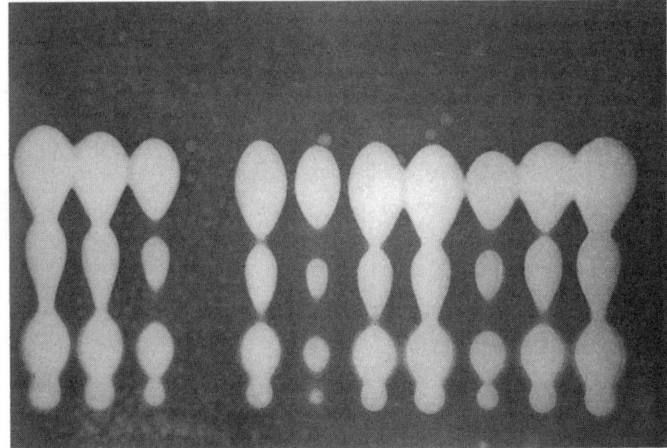

Figure 2 TLC-bioautography of fermentation extracts of *A. verrucosospora* strain ATCC 39334. (1) 3 ml of whole broth + 3 ml of ethyl acetate in a 8-ml screwcap tube. (2) Seal and place of rotater for 1 hr. (3) Centrifuge 5 min to break any emulsion. (4) Remove 0.2 ml ethyl acetate extract and evaporate to dryness. (5) Dissolve extract in 2 ml chloroform. (6) Spot 5–20 μl on Analtech GF silica gel TLC plate. (7) Develop with ether:methanol (95:5). (8) Overlay plate with Streptomycin Assay Agar with yeast extract (BBL) seeded with *Bacillus subtilus*. (9) Incubate plate overnight at 27°C. (10) Spray plate with triphenyl tetrazolium chloride solution to enhance zone distinction.

esperamicins present can then be calculated. This TLC-bioautography was shown to be extremely useful later in our screening of hyperproducer and blocked mutants.

Once a pure standard of esp A_1 was available, an HPLC assay was developed for monitoring the amount of esp A_1 in the samples. Figure 3 shows a typical HPLC chromatogram of the fermentation extract of strain ATCC 39334 growing in medium H946 (see below). The major metabolite produced in this fermentation was esp A_1, with a retention time of 8.6 min, comprising about 75% of the esperamicin complex. The second major metabolite produced by strain ATCC 39334 in medium H946 was esp A_2 with a retention time of 15.1 min. The increase in ratio of esp A_1 from 20% of the complex in the initial production medium to 75% of the complex in the improved medium facilitated the isolation of esp A_1 from the fermentation. The above assays were routinely used to evaluate the samples generated from the media development and mutation studies described in the following sections.

IV. MEDIUM-DEVELOPMENT PROGRAM

Before the development of an accurate assay for esperamicin production, we were not able to quantitate the production of the esperamicins in the early fermenta-

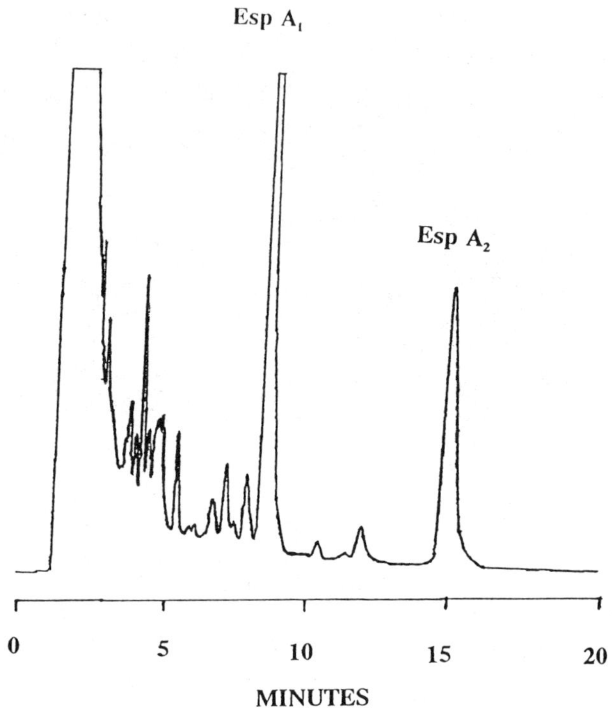

Figure 3 HPLC of a fermentation extract of *A. verrucosospora* strain ATCC 39334 grown in medium H946. Medium H946 has the following composition: 6% cane molasses, 2% cornstarch, 1.5% Pharmamedia, 0.01% $CuSO_4 \cdot 5H_2O$, 0.2% $CaCO_3$, and 0.5 mg/liter NaI.

tions. Based on a retrospective analysis of the biological data and from the plate (TLC-bioautography) assays, we have estimated that the original titer of the esperamicin complex produced by strain ATCC 39334 was about 0.1 µg/ml, with the target compound, esp A_1, accounting for approximately 20–30% of the antibiotic complex. The titer of esp A_1 was therefore about 0.02–0.03 µg/ml in the initial fermentation. In the case of the calicheamicins, the titer of calicheamicin γ_1^I in the initial fermentation was reported to be <0.05 µg/ml (14). In order to isolate enough compound from the fermentation for further chemical and biological characterization, extensive medium development was carried out to improve the production of esp A_1. Several thousand media have been tested. The following summarizes the effect of some of the medium components on the production of esp A_1.

A. Carbon Sources

The best carbon sources for esp A_1 production tested were sucrose, mannitol, and corn starch. Since molasses is an inexpensive and abundant source for sucrose, cane and beet molasses were compared as the carbon source for the production of esp A_1. It was determined that production of esp A_1 in the cane molasses medium was threefold higher than that in the beet molasses medium. Beet and cane molasses have comparable amounts of fermentable sugar, but beet molasses contains substantially higher concentrations of betaine (32), which was shown to inhibit the production of esp A_1. Supplementing cane molasses medium with cornstarch further enhanced the production of esp A_1.

B. Nitrogen Sources

Fish meal is the best nitrogen source to support the production of esp A_1. Esp A_1 production in the fish meal medium was at least twofold better than any other media containing other nitrogen sources. An interesting observation was noted when comparing the production of esperamicin in the medium containing fish meal and Pharmamedia as nitrogen source (Fig. 4). In the fish meal medium, esp A_1 is the major product of the fermentation (Fig. 3). The other major metabolite produced in this fermentation is esp A_2 with trace amounts of esp A_{1b} and esp A_{1c}. In the Pharmamedia medium, the production of esp A_1 was significantly reduced (Fig. 4). The major products of this fermentation were esp A_{1b} and esp A_{2b} (Fig. 4). Esp A_{1c}, esp A_2, and esp A_{2c} were also detected at about the same concentration of esp A_1 in the Pharmamedia medium (Fig. 4). Comparing the ingredient analysis of fish meal and Pharmamedia (33), there is a big difference in the amount of amino acids in these two nutrients. Even though the protein/amino acid content is very similar in fish meal (61%) and Pharmamedia (59%), Pharmamedia consists of 54% amino acids while fish meal consists of only 14% (33). Fish meal does not contain any hydrophobic amino acids (leucine, isoleucine, and valine) or two of the three aromatic amino acids (tyrosine and phenylalanine). These amino acids are present in quite a high concentration in Pharmamedia. We have demonstrated that when tyrosine was used as the sole nitrogen source in a defined medium for esperamicins fermentation, esp A_{1c} and esp A_{2c} but not esp A_1 and esp A_2 were detected in the fermentation (6). This suggests that certain amino acids may promote the production of certain esperamicins. For the production of esp A_1, it was determined that combination of fish meal and brewer's yeast as nitrogen and vitamin sources support the best production.

C. Metal Ions

Metal ion concentrations in media have profound effects on the growth and secondary metabolite production of microorganisms. Whereas normal growth can

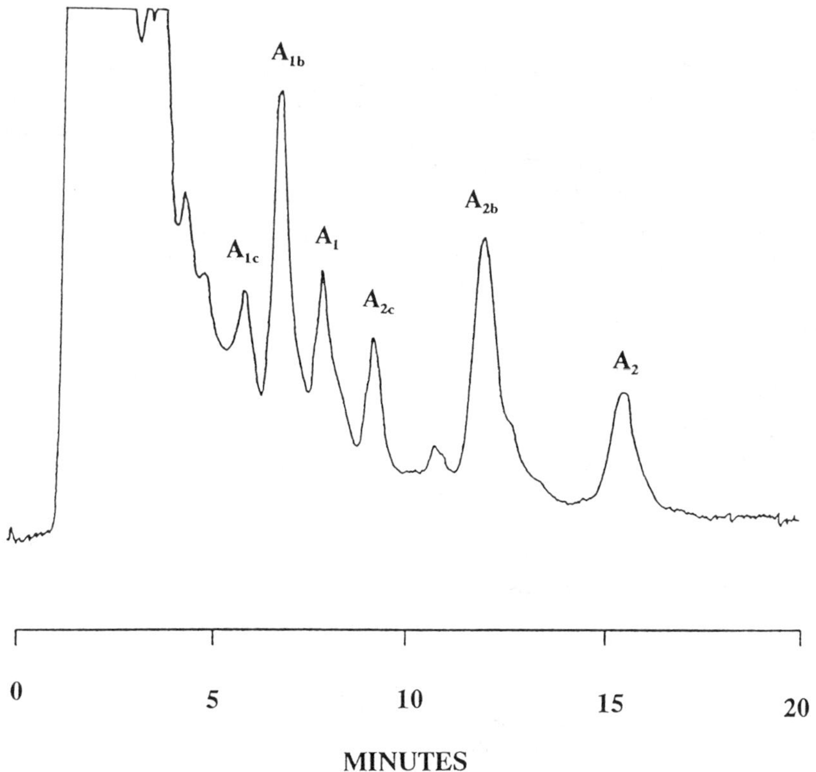

Figure 4 HPLC of a fermentation extract of *A. verrucosospora* strain ATCC 39334 grown in medium H947. Medium H947 has the following composition: 6% cane molasses, 2% cornstarch, 1.5% Pharmamedia, 0.01% $CuSO_4 \cdot 5H_2O$, 0.2% $CaCO_3$, and 0.5 mg/liter NaI.

occur within wide concentration ranges of metal ions, it has become apparent that for the synthesis of secondary metabolites, a much narrower tolerance exists in these same organisms (34,35). In a complex medium, the metal ion requirement for both growth and production of secondary products can be fulfilled by complex carbon sources (e.g., cane molasses) and nitrogen sources (e.g., fish meal and brewer's yeast) without further addition of trace metal ions into the medium. For the production of esp A_1 in the complex medium, further addition of Cu^{2+} ion enhanced the titer of esp A_1 twofold. None of the other metal ions tested showed any significant effect on the production of esp A_1 in the complex medium.

D. Iodide Ion

The addition of potassium iodide to the culture medium of *Micromonospora echinospora* NRRL 15839 significantly enhanced the production of calicheamicin

γ_1^I approximately 200-fold (14). The increase in production of calicheamicin γ_1^I can be explained by providing the precursor iodide to the organism. However, the addition of NaI to the culture medium of esperamicin-producing culture also enhanced the production of esp A_1 three- to fourfold even though iodide is not a component of esp A_1. Furthermore sodium iodide also enhanced the production (3 to 4 times) of dynemicin A, another enediyne antitumor antibiotic that does not contain iodide (36,37). We do not know the mechanism of improved production of esp A_1 and dynemicin A by iodide ion. Since there are several biosynthetic reactions of nonhalogenated metabolites derived from halogenated intermediates (38–41), the biosynthesis of esp A_1 and dynemicin A may involve iodinated intermediates. The presence of iodide ion may lead to increase in production of esp A_1 and dynemicin A by enhancing the formation of the iodinated intermediates.

E. Polypropylene Glycol (P-2000) (ppg)

Addition of antifoam, ppg (0.1%), to the shake flask culture increased the production of esp A_1 three- to fourfold. Addition of silicone-based Dow Corning antifoam (0.01–1%) to the shake flask culture has no effect on the production of esp A_1. Other surface-active agents such as cottonseed oil, lard oil, soy oil, and corn oil also have no effect on the production of esp A_1. The stimulation effect of ppg on the production of avermectin production has also been reported (42,43). Addition of 0.25% ppg to the fermentation enhanced the production of avermectin threefold and was shown to be the single most effective modification of medium for titer improvement for avermectin (42). Since ppg is not metabolized by the organism and can be quantitatively recovered from the fermentation, it cannot be a substrate or metabolic inducer for esp A_1. Esp A_1 is a highly reactive metabolite and is unstable. We have demonstrated that continuous degradation of esp A_1 occurred even during the active production phase (44). The increase in titer during the active production phase reflects the balance between synthesis and degradation of esp A_1. The rate of synthesis of esp A_1 is higher than the rate of degradation. Polypropylene glycol may sequester esp A_1 from the aqueous environment in which degradation of esp A_1 may occur. In protic solvents, esp A_1 can be readily converted to esp A_2. The action of ppg may reduce the contact of esp A_1 with its producing organism and may lead to higher production of esp A_1. The esp-producing organism is also sensitive to esp A_1 in the fermentation. In the agar culture, no growth of *A. verrucosospora* was observed when the agar was supplemented with 20 µg/ml of esp A_1 (44). In the medium containing ppg for the production of avermectin, an insoluble yellow-orange oily wax was produced during the fermentation (43). This oily wax contained a high concentration of avermectin—15–55 mg/ml of oil (43).

Based on the above findings, the medium composition of production medium H946p used for large-scale fermentation of esp A_1 was formulated as: 6% cane molasses, 2% corn starch, 2% fish meal, 0.01% $CuSO_4.5H_2O$, 0.2% $CaCO_3$, 0.5 mg/liter NaI, and 0.1% ppg.

V. MUTATION PROGRAM

A mutation program was carried out to select hyperproducer mutants and blocked mutants of esp A_1. Isolation of blocked mutants may help us to understand the biosynthetic pathway of the antibiotic (45–50), generate novel products by mutasynthesis (51–55), and clone biosynthetic genes by genetic complementation (56–60). In order to facilitate the screening for hyperproducers and blocked mutants, an agar plug screening method (61) was developed. However, one problem with this agar method is that there may only be a slight correlation between antibiotic formation in plate culture and antibiotic production in the submerged culture. Different agar media were tested for their ability to produce esp A_1 using strain ATCC 39334. An agar plug (0.5 × 0.75 cm) from each agar culture was extracted with ethyl acetate, and the extract was assayed by TLC-bioautography. It was interesting to note that using liquid medium H946 and 2% agar as an agar medium did not support the production of esp A_1. Some agar media such as ISP-2 supported the production of esp A_1 for 1–2 days. The activity of esp A_1 disappeared with additional incubation. The best agar medium found was medium 1675-2ag (7), which supported good esp A_1 production (14–15 mm inhibition zone size) over a 4- to 5-day period. Using this agar plug screening method and the TLC-bioautography assay, 300 isolates can be screened for hyperproducer and blocked mutants per day by one person.

Figure 5 summarizes the mutation program carried out in our laboratories for the isolation of hyperproducing mutants and blocked mutants. *A. verrucocospora* strain ATCC 39638 was derived from *N*-methyl-*N'*-nitro-*N*-nitrosoguanidine (NTG) treatment of the original esperamicin-producing strain, *A. verrucosospora* ATCC 39334. Strain ATCC 39638 showed improved sporulation properties and growth over the original strain. The production of esp A_1 by strain ATCC 39638 was about 2- to 2.5-fold higher than that by the original strain. Also, strain ATCC 39638 was more stable than the original strain and yielded more reproducible fermentation and production profiles. This may be attributed to the improved sporulation properties of the mutant strain. The titers of esp A_1 by strain ATCC 39638 in medium H946 and medium H946p were 5–7 μg/ml and 15–20 μg/ml, respectively. Strain ATCC 39638 was further treated with UV irradiation. The survivor single colony isolates were screened for better esp A_1 titer, and hyperproducing mutant strain MU-5019 was obtained (62). The production of esp A_1 by strain ATCC 39638 and MU-5019 in shake flask and laboratory fermenter cultures is shown in Table 2. The only difference between medium H946 and medium H946p (as described above) is that medium H946 does not contain ppg and medium H946p has 0.1% ppg. As expected, the production of esp A_1 by

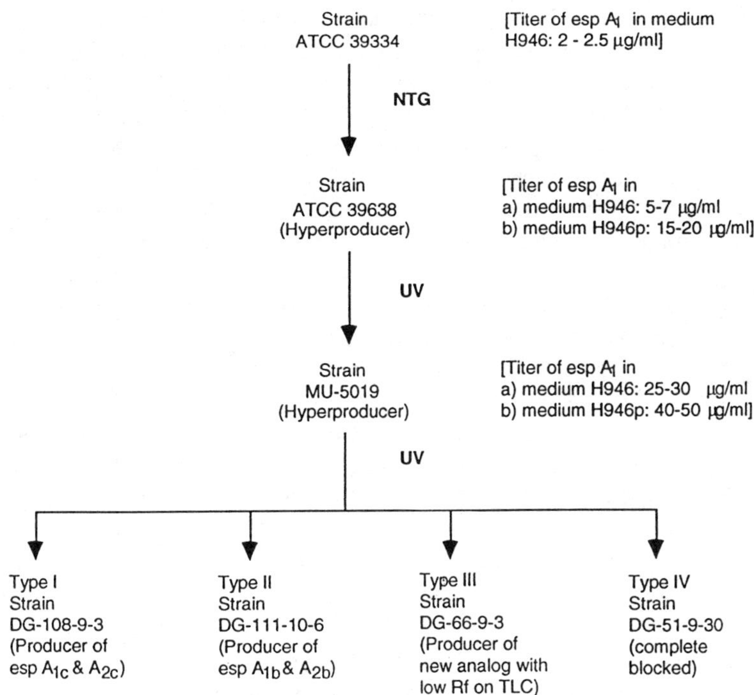

Figure 5 Hyperproducer and blocked mutants generated from *A. verucosospora* strain ATCC 39334.

strain ATCC 39638 in medium H946p (18.6 µg/ml) was 3.6-fold higher than that in medium H946 (5.1 µg/ml). The production of esp A_1 by the hyperproducing mutant MU-5019 (29.6 µg/ml) was 5.8-fold higher than the strain ATCC 39638 (5.1 µg/ml) in the medium H946. The stimulation effect of ppg on the produc-

Table 2 Production of Esp A_1 by *A. verrucosospora* ATCC 39334 and MU-5019 in Shake Flask and Laboratory Fermenter (50-liter) Cultures

	esp A_1 in shake flask culture (μg/ml)		esp A_1 in fermenter culture (μg/ml), Medium H946p
	Medium H946	Medium H946p	
Strain ATCC 39638	5.1	18.6	20.8
Strain MU-5019	29.6	50.3	43.5

tion of esp A_1 in strain MU-5019 was only 1.7-fold. The highest titer of esp A_1 in the shake flask culture detected in our laboratories was 50.3 µg/ml by strain MU-5019 in medium H946p. The scale-up production of esp A_1 by strains ATCC 39638 and MU-5019 was compared in a 50-liter laboratory fermenter containing medium H946p. The production of esp A_1 by strain MU-5019 (43.5 µg/ml) was 2.1-fold higher than that of strain ATCC 39638 (20.8 µg/ml).

Screening of the survivors from UV irradiation of MU-5019 did not yield any stable hyperproducing mutants. Several presumptive hyperproducers have been isolated (60–92 µg/ml esp A_1) from the initial screening. The production of esp A_1 in these presumptive mutants was down to 40–50 µg/ml upon retest. However, we were able to isolate several blocked mutants of esp A_1 derived from strain MU-5019. These blocked mutants do not produce esp A_1 or esp A_2 in the fermentation and can be classified into four types.

Type 1 blocked mutants do not produce esp A_1 by TLC-bioautography and HPLC assay. A representative strain of this class of mutants is DG-108-9-3, which accumulates some low Rf value active metabolites by TLC-bioautography assay (Fig. 6). HPLC analysis of the extract of strain DG-108-9-3 confirmed the production of two new esperamicin metabolites not previously isolated in our laboratories (Fig. 6). The major metabolite (RT: 6.03 min), designated esp A_{1c}, was later determined to be the same as FR-900406 reported by Fujisawa (11,12). The second major metabolite (RT: 10.07 min), designated esp A_{2c}, is a new esperamicin analog. Type II blocked mutants, represented by strain DG-111-10-6, do not produce esp A_1 but a major metabolite (RT: 6.95 min), which was identified as esp A_{1b}, previously isolated in our laboratories (3,4) (Fig. 7). Strain DG-111-10-6 also produces esp A_{1c}, esp A_{2c}, and another new esperamicin, esp A_{2b} (Fig. 7). Type III blocked mutants also produce active metabolites with low Rf values on TLC plate (Fig. 8). HPLC analysis showed that only a couple of esperamicin metabolites are produced at very low concentration (Fig. 8). A representative of this class is DG-66-9-3. Recently we isolated 2 mg of the new esperamicin congener with retention time of 9.25 minutes. Structure determination of this compound is in progress. The isolation of these blocked mutants proved to be successful in obtaining new congeners of esp A_{1c}, esp A_{2b}, esp A_{2c}, and an unknown analog in the fermentation. Blocked mutants (Type IV) that do not produce any esperamicins have also been isolated. Similar types of blocked mutants of calicheamicins have also been reported (63).

VI. LARGE-SCALE PRODUCTION OF ESP A_1

Because esp A_1 fully met our criteria of novelty, broad spectrum of activity, and novel mechanism of action, a decision was made to proceed with clinical development. Large-scale fermentation and isolation of esp A_1 was required to ensure an adequate drug supply for clinical evaluation. Esp A_1 and its congeners are

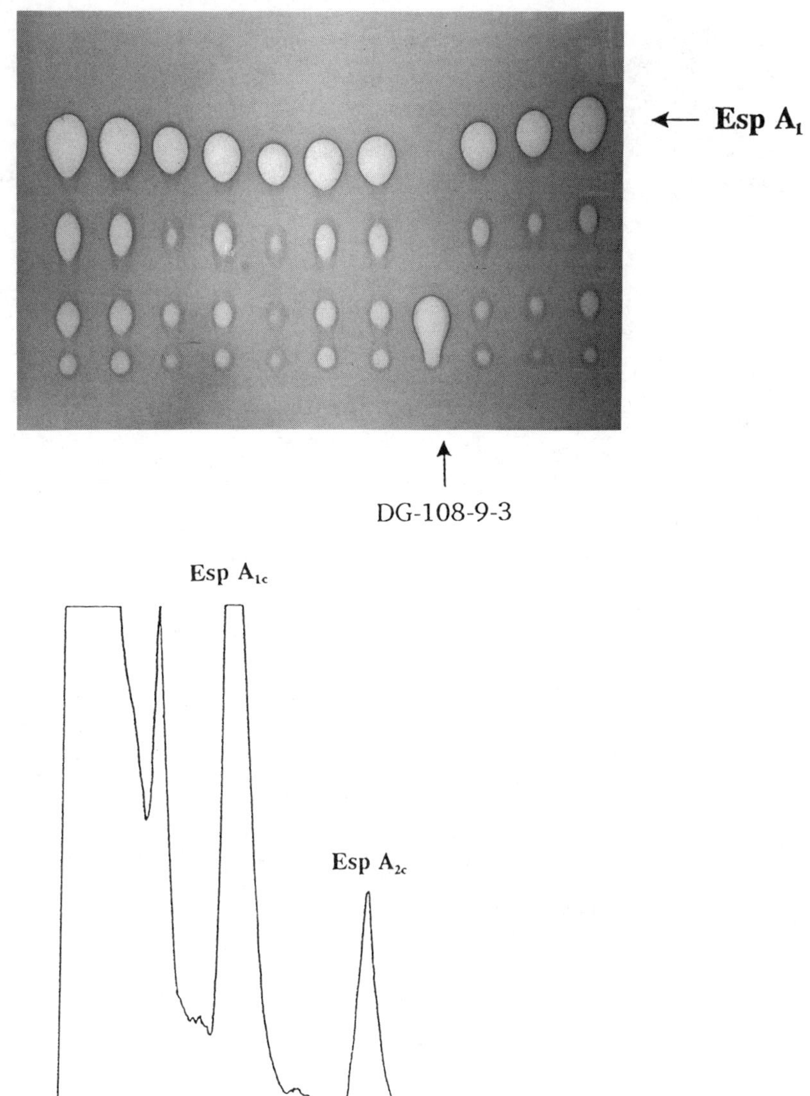

Figure 6 TLC-bioautography and HPLC of a fermentation extract of *A. verrucosospora* strain DG-108-9-3 grown in medium H946.

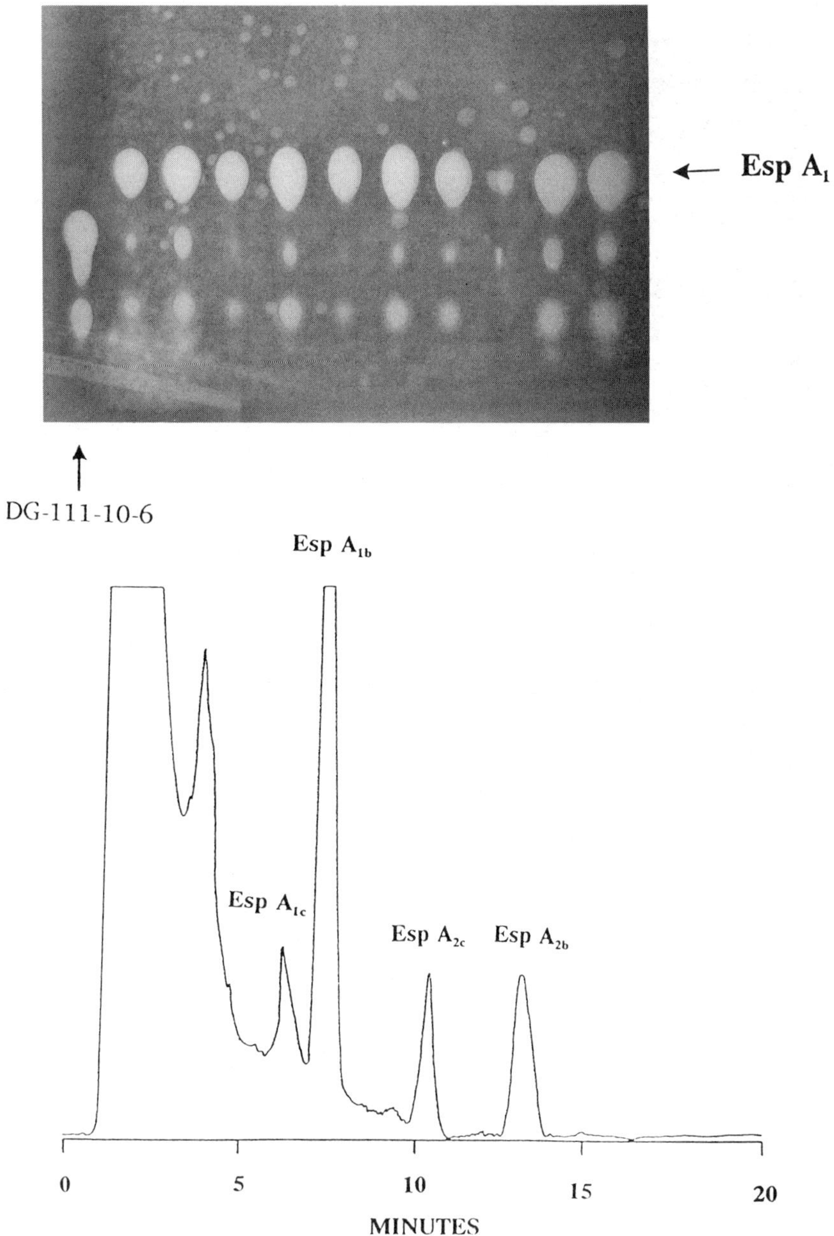

Figure 7   TLC-bioautography and HPLC of a fermentation extract of *A. verrucosospora* strain DG-111-10-6 grown in medium H946.

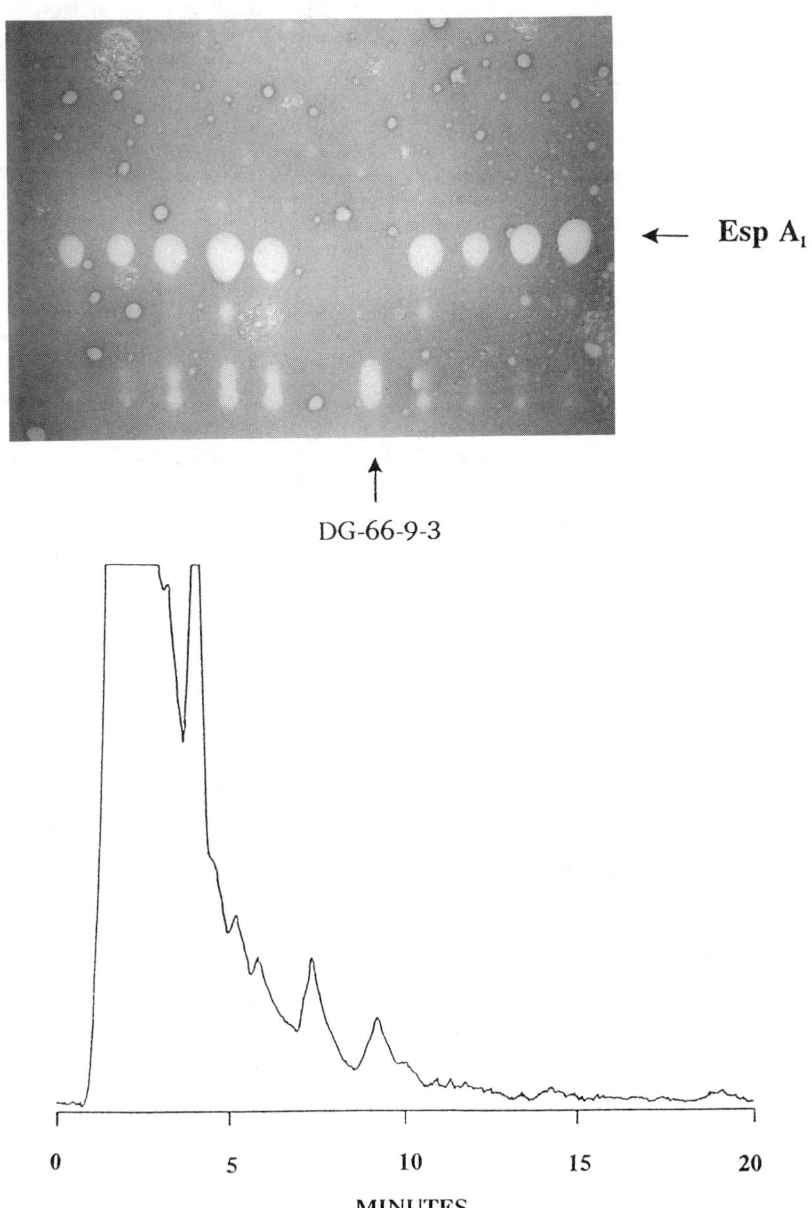

Figure 8 TLC-bioautography and HPLC of a fermentation extract of *A. verrucosospora* strain ATCC DG-66-9-3 grown in medium H946.

extremely toxic (mouse LD_{10} esp A_1 = 9 $\mu g/m^2$). Special handling and precautions are required for extracting and purifying esp A_1 and the waste generated from the large-scale fermentation process. The discovery of esperamicins in our laboratories was a collaborative effort with NCI under the NCI contract (No. 1-CM37556). The large-scale fermentation and purification of the cytotoxic anticancer drug adriamycin had been efficiently carried out in NCI's Frederick Cancer Research and Development Center (64), which was available for the esperamicin fermentation. After surveying several fermentation and production facilities, we decided that FCRDC was the most suitable site for the large-scale production of GMP grade esp A_1. The collaborative effort of FCRDC and Bristol-Myers Squibb Company has yielded more than 40 grams of esp A_1.

The isolation and purification of gram quantities of esp A_1 via large-scale fermentation process has met with several obstacles. The sensitivity of esp A_1 to light, protic solvents, and pH extremes required an approach that would avoid these adverse conditions, yet would separate esp A_1 from the cometabolites in the fermentation. The need to process large amounts of initial extracts to obtain rather modest quantities of the target compound also put constraints on the methods used. In the methods we developed, solvent extraction, elution with methylene chloride from diatomaceous earth, and four separate flash chromatography steps were used to obtain high-purity material. A final reverse-phase HPLC, back extraction, and rechromatography over silica gel yielded esp A_1 of over 95% purity.

Hyperproducing strain MU-5019 was isolated after the transfer of technology from our laboratories to FCRDC. Since a lot of fermenter-scale experiments using strain ATCC 39638 have been performed and valuable data on the fermentation and production profiles of strain ATCC 39638 have been gathered, we decided to use strain ATCC 39638 in the initial large-scale fermentation process in the 1000-liter fermenters. Good titers of esp A_1, 14.0–34.5 $\mu g/ml$, have been obtained in the 1000-liter fermenter cultures of strain ATCC 39638 growing in production medium H946p. Finally, the production of esp A_1 by strain ATCC 39638 was scaled-up in a 10,000-liter fermenter containing 6800 liters of medium H946p (Fig. 9). Four seed cultures were used to build up 680 liters of inoculum for the production tank. The fermentation and production profiles of this 10,000-liter fermenter run are shown in Figure 10. The final titer of esp A_1 in this fermentation was 17.6 $\mu g/ml$. Since the final fermentation broth (harvest volume) was 6600 liters, this fermentation yielded approximately 116 grams of esp A_1. The growth of the organism was determined by packed cell volume (PCV). The growth of the organism rapidly increased to about 25% PCV at the initial 70 hours of the fermentation. Then the growth of the organism gradually increased to about 40% at 225 hours. The increase in PCV after 70 hours may be due to thickening of the cell wall and the accumulation of assimilatory materials, such as lipids and nonstructural carbohydrates, and not a reflection of replicatory growth

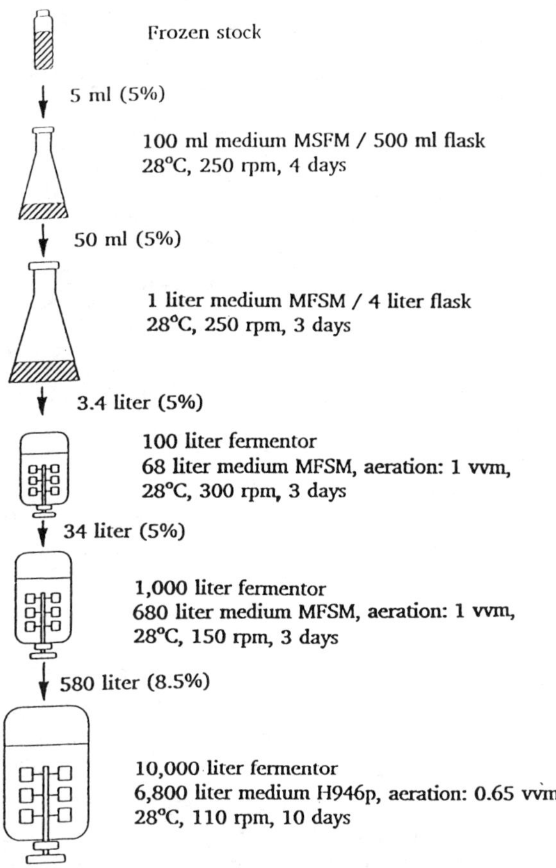

Figure 9 Scheme for scale-up production of esp A_1 by *A. verrucosospora* strain ATCC 39638 in a 10,000-liter fermenter containing 6800 liters of medium H946p.

of the organism. The culture entered the stationary phase after about 70 hours of fermentation. The onset of esp A_1 production was detected at around 105 hours, about 25 hours into the stationary phase. It is interesting to note that the production of esp A_1 began at about the same time that the CO_2 concentration in the exhaust gas began to decline rapidly (25–30 hours into the stationary phase) (Fig. 10). This correlation of drop in offgas CO_2 and initiation of esp A_1 production was also observed in the 1000-liter fermenter cultures. Therefore, the offgas CO_2 data may be used as an indicator for the estimation of the onset of esp A_1 production in the fermenter culture.

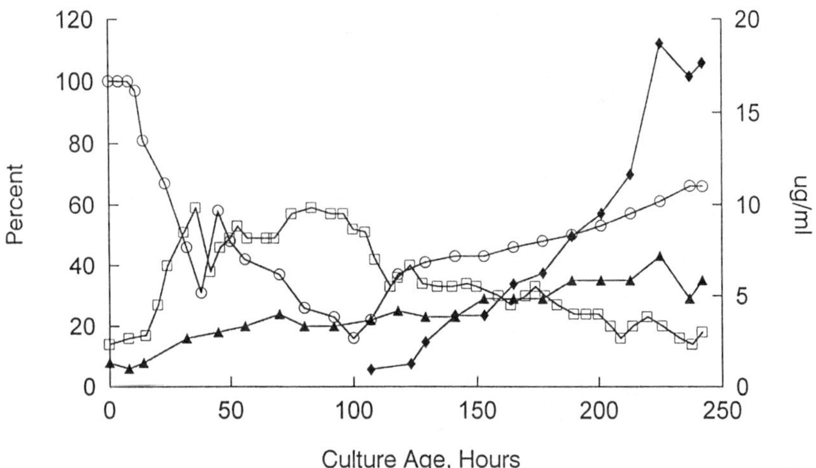

Figure 10 Time-course of esp A_1 fermentation by *A. verrucosospora* strain ATCC 39638 in a 10,000-liter fermenter containing 6800 liters of medium H946p. Symbols: ⊟, %CO_2 (×100); ⊖, % dissolved oxygen; ▲, centrifugal solids; and ◆, titer of esp A_1 (µg/ml).

Figure 11 shows a flowchart for the initial pilot plant processing of esp A_1 from the 10,000-liter fermenter culture. The first problem encountered was to concentrate approximately 6600 liters of ethyl acetate extract to a manageable size for further processing. A Wiped film evaporator was used to rapidly (18 hr) evaporate the extract down to 500 liters. The volume of the extract was further dropped to 75 liters of residue by evaporation in a Pot still (14 hr). The above evaporation processes were very efficient with good recovery of esp A_1 (about 82 g). The hexane wash of the residue followed by filtration through GAF filters precoated with Dicalite yielded both hexane filtrate and filtered cake fractions containing significant amounts of esp A_1. If the above procedure was carried out properly, one would expect most of the esp A_1 to be located in the filtered cake fraction. Significant amounts (about 33 g) of esp A_1 were found in the hexane filtrate. This may be due to presence of water in the Pot still concentrate. Also, the ratio of hexane and Dicalite used for the precipitation of esp A_1 and removal of ppg may be inadequate. Removal of water in the Pot still concentrate before mixing with hexane and using a larger volume of hexane and higher ratio of Dicalite to hexane/concentrate may enable concentration of esp A_1 to the filtered cake fraction. Both fractions were then extracted with ethyl acetate and subjected to Dicalite chromatography. Dicalite chromatography was developed with the following solvents: (1) hexane, (2) hexane/toluene (1:1), (3) CH_2Cl_2, (4) $CHCl_3$, and (5) CH_3OH. Only the CH_2Cl_2 fractions contained esp A_1 as deter-

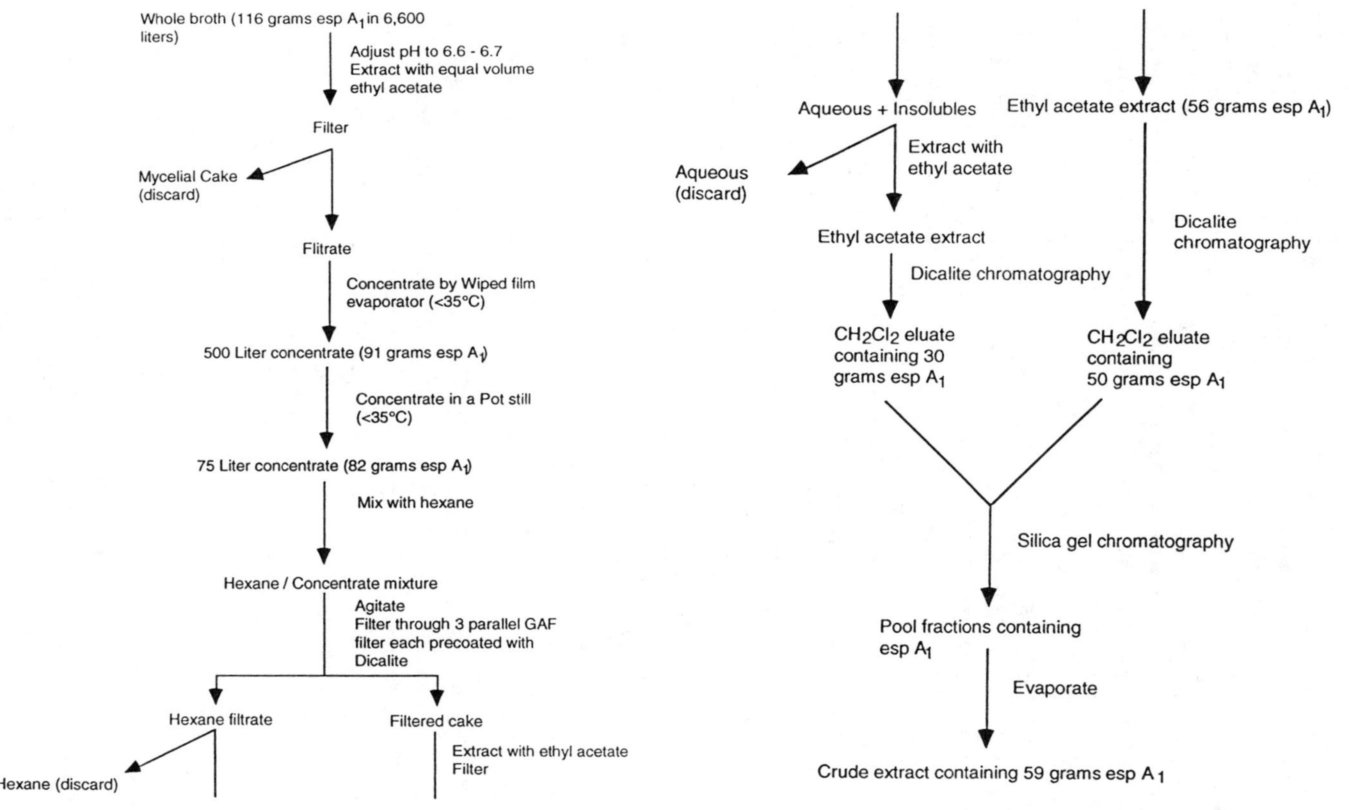

Figure 11 Pilot plant process for the recovery of crude esp A₁ from a 10,000-liter fermenter.

mined by HPLC analysis. After pooling all CH_2Cl_2 fractions containing esp A_1, the fractions were evaporated to dryness and then applied onto a silica gel column. The silica gel column was developed using the following solvents: (1) $CHCl_3$, (2) 1.8% CH_3OH in $CHCl_3$, (3) 3.6% CH_3OH in $CHCl_3$, (4) 7.2% CH_3OH in $CHCl_3$, and (5) CH_3OH. Esp A_1 was found in the fractions between the end of 1.8% CH_3OH and the beginning of 3.6% CH_3OH as determined by HPLC analysis. The fractions containing esp A_1 were pooled and evaporated to dryness and yielded about 59 g of esp A_1.

Figure 12 shows the final production process of esp A_1 on a laboratory scale. The concentrate generated from the pilot was divided into five approximately equal portions. The initial weight of one portion of the extract was 33 g with about 33% purity. Four separate silica flash column chromatographies were used to obtain esp A_1 of 97% purity. The silica flash column with a hexane/acetone wash was important to remove an unidentified metabolite that co-eluted with esp A_1 in the reverse-phase HPLC separation. The flash column with a $CHCl_3/t$-butanol wash successfully removed esp A_2 from esp A_1. A flash column with a $CHCl_3/CH_3OH/$ HOAc wash removed the undesired colored impurities from esp A_1. Final purification was carried out by reverse-phase HPLC. Back extraction of esp A_1 from the HPLC fractions and rechromatography on a silica flash column yielded 3.7 g esp A_1 of 99% purity.

Typical results of the final product specifications of esp A_1 isolated from cultures of stain ATCC 39638 using the above purification protocol is shown in Table 3. High-purity esp A_1 can be obtained from the above process. More than 40 g of esp A_1 so far has been isolated by FCDRC.

VII. SUMMARY

Several years of fermentation development in our laboratories have reliably increased the production of esp A_1 from approximately 0.02–0.03 µg/ml to 40–50 µg/ml. This corresponds to a 1000- to 2000-fold increase in the production of esp A_1. This production titer of esp A_1 was judged adequate for commercialization given the potency of esp A_1. In the original production medium, esp A_1 comprised of 20–30% of the antibiotic complex of 14–15 congeners. Extensive media development led to the formulation of the new improved production medium H946p. In medium H946p, esp A_1 is the major product of the fermentation and comprised of 75% of the esperamicin complex. The titer of esp A_1 in this new improved medium was 100- to 200-fold higher than that of the original medium.

Strain improvement programs carried out in our laboratories have yielded several hyperproducing mutants, which have improved production of esp A_1 10- to 20-fold over the original producer strain ATCC 39334. The best mutant so far isolated from our laboratories is strain MU-5019. The production of esp A_1 by

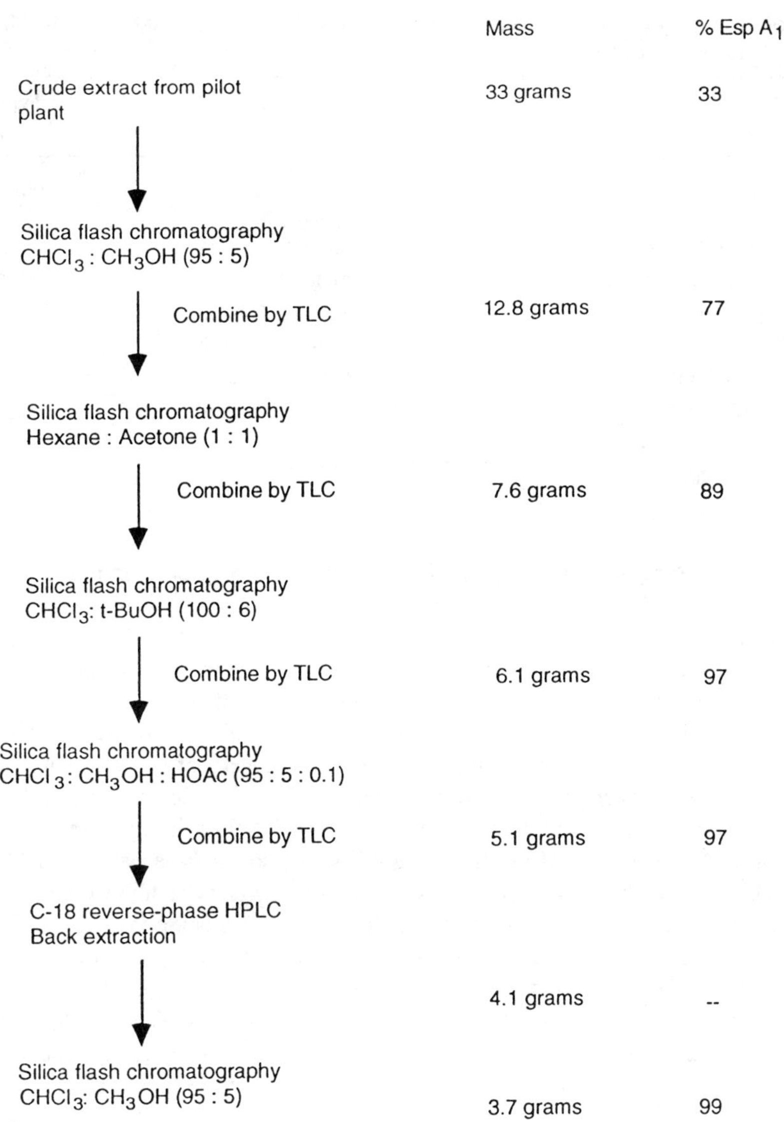

Figure 12 Laboratory-scale process for the purification of esp A_1.

strain MU-5019 in medium H946p is 40–50 µg/ml. Further improvement of esp A_1 production by *A. verrucosospora* will be involved in the isolation of deregulated mutants. Several blocked mutants of esp A_1 were also isolated in our laboratories. Isolation of these blocked mutants has resulted in the identification of

Table 3   Final Production Specifications of Esp A_1 Isolated from 1000- and 10,000-liter Fermenters at FCRDC

Test	Criterion	Typical results
Total purity	>95%	95.4%
HPLC area %	Minimum 97%[a]	97.9%[a]
Loss on drying	Maximum 3%	2.5%
Residue on ignition	Maximum 1%	0%
UV spectrum	319 nm log e 4.0–4.2	4.04
	253 nm log e 4.3–4.6	4.42
Ethanol solubility	1 mg/ml, no turbidity	passes
IR, PMR, CMR, FAB-MS, appearance, m.p.	Conforms to standard	passes

[a] No single impurity has $\geq 1\%$ area by HPLC analysis.

several new esperamicin analogs in the fermentation. These blocked mutants may be used in the cloning of the biosynthetic genes of esperamicins by genetic complementation.

The conditions for large-scale fermentation and isolation of esp A_1 by *A. verrucosospora* have been established. Reproducible fermentation and production profiles of esp A_1 have been achieved in a 10,000-liter fermenter at NCI's FCDRC. An efficient pilot plant process for the recovery of crude esp A_1 from the 6800-liter fermenter culture was developed. Final purification of esp A_1 on a laboratory scale yielded about 16 g of esp A_1 of >95% purity from a 6800-liter tank fermentation. More than 40 g of esp A_1 so far have been isolated by FCRDC. The collaborative effort of NCI and Bristol-Myers Squibb Company has ensured adequate drug supply of esp A_1 for clinical evaluation.

Dynemicin A, an enediyne class antibiotic, is produced by *Micromonospora chersina* ATCC 53710 (65). The titer of dynemicin A in the initial production medium was very low, about 0.1 µg/ml. Based on our experience in the medium development of esp A_1 fermentation, we quickly improved the production of dynemicin A to 3.5 µg/ml in the new production medium (37). We anticipate the isolation of more novel compounds in the enediyne class due to the experience we gained in working with esperamicins, calicheamicins, dynemicins, and neocarzinostatin.

REFERENCES

1.   M. Konishi, K. Saitoh, H. Ohkuma and H. Kawaguchi, U.S. Patent 4,675,187, June 23, 1987.

2. M. Konishi, H. Ohkuma, K-I. Saitoh, H. Kawaguchi, J. Golik, G. Dubay, G. Groenewold, B. Krishnan, and T. W. Doyle, *J. Antibiot., 38,* 1605 (1985).

3. J. Golik, J. Clardy, G. Dubay, G. Groenewold, H. Kawaguchi, M. Konishi, B. Krishnan, H. Ohkuma, K-I. Saitoh, and T. W. Doyle, *J. Am. Chem. Soc., 109,* 3461 (1987).

4. J. Golik, G. Dubay, G. Groenewold, H. Kawaguchi, M. Konishi, B. Krishnan, H. Ohkuma, K-I. Saitoh, and T. W. Doyle, *J. Am. Chem. Soc., 109,* 3462 (1987).

5. J. Golik, J. A. Beutler, P. Clark, J. Ross, J. Roach, G. Muschik, and W. B. Lebherz, III, U.S. Patent 5,028,536, July 2, 1991.

6. K. S. Lam, J. A. Veitch, J. Golik, S. Forenza, and T. W. Doyle, Abstract P-55, 49th Annual Meeting of Society for Industrial Microbiology, San Diego, California, August 9–14, 1992.

7. K. S. Lam, D. G. Gustavson, and S. Forenza, Abstract P-84, 46th Annual Meeting of Society for Industrial Microbiology, Seattle, Washington, August 14–19, 1989.

8. R. H. Bunge, T. R. Hurley, T. A. Smitka, N. E. Willmer, A. J. Brankiewicz, C. E. Steinman, and J. C. French, *J. Antibiot., 37,* 1566 (1984).

9. J. B. Tunac, B. D. Graham, S. W. Mamber, W. E. Dobson, and M. D. Lenzini, *J. Antibiot., 38,* 1337 (1985).

10. J. H. Wilton, G. C. Hokanson, and J. C. French, *J. Chem. Soc. Chem. Commun., 1985,* 919 (1985).

11. M. Iwami, S. Kiyoto, M. Nishikawa, H. Terano, M. Kohsaka, H. Aoki, and H. Imanaka, *J. Antibiot., 38,* 835 (1985).

12. S. Kiyoto, M. Nishikawa, H. Terano, M. Kohsaka, H. Aoki, H. Imanaka, Y. Kawai, I. Uchida, and M. Hashimoto, *J. Antibiot., 38,* 840 (1985).

13. M. D. Lee, T. S. Dunne, M. M. Siegel, C. C. Chang, G. O. Morton, and D. B. Borders, *J. Am. Chem. Soc., 109,* 3464 (1987).

14. W. B. Maiese, M. P. Lechevalier, H. A. Lechevalier, J. Korshalla, N. Kuck, A. Fanitini, M. J. Wildey, J. Thomas, and M. Greenstrin, *J. Antibiot., 42,* 558 (1989).

15. M. D. Lee, J. K. Manning, D. R. Williams, N. A. Kuck, R. T. Testa, and D. B. Borders, *J. Antibiot., 42,* 1070 (1989).

16. M. D. Lee, T. S. Dunne, C. C. Chang, M. M. Siegel, G. O. Moryton, G. A. Ellestad, W. J. McGahren, and D. B. Borders, *J. Am. Chem. Soc., 114,* 985 (1992).

17. J. E. Schurig, W. C. Rose, H. Kamei, Y. Nishiyama, W. T. Bradner, and D. A. Stringfellow, *Invest. New Drugs, 8,* 7 (1990).

18. D. W. Fry, J. L. Shills, and W. R. Leopold, *Invest. New Drugs, 4,* 3 (1986).

19. B. H. Long, J. Golik, S. Forenza, B. Ward, R. Rehfuss, J. C. Dabrowiak, J. J. Catino, S. T. Musial, K. W. Brookshire, and T. W. Doyle, *Proc. Natl. Acad. Sci. USA, 86,* 2 (1989).

20. Y. Sugiura, Y. Uesawa, Y. Takahashi, J. Kuwahara, J. Golik, and T. W. Doyle, *Proc. Natl. Acad. Sci. USA, 86,* 7672.

21. S. Kiyoto, T. Shibata, Y. Hori, O. Nakayama, H. Terano, M. Kohsaka, H. Aoki, and H. Imanaka, *J. Antibiot., 38,* 955 (1985).

22. M. Lu, Q. Quo, B. Krishnan, J. Golik, I. E. Rosenberg, T. W. Doyle, N. R. Kallenbach, *J. Biomol. Struct. Dyn., 9,* 285 (1991).

23. N. Zein, A. M. Sinha, W. J. McGahren, and G. A. Ellestad, *Science, 240,* 1198 (1988).
24. N. Zein, M. Poncin, M. Ramaswamy, and G. A. Ellestad, *Science, 244,* 697 (1989).
25. N. Zein, W. J. McGahren, G. O. Morton, J. Ashcroft, and G. A. Ellestad, *J. Am. Chem. Soc., 111,* 6888 (1989).
26. J. J. De Voss, C. A. Townsend, W. D. Ding, G. O. Morton, G. A. Ellestad, N. Zein, A. B. Tabor, and S. L. Schreiber, *J. Am. Chem. Soc., 112,* 9669 (1990).
27. G. A. Ellestad, N. Zein, and W. D. Ding, in *Advances in DNA Sequences Specific Agents* (L. Hurley, ed.), JAI Press, Greenwich, CT, 1992, pp. 293–317.
28. H. Nonomura and Y. Ohara, *J. Ferment. Technol., 49,* 904 (1971).
29. H. Nonomura, *J. Ferment. Technol., 52,* 71 (1974).
30. D. A. Scudiero, R. H. Shoemaker, K. D. Paull, A. Monks, S. Tierney, T. H. Nofziger, M. J. Currens, D. Seniff, and M. R. Boyd, *Cancer Res., 48,* 4827 (1988).
31. J. J. Catino, D. M. Francher, K. J. Edinger, and D. A. Stringfellow, *Cancer Chemother. Pharmacol., 15,* 240 (1985).
32. H. J. Peppler, in *Microbial Technology,* 2nd ed., Vol. 1 (H. J. Peppler and D. Perlman, eds.), Academic Press, New York, 1979, Chapter 5.
33. T. L. Miller and B. W. Churchill, in *Manual of Industrial Microbiology and Biotechnology* (A. L. Demain and N. A. Solomon, eds.), American Society for Microbiology, Washington, DC, 1986, Chapter 10.
34. E. D. Weinberg, in *Overproduction of Microbial Products* (V. Krumphanzel, B. Sikyta, and Z. Vanek, eds.), Academic Press, London, 1982, pp. 181–194.
35. E. D. Weinberg, in *Regulation of Secondary Metabolism in Actinomycetes* (S. Shapiro, ed.), CRC Press, Boca Raton, FL, 1989, Chapter 7.
36. K. Shiomi, H. Iinuma, H. Naganawa M. Hamada, S. Hattori, H. Nakamura, T. Takeuchi, and Y. Iitaka, *J. Antibiot., 43,* 1000 (1990).
37. K. S. Lam, J. A. Titus, T. T. Dabrah, D. L. Kimball, J. M. Veitch, D. R. Gustavson, B. J. Compton, J. A. Matson, S. Forenza, J. Ross, D. Miller, J. Roach, and J. Beutler, *J. Ind. Microbiol., 11,* 7 (1992).
38. W. Fenical, *Recent Adv. Phytochem., 13,* 219 (1979).
39. W. Fenical, *Science, 215,* 923 (1982).
40. M. A. Johnson and R. Croteau, *Arch. Biochem. Biophys., 235,* 254 (1984).
41. S. L. Neidleman, *CRC Crit. Rev. Microbiol., 5,* 333 (1975).
42. R. W. Burg, B. M. Miller, E. E. Baker, J. Birnbaum, S. A. Currie, R. Hartman, Y.-L. Kong, R. L. Monagham, G. Olson, I. Putter, J. O. Tunac, H. Wallick, E. O. Stapley, R. Oiwa, and S. Omura, *Antimicrob. Agents Chemther., 15,* 361 (1979).
43. P. A. McCann-McCormick, R. L. Monaghan, E. E. Baker, R. T. Goegelman, and E. O. Stapley, in *Advanced in Biotechnology* (M. Moo-Young, ed.), Pergamon Press, New York, 1981, pp. 63–68.
44. K. S. Lam, D. R. Gustavson, J. A. Veitch, and S. Forenza, *J. Ind. Microbiol., 12,* 99 (1993).
45. J. Sekiguchi and G. M. Gaucher, *Biochemistry, 17,* 1785 (1978).
46. J. Sekiguchi and G. M. Gaucher, *Biochem. J., 182,* 445 (1979).
47. J. Sekiguchi, G. M. Gaucher, and Y. Yamada, *Tetrahedron Lett., 41,* (1979).

48. R. H. Baltz and E. T. Seno, *Annu. Rev. Microbiol.*, *42*, 547 (1988).

49. S. W. Queener, *Annu. Rev. Microbiol.*, *32*, 593 (1978).

50. S. Omura and Y. Tanaka, in *Macrolide Antibiotics: Chemistry, Biology, and Practice* (S. Omura, ed.), Academic Press, New York, 1984, pp. 199–229.

51. O. Johdo, A. Yoshimoto, T. Ishikura, H. Naganawa, T. Takeuchi, and H. Umezawa, *Agric. Biol. Chem.*, *509*, 1657 (1986).

52. T. Oki, A. Yoshimoto, T. Matsuzawa, T. Takeuchi, and H. Umezawa, *J. Antibiot.*, *35*, 1641 (1982).

53. R. Spagnoli, L. Cappelletti, and L. Toscano, *J. Antibiot.*, *36*, 365 (1983).

54. E. J. Tynan III, T. H. Nelson, R. A. Davies, and W. C. Werman, *J. Antibiot.*, *45*, 813 (1992).

55. C. Bormann, S. Mattern, H. Schrempf, H.-P. Fiedler, and H. Zahner, *J. Antibiot.*, *42*, 913 (1989).

56. D. A. Hopwood and D. H. Sherman, *Annu. Rev. Genet.*, *24*, 37 (1990).

57. P. K. Tomich, *Antimicrob. Agents Chemother.*, *32*, 1465 (1988).

58. F. Malpartida and D. A. Hopwood, *Nature*, *309*, 462 (1984).

59. H. Motamedi and C. R. Hutchinson, *Proc. Natl. Acad. Sci. USA*, *84*, 4445 (1987).

60. K. F. Chater, *Biotechnology*, *8*, 115 (1990).

61. T. Ichikawa, M. Date, T. Ishikura, and A. Ozaki, *Folia Microbiol.*, *16*, 218 (1971).

62. K. S. Lam, J. A. Titus, and D. L. Kimball, Abstract O-40, 87th Annual Meeting of American Society for Microbiology, Atlanta, Georgia, March 1–6, 1987.

63. D. M. Rothstein and S. F. Love, *J. Bacteriol.*, *173*, 7716 (1991).

64. R. J. White and R. M. Stroshane, in *Biotechnology of Industrial Antibiotics*, Vol. 22 (Erick J. Vandamme, ed.), Marcel Dekker, Inc., New York, 1984, pp. 569–594.

65. M. Konishi, H. Ohkuma, K. Matsumoto, T. Tsuno, H. Kamei, T. Miyaka, T. Oki, H. Kawaguchi, G. D. VanDuyne, and J. Clardy, *J. Antibiot.*, *42*, 1449 (1989).

11

Structure Determination of the Esperamicins

Jerzy Golik
Bristol-Myers Squibb Pharmaceutical Research Institute,
Wallingford, Connecticut

I. INTRODUCTION

The enediynes constitute a novel class of the most potent antibacterial and anti-tumor active secondary metabolites known. Among antitumor antibiotics they are distinguished by their unique chemical structures, which upon bioactivation enable them to be extremely efficient DNA cleavers. At present the family of natural enediynes (Fig. 1) includes the neocarzinostatin chromophore (1), the esperamicins (2), the calicheamicins (3), the dynemicins (4), and, more recently, discovered, the chromophores of kedarcidin (5), maduropeptin (6), and C1027 (7).

This chapter summarizes the structure determination of the esperamicin family. As with many other natural products, the esperamicins are produced as a complex of structurally related metabolites. This complex has been resolved into a number of components, which were screened for their biological activity and submitted for structure determination. To date the structure of the major component of this complex esperamicin A_1, as well as several minor ones, A_2, A_{1b}, A_{1c}, A_{2c}, and P (8), have been elucidated as shown in Figure 2.

The esperamicins are members of the enediyne class having a 1,5-diyne-3-ene chromophore bridged in a highly strained bicyclo[7.3.1] tridecaenediyne ring system. This central unit of the esperamicins, the "core" contains also an allylic polysulfide (usually a trisulfide) and an α,β-unsaturated enone. It is the unique

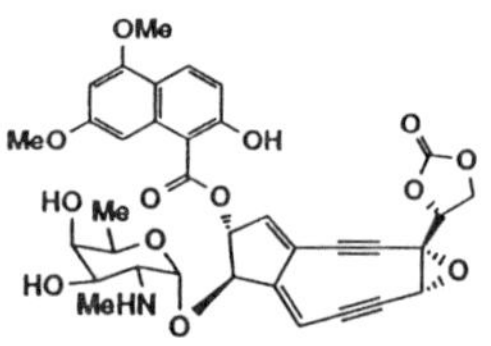

1. Neocarzinostatin Chromophore

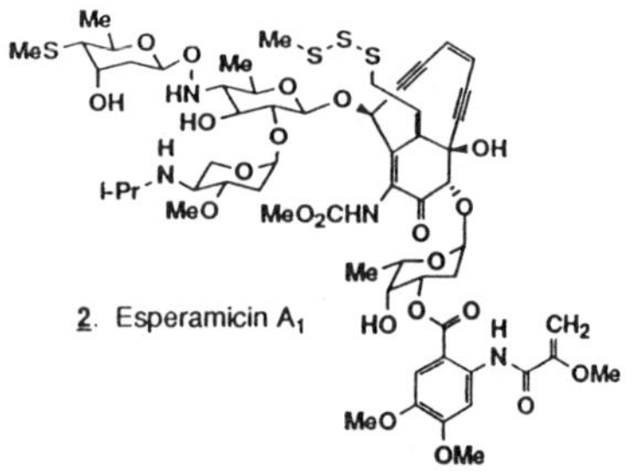

2. Esperamicin A_1

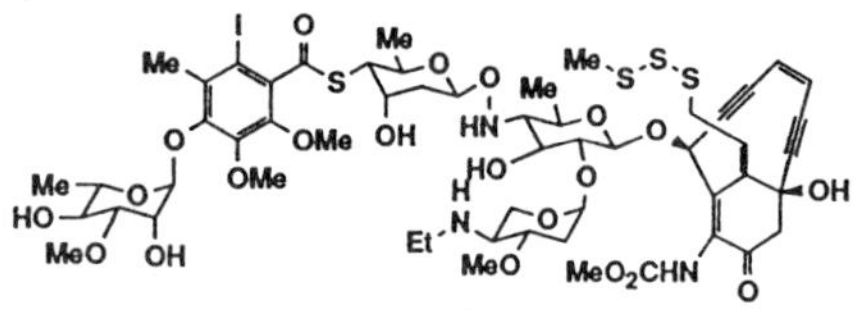

3. Calicheamicin γ^I_1

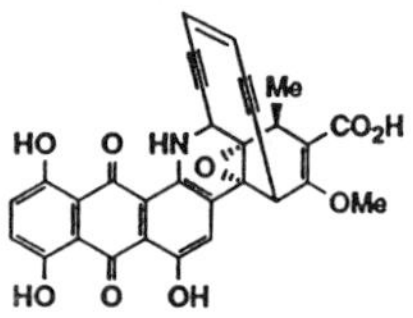

4. Dynemicin A

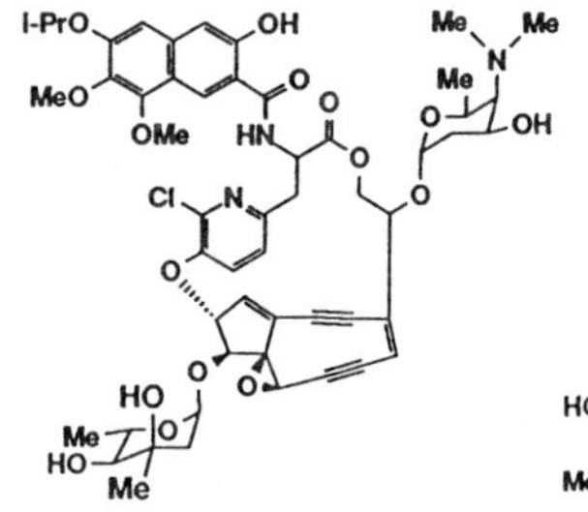

5. Kedarcidin Chromophore

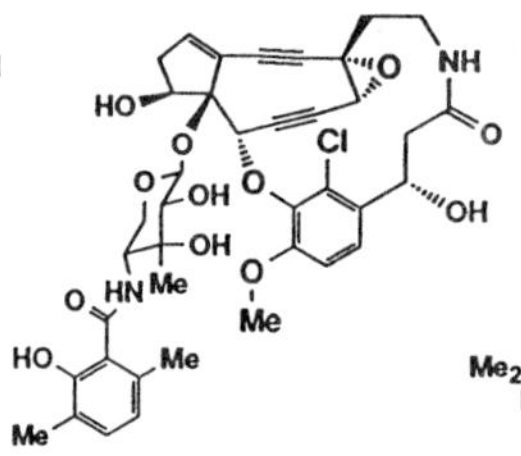

6. Maduropeptin Chromophore

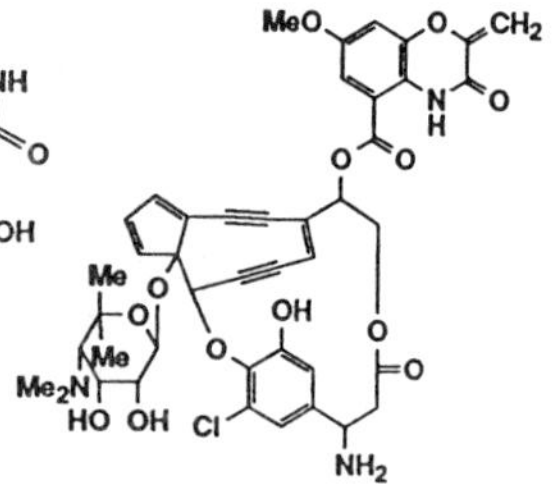

7. C - 1027 Chromophore

Figure 1 Members of the enediynes class of antibiotics.

interaction of these three functionalities triggered by bioreductive activation that results in efficient DNA cleavage. In addition to the core functional groups, the molecule also carries an unusual trisaccharide appended at the C-8 position and an acylated 2-deoxy-L-fucose moiety at C-12. These latter functional groups play important roles in the binding of the drug to DNA and in drug transport as described elsewhere in this chapter.

The crucial structural feature that results in DNA cleavage by the esperamicins is the enediyne chromophore incorporated into a 10-member ring. This ring, as a part of [7.3.1] bicyclic system, can be activated by an internal triggering mechanism in order to generate a diradical intermediate. The cascade of reactions starts with bioreductive cleavage of the methyl trisulfide side chain and formation of the sulfide anion. Intramolecular Michael addition of the sulfide to the bridgehead position of the double bond immediately follows. Saturation of this double bond

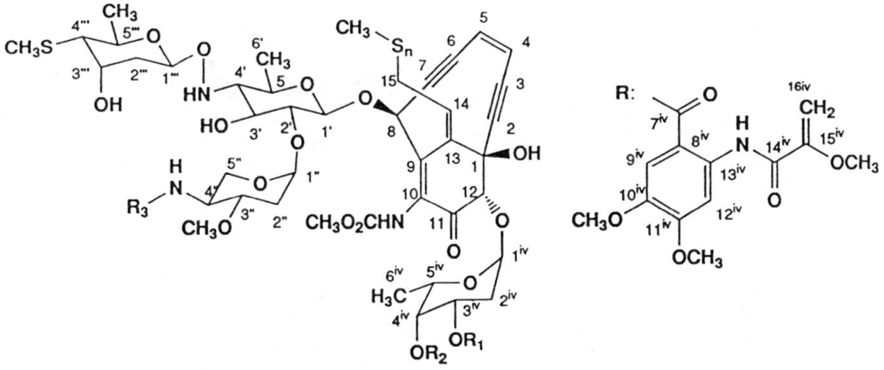

Esperamicins		R_1	R2	R3	n
2	A_1	R	H	i-Pr	3
8	A_2	H	R	i-Pr	3
9	A_{1b}	R	H	Et	3
10	A_{1c}	R	H	Me	3
11	A_{2c}	H	R	Me	3
12	P	R	H	i-Pr	4

Figure 2   Congeners of the esperamicin complex.

removes the constraints forbidding a cyclization-aromatization step and yields the benzenoid diradical. We confirmed the formation of short-lived radical intermediates upon activation of the esperamicins with thiols using electron spin resonance (ESR) spectroscopy. The presence of a 1,4-diyl in proximity to the DNA causes hydrogen atom abstraction from the deoxyribose phosphate backbone. This is the initial step for the subsequent single- and double-strand scissions of the DNA, which occur in the presence of oxygen. Figure 3 illustrates the transformations of the esperamicin molecule during this process.

II. STEPWISE METHANOLYSIS OF THE ESPERAMICINS

The complexity and novelty of the esperamicins were readily indicated by an inspection of their spectroscopic data. The instability and their low yield in the fermentation broth combined to render structure elucidation of these antibiotics very challenging. We focused our efforts on esperamicin A_1 because of its availability and superior activity against a number of tumor models. Structure determination required extensive selective degradation of esperamicin A_1 and a related molecule, esperamicin X, into fragments. Each degradation product was then fully characterized and its structure was assigned. Finally, the localization of each structural fragment in the whole molecule was determined ultimately providing the

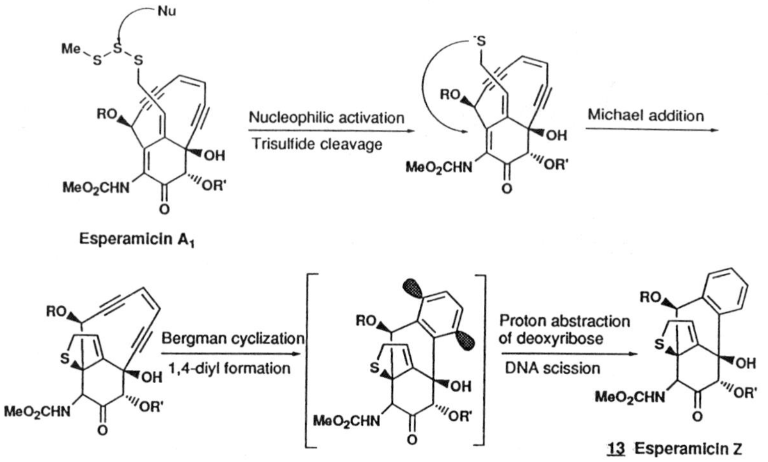

Figure 3   Mechanism of action of esperamicin A_1.

structure of the natural product. The presence of carbohydrate fragments in the esperamicins suggested methanolysis as a process to simplify spectral analysis. The methanolysis products depicted in Figure 4 were obtained by a gradual increase of the HCl concentration from 0.01 to 4.0 M, as described later. The detailed discussion of our studies presented in this chapter is based on spectral analysis of these methanolysis products, their correlation, and assignment.

III. APPLICATION OF SPECTROSCOPIC METHODS

Difficulties in obtaining crystals suitable for x-ray limited the application of this powerful technique. Although crystals of esperamicins A_1 and A_2 were obtained, they failed to give adequate diffraction before decomposition. This may have been due to the presence of the trisulfide moiety, a known radioprotective pharmacophore (9). While the structure of esperamicin X was finally determined by x-ray methods, most of the structural information on esperamicin A_1 derived from mass spectrometry (MS) (high-resolution measurements, soft ionization techniques, and secondary ion analysis), nuclear magnetic resonance (NMR) (two-dimensional homo- and hetero-nuclear correlation techniques), Fourier transform infrared (FT-IR), ultraviolet (UV) and circular dichroism (CD).

A. Ultraviolet Absorption

The characteristic UV absorption bands of the esperamicins were particularly helpful for guiding their isolation from the fermentation media. Using HPLC equipped

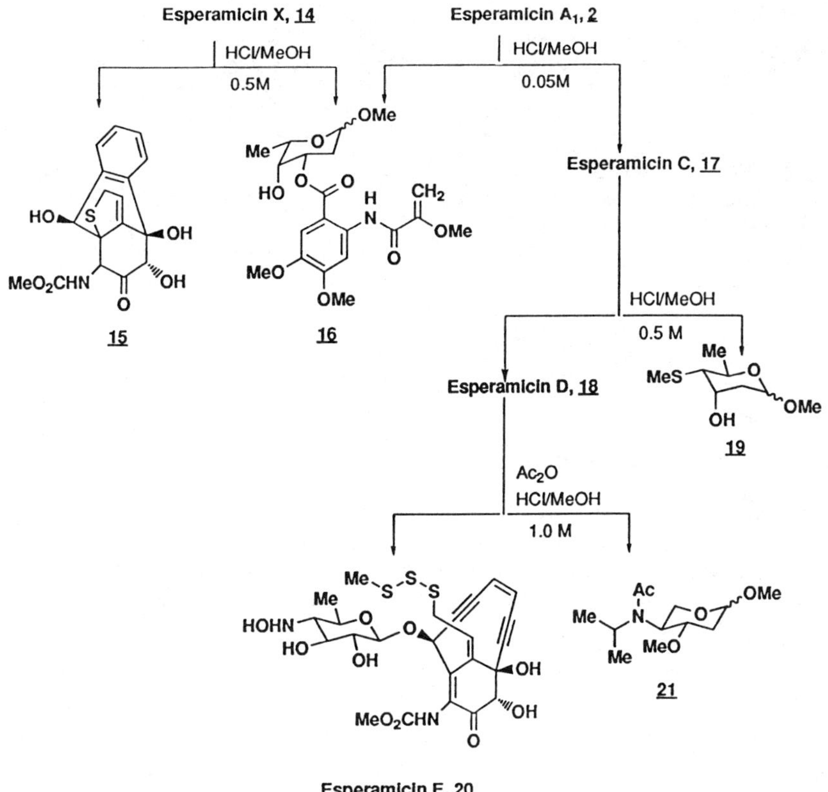

Figure 4   Stepwise methanolysis of esperamicin X and A₁.

with a diode array detector, it was possible to monitor each isolation step and to estimate the quantity of the esperamicins at any point. For practical purposes, the UV spectra of members of the esperamicin complex are superimposable due to the presence of identical chromophores. Their solutions in methanol show distinctive ε and $\Delta\varepsilon$ values in the UV and the CD, respectively.

Two chromophores can be distinguished in the esperamicin molecule: the enediyne aglycone and the anthranilate-pyruvate amide. We found that these two chromophores do not interact with each other through space. A simple additivity relationship was established after they had been separated into two primary methanolysis products and investigated by CD. The UV/CD relationship of the esperamicin chromophores is depicted in Table 1.

Table 1   UV and CD data on Esperamicins A_1, C, and Aromatic Chromophore

	Esperamicin A_1 [2]		Esperamicin C [17]		Aromatic chromophore [16]	
	γ [nm]	ϵ	γ [nm]	ϵ	γ [nm]	ϵ
UV	320	16,400	313	4,600	323	11,800
	280sh	19,500	272	10,200	284	11,500
	253	33,300			252	27,100
	210	35,900	210	23,700	210	8,100
CD	314	-37.8	313	-32.8		
	273	$+45.7$	272	$+35.7$		
	217	$+23.5$	218	$+21.9$	210	$+1.76$

B. Infrared Spectrometry

Several bands characteristic of hydroxyl groups, amide, aromatic ester, and α,β-unsaturated ketones are present in the FT-IR spectrum, but due to a massive overlapping, they cannot be definitely assigned. However, a typical IR fingerprint composed of the absorptions 3440, 3360, 2960, 2920, 1715, 1668, 1608, 1592, 1520, 1446, 1405, 1380, 1308, 1250, 1210, 1150, 1110, 1070, 1015, and 985 cm^{-1} can be useful for identification purposes. The often strong and informative absorptions of acetylenic groups in the range of 2300–2100 cm^{-1} are completely absent in the IR spectra of the esperamicins. They are also missing in the laser Raman spectra of the esperamicins. This is probably due to the rigidity and symmetry of the enediyne chromophore.

C. Mass Spectrometry

Mass spectrometric studies on the esperamicins delivered fundamental information on their structure. The molecular ions, elemental composition, fragmentation patterns, and sequence of structural subunits have been determined by MS. This was challenging due to the novelty of their structures, high molecular weight (1324 for esperamicin A_1), instability, and lack of volatility. Special precautions also had to be taken in handling samples of the esperamicins due to their extremely high toxicity.

Initial attempts to obtain molecular ions for the esperamicins using soft ionization techniques such as field desorption (FD), direct chemical ionization (DCI), and fast atom bombardment (FAB) gave inconsistent results (11). Although relatively abundant ions in the molecular regions were observed when thiols such as thioglycerol and dithiothreitol/dithioerithritol were used as a matrix in FAB mode, these ions represented the aromatization products of the esperamicins. A reduction of the allylic trisulfide chain with thiols containing matrices began the cas-

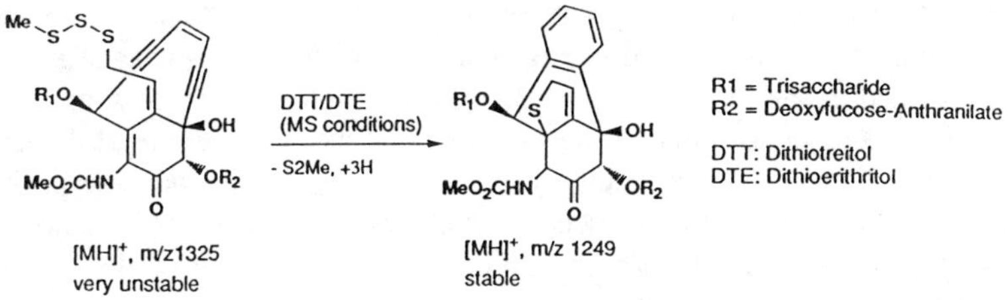

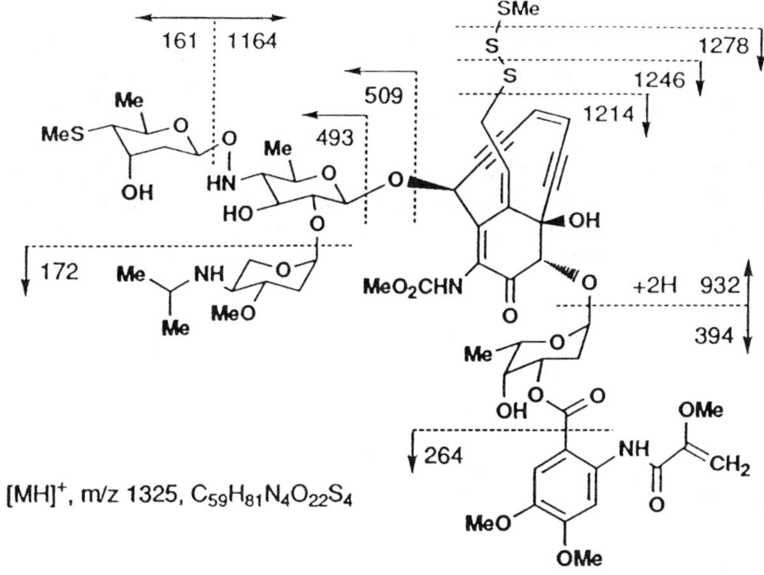

Figure 5   Aromatization of esperamicin A_1 upon FAB-MS conditions.

cade of reactions leading to aromatization of the enediyne chromophore. For instance, esperamicin A_1 (mw 1324) reacted instantaneously with thiol matrix, yielding esperamicin Z (mw 1248) (Fig. 5). Additional ions arising from thiol exchange of the trisulfide were also observed.

We obtained correct molecular ions for the esperamicins using non–thiol-containing matrices, e.g., glycerol or *p*-nitrobenzyl alcohol (12, 13). High-intensity molecular ions were also observed in the thermospray ionization (TSP) spectra of the esperamicins. In addition, clear fragmentation patterns at the ester, glycosidic, and trisulfide bonds were prominent in the TSP spectra (Fig. 6). However, due to high-pressure operation of the ion source during LC-TSP, accurate mass measurements could not be performed.

Figure 6   Mass spectrometry fragmentation pattern of esperamicin A_1.

The base peaks in the TSP spectra represented the amino sugar fragments of the esperamicins. In the case of esperamicin A_1 and A_2 they appear at m/z 172 (m/z is defined as the mass of the ion divided by its charge). Since some congeners of the esperamicins differ by the substitution at the amine group of the amino sugar fragment, they can be readily identified. For example, the base peak for esperamicin A_{1b} at m/z 158 represented the cleavage of the *N*-ethyl amino sugar and for esperamicin A_{2c} at m/z 144 represented the cleavage of the *N*-methyl amino sugar.

In order to observe the high-intensity molecular ions required for exact mass measurements, we searched for a nondestructive FAB matrix that could be used in the high-resolution instrument. Optimum performance was achieved with *p*-nitrobenzyl alcohol. A peak matching method allowed measurements at resolution as high as 7,000–10,000 using polyethylene and polypropylene glycols as standards (Table 2).

The fragmentation patterns of esperamicin C, D, and E were similar to those observed for esperamicin A_1. Cleavage of the glycosidic bonds gave highly abundant ions diagnostic for identification of the sugar fragments and their sequence. The elemental composition for these major fragmentation was determined by high-resolution measurements.

D. Nuclear Magnetic Resonance

The complexity of the esperamicin molecule precluded direct assignment of its structure by an examination of the spectra of the intact molecule. An extensive NMR study had to be correlated with the other spectroscopic data, and this correlation continued through every product obtained upon stepwise methanolysis leading to a final structure and a full assignment of all ^{1}H and ^{13}C resonances (Table 3).

The assignment of the ^{13}C chemical shifts for the quaternary carbon atoms of the esperamicin core was based on the long range ^{1}H-^{13}C heteronuclear coupling correlation spectra of esperamicin A_1, C, D, and E. Although more prominent

Table 2 HR-MS of the Esperamicins

	$[M+H]^+$	Ref. ions	Ref. accurate mass	Max. error (ppm)
Esperamicin A_1 $C_{59}H_{81}N_4O_{22}S_4$	1325.4299	$H(PEG)_{29}OH_2$	1295.7782	0.3
Esperamicin C $C_{40}H_{58}N_3O_{14}S_4$	932.2799	$H(PPG)_{15}OH_2$	889.6469	0.3
Esperamicin D $C_{33}H_{46}N_3O_{12}S_4$	772.2240	$H(PPG)_{13}OH_2$	773.5626	0.5

Table 3 ^{1}H- and ^{13}C-NMR Assignments for Esperamicin A$_1$

esp A$_1$	^{13}C (ppm)	^{1}H (ppm)	esp A$_1$	^{13}C (ppm)	^{1}H (ppm)
1	76.8	—	1″	99.5	4.98
2	98.2	—	2″	35.1	1.56, 1.96
3	83.3	—	3″	64.5	4.20
4	124.9	6.06	4″	55.6	2.37
5	123.1	5.94	5″	69.2	3.87
6	88.3	—	6″	19.8	1.38
7	98.2	—	4‴ SCH$_3$	13.7	2.14
8	68.0	6.17	1^{iv}	99.0	5.48
9	147.0	—	2^{iv}	29.0	2.15, 2.32
10	131.0	—	3^{iv}	70.2	5.48
11	191.3	—	4^{iv}	66.7	3.90
12	86.0	4.31	5^{iv}	68.8	4.62
13	135.0	—	6^{iv}	16.5	1.25
14	130.1	6.66	7^{iv}	166.4	—
15	39.5	4.11, 3.85	8^{iv}	107.6	—
S$_3$CH$_3$	22.6	2.54	9^{iv}	112.5	7.63
NHCO$_2$CH$_3$	155.0	—	10^{iv}	144.0	—
NHCO$_2$CH$_3$	52.5	3.71			
1′	99.5	4.57	12^{iv}	103.7	8.44
2′	77.0	3.56	13^{iv}	136.7	—
3′	69.5	3.93	14^{iv}	160.7	—
4′	68.1	2.26	15^{iv}	154.4	—
5′	71.7	3.62	16^{iv}	90.5	4.67, 5.38
6′	17.5	1.30	10^{iv}OCH$_3$	56.0	3.91
1″	97.2	5.54	11^{iv}OCH$_3$	56.0	3.85
2″	34.0	1.60, 2.47	15^{iv}OCH$_3$	56.0	3.79
3″	75.8				
4″	57.1	3.15			
5″	62.3	3.84, 3.70			
3″OCH$_3$	56.0	3.42			
4″NCH(CH$_3$)$_2$	47.2	3.30			
4″NCH(CH$_3$)$_2$	22.2, 22.3	1.21, 1.23			

three-bond vs. two-bond intensity of the cross peaks in the two-dimensional spectra was evident, particularly for esperamicin E, we originally switched the assignment for two vicinal quaternary carbon atoms, C-9 (147.0 ppm) and C-10 (131.0 ppm). A correction came later from our studies on biosynthesis of the esperamicins. The misassignment became obvious when we examined a set of ^{13}C-labeled NMR spectra of the esperamicins produced by fermentation using [1-^{13}C],

[2-^{13}C], and [1,2-^{13}C] acetate precursors, and we established head-to-tail sequence of the acetate units in the core (see Chapter 12). The unexpected reversed direction of the C9-C10 acetate units in the whole sequence suggested reexamination of the NMR data and led us to correct our previous assignment.

IV. ESPERAMICIN X

In addition to the bioactive metabolites depicted earlier, an inactive compound esperamicin X (Fig. 7), co-produced by the same microorganism was isolated (12). Preliminary characterization of esperamicin X by spectroscopy revealed its structural resemblance to the bioactive congeners. The relatively better stability and lower molecular weight of esperamicin X versus A_1 encouraged us to undertake a study of its structure as a means of gaining insight into the structure of the more complex esperamicin A_1.

The molecular weight of esperamicin X (756 daltons) and its elemental composition ($C_{36}H_{40}N_2O_{14}S$) were determined by high-resolution FAB mass spectrometry and by combustion analysis. Examination of the ^{1}H- and ^{13}C-NMR spectra of esperamicin X showed the presence of numerous resonances observed in the spectrum of esperamicin A_1. Among them, the four methoxy groups (δ 3.95, 3.85, 3.78, and 3.71 ppm), the geminal methylene (δ = 5.48 ppm and 4.56 ppm, J = 2.6Hz), and the deoxy sugar fragment were readily identified. Several other fragments of esperamicin X, including an allylic group =CHCH$_2$S, three isolated methines bearing heteroatoms, a ketone carbonyl, a methyl carbamate, and two heteroatom-substituted quaternary carbon atoms, were also identified by ^{1}H- and ^{13}C-NMR.

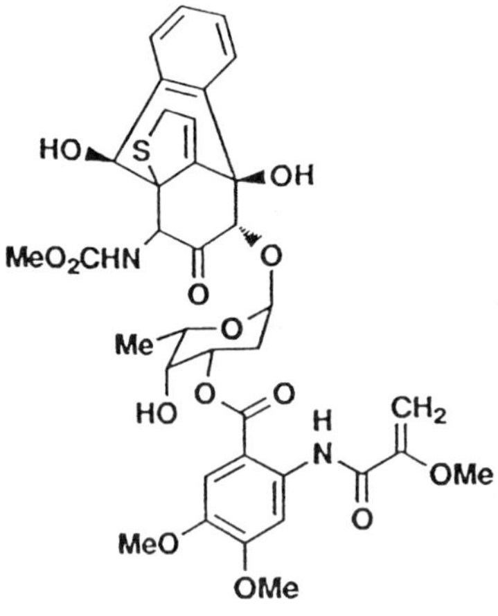

Figure 7   The structure of esperamicin X, **14**.

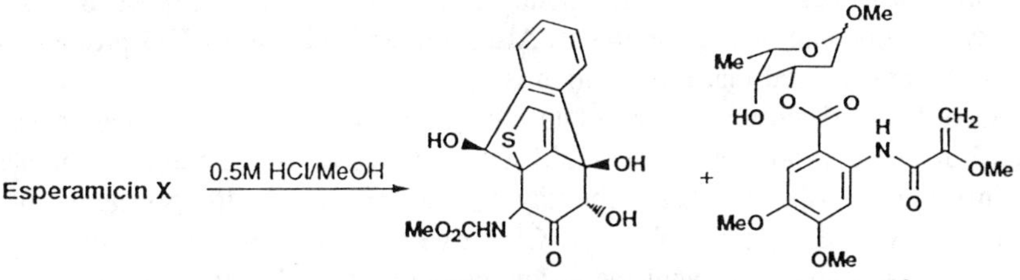

15, Esperamicin X aglycone, 16

Figure 8 Methanolysis of esperamicin X.

Despite isolation of esperamicin X in a crystalline form, our first attempts to determine its structure by x-ray analysis were unsuccessful. However, we were able to obtain x-ray–quality crystals of its tetracyclic aglycone [**15**], which we isolated as a major methanolysis product (Fig. 8). In addition to the aglycone, an anomeric mixture of 2-deoxy-L-fucoside fragments [**16**] identical with those obtained on methanolysis of esperamicins A_1, A_{1b}, and A_{1c} were obtained (12).

The evidence for the structure of the 2-deoxy fucose-anthranilate moiety [**16**] was provided by its further degradation (Fig. 9). Mild alkaline methanolysis of **16** gave a mixture of the anthranilate-pyruvate moiety [**22**] and 2-deoxy-L-fucose [**23a**]. Acidic methanolysis of **22** gave methylanthranilate [**24**] and pyruvic acid. The structure of **24** was confirmed by comparison with an authentic sample. Treatment of the hydrolysate with 2,4-dinitrophenyl hydrazine gave the hydrazone of pyruvic acid [**25**]. The relative configuration of the 2-deoxy fucopyranoside was

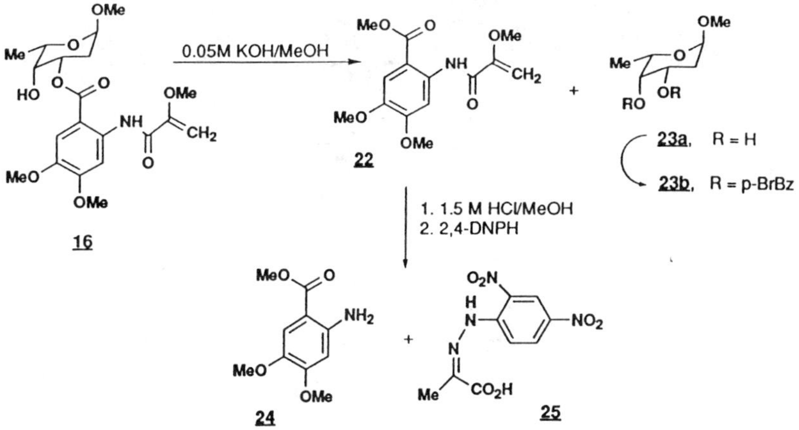

Figure 9 Degradation reactions of the anthranilate-deoxyfucose fragment.

readily determined from the ^{1}H coupling constants in the NMR spectrum of 2-deoxy fucoside-anthranilate fragment. Also, a downfield shift of H-3 proton at δ = 5.38 ppm showed that this position is acylated.

In order to determine the absolute configuration of 2-deoxy fucopyranoside [**23a**], its 3,4-di-*p*-bromobenzoate [**23b**] was synthesized and examined by circular dichroism (CD), the dibenzoate chirality method (14–16). A strong negative first Cotton effect and a typical split of its CD curve $\Delta\varepsilon_{253}$ = –20.2, $\Delta\varepsilon_{244}$ = 0, $\Delta\varepsilon_{237}$ = +11.2 was consistent with the L configuration. This determination was later confirmed by a single crystal x-ray analysis of methyl 3,4-di-*p*-bromobenzoate 2-deoxy-α-fucoside, which was crystallized from ethyl acetate in a form of long thin plates.

The point of attachment of 2-deoxy fucose (Fig. 10) was established from MS fragmentation analysis of esperamicin X and its aglycone (Fig. 11). In the EI mass spectrum of esperamicin X aglycone [**15**] two major fragments were observed at m/z 146 and 218. Similarly, in the mass spectrum of esperamicin X, fragmentation ions at m/z 540 and 216 were consistent with the analogous cleavage in which 2-deoxy-L-fucoside is glycosidically attached to the C-4 hydroxyl group. Further support for this assignment was delivered from ^{1}H- and ^{13}C-NMR. The shift of the C-4 carbon atom from 85.1 to 82.7 ppm and corresponding shift of the proton from δ = 4.68 to δ = 4.49 ppm were observed, whereas the other ^{1}H and ^{13}C signals remained unchanged going from esperamicin X to its aglycone. Crystals of the tetracyclic aglycone grown from methanol:chloroform were subjected

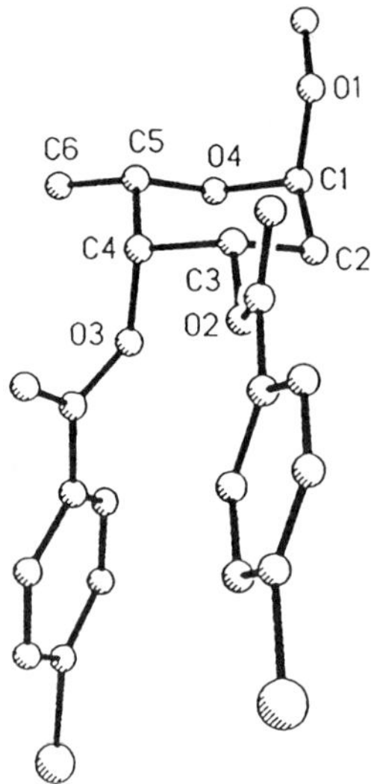

Figure 10   ORTEP drawing of 3,4-dibromobenzoate 2-deoxyfucose, **23**.

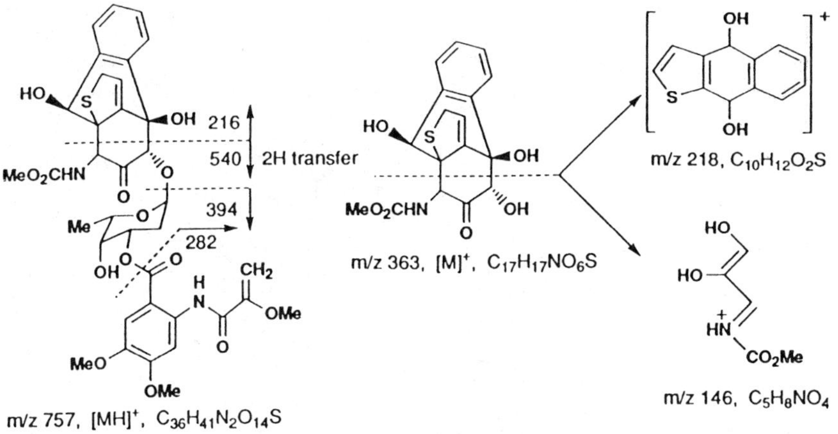

Figure 11 Mass spectrometry fragmentation of esperamicin X and its aglycone.

to single crystal x-ray analysis, revealing its structure but shedding no light on its absolute configuration.

Recently, our continuing efforts to obtain crystals of esperamicin X suitable for x-ray were successful. The crystals grown from aqueous acetonitrile as thin plates were subjected to x-ray analysis, revealing the relative configuration of the aglycone and 2-deoxy-L-fucose fragments. Although the absolute configuration could not be determined in this study, we were able to choose the right enantiomer knowing the absolute stereochemistry of the 2-deoxy-L-fucose fragment (Fig. 12).

These results completed the structure determination of esperamicin X. The information on its structure was of critical importance in our further investigation of the bioactive esperamicin congeners. It also gave us an important clue with regard to mechanism of action of the esperamicins.

V. ESPERAMICIN A$_1$ AND A$_2$

Since the complexity of the esperamicin spectra precluded direct assignment of its structure, we embarked on a series of selective degradation reactions. An indication in ^{1}H- and ^{13}C-NMR spectra of the presence of four sugar fragments attached by the glycosidic bonds suggested that a stepwise methanolysis could assure selectivity. Thus, upon mild methanolysis of esperamicin A$_1$ with 0.01 M hydrogen chloride solution, two fragments were isolated: esperamicin C [17] and the α- and β-methyl-2-deoxy-L-fucosides [16]. Under similar reaction conditions, esperamicin A$_2$ also gave esperamicin C and the anomeric mixture of α- and β-2-deoxy-L-fucosides [26] (Fig. 13).

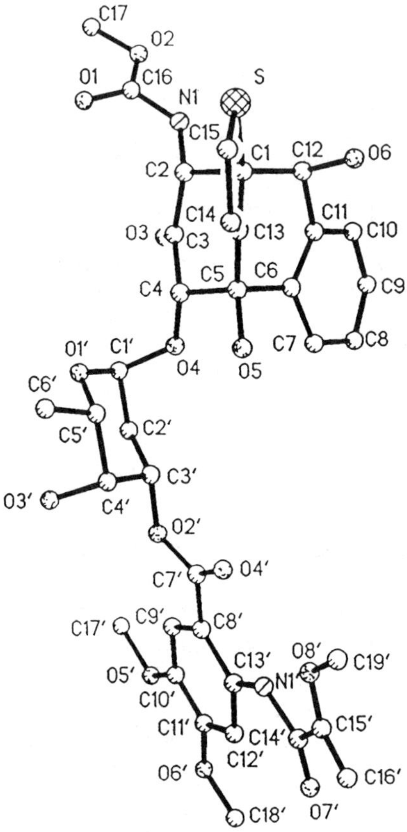

Figure 12 ORTEP drawing of esperamicin X, **14**.

A comparison of the chemical shifts for positional isomers **16** and **26** (Table 4) readily allowed us to determine that the resonances for H-3 in **16** at $\delta = 5.38$ ppm and for H-4 in **26** at $\delta = 5.27$ ppm indicated the acyloxy positions in 2-deoxy fucose in otherwise similar ^{1}H-NMR spectra. The ^{13}C resonances further supported this assignment.

Interestingly, a distinctive difference between the chemical shifts for H-3′ and H-6′ is observed for both of these methanolysis products as well as in the parent esperamicins. Since these resonances appear as singlets in the lowest field of the noncrowded region of their spectra, they are easy to localize, providing a marker for quick structural classification.

In addition to **16** and **26**, both esperamicins A$_1$ and A$_2$ produced a common product, esperamicin C [**17**], which was isolated and fully characterized by spectroscopy. Further methanolysis of **17** with 0.5 M hydrochloride solution yielded

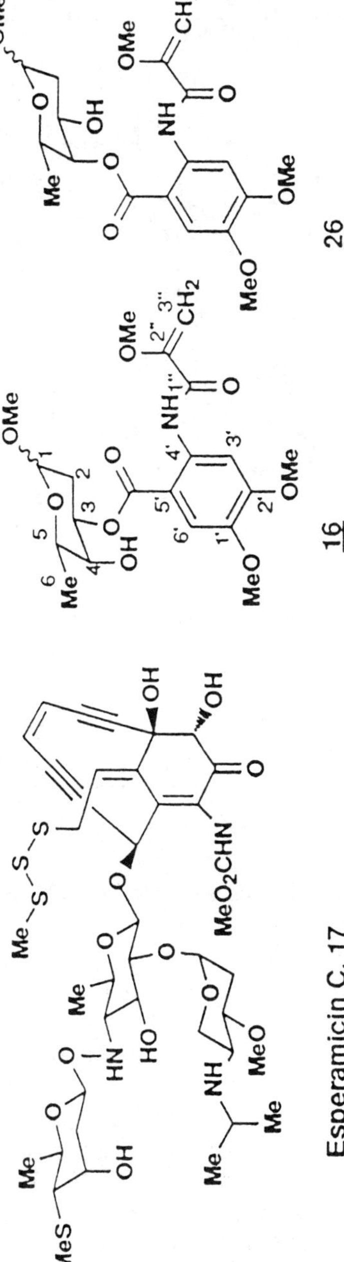

Esperamicin C, **17**

Figure 13 Primary methanolysis products of esperamicins A_1 and A_2.

Table 4 Comparison of ^{1}H and ^{13}C Chemical Shifts for Compounds **16** and **26**

	16		**26**	
	^{1}H (ppm)	^{13}C (ppm)	^{1}H (ppm)	^{13}C (ppm)
1	4.85, brd, 1.8Hz	99.0	4.9, brd, 2.9Hz	98.8
1-OMe	3.34	54.7	3.35	54.9
2	2.21, 1.97	29.0	2.00, 1.96	33.3
3	5.38	70.2	4.30	64.7
4	3.93	68.8	5.27	73.4
5	4.03	66.6		
6	1.29	16.6	1.12	16.9
1′		144.1		144.2
1′-OMe	3.93	56.0	3.93	56.1
2′		153.9		154.4
2′-OMe	3.83	56.0	3.87	56.1
3′	8.49	103.8	8.61	103.9
4′		137.5		137.5
4′-NH	11.75		11.89	
5′		107.6		107.1
5′-COO		166.5		168.0
6′	7.42	112.6	7.58	112.7
1″		160.9		160.9
2″		154.4		154.5
2″-OMe	3.74	56.0	3.76	56.1
3″	5.48, 4.50	90.6	5.45, 4.53	90.4

a mixture of α- and β-methyl glycosides of thiosugar [**27**] and esperamicin D [**18**] (17) (Fig. 14).

We continued methanolytic degradation of esperamicin D [**18**] under more vigorous conditions using hydrochloride solutions up to 4.0 M. This time degradation led to a complex mixture of products from which amino sugar **28** was isolated in a low yield. In order to improve the selectivity and yield of this step, esperamicin D was *N*-acetylated and then subsequently methanolyzed with 0.5 M hydrogen chloride/methanol solution. This additional step allowed us to isolate the mixture of the methyl glycosides of the *N*-acetylamino sugar **21** in a good yield. In addition to **21** we also isolated esperamicin E [**20**] (Fig. 15).

Our attempts to isolate the bicyclic aglycone of esperamicin E or to isolate the hydroxylamino sugar failed, presumably due to their instability and particularly resistance of the allylic-propargylic glycosidic linkage at C-8 to methanolysis. Since the further methanolytic sequencing of esperamicin E was not possible, we fo-

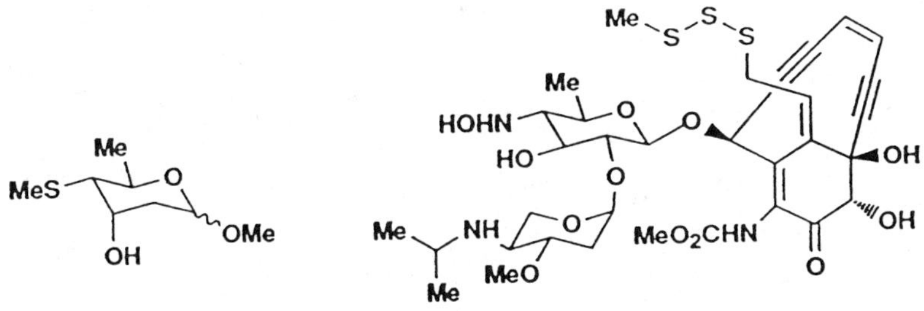

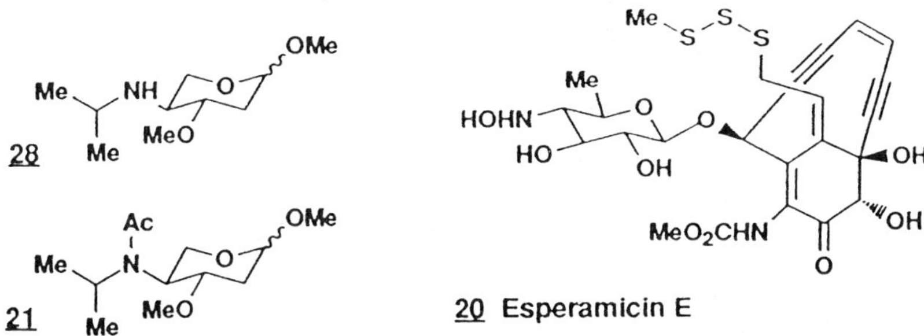

27

<u>18.</u> Esperamicin D

Figure 14 Primary methanolysis products of esperamicin C.

cused our spectroscopic studies on this compound in order to establish the structure of the aglycone.

Thermospray mass spectrometry of **20** gave the [MH]$^+$ ion at m/z 601 and a typical fragmentation for the esperamicins about the C-8 glycosidic bond. Two sets of ions were present in this case for both the sugar fragment and the agylcone, as indicated in Figure 16.

From the examination of the ^{1}H- and ^{13}C-NMR spectra of **20**, the following features of the core were readily apparent: -ROCH-C≡C-CH=, -C=CH-CH$_2$-S$_n$-CH$_3$, -NHCO$_2$CH$_3$, O=C-CX=C-, -CH(OH)-. A long-range ^{1}H-^{13}C heteronuclear correlation allowed us to assemble these units into structural fragments (Fig. 17). An important clue to this assemblage was structure elucidation of the esperamicin X core and its resemblance to esperamicin E. The similar patterns of their long range H-^{1}H and ^{1}H-^{13}C correlations supported our structural hypothesis.

Several exceptions in the structure of the esperamicin X core—replacement of the α,β-unsaturated ketone by a saturated ketone, elimination of the S$_2$CH$_3$ fragment, and replacement of the enediyne system by a 1,2-disubstituted benzene

28

21

<u>20</u> Esperamicin E

Figure 15 Primary methanolysis products of *N*-acetyl esperamicin D.

[MH]$^+$, m/z 601, $C_{24}H_{29}N_2O_{15}S_3$

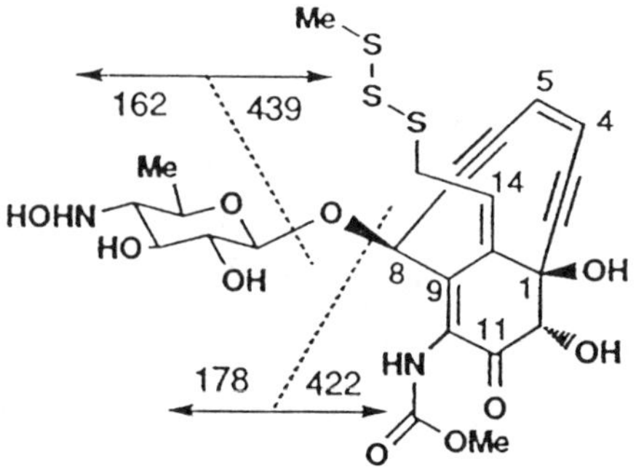

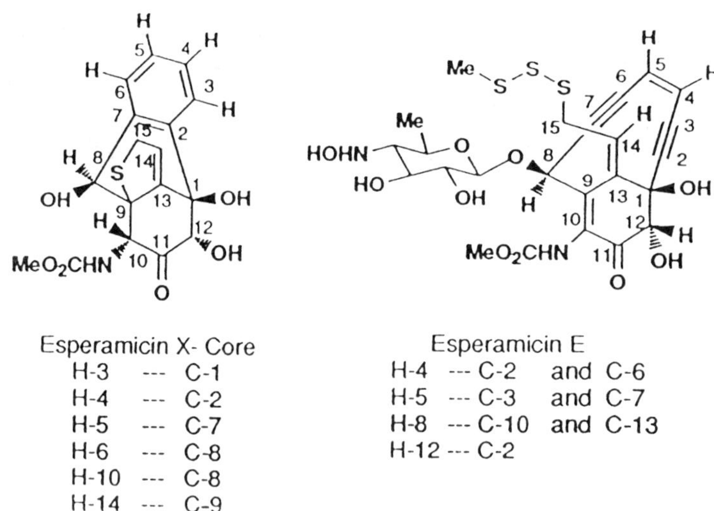

Figure 16 Mass spectrometry fragmentation of esperamicin E.

ring—indicate that it could readily have derived from esperamicin upon reductive cleavage of trisulfide, Michael addition to the bridgehead position of the double bond, and aromatization of enediyne chromophore.

The full assignment of the NMR data for esperamicin E was unequivocally established as shown in Figure 18. Localization of the glycosidic linkages between the *N*-isopropylamino sugar, thiomethyl sugar, and hydroxylamino sugar consti-

Esperamicin X- Core
H-3 --- C-1
H-4 --- C-2
H-5 --- C-7
H-6 --- C-8
H-10 --- C-8
H-14 --- C-9

Esperamicin E
H-4 --- C-2 and C-6
H-5 --- C-3 and C-7
H-8 --- C-10 and C-13
H-12 --- C-2

Figure 17 A comparison of the long-range ^1H-^{13}C heteronuclear correlation data on esperamicin E and esperamicin X core.

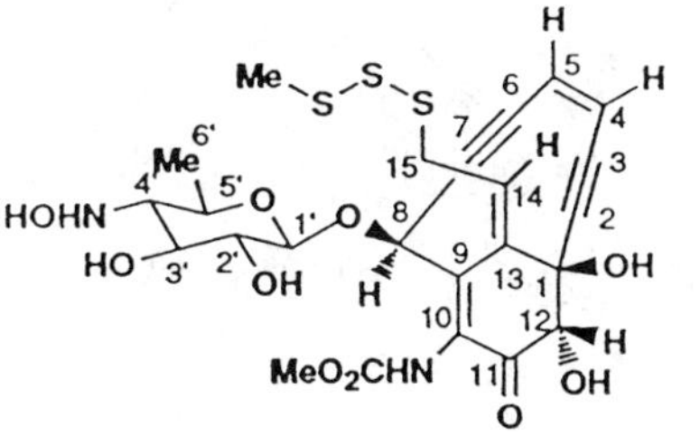

H	δ	mult	J (Hz)
H-4	5.98	d	9.6
H-5	5.90	dd	9.6, 1.8
H-8	6.03	d	1.8, LRC to H-1'
H-12	4.12	s	
H-14	6.49	dd	4.6, 10.5
H-15a	4.12	dd	10.5, 14.7
H-15b	3.84	dd	4.7, 14.7
H-1'	4.52	d	7.8 LRC to H-8
H-2'	3.35	dd	7.8, 9.2
H-3'	3.70	dd	9.2, 10.3
H-4'	2.26	dd	9.6, 10.3
H-5'	3.66	dq	6.4, 9.6
H-6'	1.36	d	6.4

C	δ	C	δ
C-1	80.6	C-1'	104.3
C-2	99.9	C-2'	76.3
C-3	84.6	C-3'	72.0
C-4	125.9	C-4'	69.6
C-5	124.2	C-5'	72.0
C-6	88.5	C-6'	18.8
C-7	99.3		
C-8	71.3		
C-9	149.0		
C-10	132.9		
C-11	194.0		
C-12	84.4		
C-13	136.8		
C-14	130.8		
C-15	40.8		

Figure 18 Assignment of ^{1}H and ^{13}C data for esperamicin E.

tuted a challenging structural problem. The connection of the amino sugar to the 2' position and the thiomethyl sugar to the oxygen atom at the 4'-hydroxylamine function was determined from a comparative analysis of the ^{1}H and ^{13}C chemical shifts in esperamicins A_1, C, D, and E and their peracetylated derivatives.

The differences in shift of the glycosidic proton H-1″ in the intact esperamicins A_1, C, and D and that observed in a methyl glycoside of the amino sugar (Δδ = 0.75 ppm) was surprisingly large (Fig. 19). We attributed this shift to the shielding effect of the enediyne in proximity to H-1″ and consequently have assigned the C-2' hydroxyl as the position of attachment of the amino sugar to the hydroxylamino sugar. This was confirmed by clearly observed long-range coupling between H-2' and H-1″. Our analysis was also supported by ^{13}C data on esperamicin D and E (Fig. 20). A Δδ = –5.5 ppm shift was observed in the resonance of C-2' going from D to E (81.8 ppm to 76.3 ppm, respectively), while other chemical shifts essentially remained unchanged.

The point of attachment of the thiosugar was established as follows: peracetylation of esperamicin C and D gave their peracetates, in which significant shifts for H-3' were observed (δ = 3.93 to 5.39 ppm and δ = 3.88 to 5.26 ppm, respectively) (Fig. 19). This ruled out the C-3' hydroxyl as a feasible attachment point of the thiomethyl sugar, leaving the hydroxylamino function as the

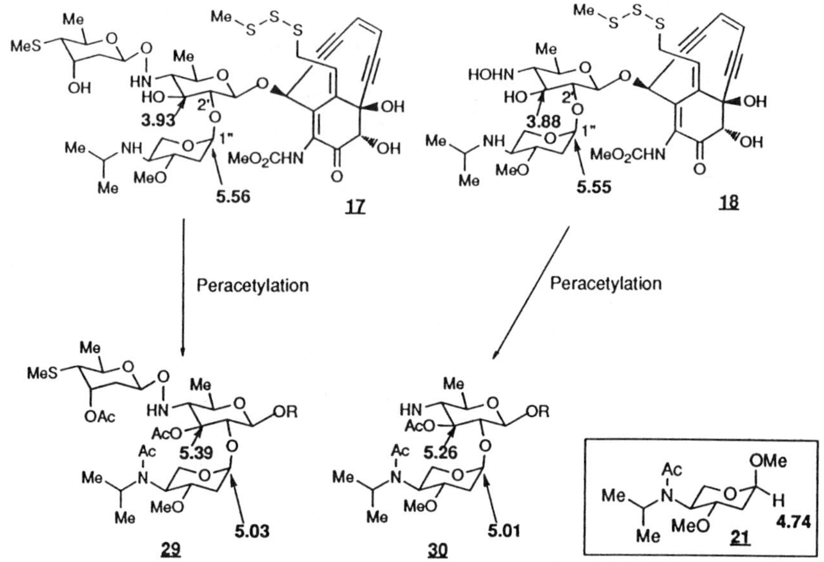

Figure 19 Acylation of the esperamicins; connectivity within the trisaccharide fragment.

only possible point for their connection. The lack of significant shifts going from esperamicin C to D ruled out possible attachment to the nitrogen of the hyroxylamine.

Comparison of the chemical shifts for H-1″, δ = 4.98 ppm in A_1 and C, vs. δ = 4.80 ppm in the β-methyl glycoside of the thiomethyl sugar obtained upon methanolysis of esperamicin C also indicated the presence of the O-glycosidic linkage. Further evidence was found from MS fragmentation of esperamicin C (Fig. 21). This MS sequencing of the glycosidic bond was confirmed by high-resolution measurements for the m/z 161 and m/z 177 ions.

	D	E	$\Delta\delta$
C-8	72.3	71.3	-1.0
C-1'	101.7	104.3	+2.6
C-2'	81.8	76.3	-5.5
C-3'	71.5	72.0	+0.5
C-4'	69.6	69.6	-
C-5'	71.6	72.0	+0.4
C-6	18.6	18.8	+0.2

Figure 20 Comparison of the ^{13}C data of esperamicins D and E.

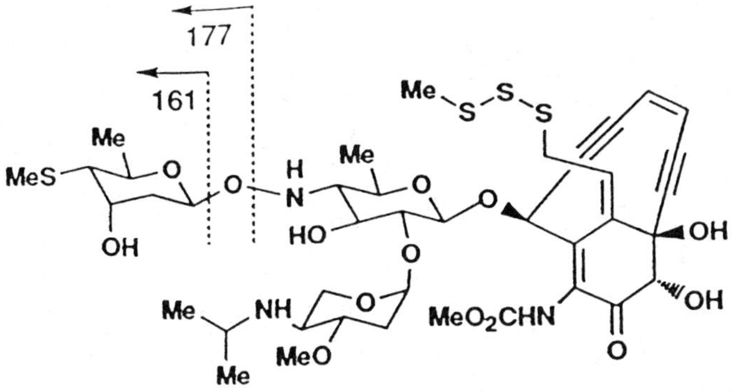

Figure 21 Mass spectrometry fragmentation of the glycosidic bond at the hydroxylamino group.

The deoxy sugar fragments that were isolated upon stepwise methanolysis of the esperamicins were subjected to detailed analysis in order to determine their stereochemistry and absolute configuration (18–20). The thiomethyl sugar [**19**] was obtained as a mixture of α and β anomers readily separable by silica gel chromatography. They were identified as methyl, 2,4,6-trideoxy-4-methylthio-ribo-hexopyranosides. Comparison of $J_{1,2}$ coupling constants to those present in esperamicins A_1 and C permitted assignment of the β configuration for the natural glycoside (Fig. 22). In order to evaluate the absolute configuration of **19**, the anomeric mixture ($\alpha:\beta$, 1:1) was oxidized with m-chloroperoxybenzoic acid in methylene chloride. The resultant sulfones were acylated with p-bromobenzoyl chloride in pyridine affording an anomeric mixture of the 3-p-bromobenzoates. The β anomer was selected for the x-ray study. The structure was solved routinely using direct and heavy atom methods revealing the D configuration for the thiomethyl sugar (18).

The isopropyl amino sugar subunit of the trisaccharide was also isolated as its α- and β-methyl glycosides upon treatment of esperamicin D (or A_1, or C) with 4.0 M hydrogen chloride solution in methanol. In an attempt to obtain crystals suitable for x-ray, the N-isopropylamino sugar was derivatized with p-bromophenyl isocyanate in pyridine (Fig. 23). This protection of the amine group provided a strong UV chromophore essential for purification, easy detection, and an acceptable derivative for use in spectropolarimetry. Unfortunately, the poor crystal quality of both urea anomers precluded their use for x-ray analysis. Alternatively, we decided to synthesize both D and L antipodes starting from naturally occurring and readily available monosaccharides and then compare their CD spectra to the authentic sample of natural origin. A small coupling constant $J_{1,2} = 2.4$ Hz (br.dd) for the anomeric proton of the α-glucoside at $\delta = 4.78$ ppm was similar to that

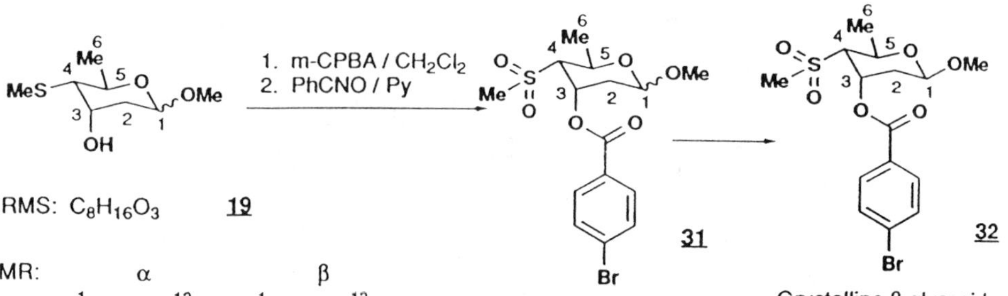

HRMS: $C_8H_{16}O_3$ **19**

NMR:	α		β	
	^1H	^{13}C	^1H	^{13}C
1	4.70	98.5	4.80	98.7
2	1.62	36.0	1.89	37.7
	2.20			2.13
3	4.10	64.0	4.06	64.6
4	2.49	55.1	2.37	56.3
5	3.70	66.7	4.01	69.0
6	1.36	19.6	1.37	20.0
SMe	2.09	15.2	2.16	13.6

Figure 22 ^1H and ^{13}C data assignment to **19** and its derivatization for the x-ray study.

observed in esperamicins A_1 and C. Accordingly, we used α-methyl glucosides in our syntheses as starting materials.

The synthesis of the D antipode was accomplished from the readily available 1-*O*-methyl-β-L-(+)-arabinoside via a four-step reaction sequence to the 2-deoxyglucoside intermediate. Partial 3-*O*-methylation was followed by phthalimidation under Mitsunobu conditions yielding the 4-phthalimidate. Hydrazinolysis of the phthalimidate afforded the 4-aminoglycoside, which was subsequently subjected to a reductive amination reaction with acetone yielding the methyl 4-*N*-isopropylaminoglycoside. Finally, the *p*-bromophenyl urea derivative

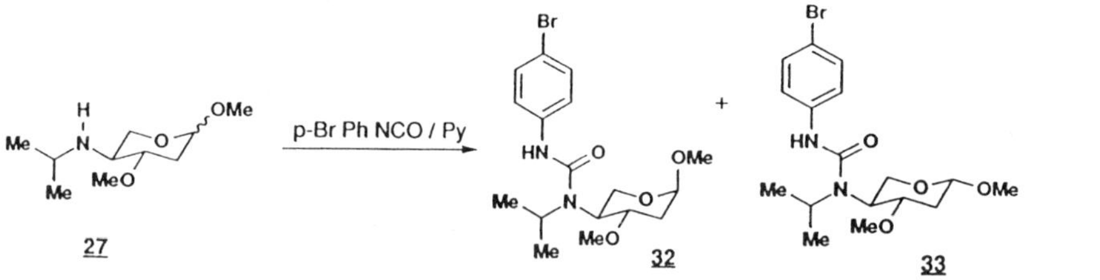

Figure 23 Derivatization of the amino sugar for the x-ray diffraction study.

38 was obtained by reaction with *p*-bromophenylisocyanate. Synthesis of the L-antipode **32** was accomplished from methyl 2-deoxy-α-D-ribo-pyranoside in a reaction sequence similar to that described above (Fig. 24).

Both synthetic epimers and the natural product exhibited identical UV, IR, MS, and NMR spectra. The CD spectra of the D and L antipodes showed Cotton effects of opposite signs at λ_{max} = 250 nm with $\Delta\varepsilon \pm 5.7$ m°/cm. The CD spectrum of the natural product was superimposable with that of the L-antipode. Thus the absolute configuration was established to be α-L-threo-pentopyranoside (19).

Our further structural studies focused on the hydroxylamino sugar fragment. Although its glycopyranoside configuration was elucidated by NMR analysis of esperamicins A_1, C, and D, its absolute configuration still remained unknown. Methanolytic conditions failed to disconnect the hydroxylamino sugar from the core. We accomplished the cleavage of this glycosidic bond in esperamicin A_1 under reductive conditions with sodium borohydride in ethanol (Fig. 25). The resulting trisaccharide upon treatment with a catalytic amount of acetic acid in methanol yielded the methyl glycoside, which was isolated and characterized spectroscopically. The assignment of the ^{1}H-NMR coupling constant data for the hydroxylamino sugar fragment indicated that its hexopyranoside ring had rearranged to the pyrrolidine form. *N*-Acetylation of this trisaccharide with acetic anhydride in methylene chloride in the presence of 4-dimethylamino pyridine and subsequent treatment with 0.5 M hydrogen chloride solution in methanol afforded a mixture of the previously characterized methyl glycosides of the thiosugar [**16**] and the *N*-acetyl-*N*-isopropylamino sugar [**21**] in addition to a novel nitrone [**41**] as shown in Figure 25. Since the configuration of the four asymmetric cen-

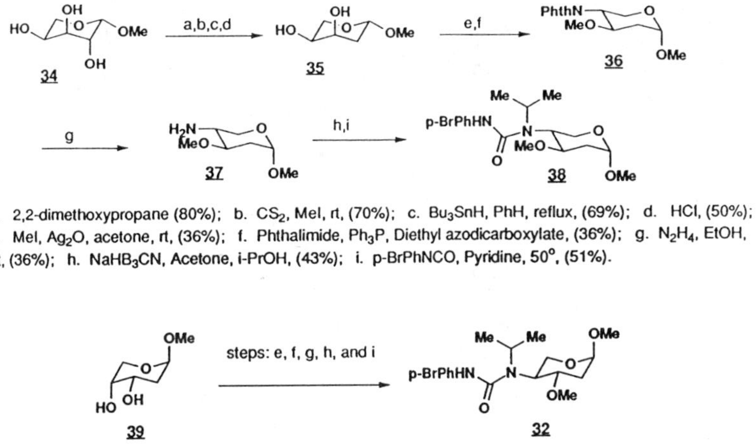
34
a,b,c,d
35
e,f
PhthN
MeO
36
OMe
g
H_2N
MeO
37
h,i
p-BrPhHN
Me
N
38
a. 2,2-dimethoxypropane (80%); b. CS_2, MeI, rt, (70%); c. Bu_3SnH, PhH, reflux, (69%); d. HCl, (50%); e. MeI, Ag_2O, acetone, rt, (36%); f. Phthalimide, Ph_3P, Diethyl azodicarboxylate, (36%); g. N_2H_4, EtOH, rt, (36%); h. $NaHB_3CN$, Acetone, i-PrOH, (43%); i. p-BrPhNCO, Pyridine, 50°, (51%).
steps: e, f, g, h, and i
39
32

Figure 24 Synthesis of the D-amino sugar [**38**] and the L-amino sugar [**32**].

ters in the hydroxylamino sugar remained unchanged during the ring rearrangement and elimination reactions, the nitrone was valuable for configurational assignment. Due to difficulties in preparation of x-ray–quality crystals of the natural nitrone, again we employed spectropolarimetry for determination of the absolute configuration. For this purpose antipodes of the nitrone were synthesized starting from commercially available D- and L- fucose. This synthesis in the case of D-fucose was accomplished as shown in Figure 26. D-fucose was glycosylated and then selectively benzoylated at both C-2 and C-3 equatorial positions. Subsequent acylation of the four-axial hydroxyl group with triflic anhydride was followed by transformation of that triflate into the equatorial azide. Hydrogenation of the azide over palladium on charcoal afforded the methyl-4-aminoglycoside, which was oxidized with dimethyldioxirane in acetone at –78°C, yielding the 4-hydroxylaminoglycoside. Formation of the 2,3-dibenzoate nitrone occurred spontaneously during demethylation with 0.1 M borone trichloride in methylene chloride at –78°C. Final deprotection of the dibenzoate with 25% sodium methoxide provided the desired nitrone. The identical synthesis was applied to L-fucose in order to provide the antipodal nitrone. Both synthetic epimeric nitrones and the one obtained from esperamicin A_1 exhibited identical spectroscopic data with the exception of the CD. The synthetic antipodes showed opposite Cotton effects at

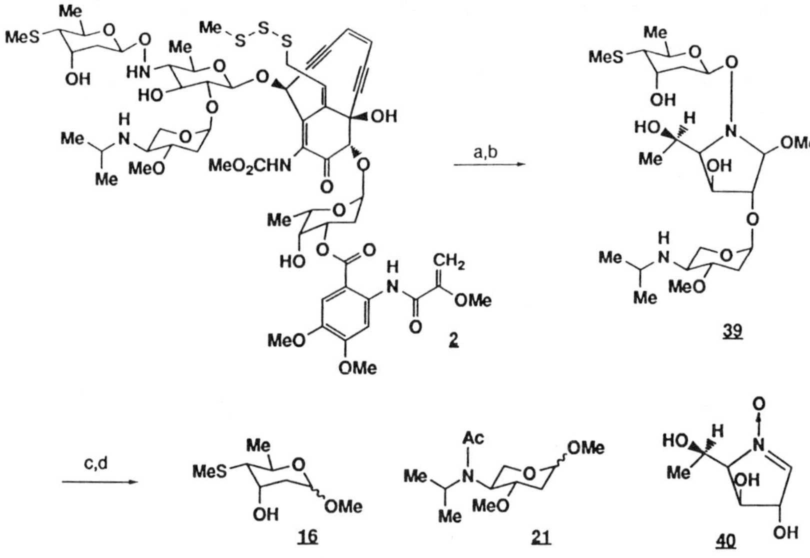

a. NaBH4, EtOH; b. MeOH, cat. AcOH; c. Ac2O, DMAP, CH2Cl2, d. 0.5 M HCl / MeOH

Figure 25 Cleavage of the trisaccharide fragment of esperamicin A_1 with sodium borohydride; isolation of the nitrone.

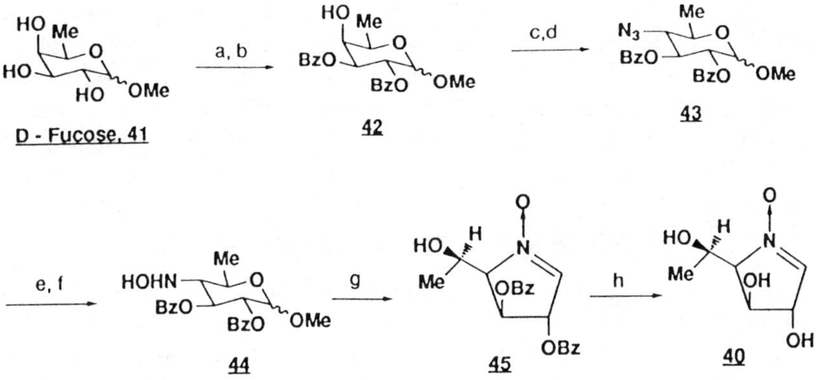

a. 0.5 M HCl - MeOH, (90%); b. 2 eq. p-BrBzCl /Py, (61%); c. Tf$_2$O / Py, (quant.); d. (Bu$_4$N)N$_3$, MeCN,(91%); e. H$_2$ / 10% Pd - C, (50%); f. Me$_2$CO$_2$, Me$_2$CO, (14%); g. 0.1 M BCl$_3$ / CH$_2$Cl$_2$, (quant.); h. NaOMe / MeOH, (quant.).

Figure 26 Synthesis of the nitrones.

λ_{max} = 271 nm $\Delta\varepsilon_{271}$ = $\pm$0.2. The CD spectrum of the natural nitrone was superimposable with that derived from D-fucose. Thus, the D-gluco configuration has been assigned to the hydroxylamino sugar (20).

Single crystal x-ray analysis of esperamicin X permitted us to assign the absolute configuration for the aromatized aglycone as C-1 (S), C-8 (S), and C-12 (S) (21). The correlation of the absolute configuration of esperamicin X and esperamicin A$_1$ was accomplished as follows: treatment of esperamicin A$_1$ with triphenylphosphine-1,4-cyclohexadiene in methylene chloride yielded the aromatized product esperamicin Z (Fig. 27).

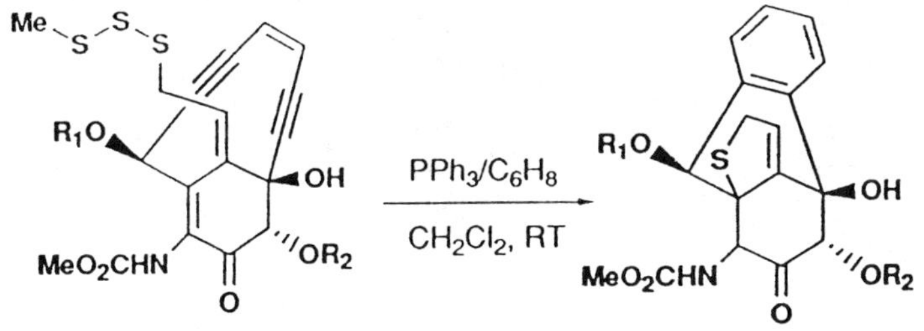

R$_1$ = Trisaccharide
R$_2$ = Deoxyfucose-Anthranilate

Figure 27 Aromatization of esperamicin A$_1$; isolation of esperamicin Z.

It is reasonable to expect that all esperamicin congeners including esperamicin X have the same absolute configuration due to their common biogenetic origins. The evidence for this was found when we compared the CD spectra of esperamicin X and esperamicin Z. Almost identical values of their molar circular dichroism ($\Delta\varepsilon$) suggested that the chiral centers around the chromophores present in the core have the same absolute configuration.

VI. MINOR CONGENERS OF THE ESPERAMICIN COMPLEX

Screening for the bioactive metabolites of *Actinomadura verrucosospora* led to the discovery of several minor congeners, designated as esperamicins A_2, A_{1b}, A_{2b}, A_{1c}, A_{2c}, and P. While esperamicins A_2 and A_{1b} were isolated in quantities sufficient for detailed assignment of their spectral data, the remaining components were obtained in only minute quantities. Although their systematic analysis was not possible, several of them were characterized and their structures assigned. Relying on reverse-phase HPLC separation, these novel esperamicin congeners were primarily identified by their retention times and characteristic UV chromophore using diode array detection. Secondary identification was performed by mass spectrometry. In this instance, the LC system was directly coupled to the thermospray ion source of the MS allowing determination of the molecular ions of each component selected in primary assay. Based on this procedure the following data set was collected using only microgram quantities of the esperamicin extract:

Esperamicin	RT (min)*	$[MH]^+$
A_1	13.15	1325
A_{1b}	10.00	1311
A_{1c}	6.50	1297
A_2	32.00	1325
A_{2b}	25.55	1311
A_{2c}	16.10	1297

*HPLC separation conditions: Nova Pak Waters C18, 5 μ, 1 = 15 cm, id = 0.4 cm analytical column; acetonitrile:methanol:water (33:33:34, v/v) solvent system, 1 ml/min flowrate.

Further structural details were obtained from the NMR data. A sufficient amount of esperamicin A_{1c} and A_{2c} (2–3 mg of each) was isolated and analyzed by ^{1}H- and ^{13}C-NMR. Unfortunately, the A_{2b} component collected in a trace quantity could not be used in this study. As mentioned before, availability of the esperamicins in small quantities, their instability, and the complexity of their NMR spectra precluded full assignment of the chemical shifts for the minor components, yet the close structural relations among them allowed us to classify them based on a few readily identifiable diagnostic peaks. In the ^{1}H spectra the lowest three singlets at 11.77 ppm (br, NH), 8.58 ppm (H-12^{iv}), and 7.47 ppm (H-9^{iv}) are indicative of the A_1 series, while the equivalent peaks for the A_2 series are found at 11.90, 8.61, and 7.57 ppm, respectively. Additional diagnostic information can be obtained by inspection of the methyl region of the ^{13}C spectra. The following ^{13}C chemical shift comparison clearly indicates structural differences among the esperamicins.

Methyl groups	A_1	A_{1b}	A_{1c}	A_2	A_{2c}
C-4‴-S<u>Me</u>	13.7	13.0	13.7	13.7	13.7
C-4″-NCH$_2$<u>Me</u>	—	14.6	—	—	—
C-6^{iv}	16.8	16.7	16.7	16.9	16.6
C-6′	17.6	17.6	17.6	17.5	17.5
C-15-S$_3$<u>Me</u>	22.6	22.8	22.7	22.6	22.7
C-4″-NCH<u>Me</u>$_2$	22.2, 22.3	—	—	22.3, 22.4	—
C-4″-NH<u>Me</u>	—	—	34.1	—	33.6

As indicated earlier in this chapter, the differences among the esperamicins are localized at the nitrogen atom of the amino sugar moiety. The MS fragmentation of the glycosidic bond of this amino sugar residue results in formation of base peaks. Their m/z value clearly points out the alkylation pattern of the analyzed congeners.

Esperamicin P differs from the other known components of the esperamicin complex by retention time (Rt) in the reverse-phase HPLC. For instance, Rt for esperamicin P is 12.9 minutes versus 8.8 minutes for esperamicin A_1 using a typical C-18 analytical column and 1 ml/min flow rate of aceto-nitrile:methanol:0.05 M ammonium acetate (32.5:32.5:35, v/v) solvent system. Elemental analysis indicates the presence of an additional sulfur atom in comparison to other esperamicins. Thermo-spray mass spectrometry of esperamicin P shows a quasi-molecular ion at m/z 1357, which is 32 daltons higher than the molecular weight of esperamicin A_1, indicating the presence of the additional sulfur atom. The fragmentation pattern of the TSP-MS allows one to localize an additional sulfur atom in the bicyclic core of esperamicin P. The UV, IR, and ^{1}H- and ^{13}C-NMR data on esperamicin A_1 and P are substantially identical, hence the only possible place for the insertion of extra sulfur atom is an extension of the trisulfide side chain of esperamicin A_1 to its tetrasulfide analog. This difference between esperamicin A_1 and P is manifested in ^{13}C-NMR spectra where a methylene carbon atom (CH$_2$-15) of esperamicin A_1 is shifted from 39.5 ppm to 40.1 ppm.

The presence of several other minor components of esperamicin complex were indicated during our isolation and purification workup. Some of these were later identified as the air oxidation products of already known congeners; the others were identified in extremely small quantities during a low-volume media study, and hence the assignments of their structures remain uncertain.

ACKNOWLEDGMENTS

We would like to express many thanks to all contributors to this work whose names precede the titles of their original publications as listed in the References. Particularly acknowledgments are due to the following individuals who directly participated in this structure determination study and without whom this work could not have been completed:

From Bristol-Myers Research Institute, Japan: H. Kawaguchi, M. Konishi, H. Ohkuma, and K. Saitoh.

From Bristol-Myers Squibb Pharmaceutical Research Institute, U.S.A.: T. W. Doyle, G. Dubay, J. Golik, G. Groenewold, B. Krishnan, D. M. Vyas, and H. Wong.

From Cornell University: J. Clardy and G. VanDuyne.

From the NCI-PRI, Frederick, MD: J. Beutler, P. Clark, W. B. Lebherz III, G. Muschik J. Roach, and J. Ross.

We acknowledge the financial support for the work summarized in this chapter provided by the Bristol-Myers Squibb Company.

REFERENCES

1. K. Edo, Y. Muzukaki, H. Seto, K. Furihata, N. Ohtake, and N. Ishida, *Tetrahedron Lett., 26,* 331 (1985).

2. J. Golik, G. Dubay, G. Groenewold, H. Kawaguchi, M. Konishi, B. Krishnan, H. Ohkuma, K. Saitoh, and T. W. Doyle, *J. Am. Chem. Soc., 109,* 3462 (1987).

3. M. D. Lee, T. S. Dunne, C. C. Chang, G. A. Ellestad, M. M. Siegel, G. O. Morton, W. J. McGahren, and D. B. Borders, *J. Am. Chem. Soc., 109,* 3466 (1987).

4. M. Konishi, H. Ohkuma, K. Matsumoto, T. Tsuno, H. Kamei, T. Miyaki, T. Oki, H. Kawaguchi, G. D. VanDuyne, and J. Clardy, *J. Antibiot., 42,* 1449 (1989).

5. J. E. Leet, D. R. Schroeder, S. J. Hofstead, J. Golik, K. L. Colson, S. Huang, S. E. Khlor, T. W. Doyle, and J. A. Matson, *J. Am. Chem. Soc., 114,* 7946 (1992).

6. D. R. Schroeder, K. L. Colson, S. E. Klohr, N. Zein, D. R. Langley, M. S. Lee, S. W. Mamber, K. S. Lam, D. R. Gustavson, J. A. Matson, and T. W. Doyle, in Third International Conference on the Biotechnology of Microbial Products. Novel

Pharmacological and Agrobiological Activities, Rohnert Park, CA, April 18–21, 1993.

7. Y. Minami, K. Yoshida, R. Azuma, M. Saeki, and T. Otani, *Tetrahedron Lett.,* *34,* 2637 (1993).

8. J. Golik, J. A. Beutler, P. Clark, J. Ross, J. Roach, W. B. Lebherz III, and G. Muschik, U.S. Patent No. 5,086,045 (1992).

9. D. L. Klayman and E. S. Copeland, *Kirk-Othmer Encycl. Chem. Technol.,* 3rd ed., John Wiley and Sons, New York, Chichester, Brisbane, Toronto, Singapore, 1982, pp. 813–814.

10. P. K. Srivastava and L. Field, *J. Med. Chem.,* *18,* 798 (1975).

11. M. Konishi, K. Saitoh, H. Ohkuma, K. Kawaguchi, J. Golik, G. Dubay, G. Groenewold, B. Krishnan, and T. W. Doyle, *J. Antibiot.,* *38,* 1605 (1985).

12. J. Golik, J. Clardy, G. Dubay, G. Groenewold, H. Kawaguchi, M. Konishi, B. Krishnan, H. Ohkuma, K. Saitoh, and T. D. Doyle, *J. Am. Chem. Soc.,* *109,* 3461 (1987).

13. G. R. Dubay, G. S. Groenewold, and J. Golik, Proceedings of the 35th Annual Conference on Mass Spectrometry and Allied Topics, Denver, CO, ASMS, East Lansing, 1987.

14. N. Harada and K. Nakanishi, *Circular Dichroic Spectroscopy—Exciton Coupling in Organic Chemistry,* University Science Books, Mill Valley, CA, 1983, pp. 164–189.

15. H.-W. Liu and K. Nakanishi, *J. Am. Chem. Soc.,* *103,* 5591 (1981).

16. H.-W. Liu and K. Nakanishi, *J. Am. Chem. Soc.,* *104,* 1178 (1982).

17. J. Golik, U.S. Patent No. 4,921,700 (1990).

18. J. Golik, T. W. Doyle, G. VanDuyne, and J. Clardy, *Tetrahedron Lett.,* *43,* 6149 (1990).

19. J. Golik, H. Wong, D. M. Vyas, and T. W. Doyle, *Tetrahedron Lett.,* *30,* 2497 (1989).

20. J. Golik, H. Wong, B. Krishnan, D. M. Vyas, and T. W. Doyle, *Tetrahedron Lett.,* *32,* 1851 (1991).

21. J. Golik, B. Krishnan, T. W. Doyle, G. VanDuyne, and J. Clardy, *Tetrahedron Lett.,* *41,* 6049 (1992).

12

Biosynthesis of Esperamicin

Kin Sing Lam and Judith A. Veitch
*Bristol-Myers Squibb Pharmaceutical Research Institute,
Wallingford, Connecticut*

I. INTRODUCTION

Epseramicin A_1 (esp A_1), one of the most potent antitumor antibiotics, was isolated from cultures of *Actinomadura verrucosospora* (1) (Fig. 1). The producing organism was isolated from a soil sample collected at Pto Esperanza, Misiones, Argentina. The isolation and the elucidation of the structure of esp A_1 have been reported (1–3). The absolute configuration of each of the sugars and the bicyclic core has also been established (4–7). Esp A_1 consists of a bicyclic core to which are attached a trisaccharide and a substituted 2-deoxy-L-fucose, with an aromatic chromophore attached to the sugar 3 position. The individual sugars of the trisaccharide are novel sugars and contain an unusual hydroxylamino sugar linked to a thiomethyl sugar via an *O*-glycosidic linkage at the 4 position. The hydroxylamino sugar is further attached to an isopropyl sugar at the 2 position. The bicyclic core contains the very unusual enediyne, an allylic trisulfide, and a bridgehead enone. Detailed structure and activity studies have established that the interaction of these three functionalities results in a bioreductively activated, highly efficient, DNA strand scission (8,9).

We believe that knowing the biosynthesis of the antibiotic can be used to (1) provide information leading to increase in production of the target antibiotic, (2) exploit fermentation possibilities leading to the production of novel analogs, and (3) provide an optimal route for the preparation of isotopically labeled drug, which

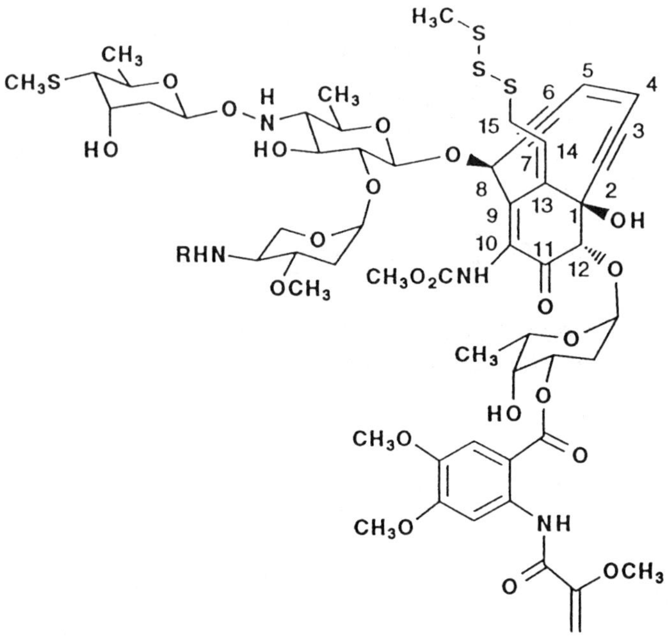

Esperamicin A_1 R = CH(CH$_3$)$_2$

Esperamicin A_{1b} R = CH$_2$CH$_3$

Esperamicin A_{1c} R = CH$_3$

Figure 1 Structures of esperamicin A_1, esperamicin A_{1b}, and esperamicin A_{1c}.

could yield important pharmacokinetic data for the compounds in clinical studies. Not much work has been done in the area of biosynthesis of the enediyne class compounds. There are only two published reports in this area: on the biosyntheses of the chromophore of neocarzinostatin (NCS Chrom A) (10) and dynemicin A (DNM-A) (11). The study of the biosynthesis of esp A_1 is of great interest because of its extreme potency against tumors in animal model (12), its unique mechanism of action (8,9), and its complex structure. In this chapter, we present some of the data from our studies on the biosynthesis of esp A_1.

II. RADIOACTIVE PRECURSOR LABELING STUDY

The major problem in elucidating the biosynthesis of esp A_1 is due to its low production in the fermentation. The estimated titer of esp A_1 by the original strain

SA-24868 was about 0.05 µg/ml. Through extensive media development and strain-improvement studies, the titer of esp A_1 was increased to 5 µg/ml in the complex medium by the new strain SA-25262, which was derived from strain SA-24868 (13). When shifting the fermentation from the complex medium to a defined medium, which is more suitable for biosynthetic studies because of a lower dilution effect, the production of esp A_1 dropped 5- to 10-fold. Table 1 summarizes the results obtained from the incorporation studies with ^{14}C-labeled and ^{35}S-labeled precursors.

The rates of incorporation of the metabolites ranged from 0.0037 to 0.11%. Metabolites with such low rates of incorporation are not usually considered to be genuine precursors. Acceptable rates of incorporation of precursors into secondary metabolites in microorganisms usually are above 1% (14). However, the low rates of incorporation of the above metabolites into esp A_1 are due to the low production in the fermentation. The specific activities of esp A_1 obtained from the above experiment ranged from 16,200 to 473,800 dpm/mg. These values of specific activity are acceptable considering the amount of radioactivity (0.25–1 µCi/ml) that was fed into the cultures. Therefore, we can confidently draw the conclusion that sodium acetate, sodium pyruvate, L-methionine, and D-glucose are the precursors of esp A_1, while the sulfur from L-methionine, L-cysteine, and sodium sulfate provide the sulfur source for esp A_1 production. In order to determine the exact sites of incorporation into esp A_1 by some of the above precursors, stable isotopes of these precursors were used in the feeding experiments.

III. BIOSYNTHESIS OF THE ENEDIYNE RING

From Table 1, the rate of incorporation of sodium [1-^{14}C]acetate into esp A_1 (0.0037%) was the lowest among the precursors tested. With such a low rate of incorporation, we were not sure that by replacing the radioactive isotope with the

Table 1 Incorporation of Radiolabeled Precursors into Esperamicin A_1

Radiolabeled precursor	Amount radioactivity added (dpm)	Radioactivity incorporated into esperamicin (dpm)	% Incorporation
Sodium [1-^{14}C]-acetate	2.22×10^8	8,100	0.0037
Sodium [1-^{14}C]-pyruvate	5.55×10^7	19,300	0.035
L-[Methyl-^{14}C]-methionine	2.22×10^8	236,900	0.11
D-[U-^{14}C]-Glucose	2.22×10^8	9,200	0.0041
L-[^{35}S]Methionine	2.22×10^8	210,400	0.095
L-[^{35}S]Cysteine	2.22×10^8	41,000	0.019
Sodium [^{35}S]sulfate	2.22×10^8	74,600	0.034

Radiolabeled precursors were added to the culture growing in the medium H946 at day 3 of the fermentation.

^{13}C-labeled acetate, the enrichment of the corresponding carbons could be detected by NMR analysis, which is much less sensitive than the method used to assay radioactivity. Adding high concentrations of ^{13}C-labeled acetate to the culture in order to achieve high enrichment may disturb the normal metabolism of the microorganism under study, resulting in a false conclusion. In addition, due to the low production of esp A_1 in the culture, large-volume fermentations are required and hence large quantities of ^{13}C-labeled acetate are needed in order to obtain enough ^{13}C-labeled esp A_1 for NMR analysis. Without further evidence that esp A_1 was indeed derived from acetate, we hesitated to proceed with the ^{13}C-labeled acetate feeding experiments.

Cerulenin is a fungal antibiotic that inhibits the condensing enzyme involved in fatty acid and polyketide biosynthesis (15–17). We decided to determine the effect of cerulenin on the production of esp A_1. If the biosynthesis of esp A_1 is derived from head-to-tail condensation of acetate units, i.e., via the polyketide pathway, cerulenin should inhibit its production. The effect of cerulenin on the production of esp A_1 is shown in Table 2. At all concentrations tested, cerulenin did not affect the growth of the organism or the pH of the fermentation. Significant inhibition of esp A_1 production (61.5%) was observed when 0.25 mM cerulenin was added to the culture. At 1 mM cerulenin concentration, no esp A_1 can be detected in the culture. This indicated that esp A_1 is biosynthesized in part by the polyketide pathway. At about the same time of this finding, Hensens et al. (10) reported that the C_{14} dienediyne ring system of NCS Chrom A is derived from head-to-tail condensation of acetate units. Given the similarities between the C_{15} enediyne ring system of esp A_1 and the C_{14} ring system of NCS Chrom A and our finding that cerulenin inhibits the formation of esp A_1, the enediyne moiety of esp A_1 should also be derived from acetate units.

During the above studies, we isolated a hyperproducer mutant of esp A_1 from strain SA-25262 in our laboratory. The production of esp A_1 in this mutant strain,

Table 2 Effect of Cerulenin on Esperamicin A_1 Production by *Actinomadura verrucosospora* SA-25262 in Medium H946

[Cerulenin][a] (mM)	[Esperamicin A_1][b] (μg/ml)	% Inhibition	% Sediment
0	5.2	—	25
0.10	4.2	19.2	27
0.25	2.0	61.5	25
0.50	1.4	73.1	25
1.0	0	100	25

[a] Cerulenin was added to the culture at day 3 of the fermentation.
[b] The tiers of esperamicin A_1 and the % sediment of the culture were determined at day 10 of the fermentation.

designated strain MU-5019, is about 25–30 µg/ml, five- to sixfold higher than the production of esp A_1 in strain SA-25262 (18). With the improvement in production of esp A_1 by the mutant strain, feeding experiments could be carried out in a 5- to 10-liter scale to obtain enough ^{13}C-enriched esp A_1 for NMR studies. The feeding experiments were then carried out by feeding 0.2% sodium [1-^{13}C]acetate, sodium [2-^{13}C]acetate, and sodium [1,2-^{13}C]acetate to the cultures of strain MU-5019. Usually we could isolate 25–30 mg pure ^{13}C-enriched esp A_1 from a 10-liter fermentation. Since esp A_1 is very soluble in chloroform but has limited solubility in methanol, $CDCl_3$ was used as the solvent for ^{13}C-enriched esp A_1 in NMR analysis. The signals of carbons 8, 9, and 10 of the enediyne ring were difficult to quantitate because they are broadened in $CDCl_3$. The signal of carbon 1 of the enediyne ring was also buried underneath the $CDCl_3$ signal. In order to obtain the accurate integration of the signals for the above carbons, ^{13}C-enriched esp A_1 was first converted to its diacetyl derivative and CD_3OD was used as the solvent for NMR analysis. Diacetyl-esp A_1 is very soluble in methanol. Sharp signals for all 15 carbons of the enediyne ring of the diacetyl-esp A_1 were obtained in the NMR spectrum (Table 3). Figure 2 summarizes the ^{13}C-labeling pattern of esp A_1 for the ^{13}C-acetate supplemented cultures. Feeding the culture with sodium [1-^{13}C]acetate, we have demonstrated that carbons 1, 3, 5, 7, 9, 11, and 14 of the enediyne ring were enriched (Fig. 2a). The inten-

Table 3 ^{13}C-NMR Assignments of [1-^{13}C]- and [2-^{13}C]-Acetate–Labeled Diacetyl-Esperamicin A_1 and J_{cc} of [1,2-^{13}C$_2$]-Acetate–Labeled Diacetyl-Esperamicin

Carbon	δ (ppm)	[1-^{13}C]acetate (relative intensity)	[2-^{13}C]acetate (relative intensity)	[1,2-^{13}C$_2$]acetate J^{13}C1-J^{13}C2	Satellites
1	77.7	4.5	1	79.9	45.1
2	99.9	1	3.0	80.2	186
3	84.2	4.2	1	89.4	187
4	126.8	1	3.8	90.3	72.2
5	123.5	4.1	1	89.7	72.1
6	88.9	1	3.5	89.8	—
7	98.1	4.2	1	74.4	165
8	72.5	1	4.7	74.0	—
9	148.8	4.3	1	76.7	52.2
10	134.4	1	3.0	77.0	—
11	194.8	2.0	1	45.2	Broad
12	84.3	1	3.3	45.5	Obscured
13	136.7	1	4.7	80.7	45.0
14	131.8	5.8	1	80.5	45.4
15	41.0	1	6.0	—	45.2

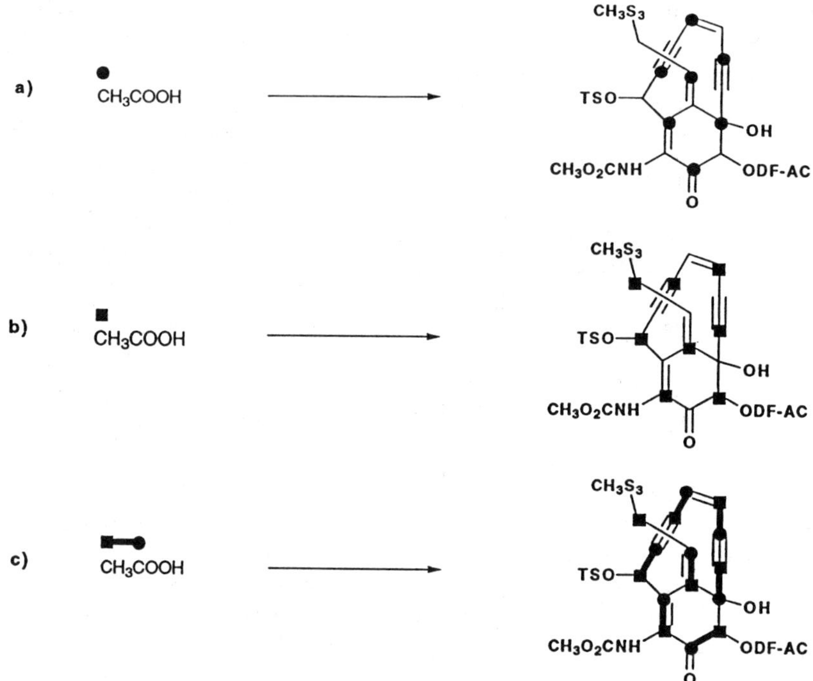

Figure 2 ^{13}C enrichment pattern of esperamicin A_1 from cultures of *Actinomadura verrucosospora* supplemented with (a) sodium [1-^{13}C]acetate, (b) sodium [2-^{13}C]acetate, and (c) sodium [1,2-[13]C$_2$]acetate.

sity of the signals of these seven carbons were 2.0- to 5.8-fold the intensity of the signals of the control (culture without addition of sodium [1-^{13}C]acetate) (Table 3). Using sodium [2-^{13}C]acetate, we have demonstrated that carbons 2, 4, 6, 8, 10, 12, 13, and 15 were enriched (Fig. 2b). The intensity of the signals of these eight carbons were 3.0- to 6.0-fold the intensity of the signals of the control (culture without addition of sodium [2-^{13}C]acetate) (Table 3). We have clearly shown that all 15 carbons of the enediyne ring portion of esp A_1 were derived from acetate. In order to determine the connectivity of the carbon units of the enediyne ring, doubly enriched sodium [1,2-[13]C$_2$]acetate was fed to the esperamicin-producing culture. The resulting enrichment pattern is shown in Figure 2c. The values of the J_{cc} coupling constants clearly showed that seven pairs of carbon were coupled to each other, with C-15 being the only carbon that is uncoupled.

There are only four possible folding patterns for a linear C_{15} unit of esperamicin's enediyne ring system, as shown in Fig. 3. Based on the result of the connectivities of the carbons in Figure 2c, folding patterns a and d can be

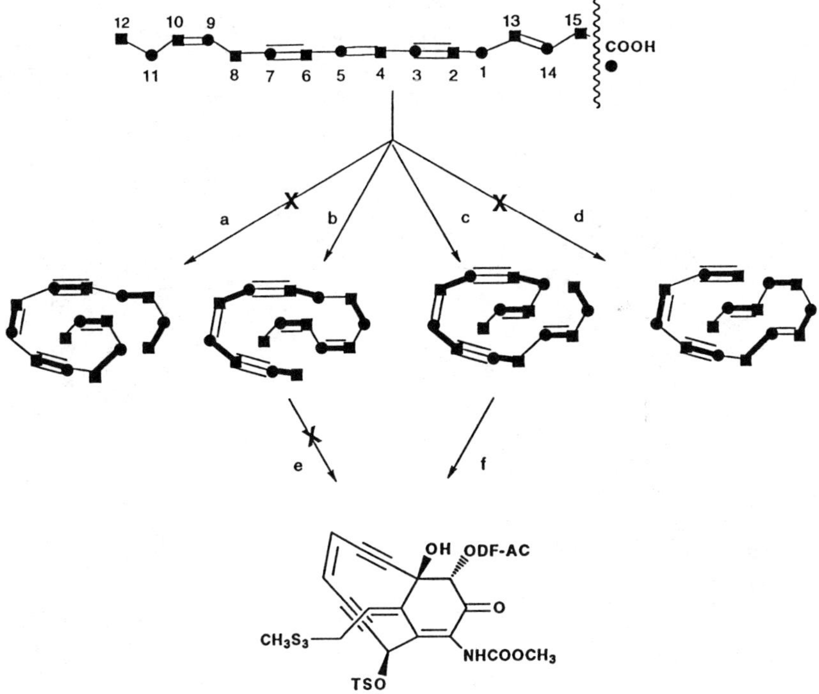

Figure 3   Possible folding patterns of the C_{15} enediyne ring of esperamicin A_1.

eliminated from consideration. From Table 3, C-14 and C-15 have the highest peak intensity enhancements at 5.8- to 6.0-fold, while C-11 and C-12 have the least peak intensity enhancements at 2.0- to 3.3-fold. It is reasonable to assume that C-11 and C-12 may be the chain-termination unit, while C-15 is part of the starter acetate unit. If this is true, the C_{15} chain can then be folded as in path c, and further reaction (path f) would lead to the formation of the enediyne ring of esp A_1. Alternatively, chain folding could proceed as in path b and e. Tokiwa et al. (11) have demonstrated that DNM-A is biosynthesized from two heptaketide chains, which form the enediyne ring and anthraquinone moiety, respectively. Both the enediyne and anthraquinone moieties are derived from seven head-to-tail coupled acetate units. They further proposed a biosynthetic scheme involving a common octaketide intermediate for the formation of the enediyne ring of the esperamicin/calicheamicin/dynemicin class of antibiotics (Fig. 4). Our ^{13}C-acetate enrichment data of the enediyne ring of esp A_1 supported the above hypothesis. The labeling patterns of the diyne moieties of esp A_1 and DNM-A are the same. The two carbons comprising the respective yne moieties are derived from separate acetate units.

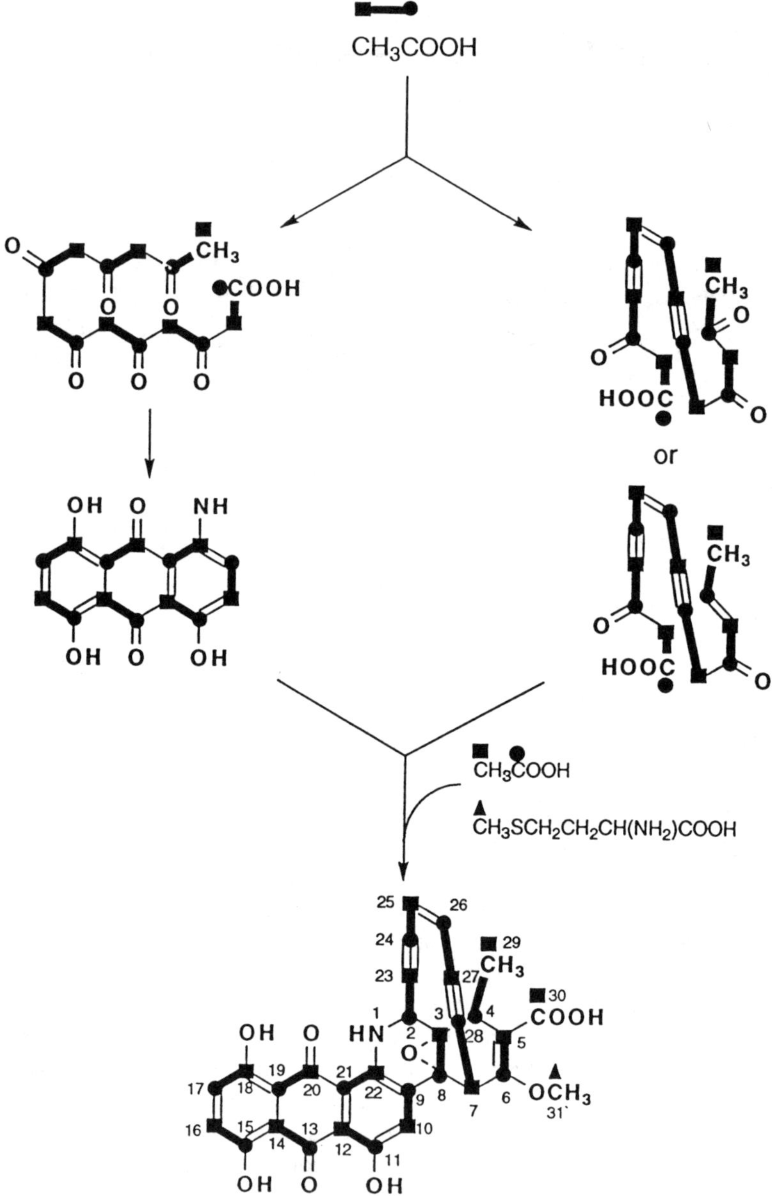

Figure 4 Proposed biosynthetic pathways of the esperamicin/calicheamicin and dynemicin class of antibiotics. (From Ref. 11.)

Hensens et al. (10) have proposed that the C_{14} chain of NCS Chrom A is derived from degradation of oleate via the oleate-crepenynate pathway (19–24) for polyacetylenes rather than by de novo synthesis from acetate. Hensens et al. (10) further postulate that the C_{15} enediyne ring of esperamicin/calicheamicin can similarly be derived via the oleate-crepenynate pathway (Fig. 5). However, the oleate-crepenynate pathway has so far been shown to be present only in higher plants and fungi (19–24). Our data on esp A_1 production from cultures supplemented with cerulenin and sodium oleate are at variance with the above hypothesis. Sodium oleate (0.1–0.5%) did not reverse the inhibitory effect of cerulenin on esp A_1 production by *A. verrucosospora* SA-25262 (Table 4). Cerulenin specifically inhibits the β-ketoacyl-acyl carrier protein synthase (condensing enzyme) of fatty acid and polyketide biosynthesis and has no effect on the performed fatty acid. If esp A_1 is derived from the oleate-crepenynate pathway, adding sodium oleate

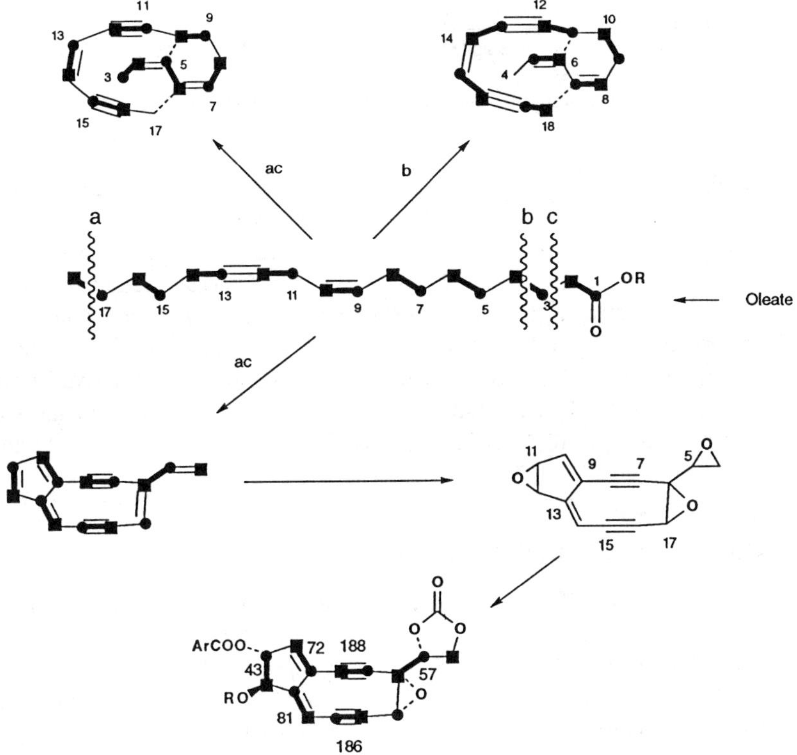

Figure 5 Proposed biosynthetic pathway of C_{14} substructure of neocarzinostatin chromophore and biosynthetic pathways of C_{15} substructure of esperamicin/calicheamicin. (From Ref. 10.)

Table 4 Effects of Cerulenin and Sodium Oleate on Esperamicin A_1
Production by *Actinomadura verrucosospora* SA-25262

Culture condition[a]	[Esperamicin A_1][b] (μg/ml)	% Inhibition
Control (no addition)	4.6	—
0.5 mM cerulenin	1.0	78.3
0.5 mM cerulenin + 0.1% sodium oleate	0.93	79.8
0.5 mM cerulenin + 0.5% sodium oleate	0.81	82.4
1.0 mM cerulenin	0	100
1.0 mM cerulenin + 0.1% sodium oleate	0	100
1.0 mM cerulenin + 0.5% sodium oleate	0	100

[a] Cerulenin and/or sodium oleate were added to the culture at day 3 of the fermentation.
[b] The titers of esperamicin A_1 were determined at day 10 of the fermentation.

to the cerulenin-supplemented culture should relieve its inhibition effect by providing precursor for esp A_1. However, we did not observe any improvement in esp A_1 production when adding sodium oleate to the cerulenin-supplemented cultures of *A. verrucosospora* SA-25262 (Table 4). The ^{14}C-acetate–labeling pattern of esp A_1 in the cultures with or without cerulenin at the active production phase have demonstrated that esp A_1 is synthesized de novo from acetate (25). Furthermore, the two carbons of the yne moieties of NCS Chrom A are derived from the same acetate units (10), indicating that the biosynthetic pathway of the C_{14} dienediyne ring structure of NCS Chrom A is different from those of esp A_1 and DNM-A.

IV. BIOSYNTHETIC ORIGIN OF SULFUR

Esp A_1 contains four sulfur atoms. It contains a thiomethyl sugar in the trisaccharide moiety and an allylic trisulfide in the bicyclic core (Fig. 1). Understanding the biosynthesis of the allylic trisulfide is very important. Mechanisms of action studies indicated that the reduction of the methyl trisulfide group to form a thiolate anion and its subsequent interaction with the bridgehead enone and the enediyne moiety results in highly efficient DNA strand scission (8,9). Feeding ^{35}S-labeled precursors to the culture, we were able to detect the incorporation of $Na_2^{35}SO_4$, L-[^{35}S]cysteine, and L-[^{35}S]methionine into esp A_1 in the complex medium (Table 1). The rates of incorporation of these three radiolabeled precursors were very low (0.019–0.095%). In an attempt to increase the rate of incorporation of ^{35}S-precursors into esperamicins, the above experiment was repeated by growing the culture in a defined medium. Defined medium DF-15, using sodium sulfate as the sole source of sulfur, supports the production of esp A_{1c} and esp A_{2c} but not esp A_1 in the fermentation (26). Adding $Na_2^{35}SO_4$ into this defined medium yielded 1.7% incorporation of radioactivity into esp A_{1c}. L-[^{35}S]Methionine and L-[^{35}S]-cysteine were also incorporated into esp A_{1c} at about the same efficiency as $Na_2^{35}SO_4$. When L-methionine or L-cysteine was substituted for sodium sulfate as the sole sulfur source in the defined medium DF-15, we could not detect any production of esperamicins even though the growth of the organism and pH of the fermentation were the same as those in medium DF-15. The above data suggested that the sulfur form L-methionine or L-cysteine can only be incorporated into a certain subunit of esperamicin and cannot provide all four sulfur atoms. The sulfur from L-methionine or L-cysteine can only be incorporated into either the thiomethyl sugar or the trisulfide moiety. Since sulfur from L-methionine has been shown to be efficiently incorporated into the thiosugar moieties in actinomycete fermentations (27), this may suggest that the allylic trisulfide cannot be derived from L-methionine or L-cysteine.

The above hypothesis can be tested by preparing $Na_2^{35}SO_4$-labeled- and L-[^{35}S]-methionine–labeled esperamicin with high specific activity. Degradation studies can then be carried out to determine which moieties of esperamicin contain the radioactivity. Alternatively, we can use $Na_2^{34}SO_4$ stable isotope to label esperamicin and evaluate the incorporation of ^{34}S isotope by mass spectrometry. Comparison of the substructures generated by mass spectrometry from the natural esperamicin (^{32}S) with those of the labeled species (^{34}S) allowed for the rapid quantitation and location of the incorporated ^{34}S atoms. We have applied this method to show that all four sulfur atoms in esperamicin can be derived from $Na_2^{34}SO_4$ using microgram quantities of ^{34}S-labeled esperamicin (28). ^{34}S-Esp A_{1c} was prepared by growing the culture in defined medium DF-15 using $Na_2^{34}SO_4$ as the sole sulfur source. The full-scan fast atom bombardment mass spectrum of ^{34}S-esp A_{1c} showed a molecular weight of 1304 daltons. This molecular weight is 8 daltons greater than native esp A_{1c}, suggesting the incorporation of four atoms of ^{34}S. The presence of the four ^{34}S atoms was confirmed by high-resolution fast atom bombardment mass spectrometry ([M + H]$^+$ m/z 1305.7708, calcd. for $C_{57}H_{77}N_4O_{22}^{34}S_4$ 1305.3743). The location of the labeled atoms is determined by comparison of the substructures of the native and labeled compounds (Fig. 6). The increase of 6 daltons for the neutral loss of the allylic trisulfide in the labeled compound confirms that all three sulfur atoms of the trisulfide are ^{34}S atoms. The difference of 2 daltons observed with the trisaccharide substructures confirm the presence of ^{34}S in the thiosugar. Further work will be carried out to elucidate the biosynthesis of sulfur in esperamicin using the combination of ^{34}S-precursors, the blocked mutants of the sulfur pathway, and mass spectrometry.

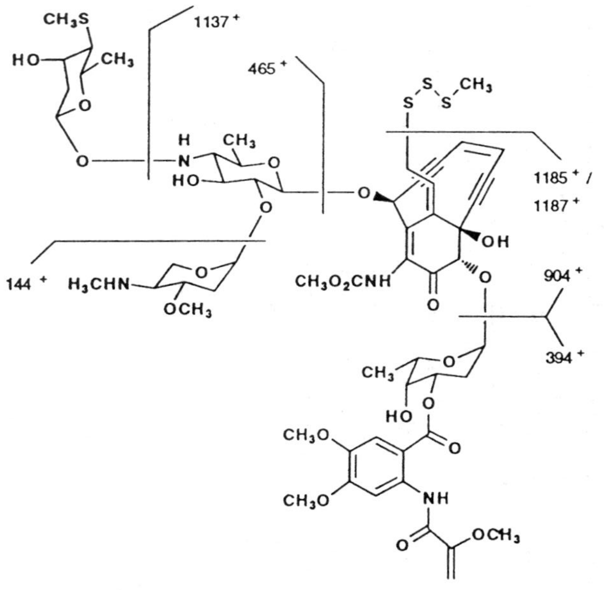

^{32}S - Esperamicin A_{1c}

Accurate Mass : 1296.3860 ($C_{57}H_{76}N_4O_{22}S_4$, 2.0 ppm)

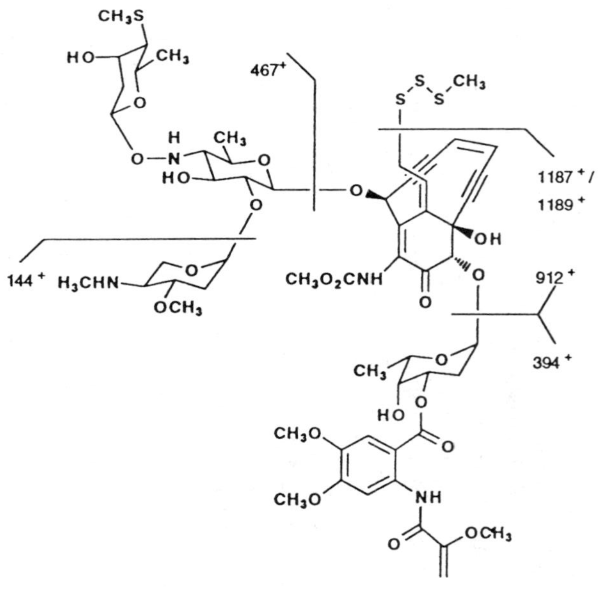

^{34}S - Esperamicin A_{1c}

Accurate Mass : 1304.3630 ($C_{57}H_{76}N_4O_{22}{}^{34}S_4$, 2.6 ppm)

Figure 6 Summary of ions observed in the full-scan FAB mass spectra of ^{32}S-esperamicin A_{1c} (MW 1296) and ^{34}S-esperamicin A_{1c} (MW 1304).

In the literature, a large number of bacteria and some fungi have been shown to oxidize thiosulfate to tetrathionate by virtue of processing the thiosulfate-cytochrome c oxidoreductase type of enzyme (29–33). The hydrolysis of tetrathionate to yield $HS_2SO_3^-$ can be the precursor of the trisulfide in esperamicin:

$$S_4O_6^{2-} + H_2O \rightarrow HS_2SO_3^- + HSO_4^-$$

The enzyme that catalyzes the above reaction has been detected in thiobacilli (34–37). Whether the same enzyme exists in actinomycete or not needs to be proven.

V. BIOSYNTHETIC ORIGIN OF THE METHYL GROUPS

C-, *N*-, and *O*-methyl groups are frequently found in natural products. Most biological methylation in bacteria involves L-methionine, the methyl group of which is activated by S-adenosylation with ATP (38). Table 1 shows that the most efficient precursor of esp A_1 is L-[methyl-^{14}C]methionine. The rate of incorporation of L-[methyl-^{14}C]methionine is 30-fold higher than that of sodium [1-^{14}C]acetate. Based on our experience in the biosyntheses of antitumor antibiotics elsamicin A and rebeccamycin, we observed a significant inhibitory effect on antibiotic production by L-methionine in the ^{13}C-enrichment studies even though L-methionine is the biosynthetic precursor (as methyl donor) for the antibiotic (39,40). We decided to examine the effect of L-methionine on the production of esp A_1 before we carried out the feeding experiment. L-Methionine, at a concentration as low as 0.02%, inhibited the production of esp A_1 by 36.6% (Table 5). At 0.1% L-methionine concentration, no esp A_1 can be detected in the fermentation even though there was no effect on growth of the organism and the pH of the culture. We do not know why L-methionine at such a low concentration inhibits esp A_1 production even though L-methionine is the biosynthetic precursor of esp A_1. The only report we can find in the literature of a L-methionine inhib-

Table 5 Effect of L-Methionine on the Production of Esperamicin A_1 by *Actinomadura verrucosospora* SA-25262

[L-Methionine]	[Esperamicin A_1] (μg/ml)	% Inhibition
0	4.1	—
0.02%	2.6	36.6
0.05%	1.5	63.4
0.10%	0	100
0.20%	0	100

L-Methionine was added to the culture growing in medium H946 at day 3 of the fermentation.

itory effect on antitumor antibiotic production without effect on the growth of the microorganism is that reported by Gairola and Hurley (41) on anthramycin production in *Streptomyces refuineus*. Experiments with radiolabeled anthramycin have demonstrated that reduced yields of anthramycin production are due to the interaction of the anthramycin with reactive metabolites produced in the methionine-supplemented cultures. At 0.03% L-methionine concentration, 56% inhibition of anthramycin production was observed. The inhibitory effect of L-methionine is very similar on anthramycin and esp A_1 production. The thiol of L-methionine or its reactive metabolites generated in the fermentation may react with the trisulfide of esp A_1 and convert esp A_1 to its aromatized derivative. The above findings indicated that we could not add a high initial concentration of L-[methyl-^{13}C]methionine to the culture for the labeling study. Consequently L-[methyl-^{13}C]methionine was added to the culture on two different days to yield a final concentration of 0.05%. Even though the production of esp A_1 was significantly decreased with the addition of L-methionine, adequate amounts of ^{13}C-enriched esp A_1 were obtained for NMR analysis. Figure 7 shows the ^{13}C-enrichment pattern of esp A_1 isolated from the L-[methyl-^{13}C]methionine feeding study. The carbons of seven methyl groups were clearly enriched by L-[methyl-^{13}C]methionine. We also observed small enrichment of the three carbons of the isopropyl group of the aminosugar. This observation is very unusual. Formation of an ethyl group from two methyl groups is unusual but not unique. The methyl group of L-methionine has been shown to be the precursor of the two carbons of the hydroxyethyl group attached to C-6 of thienamycin (42). Weller and Rinehart (43) have demonstrated that both carbons and all hydrogens of the hydroxyethyl group of pectamycin derived from the methyl of L-methionine. It has been reported that the C-24 ethyl group of certain plant sterols is synthesized from the methyl of L-methionine (44,45). However, formation of an isopropyl group from the methyl group of L-methionine has not been reported. We need to obtain more L-[methyl-^{13}C]methionine–enriched esp A_1 in order to obtain better integration of ^{13}C-NMR data to confirm the enrichment observed in the carbons of the isopropyl group of the amino sugar. The possible incorporation of the methyl of L-methionine into the isopropyl group of esp A_1 is further suggested by our results from blocked mutants study. We isolated two blocked mutants of esp A_1 in our laboratory. These blocked mutants, DG-111-10-6 and DG-108-9-3, do not produce any esp A_1. Mutant DG-111-10-6 and DG-108-9-3 each produces one major product in the fermentation, esp A_{1b} (Fig. 1) and esp A_{1c} (Fig. 1), respectively (46). Esp A_{1b} and esp A_{1c} differ from esp A_1 only in the *N*-alkyl substitution of the amino sugar. The presence of these blocked mutants may suggest that the conversion of esp A_{1c} (methyl), esp A_{1b} (ethyl), and esp A_1 (isopropyl) involves the sequential addition of methyl groups onto the nitrogen of the amino sugar. Similar blocked mutants of the related enediyne antitumor antibiotic calicheamicin have recently been reported (47).

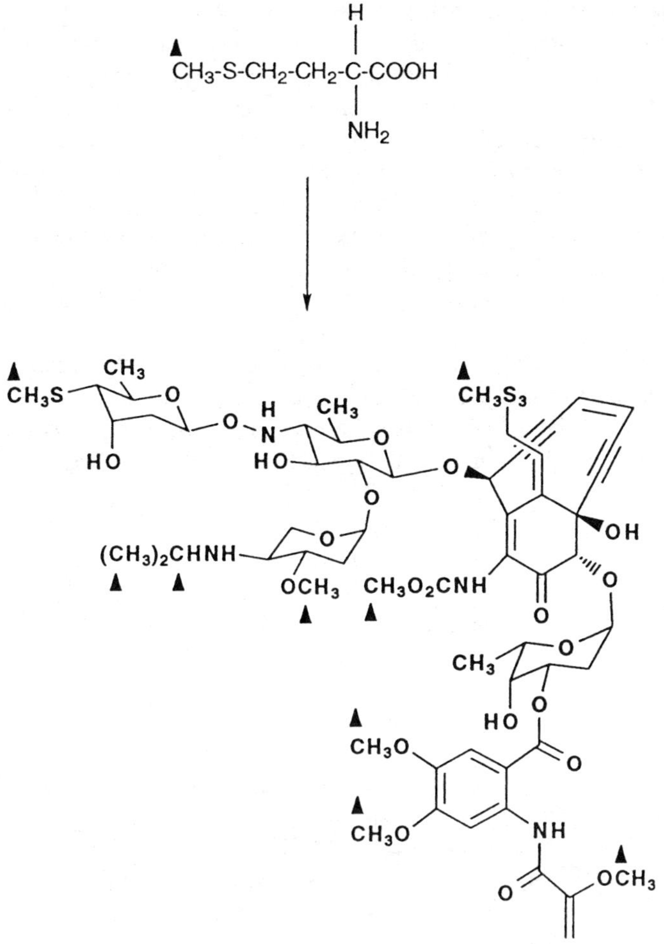

Figure 7 ^{13}C enrichment pattern of esperamicin A_1 from culture of *Actinomadura verrucosospora* supplemented with L-[methyl-^{13}C]methionine.

VI. BIOSYNTHESES OF THE AROMATIC AGLYCONE AND SUGARS

We have not made a great effort to elucidate the biosyntheses of the aromatic aglycone and the sugar moieties of esp A_1. Table 1 shows that sodium [1-^{14}C]pyruvate is incorporated into esp A_1. Since pyruvate is the precursor of acetate, ^{14}C-pyruvate can be converted into ^{14}C-acetate, which may in turn incorporate into esp A_1. However, the rate of incorporation of sodium [1-^{14}C]pyruvate is about 10-fold higher than that of sodium [1-^{14}C]acetate. If ^{14}C-pyruvate is first converted into ^{14}C-acetate before the incorporation of esp A_1, the rate of incorporation of sodium [1-^{14}C]pyruvate into esp A_1 should be lower than that of sodium [1-^{14}C]acetate due to the dilution effect. Konishi et al. (1) have demonstrated that the sugar-aromatic aglycone moiety can be hydrolyzed to yield pyruvate as one of the final products. The data support the incorporation of pyruvate into the aromatic aglycone moiety. From Figure 7, the three methyl groups of the anthranilic aglycone of esp A_1 are derived from L-methionine. The similarity in structure between the anthranilate portion of esp A_1, tomaymycin, and anthramycin indicates that the anthranilate ring of esp A_1 may be derived from L-tryptophan (Fig. 8) (48–51).

In Table 1, D-[U-^{14}C]glucose was incorporated into esp A_1. Since D-glucose is the precursor for both pyruvate and acetate, we would expect some of the D-[U-^{14}C]glucose to be converted to ^{14}C-acetate and ^{14}C-pyruvate and then incorporated into the enediyne ring and the aromatic chromophore moiety, respectively.

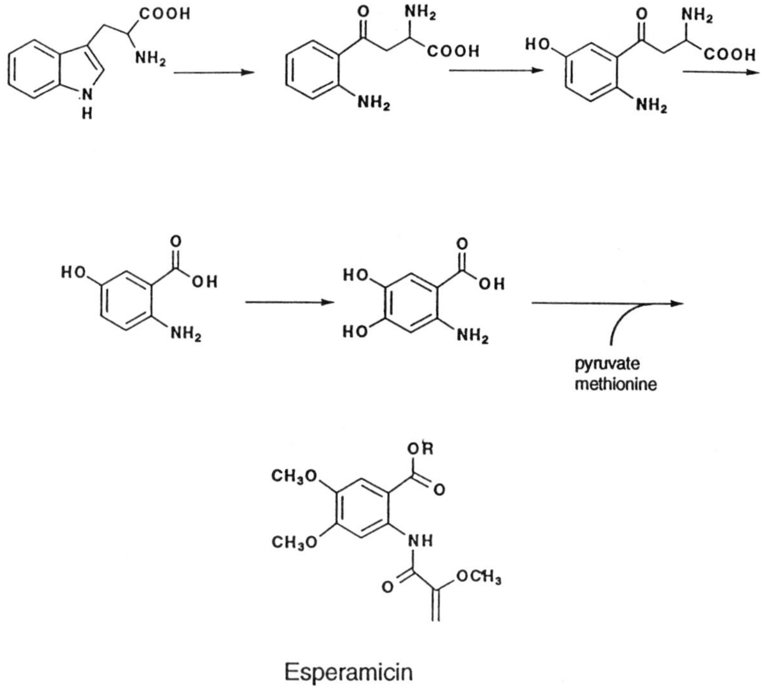

Figure 8 Proposed pathway from L-tryptophan to the anthranilate moiety of esperamicins.

From Table 1, the specific activities of ^{14}C-esp A_1 in the cultures supplemented with sodium [1-^{14}C]acetate and D-[U-^{14}C]glucose are very similar. This indicated that the majority of the incorporated radiolabeled glucose is at the sugar moieties instead of the enediyne ring of esp A_1. Esp A_1 contains four sugars: two deoxysugars and two amino deoxysugars. These four sugars should be derived from D-glucose.

VII. SUMMARY

We have initiated studies on the biosynthesis of esperamicin, demonstrating that the enediyne ring of esp A_1 is derived from head-to-tail condensation of seven acetate units and that the uncoupled carbon is derived from the C-2 of an acetate unit. The two carbons of the yne moieties of esp A_1 are derived from separate acetate units, which is in good agreement with that of DNM-A. Based on the ^{13}C-labeled acetate-enrichment pattern, we propose that the enediyne ring moiety of esp A_1 is derived from an octaketide with the loss of the C-1 of the end acetate unit, as shown in Figure 3. The formation of this enediyne ring is inhibited by cerulenin. Our data on the production of esp A_1 from cultures of *A. verrucosospora* supplemented with cerulenin and sodium oleate rule out the possibility that the enediyne moiety of esp A_1 is derived from oleate-crepanynate catabolic pathway. Since the labeling pattern of the two carbons of the yne moieties of NCS Chrom A is different from those of esp A_1 and DNM-A, this may suggest that enediyne cores of esp A_1 and DNM-A are biosynthesized from a common precursors while NCS Chrom A is biosynthesized via a different process. In order to fully understand the mechanism of the formation of this unusual C_{15} chain, isolation of the polyketide synthase and/or the gene coding for this enzyme may be required.

Identification of the biosynthetic origin of the four sulfur atoms is important. In initial studies carried out in our laboratory using $Na_2^{34}SO_4$ as the sole sulfur source in the fermentation and by mass spectrometric analysis, we have demonstrated that all four sulfur atoms in esperamicin can be derived from $Na_2^{34}SO_4$. The above method requires only microgram quantities of ^{34}S-labeled esperamicin. We may be able to use the combination of ^{34}S-precursors, the blocked mutants of sulfur metabolism of *A. verrucosospora*, and mass spectrometry to study the biosynthesis of sulfur in esperamicin. The information concerning the sulfur metabolism in actinomycete is scarce. It would be valuable to provide information about the biosynthetic pathway leading from sulfate to the allylic trisulfide and the thiosugar in esperamicin from *A. verrucosospora*.

The L-[methyl-^{13}C]methionine incorporation result shows that S-methyl groups of the trisulfide and the thiosugar and the O-methyl groups of the amino sugar, the aromatic chromophore, and the carbamate moiety are derived from L-methionine via S-adenosylmethionine. Further work will be carried out to confirm the formation of the isopropyl group of the aminosugar from L-methionine. The inhibitory effect of L-methionine on the production of esperamicin makes this project more difficult. We consider to use a slow feeding of L-[methyl-^{13}C]methionine into a fermenter culture to keep the concentration of L-methionine low at all times but with enough L-methionine over a period of time for the labeling of esperamicin. We will also determine the biosynthetic origin of the methyl and ethyl of the amino sugar of esp A_{1c} and esp A_{1b} from the blocked mutants. Understanding the mechanism of inhibition of esperamicin production by L-methionine may help us to design a way to relieve this inhibitory effect and controlling the formation of esp A_{1c}, esp A_{1b}, and esp A_1 in the fermentation.

The most effective way to examine the precursor role of L-tryptophan for the formation of anthranilate ring of esp A_1, in our opinion, is to use L-[indole-^{15}N]tryptophan for the labeling of esp A_1 and determining the incorporation of ^{15}N by NMR or mass spectrometry. Since we only need microgram quantities of ^{15}N-labeled esp A_1 for mass spectrometric analysis, the labeling experiment can be carried out in small scale. Using LC-MS analysis, no extensive purification of the labeled metabolite is required.

Although we have not carried out any experiments to study the biosynthesis of the four sugars in esp A_1, the data obtained from the biosynthesis of deoxysugars and amino sugars of macrolides in actinomycetes (52–55) may provide information on the probable biosynthetic pathway of the sugars in esp A_1. The first step in the biosynthesis of deoxysugar of macrolide is to convert D-glucose to its nucleoside diphosphate derivative TDP-D-glucose. TDP-D-Glucose is then converted to TDP-4-keto-6-deoxyglucose before conversion to the desired deoxysugar. For the biosynthesis of the amino-deoxysugar, TDP-4-keto-6-deoxyglucose is transaminated to form TDP-4-amino-4,6-dideoxy-D-glucose before the conversion to the desired amino-deoxysugar. The four sugars of esp A_1 can be biosynthesized from the above pathways. Searching for the nucleotidulated sugars in esperamicin fermentation may provide the sequence of pathway leading to the formation of the deoxysugars and amino-deoxysugars of esperamicin.

REFERENCES

1. M. Konishi, H. Ohkuma, K-I. Saitoh, H. Kawaguchi, J. Golik, G. Dubay, G. Groenewold, B. Krishnan, and T. W. Doyle, *J. Antibiot., 38,* 1065 (1985).
2. J. Golik, J. Clardy, G. Dubay, G. Groenewold, H. Kawaguchi, M. Konishi, B. Krishnan, H. Ohkuma, K-I. Saitoh, and T. W. Doyle, *J. Am. Chem. Soc., 109,* 3461 (1987).
3. J. Golik, G. Dubay, G. Groenewold, H. Kawaguchi, M. Konishi, B. Krishnan, H. Ohkuma, K-I. Saitoh, and T. W. Doyle, *J. Am. Chem. Soc., 109,* 3642 (1987).

4. M. D. Wittman, R. L. Halcomb, S. J. Danishefsky, J. Golik, and D. Vyas, *J. Org. Chem., 55,* 1979 (1989).

5. J. Golik, H. Wong, D. M. Vyas, and T. W. Doyle, *Tetrahedron Lett., 30,* 2497 (1989).

6. J. Golik, T. W. Doyle, G. VanDuyne, and J. Clardy, *Tetrahedron Lett., 31,* 6194 (1990).

7. J. Golik, H. Wong, B. Krishnan, D. M. Vyas, and T. W. Doyle, *Tetrahedron Lett., 32,* 1851 (1991).

8. B. H. Long, J. Golik, S. Forenza, B. Ward, R. Rehfuss, J. C. Dabrowiak, J. J. Catino, S. T. Musial, K. W. Brookshire, and T. W. Doyle, *Proc. Natl. Acad. Sci. USA, 86,* 2 (1989).

9. Y. Sugiura, Y. Uesawa, Y. Takahashi, J. Kuwahara, J. Golik, and T. W. Doyle, *Proc. Natl. Acad. Sci. USA, 86,* 7672 (1989).

10. O. D. Hensens, J-L. Giner, and I. H. Goldberg, *J. Am. Chem. Soc., 111,* 3295 (1989).

11. Y. Tokiwa, M. Miyoshi-Saitoh, H. Kobayashi, R. Sunaga, M. Konishi, T. Oki, and S. Iwasaki, *J. Am. Chem. Soc., 114,* 4107 (1992).

12. J. E. Schurig, W. C. Rose, H. Kamei, Y. Nishiyama, W. T. Bradner, and D. A. Stringfellow, *Invest. New Drugs, 8,* 7 (1990).

13. K. S. Lam, S. Forenza, J. A. Veitch, D. R. Gustavson, J. Golik, and T. W. Doyle, in *Microbial Metabolites* (C. Nash, J. C. Hunter-Cereva, R. Cooper, D. E. Eveleigh and R. Hamill, eds.), William C. Brown, Publishers, Arlington, VA, 1993, pp. 261–274.

14. R. B. Herbert, in *The Biosynthesis of Secondary Metabolites* (R. B. Herbert, ed.), Chapman and Hall, New York, 1989, p. 18.

15. S. Omura, *Bacteriol. Rev., 40,* 681 (1976).

16. C. Kitao, H. Tanaka, S. Minami, and S. Omura, *J. Antibiot., 34,* 711 (1980).

17. S. Omura, *Methods Enzymol., 72,* 520 (1981).

18. K. S. Lam, J. A. Titus, and D. L. Kimball, Abstract O-40. 87th Annual Meeting of American Society for Microbiology, Atlanta, GA, March 1–6, 1987.

19. J. D. Bu'Lock, in *Comparative Phytochemistry* (T. Swain, ed.), Academic Press, New York, 1966, Chapter 5.

20. G. C. Barley, A. C. Day, U. Graf, E. R. H. Johns, I. O'Neill, R. Tachikawa, V. Thaller, *J. Chem. Soc. Commun.,* 1971, 3308 (1971).

21. F. Bohlmann, T. Burkhardt, and C. Zdero, in *Naturally Occurring Acetylenes,* Academic Press, New York, 1973.

22. E. R. H. Jones, C. M. Piggin, V. Thaller, and J. L. Turner, *J. Chem. Res. Synop.,* 1977, 68 (1977).

23. M. Ahmed, M. Hearn, E. R. H. Jones, and V. Thaller, *J. Chem. Res. Synop.,* 1977, 125 (1977).

24. G. C. Barley, U. Graf, C. A. Higham, M. Y. Jarrah, E. R. H. Jones, I. O. O'Neill, R. Tachikawa, V. Thaller, J. L. Tuner and A. Hodge, *J. Chem. Res. Synop.,* 1987, 232 (1987).

25. K. S. Lam, D. R. Gustavson, J. A. Veitch and S. Forenza, *J. Ind. Microbiol., 12,* 99 (1993).

26. K. S. Lam, J. A. Veitch, J. Golik, S. Forenza, and T. W. Doyle, Abstract, 49th Annual Meeting of Society for Industrial Microbiology, San Diego, CA, August 9–14, 1992.

27. A. D. Argoudelis, T. E. Eble, J. A. Fox, and D. J. Mason, *Biochemistry, 8,* 3408 (1969).

28. S. E. Klohr, K. J. Volk, M. S. Lee, K. S. Lam, J. A. Veitch, E. H. Kerns, S. Forenza, and I. E. Rosenberg, Proceedings 40th ASMS Conference Mass Spectrometry and Allied Topics, 1992.

29. P. A. Trudinger, *J. Bacteriol., 93,* 550 (1967).

30. L. B. Schook and B. S. Berk, *J. Bacteriol., 140,* 306 (1979).

31. E. Kurek, *Arch. Microbiol., 134,* 143 (1983).

32. J. H. Tuttle, J. H. Schwartz, and G. M. Whited, *Appl. Environ. Microbiol., 46,* 438 (1983).

33. J. Mason and D. P. Kelly, *Microbial Ecol., 36,* 51 (1987).

34. P. A. Trudinger, *Rev. Pure Appl. Chem., 17,* 1 (1967).

35. D. P. Kelly, *Philos. Trans. R. Soc. London Ser. B, 298,* 499 (1982).

36. D. P. Kelly, *Microbiol. Sci., 2,* 105 (1985).

37. R. Steudel, G. Holdt, T. Gobel, and W. Hazeu, *Angew. Chem. Int. Ed. Engl., 26,* 151 (1987).

38. K. G. B. Torssell, in *Natural Product Chemistry: A Mechanistic and Biosynthetic Approach to Secondary Metabolism* (K. G. B. Torssell, ed.), John Wiley and Sons, New York, 1981, p. 19.

39. K. S. Lam, J. A. Veitch, and S. Forenza, Abstract, 46th Annual Meeting of the Society for Industrial Microbiology, Seattle, WA, August 13–18, 1989.

40. K. S. Lam, S. Forenza, D. R. Schroeder, T. W. Doyle, and C. J. Pearce, in *Novel Microbial Products for Medicine and Agriculture* (A. L. Demain, G. A. Somkuti, J. C. Hunter-Cevera, and H. W. Rossmore, ed.), Elsevier, Amsterdam, 1989, pp. 63–66.

41. C. Gairola and L. Hurley, *Eur. J. Appl. Microbiol., 2,* 95 (1976).

42. J. M. Williamson, E. Inamine, K. E. Wilson, A. W. Douglas, J. M. Liesch, and G. Albers-Schonberg, *J. Biol. Chem., 260,* 4637 (1985).

43. D. D. Weller and K. L. Rinehart, Jr., *J. Am. Chem. Soc., 100,* 6757 (1978).

44. M. Castle, G. Blondin, and W. R. Nes, *J. Am. Chem. Soc., 85,* 3306 (1963).

45. L. J. Goad, A. S. A. Hamman, A. Dennis, and T. W. Goodwin, *Nature, 210,* 1322 (1966).

46. K. S. Lam, D. G. Gustavson, and S. Forenza, Abstract P-84, 46th Annual Meeting of Society for Industrial Microbiology, Seattle, WA, August 14–19, 1989.

47. D. M. Rothstein and S. F. Love, *J. Bacteriol., 173,* 7716 (1991).

48. L. Hurley, N. Des, C. Gairola, and M. Zmizewski, *Tetrahedron Lett., 18,* 1419 (1976).

49. L. H. Hurley and C. Gairola, *Antimicrob. Agents Chemother., 15,* 42 (1979).

50. J. M. Ostrander and L. H. Hurley, *J. Antibiot., 33,* 1167 (1980).

51. L. H. Hurley, *Acc. Chem. Res., 13,* 263 (1980).

52. J. F. Martin, *Ann. Rev. Microbiol., 31,* 13 (1977).

53. S. Omura and Y. Tanaka, in *Biochemistry and Genetic Regulation of Commercial-*

ly Important Antibiotics (L. C. Vining, ed.), Addison-Wesley, Reading, MA, 1983, p. 187.

54. J. F. Martin, in *Macrolide Antibiotics: Chemistry, Biology and Practice* (S. Omura, ed.), Academic Press, New York, 1984, pp. 416–417.

55. S. Shapiro, in *Regulation of Secondary Metabolism in Actinomycetes* (S. Shapiro, ed.), CRC Press, Boca Raton, FL, 1989, p. 177.

13

Mechanism of Action and Molecular Modeling for Esperamicin A_1, Calicheamicin γ_1^I, and Dynemicin A

David R. Langley
*Bristol-Myers Squibb Pharmaceutical Research Institute,
Wallingford, Connecticut*

I. INTRODUCTION

The 1,5-diyn-3-ene–containing class of natural products—the esperamicins [1] (1–11), calicheamicins [2] (12–15), and dynemicins [3] (16–19)—represent some of the most potent antitumor antibiotics (Fig. 1). Their high potency and unique structures have catapulted them into the limelight of the chemical community. Their unusual structures have presented new challenges to the synthetic organic chemist as well as the promise of a novel mechanism of action for fighting cancer. In order to gain a deeper insight into the mechanism of action of these compounds, a number of organic, biophysical, and theoretical groups have focused on this new class of natural products.

The neocarzinostatin chromophore [4] (20–27), kedarcidin chromophore [5] (28–34), C-1027 chromophore [6] (35–38), and maduropeptin chromophore [7] (39,40) also contain an enediyne system that imparts high antitumor potency (Fig. 2). The above chromophores are initially isolated as haloprotein complexes. The high sequence homology between the apoproteins of neocarzinostatin, kedarcidin, macromomycin, actinoxanthin, and C-1027 suggests that the associated chromophores may also be structurally similar. The similarities in the biosynthetic pathways for the neocarzinostatin chromophore, esperamicin A_1, and dynemicin A strongly suggests that the two classes are genetically related.

239

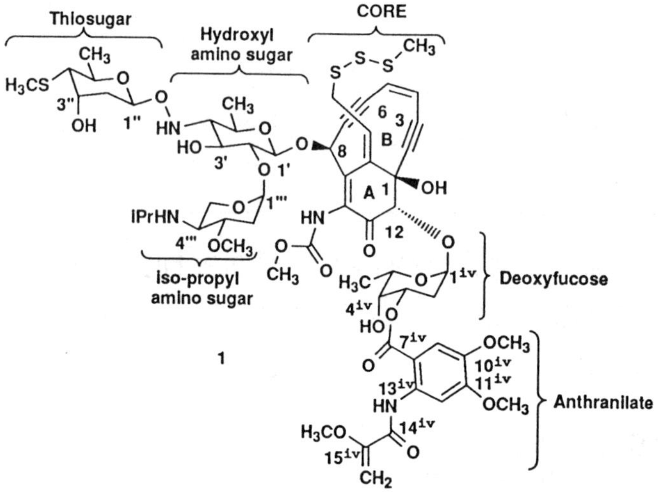

1

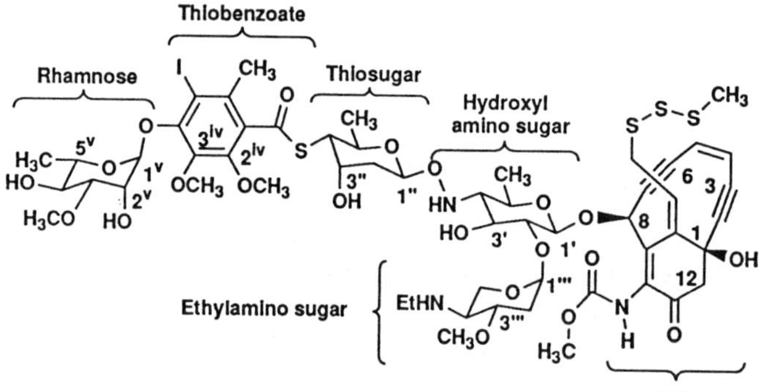

2

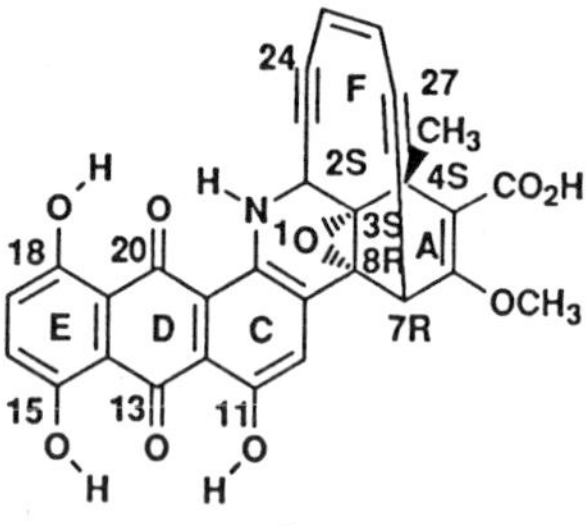

3

Figure 1 Esperamicin A_1 [**1**], calicheamicin γ_1^I [**2**], and dynemicin A [**3**].

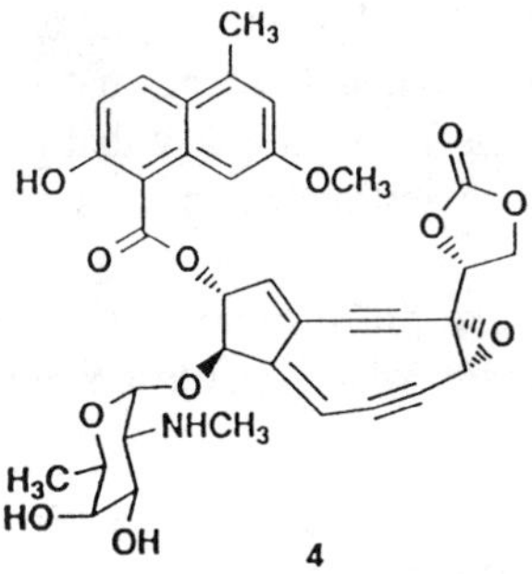

4

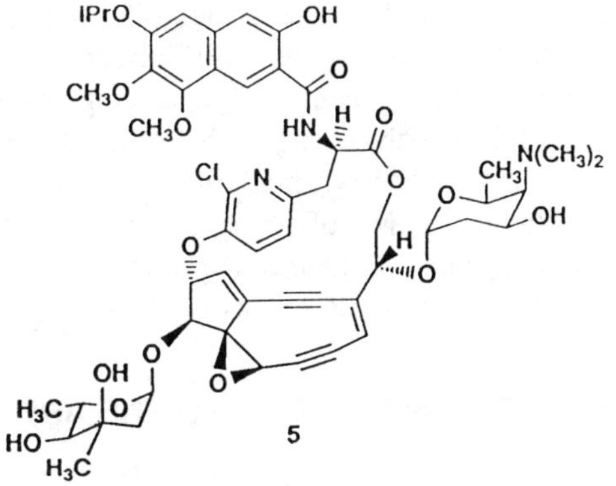

5

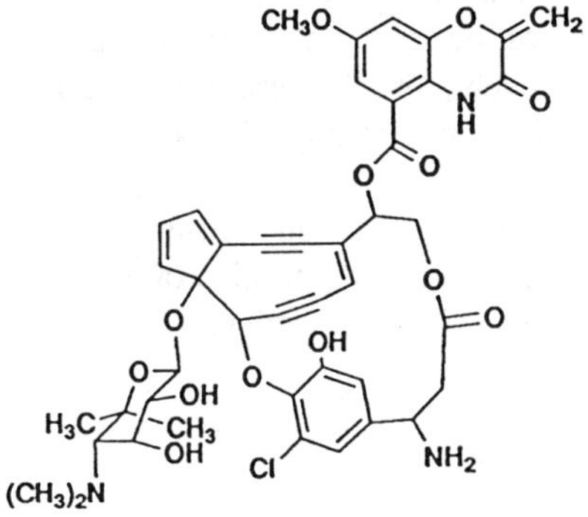

6

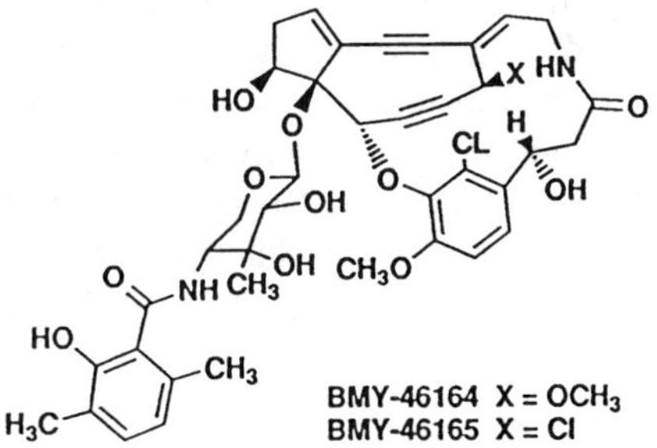

BMY-46164 X = OCH_3
BMY-46165 X = Cl

7

Figure 2 Neocarzinostatin chromophore [**4**], kedarcidin chromophore [**5**], C-1027 chromophore [**6**], and maduropeptin chromophore [**7**].

The structure of enediyne-containing compounds can be divided into three domains: (1) the diradical generator, (2) the trigger, and (3) the DNA recognition and binding elements. The core structure of the esperamicin and calicheamicin warhead is a bicyclo[7.3.1] ring system. Housed within or attached to the bicyclic system are the integral parts of the warhead. The 1,5-diyn-3-ene system contained within the larger of the two rings (B-ring) (**1**, Fig. 1) is a diradical generator (the charge). The allylic methyl trisulfide attached to the bridging atom and the bridgehead α,β-unsaturated ketone make up the hammer and pin of the trigger, respectively. The aryl-polysaccharide tail(s) appended to the core make up the DNA recognition and binding domain. Dynemicin A is composed of a heptacyclo-1,5-diyn-3-ene ring system. This ring system is a hybrid of an anthraquinone [DNA intercalator (41–44)], a 1,5-diyn-3-ene [diradical generator (4,45,46)], and a strategically located epoxide (trigger). It is believed that the DNA-binding element(s) of these drugs interact with the DNA in a way that positions the enediyne ring so that efficient DNA hydrogen abstraction occurs when it is fired to the aryl diradical.

The mechanism of action by which the enediynes exert their biological activity is attributed to their ability to produce aryl diradicals, which lead to a single and/or double strand breaks in DNA.

II. DRUG ACTIVATION TO THE ARYL DIRADICAL

Esperamicin X [8] (Fig. 3) provided valuable insight into the mechanism of activation of esperamicin and calicheamicin. The core of esperamicin X has all the structural features of esperamicin A_1 with the following exceptions: the allylic methyl trisulfide and the bridgehead α,β-unsaturated ketone are replaced by a dihydrothiophene and saturated ketone, respectively, and the enediyne is replaced with a 1,2-disubstituted benzene ring. It is apparent that the aglycone of esperamicin X could be derived from esperamicin A_1 in a four-step reaction sequence (Scheme 1), namely: (1) reductive cleavage of the allylic methyl trisulfide; (2) Michael addition of the resulting thiolate [9] to the β-position of the enone (concomitantly forming the dihydrothiophene ring [10] while removing the bridge-

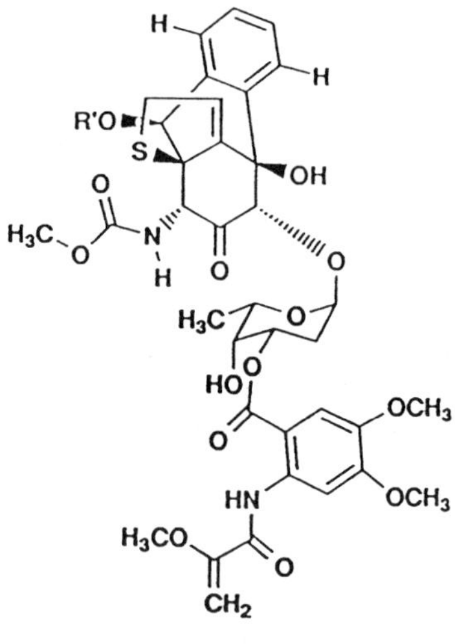

Figure 3 Esperamicin X [8].

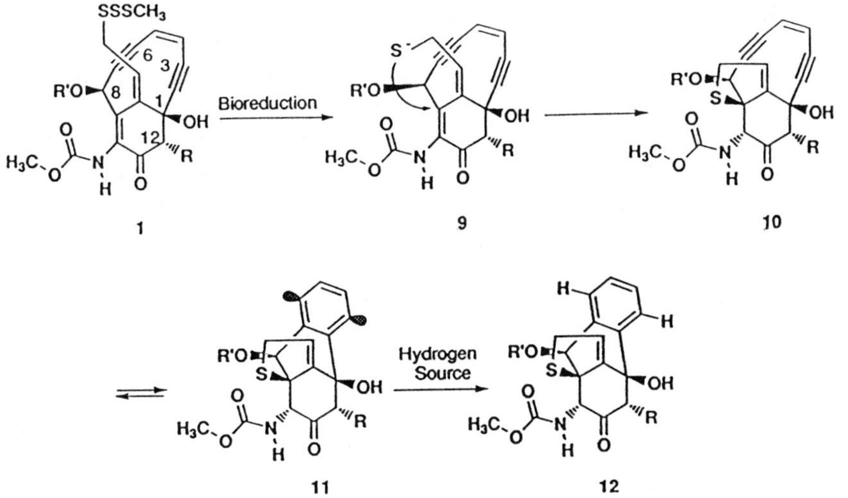

Scheme I Mechanism of activation for esperamicin and calicheamicin.

head double bond); followed by (3) the conversion of the A-ring boat to chair conformation (47) and then aromatization of the enediyne to an aryl diradical [11] and (4) hydrogen abstraction from the environment (DNA, esperamicin itself, or solvent) to quench the diradical producing esperamicin Z [12]. Due to the similarities between the esperamicin A_1 and calicheamicin γ_1^I aglycone, the same mechanism of activation applies.

Using simple models, Golik and coworkers (4) proposed that the bridgehead double bond prevented the ends of the *cis*-1,5-diyn-3-ene (C-2 and C-7) system from coming close enough together for aromatization to occur and that saturation of the bridgehead should permit geometries suitable for ring closure. Nicolaou and coworkers (48) expanded on this by synthesizing and evaluating the rate of cycloaromatization for several mono-carbocyclic *cis*-1,5-diyn-3-ene–containing molecules. Using molecular mechanics calculations the distance between the enediyne ends for their synthetic compounds as well as other known systems including the esperamicin/calicheamicin aglycones (before and after conjugate addition) was determined. They found that the end-to-end enediyne distance showed a good correlation with the rates of cycloaromatization, which led them to conclude that at least for these simple systems (48) the ground state enediyne end-to-end distance could be used to predict the stability of simple mono-carbocyclic *cis*-1,5-diyn-3-ene–containing molecules. The ground state end-to-end enediyne distance at which a molecule crosses over from stable to spontaneous cyclization was predicted to be within the range of 3.31–3.20 Å. Notably, they found the enediyne end-to-end distance to be 3.35 Å for the esperamicin/calicheamicin aglycon and 3.16 Å for the aglycon product after Michael addition. Snyder (49) took this a step further by developing a model for the cyclization pathway for *cis*-4-octene-2,6-diyne using PRDDO-GVB-CI level calculations. The calculations predict the transition state to have 35% biradical character, suggesting a least-motion cyclization pathway and an enediyne end-to-end distance of 2.06 Å. The MM2 force field was parameterized to reproduce the PRDDO-GVB-CI transition state and was used in conjunction with fixed-point PRDDO calculations on the ground (PRDDO-SCF) and transition state (PRDDO-GVB-CI) to predict the relative transition state energies for more complex systems. Using the MM2/PRDDO technology the relative transition state energies for a number of diverse enediyne systems were calculated (47,49–51). The calculations showed, as expected, that the rate of cycloaromatization is governed by the energy developed in the transition state (ΔE^*) and not the enediyne end-to-end distance. Additionally, Magnus and co-workers (47) synthesized an enediyne-containing bicyclo[7.2.1] and bicyclo[7.3.1] ring system with very similar enediyne end-to-end distances and showed that they aromatize with vastly different rates, clearly demonstrating that the ground state enediyne end-to-end distance is not a reliable predictor of cycloaromatization rates.

In dynemicin A the opening of the epoxide is the key step in the activation to its aryl diradical (50,52) intermediate. The epoxide, like the bridgehead double bond in esperamicin A_1 (53), locks the conformation of the 1,5-diyn-3-ene system so that C23 and C28 are too far apart for bonding interaction (47–49,51). The CHARMM (18,54) force field predicts the distance from C23 to C28 to be 3.53 Å in dynemicin A. The opening of the epoxide in dynemicin relieves the ring strain and allows the ends of the enediyne system to move closer together (3.16 and 3.19 Å apart for dynemicin diol and alcohol forms, respectively). This in turn reduces the strain energy required in the diradical transition state (47,49–51) and allows for the formation of the aryl diradicals via a Berman (45,46) -type reaction at ambient temperatures. The diradical intermediate is then quenched by abstracting hydrogens from its environment, producing the aromatized form of dynemicin.

Epoxides are relatively stable at physiological pH. However, the work of Koch (55–58) and Fisher (59) suggests a reasonable mechanism for the epoxide ring opening reaction. This mechanism requires the reduction of dynemicin A [13] (Scheme 2) to the hydroquinone [14] and rearrangement to open the epoxide ring producing the quinone-methide [15]. The quinone-methide can now undergo nucleophilic attack by water or be protonated giving the diol [16] or the alcohol [17], respectively. Compounds 16 and 17 can now undergo the Bergman reaction and aromatize to the diradical, via an energy barrier of $\Delta E^* = \sim 19.2$ kcal (50), followed by hydrogen abstraction from the DNA or environment affording dynemicin

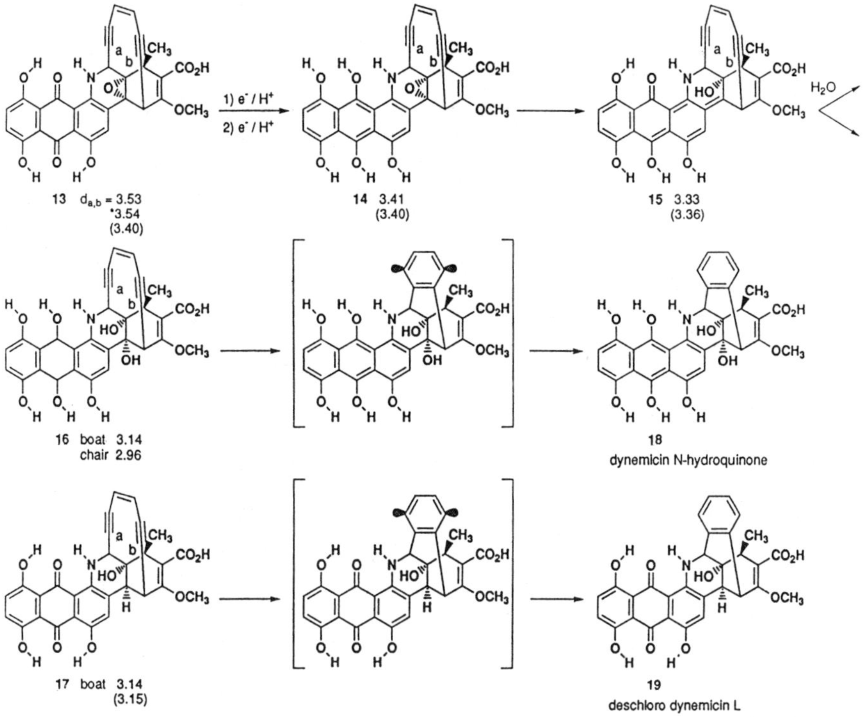

Scheme II Mechanism of activation for dynemicin A.

N hydroquinone [18] and deschloro dynemicin L (dynemicin H) [19] (T. T. Dabrah and J. A. Matson, personal communication).*

III. DNA CLEAVAGE

A number of studies have focused on the ability of esperamicin, calicheamicin, and dynemicin to cleave DNA. DNA-nicking experiments have shown that calicheamicin γ_1^I (61,62) and esperamicin C (**20**, Fig. 4) (53) produce concomitant DNA double strand breaks converting from I DNA directly into form III DNA. Esperamicin A_1 (53,62) and dynemicin A (63,64), on the other hand, cause the conversion of form I DNA into forms II and III DNA. The proportion of

*Deschloro dynemicin L has been isolated from the *Micromonosporqa chersina* sp. Nov. N956-1 fermentation broth along with dynemicin A and dynemicin N. Deschloro dynemicin L (dynemicin H) was found to be the major product formed when dynemic A was activated with visible light (60).

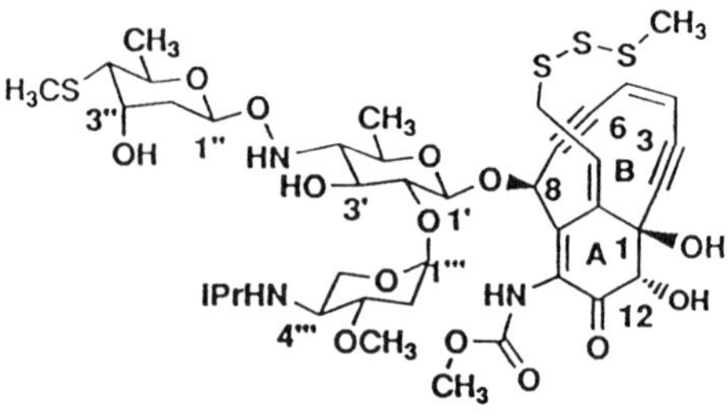

20

Figure 4 Esperamicin C [20].

form II to III is dependent on the rate of drug activation and the amount of drug in the reaction. This strongly suggests that a given molecule of esperamicin A_1 or dynemicin A causes DNA single strand breaks. The cleavage of form I DNA by esperamicin A_1, esperamicin C, and calicheamicin γ_1^I has been analyzed by coupled kinetics (62,65). These studies showed esperamicin A_1 to produce predominantly DNA single strand breaks. However, the ratio of the rate constants, k_1'/k_2', for the conversion of form I to form II, k_1', and form II to form III, k_2', is not consistent with completely random nicking, suggesting that some DNA double strand cleavage may occur. Esperamicin C and calicheamicin γ_1^I, however, were found to produce mainly DNA double strand breaks. Interestingly, the rate constant for the introduction of the first DNA break is faster for esperamicin C, whereas the second break (in the opposite strand) is faster for calicheamicin.

IV. DNA SEQUENCE SPECIFICITY

DNA affinity cleavage studies have been employed to investigate the pattern and sequence specificity of cleavage. Interestingly, all three of the parent natural products and a number of their analogs exhibit cleavage sites in one strand of the DNA accompanied by a cleavage site in the opposite strand that is staggered by three base pairs in the 3'-direction (53,61,63,66). This indicates that the diradical is being generated within the minor groove (67) of the DNA and is supported by the fact that minor groove binding drugs inhibit the ability of esperamicin A_1, calicheamicin γ_1^I, and dynemicin A to cause DNA strand breaks (61,63,66). In addition, calicheamicin has been shown to be one of the most sequence-specific nonprotein DNA-cleaving molecules reported to date. It has a cleavage preference for 5'-TCCT sites, however, other sties such as (5'-TCCC, TCCA, ACCT, TCCG, GCCT, CTCT, TCTC) (61,68) and (5'-TTTT, TTCA, and TTGT) (69) are also cleaved. In addition, the DNA breaks always occur at the 5' end of the sequence-specific site, clearly demonstrating a mono-directional mode of binding. Esperamicin A_1 and its degradation products (53,62,65,66,70–75) as well as dynemicin A (63,64,76,77) have weak absolute cleavage sequence specificity. Analyses of the strongest cleavage sites from a number of different studies have revealed that both esperamicin and dynemicin have an underlying sequence preference.

At low concentrations of drug the strongest cut sites (highest-affinity cleavage sites) will be produced first. If the drug concentration is sufficiently high, then secondary and finally tertiary cut sites will be produced. With drugs as potent as esperamicin A_1 and dynemicin A, the intercellular drug concentration can be assumed to be very low, therefore, only the highest-affinity sites are expected to produce the cuts that lead to the biological response. For this reason only the strong cleavage sites were used in the determination of the sequence specificity for esperamicin A_1 and dynemicin A.

Based on modeling studies (78), the esperamicin A_1-binding domain covers seven to eight base pairs in length (Fig. 5, see color plate; Table 1A). To determine the base preference at a particular location within the binding site, a population analysis was performed (Table 1B,C). The strong esperamicin A_1 cut sites, as determined by the original researchers, were collected from the literature (53,62,65,66,70–75) and analyzed. The strong cut sites were categorized into

Table 1 Population Analysis

		5'-	(-B4	-B3	-B2	-B1	Ct	B1	B2)	-3'
A.		11	12	13	14	15	16	17	18	19	20
	5'-	C	A	**G**	**G**	**A**	**T**	**T**	**G**	**C**	G
	3'-	G	T	**C**	**C**	**T**	**A**	**A**	**C**	**G**	C
		10	9	8	7	6	5	4	3	2	1
B.											
		Pu	30	51	58	16	7	33	44	
		Py	37	16	9	51	60	34	23	
C.											
		A	14	29	26	10	4	18	21	
		G	16	22	32	6	3	15	23	
		C	20	10	2	21	26	16	11	
		T	17	6	7	30	34	18	12	

(A) The DNA sequence used in this study is aligned with the population analysis. The bold DNA bases make up the esperamicin-binding site. One atom or more of the highlighted base is $\leqslant 4.5$ Å from esperamicin. Esperamicin makes direct contact with the floor of the <u>minor</u> and <u>major</u> groove at the underlined bases. Population analysis of the DNA bases within the 67 strong cut sites. (B) Base family: purine (Pu) or pyrimidine (Py). (C) Base type: adenine (A), guanine (G), cytosine (C), and thymine (T).

5'-(-B4 -B3 -B2 -B1 Ct B1 B2) domains where B# is a purine (Pu) or pyrimidine (Py) base and Ct is the cut site. Table 1B indicates that 5'-*N*-Pu-Pu-Py-Py-*N*-Pu sequences, where *N* is either Pu or Py, are highly reactive sites toward esperamicin A_1 cleavage. Sixteen (23.9%) of the 67 strong cut sites agree with this finding, while 32 (47.8%), 18 (26.9%), and 1 (1.5%) contain single, double, or triple position mismatches, respectively. The 32 single mismatches are nearly equally distributed through the binding domain. The double mismatches are distributed into nonequal groups of -B1, B2 (7) > -B3, B2 (5) > -B2, B2 (3) > -B3, -B1 (2) > -B1, Ct (1). The single triple mismatch is at -B3, -B2, and B2. When the sequences were broken down into their respective bases, no particular sequence stands out. Despite esperamicin's low sequence specificity there appears to be an underlying preference for 5'-*N*-Pu-Pu-Py-Py*-*N*-Pu sequences, where *N* is either Pu or Py and Py* is the cut site. A single position mismatch at any location within the domain is well tolerated, however, esperamicin A_1 shows more sensitivity to double and triple site mismatches. The least tolerated multiple mismatches are the ones at the -B1 Ct sites.

The pattern of DNA cleavage is directly related to the drug's sequence specificity and mode of cleavage. A given DNA cleavage site is often accompanied by a cleavage site on the opposite strand that is staggered by three bases in the 3' direction. These staggered cut sites can be explained by considering the symmetry of -B3 -B2 -B1 Ct within the 5'-*N*-Pu-Pu-Py-Py*-*N*-Pu/3'-Pu-N-Py*-Py-Pu-Pu-*N* binding domain and a bidirectional mode of binding (75,78). If the drug binds to the DNA with its trisaccharide tail pointing in the 5' direction relative to the CORE and top strand of the DNA, then a cut site at the 3'-Py* in the top strand will occur. However, if the drug binds with the trisaccharide pointing in the 3' direction relative to the top strand, the cut site will occur at the 3'-Py* of the bottom strand.

Modeling studies from our laboratory (18) and others (79–81) suggest that dynemicin A intercalates between the two bases immediately to the 5' side of the cut site (Fig. 6, see color plate). To determine its sequence specificity, the cleavage affinity data from Sugiura's laboratory (63) (Fig. 7) was categorized into 5'-B2-B1-Ct domains and analyzed, where B1 and B2 are purine (Pu) or pyrimidine (Py) bases and Ct is the cut site. The domains were then divided into strong, medium, and weak cuts based on their height relative to the strongest cut site (Table 2), as determined by densitometric scanning. Intensities equal to or greater than 40% of the strongest cut size (*) were assigned as strong cut sites (Fig. 7). All sites with intensities less than 20% of the strongest cut site were assigned to weak or background cuts.

Dynemicin exhibits a sequence specificity for cleaving DNA of 5'-B2-B1-Ct in which the B2-B1 site makes up the intercalation cleft. The drug preference for the B-2B1 site is 5'-Py-Pu >>> Py-Py > Pu-Py > Pu-Pu. When the sequences were broken down into their respective bases, a preference of TACT = TGCt

```
    .|:......||  ....  ...|..:::.|:    |:...::|..|:::.
5'-GTGCTCAACGGCCTCAACCTACTACTGGGCTGCTTCCTAATGCAGGAGT
3'-CACGAGTTGCCGGAGTTGGATGATGACCCGACGAAGGATTACGTCCTCA
  .  :  ..   ...:  .|:.|:.|..  ....:: .||:| |.::..
                        *
```

Figure 7 Histogram of cleavage sites on the 5'-^{32}P–labeled (SalI-DraII) pBR322 DNA restriction fragment produced by NADPH/dynemicin A (63). Strongest *, strong (|), medium (:), and weak (.) cleavage sites.

> CGCt > CACt > TTCt > GGCt was found. For example, 83.3% of 5'-TA and 71% of 5'-TG sites resulted in strong cuts, with little or no regard for the type of bases at positions B3 or Ct. Furthermore, 80.0% of the 5'-Py Pu and 100% of 5'-TA cut sites have a strong or medium cleavage site on the opposite

Table 2 Statistical Analysis of Dynemicin A DNA Cleavage Histogram (Fig. 7)

5'-B2-B1-CT domain	Possible binding sites	Strong cuts (%)	Medium cuts (%)	Weak cuts (%)
Pu Pu Ct	23	1 (4.3)	4 (17.4)	12 (52.2)
Pu Py Ct	21		7 (33.3)	7 (33.3)
Py Pu Ct	21	13 (61.9)	2 (10.0)	5 (23.8)
Py Py Ct	25	1 (4.0)	6 (24.0)	17 (68.0)
A A Ct	4		1 (25.0)	2 (50.0)
A G Ct	9		1 (11.1)	8 (88.9)
G A Ct	3		1 (33.3)	1 (66.7)
G G Ct	7	1 (14.3)	1 (14.3)	1 (14.3)
A T Ct	2		1 (50.0)	1 (50.0)
A C Ct	5		1 (20.0)	4 (80.0)
G T Ct	5		2 (40.0)	1 (20.0)
G C Ct	9		3 (33.3)	1 (11.1)
T A Ct	6	5 (83.3)	1 (16.7)	
T G Ct	7	5 (71.4)		1 (14.3)
C A Ct	6	2 (33.3)	1 (16.7)	3 (50.0)
C G Ct	2	1 (50.0)		1 (50.0)
T T Ct	4	1 (25.0)	2 (50.0)	1 (25.0)
T C Ct	4		1 (25.0)	3 (75.0)
C C Ct	7		2 (28.6)	5 (71.4)
C T Ct	10		1 (10.0)	8 (80.0)

strand staggered by three base pairs in the 3′ direction. These staggered cut sites can be explained by considering the symmetry of the 5′-Py-Pu-Ct/3′-Ct-Pu-Py double-stranded dinucleotide and the drug's low specificity for the B3 and Ct bases. If the drug intercalates into the 5′-Py-Pu sequence with the enediyne ring pointing in the 3′ direction (relative to the top strand), then the top strand is cut and the 5′-Py-Pu-Ct site results. However, if the drug intercalates with the enediyne pointing in the 5′ direction, the bottom strand is cut and the 3′-Ct-Pu-Py site is produced.

V. DNA HYDROGEN ABSTRACTION

The identity of the DNA hydrogen(s) abstracted by a radical-producing drug can be deduced by comparing the migration of the cleaved DNA fragment with Maxam-Gilbert (82) sequencing markers. The Maxam-Gilbert sequencing reactions cleave out the target DNA base and leave 3′- and 5′-phosphate termini. The abstraction of a hydrogen from the DNA backbone at C5′ was first shown by neocarzinostatin (83) to produce 5′-aldehyde and 3′-phosphate ends that run almost two bases behind and with their Maxam-Gilbert counterpart, respectively. The abstraction of the C4′ DNA hydrogen has been demonstrated with bleomycin to generate 5′-phosphate and 3′-phosphoglycolate termini (84) (which run with or slightly ahead of their Maxam-Gilbert marker) or a 4′-hydroxylated abasic site (85). The abasic product when treated with base (piperdine) produces 5′-phosphate and 3′-(3-hydroxy-5-oxo-1-cyclopentenyl) ends. The 3′-(3-hydroxy-5-oxo-1-cyclopentenyl) end moves slower than the Maxam-Gilbert marker and can be converted to a 3′-phosphate termini by treatment with warm base (75). An abasic site lactone is produced by the abstraction of the DNA 1′-hydrogen (86,87). Base treatment of the lactone abasic site produces 3′- and 5′-phosphate termini.

Comparison of the migration of the drug-induced DNA bands with Maxam-Gilbert sequencing markers after gel electrophoresis has uncovered the identity of the hydrogens abstracted by esperamicin A_1, calicheamicin γ_1^I, and dynemicin A. Calicheamicin γ_1^I generates cleavage sites in 3′- and 5′-^{32}P-labeled oligonucleotides that are consistent with a C5′ (61) and C4′-hydrogen (68) abstraction. Furthermore, it was shown that the diradical intermediate of calicheamicin concomitantly cleaves each strand of the DNA by abstracting the C5′-hydrogen from the 5′-C of 5′-TCCT sequences and the H4′ from the base on the opposite strand that is staggered in the 3′ direction by three bases from the 5′-C (Fig. 8). Using molecular modeling techniques, the carbon-centered radical at C6 of calicheamicin was predicted to abstract the H5″ (pro-S) hydrogen from the 5′-C of the 5′-B_3B_2TCCT/3′-B_3B_2AGGA preferred cleavage site (88). Using site-specific deuterium-labeled oligonucleotides it has been proven that the carbon-centered radical at C6 abstracts the H5″ (pro-S) hydrogen from the 5′-C of 5′-TCCT with ~89% efficiency and the radical at C3 is quenched by H4′ (~63%) or H5″ (pro-S) (~2%) from the 3′-B_3 base on the opposite strand or solvent (~10%) (89,90).

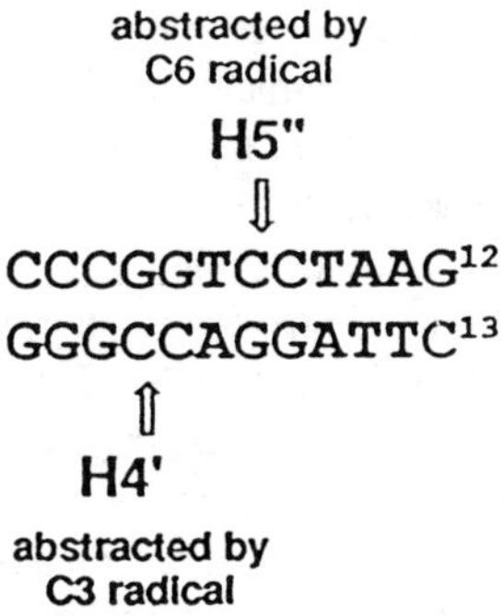

abstracted by
C6 radical

H5"

⇓

CCCGGTCCTAAG[12]
GGGCCAGGATTC[13]

⇑

H4'

abstracted by
C3 radical

Figure 8 Calicheamicin-DNA cutting pattern (see Ref. 90).

The lower sequence specificity expressed by esperamicin A_1 and its analogs has hampered the identification of the DNA hydrogens abstracted by these drugs. Additionally, slight changes occurred in the electrophoretic mobility of the esperamicin C (**20**, Fig. 4), D (**21**, Fig. 9), and E [**22**] bands compared to esperamicin A_1. These changes suggest that the esperamicin A_1 analogs cause

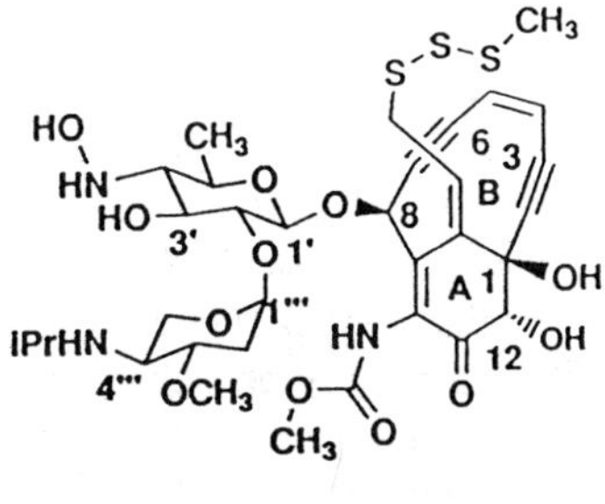

21

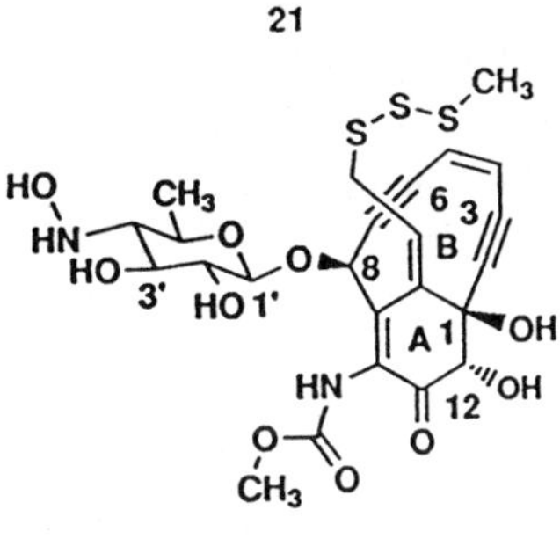

22

Figure 9 Esperamicin D [**21**] and esperamicin E [**22**].

DNA breaks through additional cleavage mechanisms. It was first predicted by Long and coworkers (53) that esperamicin A_1 abstracts a hydrogen from C5′ of the DNA backbone. It should be noted that the esperamicin A_1 analogs have the same but broader sequence specificity (53,62,65,66,70–75). The specific hydrogen abstraction chemistry has been determined for the esperamicins using short DNA fragments (29 base pairs) and analysis by high-resolution gel electrophoresis (20% polyacrylamide) (75). The cleavage of 5′-^{32}P–labeled DNA with esperamicin A_1 under neutral conditions produced only fragments that comigrated with the Maxam-Gilbert markers indicating the formation of a 3′-phosphate termini and therefore C5′-hydrogen abstraction chemistry. Treatment with piperidine did not produce additional lesions or change the relative intensities of the lesions observed under neutral conditions. Esperamicin C, D, and E also produced 3′-phosphate termini as well as additional faster- and slower-migrating bands. The new bands are consistent with C4′-hydrogen abstraction with the production of a 3′-phosphoglycolate terminus (faster bands) and a 3′-(3-hydroxy-5-oxo-1-cyclopentenyl) end (slower band). The conversion of the slower-moving bands to 3′-phosphate termini under warm basic conditions further supports the C4′-hydrogen abstraction chemistry. The C5′-hydrogen abstraction mechanism was further validated by analyzing the esperamicin cleavage of 3′-^{32}P–labeled DNA fragments. Under neutral conditions esperamicin A_1 produced only the expected 5′-aldehyde termini consistent with a C5′-hydrogen abstraction mechanism. The treatment of the 5′-aldehyde termi with $NaBH_4$ or piperidine caused its conversion to a 5′-hydroxyl termini or 5′-phosphate termini, respectively, confirming the identity of the 5′-aldehyde. Analysis of the esperamicin C–, D–, or E–cleaved 3′-^{32}P–labeled DNA fragments revealed that both 5′-aldehyde and 5′-phosphate termini were produced. Treatment with $NaBH_4$ or piperidine caused the conversion of the 5′-aldehyde to the expected 5′-alcohol or 5′-phosphate termini as expected. It should be noted that while esperamicin D and E produce results comparable with esperamicin C, they required higher drug–to–DNA base pair ratios and their sequence specificity was broader (75). Despite the low sequence specificity exhibited by the esperamicins, they appear to possess a high degree of precision in DNA hydrogen abstraction. It has been demonstrated that the degree of precision can be altered for neocarzinostatin by a sequence-specific isotope effect, which leads to the partitioning between C4′- and C5′-hydrogen abstraction at the T of 5′-GT sites (91,92). However, no isotope effect was observed at C4′ (70,75) or C5′ (75) for esperamicin A_1 or C. The absence of an isotope effect illustrates the precision of hydrogen abstraction and suggests that hydrogen abstractions occur through distinct binding modes and distinct radical centers. The similarity in the DNA double strand cleavage, pattern of cleavage, identity of the abstracted hydrogens, and structure between esperamicin C and calicheamicin γ_1^I suggests that the C3 and C6 radical centers in esperamicin C, like calicheamicin, abstract the H4′ and H5″ (pro-S) from opposite strands of the DNA, respectively.

Dynemicin preferentially cuts the DNA at the base immediately to the 3' side of purines, and these cut 5'-^{32}P–labeled oligomers produced radioactive bands that were electrophoretically identical to the Maxam and Gilbert products (82), indicating that the drug abstracts a C5'-hydrogen from the DNA backbone (93). More recently (77), it has been shown that dynemicin A–cleaved 3'-^{32}P–labeled oligomers also migrate with their respective Maxam and Gilbert products (82). Additionally, certain cleavage sites such as 5'-CT and 5'-GA produce two bands, which comigrate with its 3'-phosphate termini product or its 3'-phosphoglycolate termini. The labeling studies taken as a whole suggest that dynemicin A abstracts C1'- and C4'-hydrogens from the DNA backbone. The cleavage of branched DNA molecules by dynemicin A has revealed hypersensitive spots near the branch point (76). Hypersensitive spots within the B-Z junction (94) have also been reported. The hyperactive sites at branch points were eliminated by competitive binding of propidium diiodide (76) [an intercalative drug (95)] suggesting that the anthraquinone portion of dynemicin A intercalates into the DNA and controls the sequence specificity. The migration of the dynemicin A–induced fragments from the branched DNAs also indicates the partitioning between C5'-, C1'-, and C4'-hydrogen abstraction chemistry at certain hypersensitive sites. The preferential binding to unusual DNA structure has also been reported for other intercalative drugs (95–97). The hypersensitivity of branch points and B-Z junctions to dynemicin A cleavage suggests that unusual DNA structures may be the biological target of dynemicin A, which leads to its in vivo antitumor activity.

VI. REACTION WITH CT-DNA

Esperamicin A_1 and calicheamicin γ_1^I share a common mechanism of activation (Scheme I). However, the fate of the diradical intermediates are different. For example, in calicheamicin γ_1^I both radicals result in DNA strand breaks, while in the case of esperamicin A_1 only one radical is productive.

The aromatization of calicheamicin γ_1^I in a solution of deuterated buffer, deuterated methylthioglycolate, and excess calf thymus DNA produced calicheamicin ϵ in 65% yield (98). The lack of deuterium incorporation into the C3 and C6 of calicheamicin ϵ, the radical-bearing carbons, indicates that the calicheamicin diradical intermediate abstracts hydrogen atoms almost exclusively from the carbohydrate backbone of the DNA. When the reaction was repeated in the absence of CT-DNA, calicheamicin ϵ was produced in ~20% yield, but with over 98% deuterium incorporation at C3 and C6. These results suggest that DNA may serve as a catalytic template for quenching the diradical intermediate (89,90,99) and to protect calicheamicin from self-destruction.

Under analogous reaction conditions with CT-DNA, esperamicin A_1 produced no detectable quantity of esperamicin Z (78). Instead, the cleavage of the glycosidic bond at the C8 was observed (Scheme III), producing as the major isolated product the trisaccharide fragment [24] in 60% yield. The cleavage of the trisaccharide fragment has been previously observed from esperamicin A$_1$ following its reduction with sodium borohydride (10). It should be noted that the trisaccharide fragment undergoes spontaneous rearrangement of the pyranose form of the hydroxylamino sugar [23] to its furanose carbinolamine equivalent [24]. Traces of the aromatized core were detected in the ^{1}H-NMR spectra of the crude reaction mixtures, however, the aromatized core fragment has not yet been isolated and completely characterized.

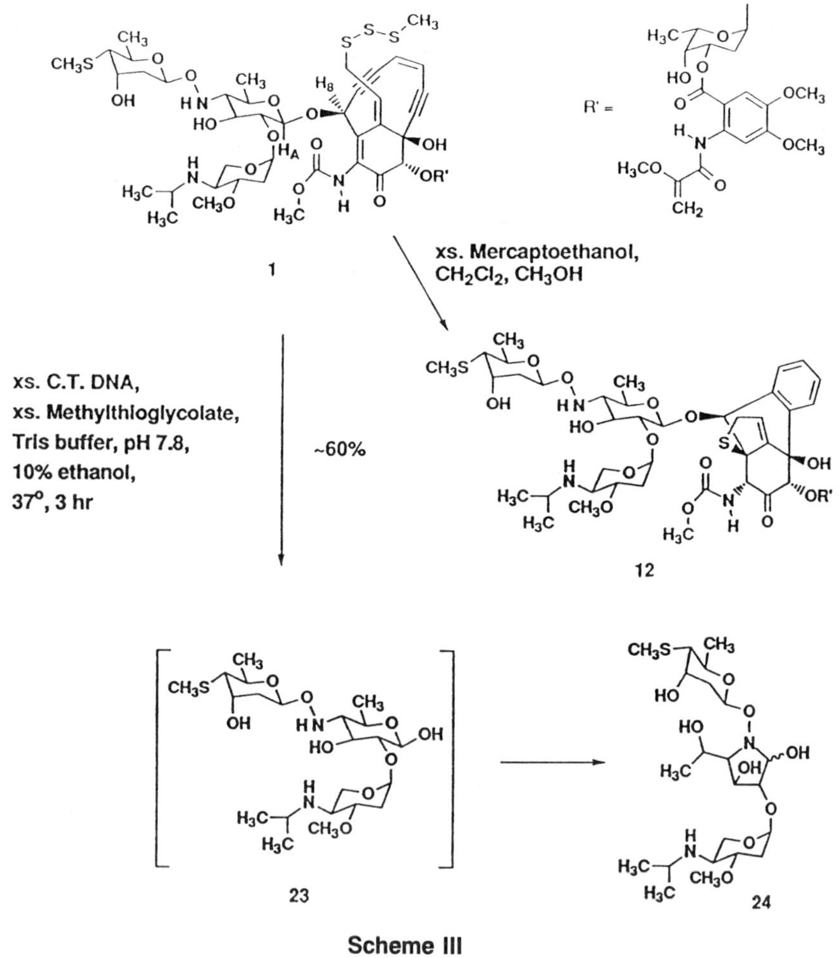

Scheme III

The base sensitivity of both esperamicin A_1 (10) and calicheamicin γ_1^I (15) has been demonstrated but appears inadequate to explain the differences observed between the reactions of esperamicin A_1 and calicheamicin γ_1^I with CT-DNA under analogous reaction conditions. Additionally, when the reaction between esperamicin A_1 and CT-DNA was repeated at lower pH (7.0, 7.2, and 7.4), only minor variations in the yield of the rearranged trisaccharide fragment [24] were observed.

VII. DNA RECOGNITION, BINDING, AND CLEAVAGE

The ability to cleave DNA by a carbon-centered radical depends on the drugs ability to recognize and bind with DNA. Equally important is the orientation of the radical relative to the DNA-abstractable hydrogens. Recognition can be divided into two categories: detailed and general. Calicheamicin γ_1^I recognizes the DNA fine structure, which allows it to discriminate between different sequences as well as the directionality of a preferred sequence. Esperamicin A_1 and dynemicin A more or less only recognize the general characteristics of DNA, making them considerably less sequence specific. It is commonly believed that high sequence specificity is preferred and that double strand breaks result in greater potency. However, esperamicin A_1 is active across a broad range of cancer types (53) and is equally as potent as calicheamicin γ_1^I. Dynemicin A, like esperamicin A_1, causes predominantly single strand breaks but is considerably less potent than either esperamicin A_1 or calicheamicin γ_1^I.

In DNA nicking (53) and affinity cleavage (65,66,73,75) experiments, the potency of cleavage for esperamicin A_1 and its degradation products were found to be esperamicin $A_1 > C > D > E$. The cytotoxic potency in eukaryotic cancer cells (53) of the esperamicins mirrors the cleavage potencies. In esperamicin A_1 the recognition and binding elements orient the diynene in a way that makes one of the radicals inefficient at abstracting a hydrogen, leading to DNA cleavage. In esperamicin C, D, and E, the recognition element is unchanged (65,66,73,75), but the binding and orientation elements have changed compared to esperamicin A_1. The orientation of the diynene relative to the DNA has changed so that both radicals are productive, resulting in concomitant DNA double strand breaks. However, for the simpler analogs the number of binding interactions is decreased, which reduces their binding constants and allows more of the drug to aromatize in the nonbound form, resulting in lower potency.

In calicheamicin the deoxyfucose and anthranilate are missing from the core and are replaced by the thiobenzoate and rhamnose sugar on the end of the carbohydrate tail. The removal of the rhamnose sugar [25] (Fig. 10) or the ethylamino sugar [26 from calicheamicin γ_1^I reduced its DNA cut efficiency 50–100 times and 2000–3000 times, respectively, but did not alter its sequence specificity (68). Additionally, acetylation of the ethylamino sugar reduced the DNA cutting

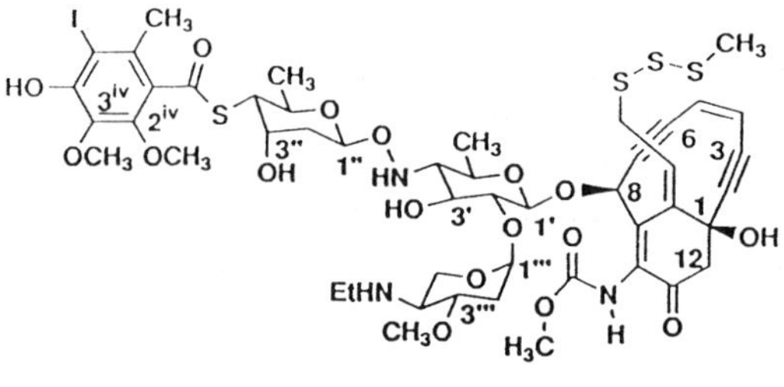

Figure 10 Calicheamicin analogs calicheamicin T [27] and aglycone [28].

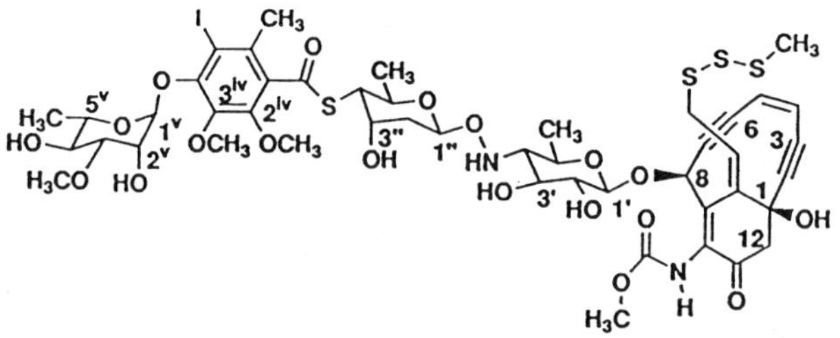

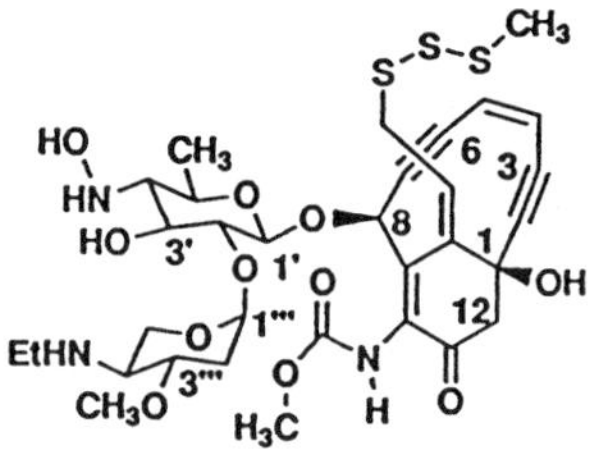

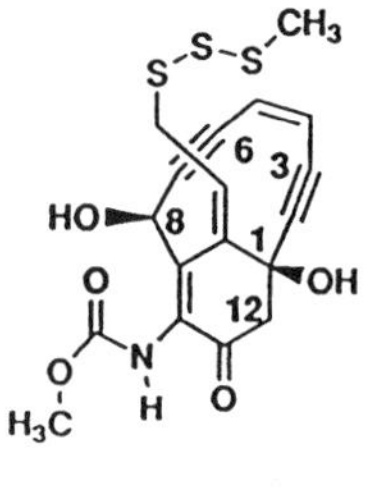

efficiency without affecting the specificity, suggesting that the ethylamino sugar provides an energetically favorable ionic intercation between the drug and the DNA (100). However, the removal of the thio sugar, thiobenzoate, and rhamnose sugar gives calicheamicin T [27], which exhibits reduced DNA cutting and sequence specificity (69). The calicheamicin aglycone [28] also exhibits reduced DNA cutting and sequence specificity, producing mostly DNA single strand nicks (101). DNA footprinting studies carried out on the aryl tetrasaccharide portion of calicheamicin (102,103) have shown it to exhibit similar but broader sequence specificity when compared to calicheamicin γ_1^I. Furthermore, esperamicin C can be thought of as an analog of calicheamicin (69,101,104) with a hydroxyl at C12 and thiomethyl and isopropylamino groups in place of the thiobenoate-rhamnose moieties and ethylamino group, respectively. Esperamicin C, like calicheamicin, binds in the minor groove of DNA (53,66) and causes double strand DNA breaks by simultaneously abstracting the H5″ from one strand and a H4′ from the opposite strand (75,78), however, it is considerably less sequence specific and its cleavage pattern indicates a bidirectional mode of binding (75,78).

Collectively, the above results strongly suggest that the deoxyfucose and anthranilate moieties in esperamicin A_1 strongly influence the drug's ability to bind with DNA and the orientation of the enediyne within the DNA minor groove. On the other hand, the thiobenzoate plays a major role in determining the sequence specificity and binding directionality exhibited by calicheamicin γ_1^I but has little or no effect on orienting the core within the DNA for hydrogen abstraction.

VIII. FOOTPRINTING OF BOUND ESPERAMICIN A_1 AND C

The reactive probe osmium tetroxide (OsO_4) (105) has proven useful in monitoring features of the groove structure in duplex DNA. OsO_4 oxidizes the thymine C5-C6 double bond, which lies in the major groove. The oxidation preferentially occurs in the open rather than the base-paired state but has been observed in B-DNA (106). Unactivated esperamicin A_1 when bound with DNA reduces the ability of OsO_4 to oxidize thymine residues (78) when compared to the oxidation of naked DNA (Fig. 11). In contrast, the oxidation of the unactivated DNA–esperamicin C complex produced oxidation levels comparable to that of naked DNA. This suggests that the groove structure of the DNA–esperamicin A_1 complex is close to that of regular B-DNA (105) and possibly that a portion of the deoxyfucose and/or anthranilate moieties are bound in the major groove.

IX. MOLECULAR MODELING

A wealth of experimental data characterizing the mechanism of activation of the aglycons of esperamicin A_1 and calicheamicin γ_1^I and dynemicin A are available, and the process of DNA hydrogen atom abstraction also exists. These results can

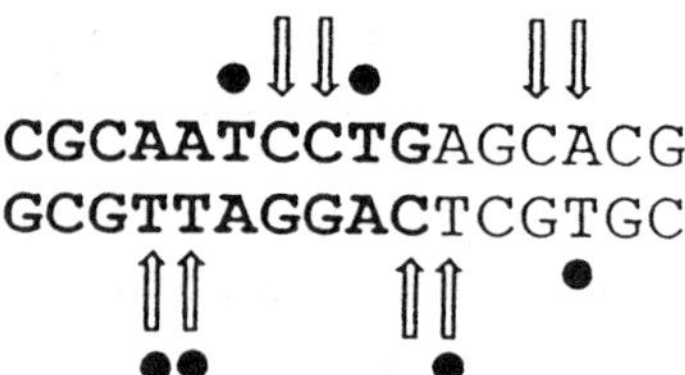

Figure 11   The oligonucleotide used in the affinity cleavage and osmium tetroxide experiments (73,78). The arrows mark the strong esperamicin A$_1$ cleavage sites. The dots mark the sites that were protected by esperamicin A$_1$ during OsO$_4$ oxidation. The 10-base-pair sequence in bold type was used in the modeling study.

be used to infer the relative orientation of the activated diradicals within their respective DNA-cleavage sites. However, very little is known about the three-dimensional structure of the DNA-drug complex, specifically, the molecular bases for their cleavage sequence specificity.

Using the x-ray crystal structure of dihydrocalicheamicin pseudoaglycon (13), esperamicin X (11), and dynemicin A triacetate (17) and NMR COSY and ROESY data on calicheamicin ε (107) as references, models for esperamicin A$_1$ (78), calicheamicin γ_1^I (104), and dynemicin A (18) were constructed in our laboratory using the CHARMM (54) force field and parameter set (108). DNA docking studies for each drug were carried out with a sequence of DNA that has been experimentally shown to contain a cleavage hot spot for that drug. The viability of each model was then tested using in vacuo and/or solvated molecular dynamics. The results from each simulation were compared with experimental data, and only those runs that were consistent with all of the available experimental data were considered. Additionally, models of the DNA–calicheamicin γ_1^I (68,68) and DNA–dynemicin A (79–81) complexes have been produced by other laboratories.

A. DNA–Dynemicin A Complex

Different modes of binding dynemicin A with DNA (major and minor groove intercalation, groove and backbone binding) have been investigated (18,79,80). The docking of dynemicin A as a major groove intercalator was found to be inconsistent with the experimental data in that H5′, H4′, and H1′ point into the minor groove, while H5′ points straight out into the bulk solvent and not into the major groove. Additionally, intercalation into the minor groove is favored by about 10 kcal/mol over the major groove (80). Furthermore, the L-shaped geometry of dynemicin makes for a poor fit for groove binding along the straight and narrow major or minor groove (18). Consistent with the intercalation mode of binding, the calculations (80) predict that the intercalation of dynemicin A into a 5′-CG site is favored by about 9 kcal/mol over intercalation into 5′-TA sites. Interestingly, the major DNA-cleavage sites occur at 5′-PyPuCt sites, where Ct is the cleavage site, the 5′-TACt sequence appears to be preferred (18,63). This suggests that equilibrium binding thermodynamics does not control the hydrogen abstraction reaction (80) and may in part explain the diminished potency exhibited by dynemicin A. However, it should be noted that the diradical intermediate formed from dynemicin A is responsible for cleaving the DNA and not unactivated dynemicin A.

In the two-electron reducing environment of the NADPH–dynemicin DNA system (63), dyemicin A is presumably reductively activated to the hydroquinone (**14**, Scheme II) prior to intercalation. Its rearrangement to the quinone methide [**15**] followed by nucleophilic attack and/or protonation would produce the diol [**16**] and/or alcohol [**17**], respectively. The relaxed ring strain allows the diol and/or alcohol to undergo conformational changes leading to the diradical intermediate. The most dramatic conformational change occurs when going from the diol or alcohol to dynemicin N hydroquinone [**18**] or deschloro dynemicin L [**19**], respectively. The A-ring flips from a quasi-boat to a quasi-chair, placing the C4 methyl group in an equatorial position. The quasi-boat to -chair transition twists the aromatic ring away from and to one side of the hydroquinone or quinone ring system giving the (2S,7R)-enantiomers a right-handed conformation. The right-handed twist of the (2S,7R)-enantiomer for **15** and **16** is amplified as the ends of the enediyne are pulled together to their aromatic forms. The right-handed twist makes the molecules more complementary to the minor groove of the right-handed B-DNA (Fig. 12, see color plate) (18,79).

The actual dynemicin intermediate that intercalates into the DNA and leads to DNA strand breaks is unclear. In the two-electron reducing environment of the DNA–NADH–dynemicin A experiments by Sugiura (66), dynemicin A must be reduced prior to intercalation into the DNA. However, it is also certain that the diol [**15**] or alcohol [**16**] must be intercalated prior to aromatization for DNA cleavage to occur (63). The slight left-handed twist of unactivated dynemicin A leads one to predict that the dynemicin A has a lower DNA binding constant than its activated form (Fig. 12). If this is true, dynemicin A represent a highly tuned prodrug that finds its target and becomes sequestered loosely in or near the DNA until a reducing agent (NADH) comes along and activates it.

Only the minor groove intercalated (2S,7R)-dynemicin *N*-hydroquinone and deschloro dynemicin L-enantiomers (18) or their diradical equivalent (79,81) produced a dynamically stable model (Fig. 13, see color plate) that is consistent with the affinity cleavage results. Furthermore, the (2S,7R)-enantiomers intercalate in the DNA with the long axis of dynemicin perpendicular to the intercalation cleft base pairs, and the helix twist and base pair rise of the MD-equilibrated complexes (18) are consistent with the intercalation mode, helix twist, and base pair rise found in the daunomycin- (41–44) and adriamycin-DNA (44) crystal complexes. These results strongly predict that the (2S,7R)-enantiomer is the correct absolute stereochemical form of dynemicin. A synthetic analog of dynemicin A was recently reported that supports this stereochemical prediction (109).

The intercalation of dynemicin N hydroquinone [**18**], deschloro dynemicin L [**19**] the epoxide hydroquinone [**14**] is stabilized by strong van der Waals and hydrogen-bonding interactions between the 5'-Py-Pu intercalation cleft and the diol hydroquinone or the alcohol quinone ring systems, which provide the binding energy to anchor the activated drug in or near the proper reading frame for efficient DNA hydrogen abstraction. Changing the bases in the preferred sequence would reduce the number of hydrogen bonds (decrease the binding energy) and/ or change the reading frame, making DNA hydrogen abstraction less efficient (18,81). The intercalation of the quinone methide [**15**] is also stabilized by van der Waals and electrostatic interaction.

The position of the quinone methide in the intercalation cleft places C8 up off of the floor and in about the center of the minor groove of the DNA, which makes it highly accessible and directionally correct for nucleophilic attack by bulk water (18,79) or other nucleophiles (110) (Figs. 6, 12, 13). On the other hand, the hydrogen bonds observed between the quinone methide and the DNA backbone could assist in the rearrangement to the alcohol [**17**] (18). In addition, as dynemicin A is activated to the diradical intermediate, it develops a right-handed twist and becomes more complementary to the right-handed B-DNA. This suggests that the DNA may be acting as a self-immolative catalyst by way of deprotonation and/or reprotonation and as a chiral catalyst (18,99,111,112) leading to the diradical transition state and DNA hydrogen abstraction.

B.   DNA–Esperamicin A₁ Complex

In constructing the model of the DNA-esperamicin complex, several modes of binding were considered, including a minor groove binder, four different intercalation modes, and minor-major groove binder as well as several variations of both the minor and major-minor groove binders (78). However, only two of the models warrant further discussion.

Of the four different intercalation models, only the model based on the d(CG)-proflavine intercalation cleft geometry (113) produced a model that correctly predicted the abstraction of a C5'-hydrogen (Fig. 14, see color plate). In this model the anthranilate moiety is intercalated into the binding cleft, where its aromatic ring sets between A:4 and A:5 of the upper strand of the d(CGCAATCCTG) · d(CAGGATTGCG) (Fig. 11) (73) oligonucleotide, and the long axis of the anthranilate is approximately parallel with the long axis of the DNA base pairs. The deoxyfucose sets in the minor groove, closer to the lower strand, with its 1^{iv},4^{iv}-axis approximately perpendicular to the groove. Its 4^{iv}-hydroxyl forms a hydrogen bond with the 2-carbonyl of T:17, and C6^{iv} is located almost equally distant from C5′ of G:18 and C4′ of T:17. The core is bound across the minor groove positioning the radicals at C3 and C6 close to and directionally aligned to abstract H1′ of T:16 and H5″ (pro-S) of C:8, respectively. The orientation of the core within the minor groove is stabilized by hydrogen bonds between its C10NH and C1-hydroxyl to O3′ of C:7 and T:16, respectively. The hydroxylamino sugar, unexpectedly, lies flat in the minor groove one water molecule above the floor. Its C3′-hydroxyl hydrogen bonds with O2P of T:9, and C6′ is positioned near C4′ and C5′ of the deoxyribose of T:16 on the opposite strand. The thiomethyl sugar is sandwiched in the minor groove between the DNA backbones where its 3″-axial hydroxyl group can form a hydrogen bond with N3 of G:14 or O4′ of A:15. The isopropylamino sugar is located near the lip of the minor groove so that the ammonium group can form a salt bridge (100) with O2P of the C:8 phosphate group.

The esperamicin minor-major groove model also proved to be of interest. It places the radicals at C3 and C6 near and directionally aligned to abstract DNA hydrogen from C5′ of T:17 and C:8, respectively (Fig. 15, see color plate). This model has a lot in common with the intercalation model. The placement of the trisaccharide (thiomethyl, hydroxylamino, and isopropylamino sugars) with respect to the DNA is for the most part unchanged, however, the orientation of the core within the minor groove and position of the deoxyfucose and anthranilate moieties has changed. In the minor-major groove complex the thiomethyl sugar and hydroxylamino sugar interact with the DNA floor and backbone, respectively, as described for the intercalation model with the exception that the hydroxylamino sugar does not penetrate as deeply into the minor groove. Due to the shallow binding of the hydroxylamino sugar, the isopropylamino sugar develops greater VDW contact with the deoxyribose of C:8 when forming a salt bridge (100) between its C4‴ ammonium group and O1P of the T:9 phosphate group. The core occupies the space in the minor groove approximately equally distant between C5′ and C:8 and T:17 and the tertiary hydroxyl at C1 hydrogen bonds with O3′ of T:16. The bulky deoxyfucose group and the stereochemistry at C12 forces the diradical-containing ring to point into and slightly down the minor groove (in the 3′ direction relative to C5′ of T:17 and away from the trisaccharide group). The deoxyfucose forms a bridge across the DNA backbone between the core in the minor groove and the anthranilate moiety in the major groove. The deoxyfucose resides over the deoxyribose of T:17 between the two phosphate groups of T:17 and G:18. The anthranilate moiety lies to one side of the major groove interacting predominantly with the major groove side of the DNA backbone. The pyruvate group sits within 3.5–4.0 Å of the T:17 C5-methyl and hydrogen bonds and O1P of T:17 via its amide hydrogen. At the other end of the anthranilate, the methoxy group at C11^{iv} accepts a hydrogen bond from the 4-amino group of C:19 and its methoxy group at C10^{iv} is approximately 3.15 Å from C2′ of G:18. The anthranilate aromatic ring hovers over the major groove face of G:18. The C8 hydrogen of G:18 and C2′ hydrogens of T:17 are within the anthranilate shielding cone.

In both binding modes the conformation and geometric relationship between the bound core, deoxyfucose, and anthranilate moieties very closely mimic that found in the x-ray structure of esperamicin X (11). Only slight tweaking of the C12-O12 and O12-C1^{iv} dihedral angles is needed to convert the x-ray conformation into either the intercalation or minor-major groove-binding conformation. Additionally, the geometry of the hydroxylamino and thiomethyl sugars and their arrangement relative to one another is very similar to that found in the crystalline environment of dihydrocalicheamicin pseudoaglycon (13), i.e., their planes, defined by C2, C3, C5, and O5, are approximately perpendicular to one another (Fig. 16, see color plate).

The only problem with the energy-minimized intercalation and minor-major groove models is that they portray esperamicin A$_1$ as a double-strand–cleaving molecule that produces cut sites staggered by three (intercalation) or four (minor-major) base pairs in the 3′ direction. While esperamicin has been shown to produce strong cuts at all of these sites (Fig. 11) (73,78), these cuts presumably occur via different molecules, as esperamicin causes predominantly single strand breaks.

Due to the multiminima problem often associated with energy-minimization studies, each model complex was subjected to both vacuum and solvated molecular dynamics of 100 psec or more. None of the vacuum simulations provided a stable molecular dynamics run that was consistent with the available experimental data, suggesting the importance of structural water molecules for stabilizing the DNA-esperamicin complex. The distance and angle between the radical centers and the three closest abstractable hydrogens were monitored (18,78) to determine which, if any, of the models would fit the experimental data.

The greatest changes occurred in the minor-major groove-binding complex at the onset of the dynamics simulation demonstrating how easy it is to get trapped in a local minima using energy-minimization techniques (18,114,115). While most of the individual DNA conformational and helicoidal parameters stabilized by the end of the equilibration phase (first 15 psec) of the calculation, a gradual change occurred in the complex throughout the first 65 psec of the dynamics trajectory. By the end of the equilibration phase the drug had settled into the binding pocket. The combined minor conformational changes in the DNA and drug that occurred during the dynamic dance at the onset of the run repositioned the C6 radical so that it no longer was correctly positioned for DNA hydrogen abstraction. The radical at C3, however, remained firmly planted for the abstraction of a C5′ hydrogen from T:17 (Fig. 17, Tables 3 and 4). The intercalation model, on the other hand, was found to be quite stable throughout the molecular dynamics simulation, and, contrary to the experimental data, this model strongly predicts that esperamicin A$_1$ should cause a double strand break by abstracting a C5′ hydrogen from one strand and a C1′ hydrogen from the opposite strand that is staggered by three base pairs in the 3′ direction (Fig. 17, Tables 3 and 4).

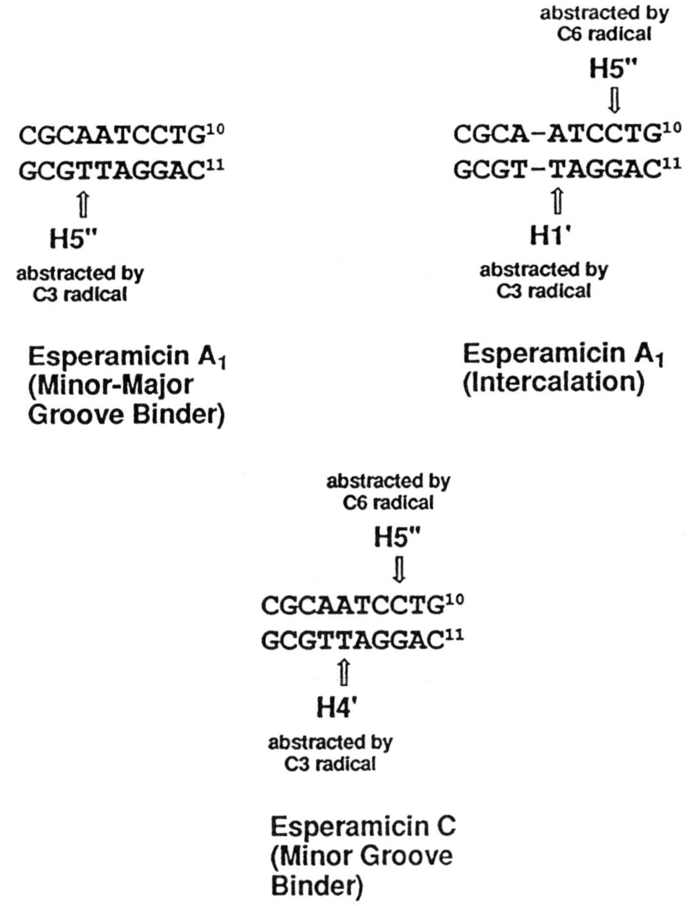

Figure 17 Predicted hydrogen atom abstraction pattern by the esperamicin A₁ (minor-major and intercalation binding modes) and esperamicin C when bound with their trisaccharide tails pointing in the 3′ direction relative to the top strand.

The minor-major groove-binding motif is further supported experimentally by the osmium tetraoxide experiments (78). In this binding mode the drug binds to B-form double-stranded DNA and causes only minor perturbations in the DNA groove structure. While one face of the thymine C5-C6 double bond is sterically blocked by the DNA base to its 5′ side, due to DNA's right-handed helical twist, the 3′ face is approachable from the major groove in both naked and esperamicin C–complexed DNA. However, in the DNA–esperamicin A₁ complex the approach to both the 5′ and 3′ faces of T:17 is completely blocked (Fig. 18,

Table 3 Average Distance (Å) Between the Esperamicin Radical Centers and Closest Three Abstractable Hydrogens

	A	B
C6-H5″/C:8	4.20	2.83
C6-H5′/C:8		4.08
C6-H1′/C:7		3.25
C6-H8/esp	2.70	
C6-H1′/esp	2.80	
C6-WH1	3.04	
C6-WH2	3.28	
H8/esp-WO	2.83	
C3-H5″/T:17	2.81	
C3-H5′/T:17	2.83	
C3-H4′/C:17	3.11	
C3-H1′/T:16		2.68
C3-H4′/T:16		3.19
C3-H3^{iv}/esp		3.82

(A) From the minor-major groove binding model. (B) From the intercalation model. WH1, WH2, and WHO are from an ordered water molecule.

Table 4 Average Angle (degree) Between the Esperamicin Radical Centers and Closest Three Abstractable Hydrogens

	A	B
C6-H5″/C:8	141.8	163.9
C6-H5′/C:8		144.2
C6-H1′/C:7		126.5
C6-H8/esp	104.0	
C6-H1′/esp	110.0	
C6-WH1	150.6	
C6-WH2	151.5	
H8/esp-WO	153.0	
C3-H5″/T:17	159.0	
C3-H5′/T:17	163.5	
C3-H4′/C:17	128.2	
C3-H1′/T:16		142.8
C3-H4′/T:16		144.7
C3-H3^{iv}/esp		124.8

(A) From the minor-major groove binding model. (B) From the intercalation model. WH1, WH2, and WHO are from an ordered water molecule.

see color plate). The intercalative mode of binding, on the other hand, offers little or no protection to the thymine double bond. In addition, the intercalative mode of binding disrupts the DNA groove structure in the vicinity of the intercalation site causing both the major and minor grooves to widen. The intercalation of esperamicin A_1 into the 5'-ApA/3'-TpT step increases the exposure of the 3' face of T:16 and T:17 to the surrounding environment. Due to this disruption in the groove structure, one would not expect reduced levels of oxidation for the DNA–esperamicin A_1 complex but instead would predict higher or at best equal levels of oxidation when compared with naked DNA.

The minor-major groove-binding model also suggests a plausible explanation as to how esperamicin A_1 is degraded during the CT-DNA cleavage reaction. The core, deoxyfucose, and anthranilate act as a C-clamp around the deoxyribose of T:17, firmly planting the radical at C3 of the core for highly efficient DNA hydrogen abstraction from C5' of T:17. However, the C6 radical is ill positioned for DNA hydrogen abstraction and is exposed to the solvent. The closest and most directionally aligned hydrogen is from an ordered water molecule (Fig. 19, see color plate; Tables 3 and 4). The quenching of the C6 radical (**29**, Scheme IV) to produce the hydroxyl radical [**30**] is energetically disfavored by 4.22 kcal/mol (AM1-CI) (116,117), however, the caged hydroxyl radical is well positioned for abstraction of the C8 hydrogen producing **31**. The overall reaction (**29** → **31**) is favored by –28.94 kcal/mol. Oxidation of the C8 radical [**31**] followed by homolytic cleavage of the core C8-O-glycosidic linkage would generate the hemiacetal [**23**] and after rearrangement to an aldehyde and a Schiff base reaction with the NO-glycosidic linkage would produce the carbinolamine [**24**] form of the trisaccharide, the major isolated esperamicin product from the CT-DNA-esperamicin cleavage reaction.

While the intercalation model does not appear to fit the current experimental data, we are reluctant to exclude it as a possible mode of binding. The coupled kinetics analysis (62,65) of the DNA cleavage by esperamicin A_1 showed predominantly single-strand cleavage. However, the ratio of the rate constants suggests that some double-strand cuts may take place. Additionally, it should be noted that the OsO_4 experiments only provided information about the region of the DNA-esperamicin complex around thymine residues. Finally, the modeling study focused on a single esperamicin-binding site (a site that placed the intercalation cleft at a 5'-AA step) (78). Given the existence of sequence-dependent DNA structure and the preference for Gs and/or Cs at intercalation sites, we cannot rule out the possibility of the intercalation mode of binding or sequence-dependent modes of binding.

In the model of the DNA–esperamicin C complex (Fig. 20, see color plate) the core is positioned in the minor groove of the DNA so that the radicals at C3

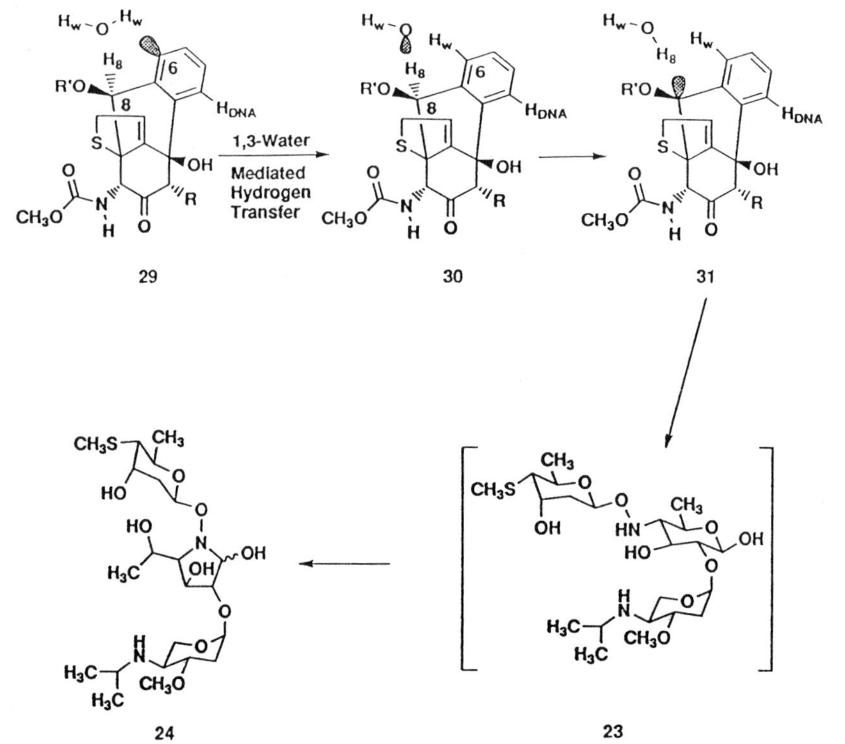

29   30   31

24   23

Scheme IV Proposed mechanism for the homolytic cleavage of the C8-O-glycosidic bond of esperamicin observed in the DNA cleavage experiments.

and C6 are near and directionally aligned for the abstraction of the 4′ hydrogen from T:16 and 5″ hydrogen (pro S) from C:8, respectively (Fig. 17). The concomitant abstraction of H4′ and H5″ would produce a DNA double-strand break with a 3-base-pair stagger in the 3′ direction, which is consistent with the observed cleavage pattern for esperamicin C (65,72–75) and calicheamicin (61,68, 69,89,90,101). The diradical-containing ring of esperamicin C is pointed almost directly into the minor groove of the DNA (Fig. 20), but more importantly the C12 hydroxyl is hydrogen bonding with O2P of T:17. For esperamicin A_1 to cause concomitant double-strand breaks with the same cutting pattern as esperamicin C, the deoxyfucose would have to occupy the same space as the T:17 phosphate group. Instead, the core of esperamicin A_1 is turned slightly in the minor groove, relative to esperamicin C, so that the deoxyfucose can sit between the phosphate groups of G:18 and T:17 and over the deoxyribose of T:17. The binding orientation of the esperamicin A_1 core within the minor groove positions the C3 radical for highly efficient hydrogen abstraction from C5′ of T:17 (Fig. 17), while the C6 radical is ill positioned for DNA hydrogen abstraction and ultimately leads to the fragmentation of esperamicin.

The short lifespan of the diradical (112) suggests that only the activation of enediyne-containing drug bound to or at least very near the DNA will produce DNA strand breaks. An examination of the DNA–esperamicin A_1 model (Fig. 15) shows that the methyl trisulfide is pointing into the surrounding environment, making it highly accessible for reductive activation. This suggests that esperamicin can bind with DNA prior to activation.

C. DNA–Calicheamicin γ_1^I Complex

Two modeling studies (68,88) were reported previous to our work (104) that describe the DNA-calicheamicin complex. However, both of these models have been found (at least in part) to be inconsistent with the experimental evidence available prior and subsequent to their publication. The Schreiber model (88) places the drug along the minor groove so that the polysaccharide tail is bound within the 5′-TCCT preferred binding sequence but uses a boat conformation for the hydroxyamino sugar. The crystal structure of dihydrocalicheamicin pseudoaglycon (13) (Fig. 16) had previously shown this sugar to exist in the expected chair conformation. More recently, NMR studies (107) have confirmed the chair conformation for all of the calicheamicin sugars in three different solvents and at different temperatures. However, it should be noted that the model correctly predicted the correct absolute stereochemistry at C8 of the aglycone and the abstraction of the H5″ (pro-S) hydrogen from the 5′-C of the TCCT-binding site. In the second model, reported by the Lederle group (68), calicheamicin is docked into the minor groove, but resides almost entirely to the 5′ side and out of the preferred binding sequence. While the two models differ in several ways, they both place the iodine of the thiobenzoate near the floor of the minor groove. Both of these models may contain valuable insights into the DNA-calicheamicin complex, but because of their inconsistencies with the experimental data and each other it is difficult to know what to take from them. This prompted our study (104) of the DNA-calicheamicin complex.

The initial docking of the core, hydroxylamino sugar, and ethylamino sugar residues was based on our DNA–esperamicin C model (78). The CORE sets in the minor groove positioning C3 and C6 (radical-bearing carbons) for the abstraction of the DNA H4′ of T:18 and H5″ of C:6 of the oligonucleotide (d(CGA-CTCCTGC) · d(GCAGGAGTCG), respectively (Fig. 21). Additionally, the C1-hydroxyl hydrogen bonds with O3′ of T:18. The hydroxylamino sugar lies flat in the mouth of the minor groove approximately one or two water layers above the floor with its 1′,4′-axis parallel with the groove floor. Its methyl group (C6′) sits near the deoxyribose of T:18 and its C3′-hydroxyl hydrogen bonds with O2P

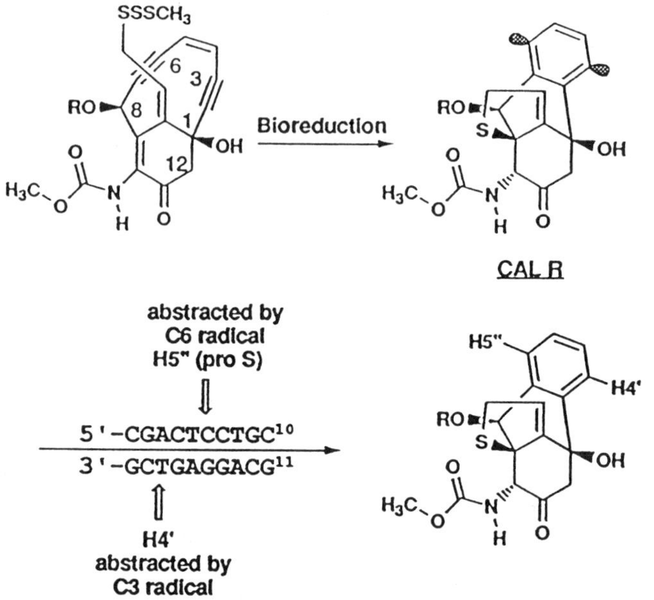

Figure 21 Mechanism of activation for calicheamicin and predicted cleavage sights within the modeled DNA sequence.

of C:7. The ethylamino sugar hovers at the lip of the minor groove over the deoxyribose of C:6 and forms a hydrogen bond/salt bridge (100) with O5′ and O2P of the C:6 phosphate group. The differences in the models were designed to systematically investigate the interactions of the thiosugar, thiobenzoate, and rhamnose moieties with the minor groove of the DNA. In the first four models the rhamnose moiety was docked into the DNA with its methyl group (C6^v) pointing into the groove and is positioned near O2 of T:8 and H2 of A:13. The first four models are (1) the IH_in model (Fig. 22), which places both the iodine and 3″ hydroxyl near the floor of the minor groove, (2) the IH_out model, which points both groups out of the minor groove, (3) the I_out/H_in model, and (4) the I_in/H_out model, which alternately points one group in and the other out of the minor groove. In the last two models the rhamnose moiety was docked into the DNA with its methoxy group at C3^v pointing into the minor groove and the hydroxyl groups at C2^v and C4^v set near and hydrogen bonded with O4′ of G:15 and O3′ of G:9, respectively. Additionally, the thiosugar was docked with its 3″ hydroxyl near the floor of the minor groove where it hydrogen bonds with N3 of A:17. In models (5) the I_in model and (6) the I_out model, the iodine is alternately placed pointing in or out of the minor groove as their names imply. The last two possibilities, I_in′ and I_out′ (Fig. 22a), were not modeled due to

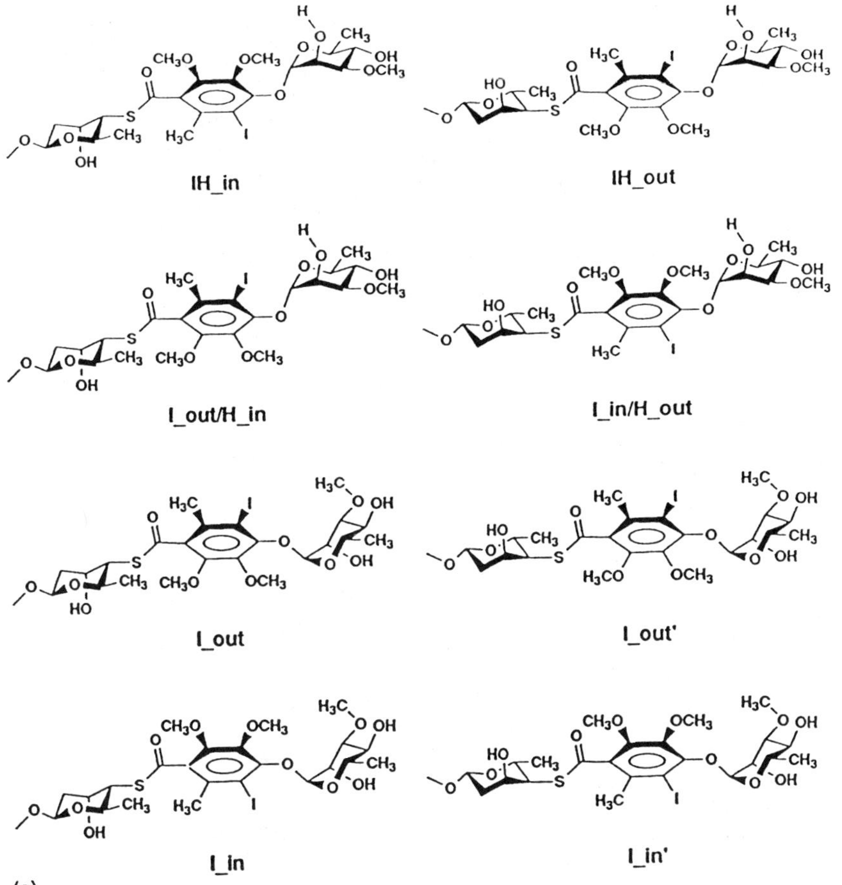

Figure 22 (a) Eight possible models resulting from the binding perturbations of the thiosugar, thiobenzoate, and rhamnose. (b) Graphical representation of the DNA-calicheamicin (I_out) model. (c) Graphical representation of the DNA minor groove width for the I_out model over the last 400 psec. The width is determined by monitoring the closest interstrand phosphate distances as determined from canonical B-form DNA. The lower (nonattached) horizontal bars are the phosphate distances (11.46 Å) from canonical B-form DNA.

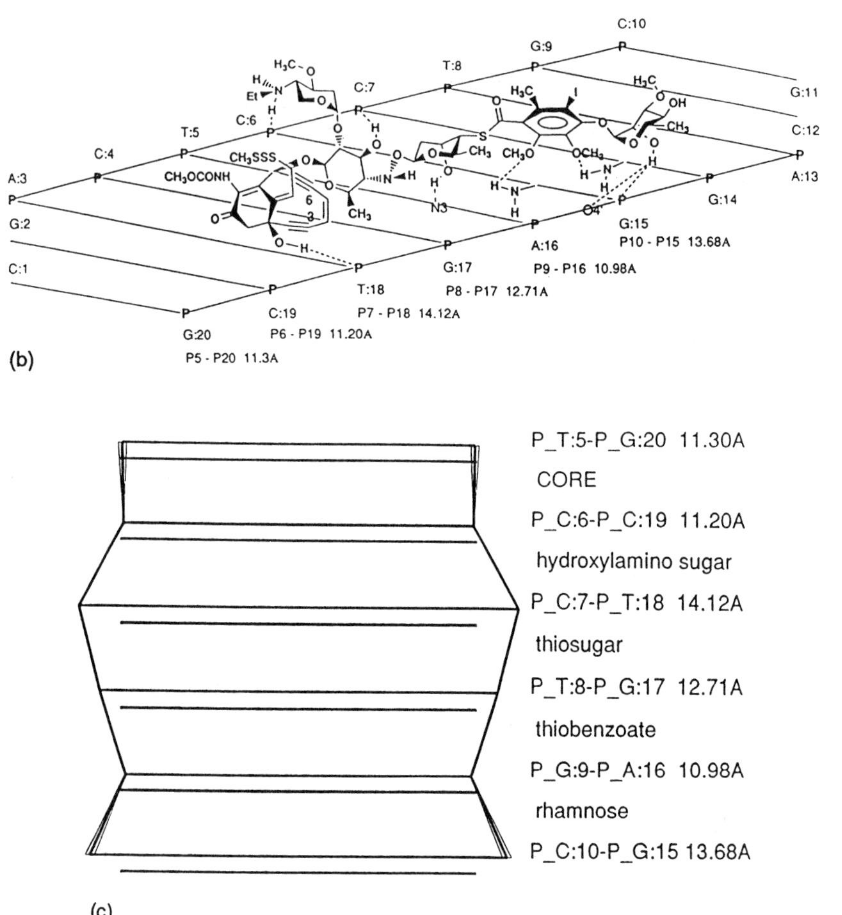

Figure 22 Continued.

the instability of the IH_out and I_in/H_out models and their lack of consistency with either the x-ray crystal structure of dihydrocalicheamicin pseudoaglycon (13) or our DNA-esperamicin (78) model.

Each complex was submitted to 515 psec of solvated molecular dynamics. In the first 115 psec, a soft distance constraint (118) of 2.7(+0.1 or –2.7) Å with a 1 kcal/mol at 300 K force constant was used between the calicheamicin radicals at C3 and C6 and the DNA H4′ of T:18 and H5″ of C:6, respectively, to equilibrate the complexes with experimental points of reference. The final 400 psec of the MD runs were conducted without constraints.

The distance and angle (18,78,104) between the carbon-centered radicals and the three closest DNA hydrogens were monitored as a function of time to determine which if any of the models would remain consistent with the experimental hydrogen abstraction data. The average distance and angle between the radical centers and the three closest DNA hydrogens with respect to each radical are presented in Tables 5 and 6, respectively.

All six models, like the Schreiber model (88), correctly predict the H5″ (pro-S) of C:6 as the prime candidate for abstraction by the radical at C6 (Tables 2 and 3). However, the prediction of which DNA hydrogen will be abstracted by the C3 radical varies between models. Only the IH_out model clearly does not correctly predict the abstraction of the H4′ of T:18. The IH_in model equally predicts the H4′ and H5″ of T:18, however, since the H4′ is tertiary it should be energetically easier to abstract. The I_out/H_in, I_in/H_out, I_in, and I_out models all cleanly predict the correct abstraction of the H4′ of T:18. Therefore, all but the IH_out model must be considered as possible modes of binding solely based on the hydrogen abstraction data. While the minor groove width, within the drug-binding site, for all of the DNA-calicheamicin (Fig. 22b) and DNA-esperamicin models is larger than that found in canonical B-form DNA, only the I_out/H_in, I_in/H_out and IH_in models produce large to very large bulges in the DNA around the thiobenzoate and rhamnose, thio, and rhamnose sugars and rhamnose moiety, respectively. This leaves the I_in and I_out models as primary candidates for the DNA-calicheamicin complex.

The molecular interactions between 5′-TCCT/3′-AGGA sequence and calicheamicin from the I_out model provide a clear and simple rational for the observed 5′-TCCT sequence specificity (Fig. 23, see color plate). The thiosugar C3″-hydroxyl hydrogen bonds with N3 of the A:16. Additionally, the thiosugar C2″-methylene sets near the C2 methine of A:16 sterically selecting against a guanine at this site. The thiobenzoate methoxy groups at C2^{iv} and C3^{iv} set near the floor of the minor groove and accept a hydrogen bond from the 2-amino group of G:15 and G:14, respectively. The rhamnose binds in the minor groove in a way that places its C3^{v}-methoxy approximately an equal distance between the 2-carbonyl of T:8 and the C2-methine of A:13, which sterically selects for the T/A base. This binding orientation of the rhamnose sugar is further stabilized by a hydrogen bond between the C2^{v}-hydroxyl groups and O4′ of G:15. The carbohydrate-thiobenzoate tail reads the DNA-recognition elements along the floor of the 3′-AGGA strand. Since the binding site is not palindromic, the recognition elements are different when viewed from different directions, resulting in the observed unidirectional mode of binding. While this model provides a straightforward explanation for 5′-TCCT sequence specificity, it does not explain the high specificity for 5′-TTTT sequences.

In the I_in model (Fig. 24, see color plate), the nonbonded interactions between the core and hydroxylamino, thio, and ethylamino sugars of calicheamicin

Table 5 Average Distance (Å) Between the Calicheamicin Radical Centers and Closest Three DNA Hydrogens

	L_out/H_in	IH_in	L_in/H_out	IH_out	L_in	L_out
C6-H5″/C:6	2.79	3.05	2.87	2.73	2.61	2.65
C6-H5′/C:6	3.88	3.61	3.71	3.82	3.55	3.66
C6-H4′/C:5	4.33	4.56	4.14	4.29	4.13	4.38
C3-H4′/T:18	2.74	3.10	2.80	7.65	2.68	2.81
C3-H1′/T:18	3.45	5.61	3.47	7.79	3.43	3.30
C3-H5″/C:19	3.03	3.10	3.12	8.24	3.15	3.23

In some of the models the C6-H1′/C:6 distance was found to be slightly closer than C6-H4′/C:5.

COLOR PLATES

Figure 5 Stereo views of energy-minimized complex between esperamicin diradical intermediate and d(CGCAATCCTG)·d(CAGGATTGCG) duplex oligonucleotide. The coloring scheme for the DNA is blue for carbon, light green for nitrogen, yellow for oxygen, and amber for phosphate. The coloring scheme for esperamicin is green for carbon, red for oxygen, blue for nitrogen, and yellow for sulfur. All polar hydrogens are white. Nonpolar hydrogens were omitted for the sake of clarity. The DNA C:8 C5′-hydrogens and T:17 C5′-hydrogens as well as esperamicin C6 and C3, upper and lower, respectively, are purple. The white dotted lines depict hydrogen bonds. TMS = thiomethyl sugar; HAS = hydroxylamino sugar; IAS = isopropylamino sugar; CORE = aglycone; DF = deoxyfucose; AC = anthranilate.

Figure 6 Stereo view of the EM complex between (2S,7R)-dynemicin N-hydroquinone and the d(CTACT_ACTGG)·(CCAGT_AGTAG) duplex oligonucleotide. The coloring scheme for the DNA is the same as in Figure 5: carbon (green), nitrogen (blue), oxygen (red), hydrogen (white), and C27-H (left) and C24-H (right) bonds (violet). The white dotted lines represent hydrogen bonds.

Figure 12 The superimposed EM form of the diol [16] quasi-boat (green), quasi-chair (purple), and dynemicin N hydroquinone [18] (red) intercalated into the d(CTACT_ACTGG)·d(CCAGT_AGTAG) duplex DNA. The coloring scheme for the DNA is the same as in Figure 5. The red and white hydrogens of guanine 17 are H5" and H1′, and the yellow and green hydrogens of thymine 5 are H1′ and H2′, respectively. All polar hydrogens are white. Nonpolar hydrogens were omitted for the sake of clarity.

Figure 13 Composite of seven snapshots taken every 5 psec from the end of the molecular dynamics simulation.

Figure 14 Minimized average structure from the molecular dynamics simulation on the DNA-esperamicin intercalation complex. The color scheme is the same as in Figure 5. The C1′-hydrogen of T:16 is red (lower strand).

Figure 15 Energy-minimized structure of the DNA–esperamicin A_1 complex. The coloring scheme is the same as in Figure 5.

Figure 16 X-ray conformation of esperamicin X (11) and the hydroxylamino sugar, thiosugar, and thiobenzoate portion of dihydrocalicheamicin pseudoaglycon (13).

Figure 18 Major groove view of the DNA-esperamicin complex showing the protection of the 3′ face of T:17 by the anthranilate moiety. Coloring scheme is the same as in Figure 5. The C4-C5 double bond of T:16 and T:17 are colored red.

Figure 19 DNA-esperamicin–ordered water molecule complex, a snapshot of the 160-psec frame of the molecular dynamics simulation.

Figure 20 The DNA–esperamicin C complex. The color scheme is the same as in Figure 5, with the addition of the green H4′ T:16 hydrogen on the lower strand.

Figure 23 Stereo view of the average structure from the free molecular dynamics simulation on the I_out model. Coloring scheme for the DNA is the same as in Figure 5, except the calicheamicin radical centers at C3 (lower) and C6 (upper) are violet. H4′/ T:18 is red (lower strand), H5′ and H5″ of C:6 (upper strand) and C:19 (lower strand) are violet.

Figure 24 Stereo view of the average structure from the free molecular dynamics simulation on the I_in model. Coloring scheme for the DNA is the same as in Figure 5, except the calicheamicin radical centers at C3 (lower) and C6 (upper) are violet. H4′/ T:18 is red (lower strand), H5′ and H5″ of C:6 (upper strand) and C:19 (lower strand) are violet.

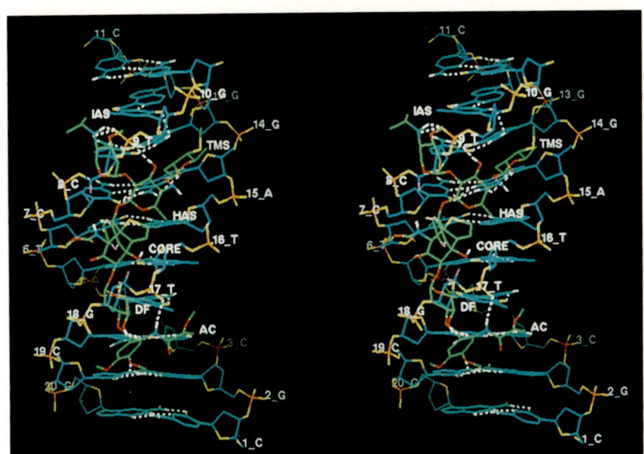

Figure 5

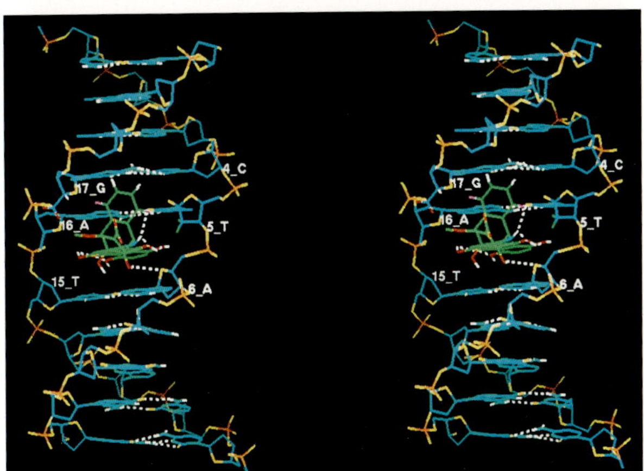

Figure 6

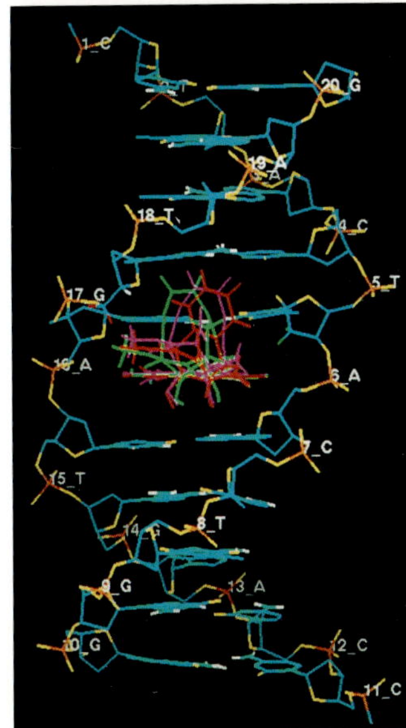

Figure 12

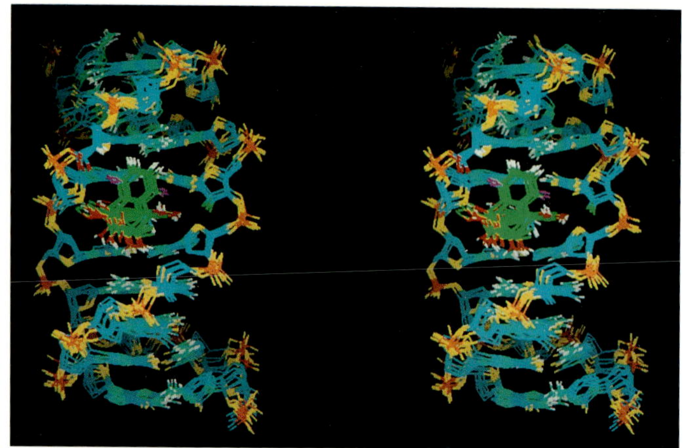

Figure 13

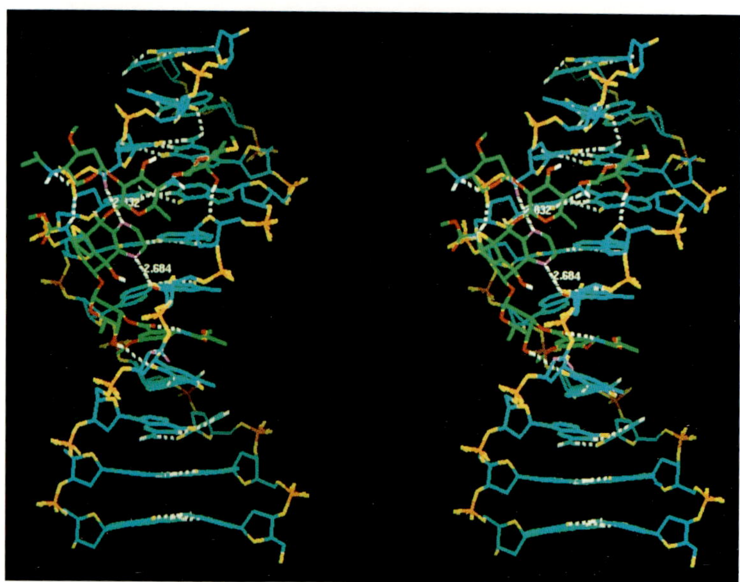

Figure 14

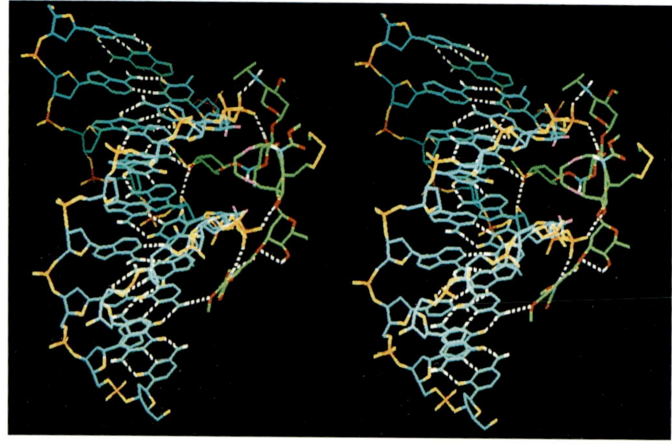

Figure 15

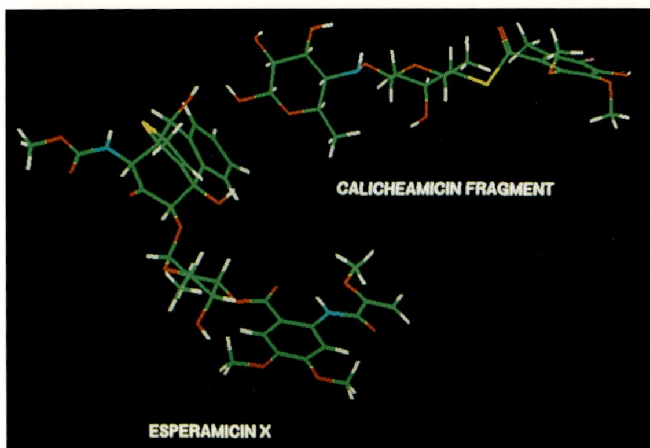

Figure 16

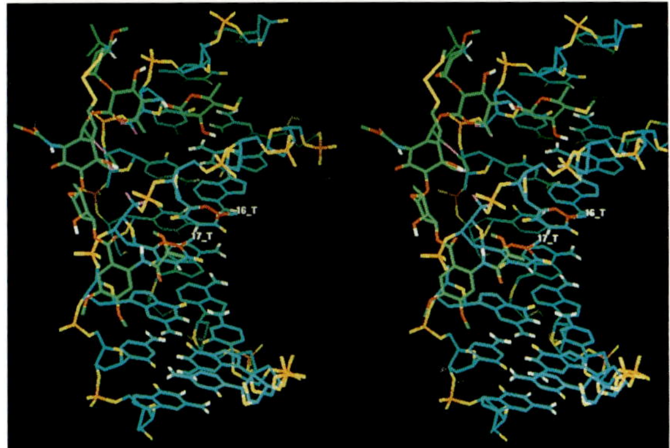

Figure 18

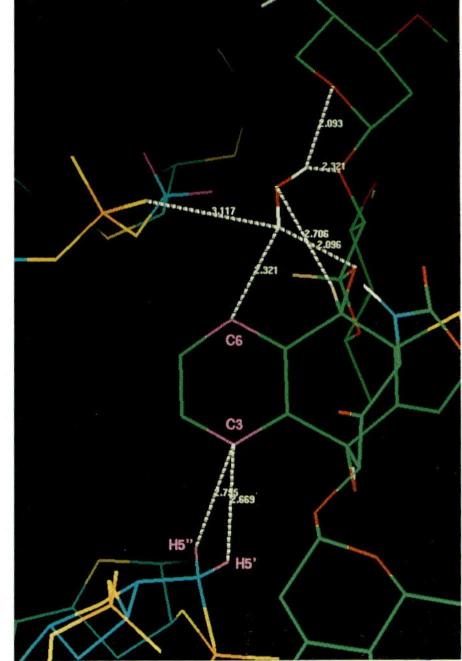

Figure 19

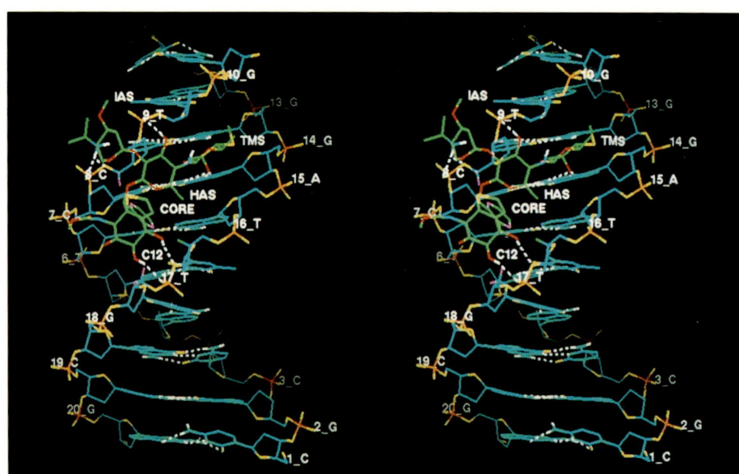

Figure 20

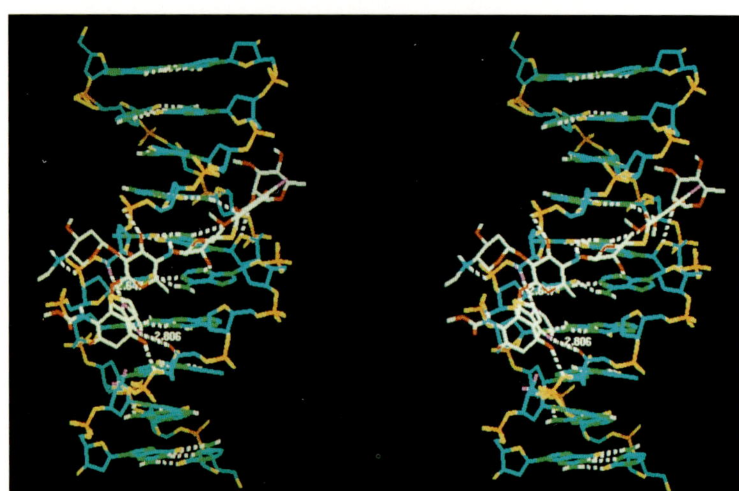

Figure 23

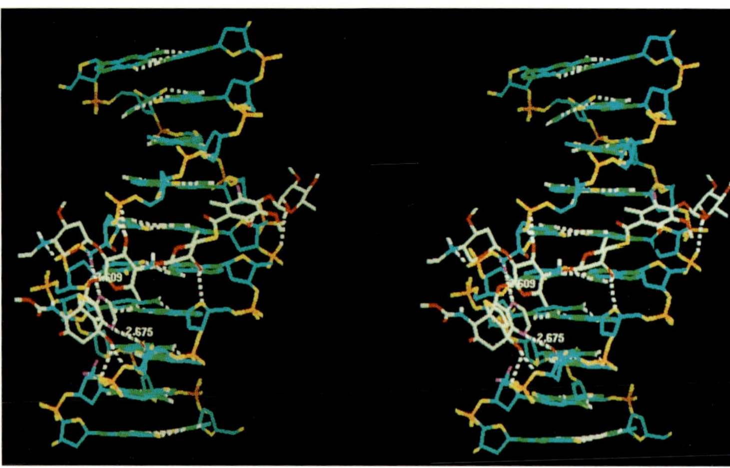

Figure 24

Table 6 Average Angle (degree) Between the Calicheamicin Radical Centers and Closest Three DNA Hydrogens

	I_out/H_in	IH_in	I_in/H_out	IH_out	I_in	I_out
C3-C6-H5″/C:6	153.9	142.9	155.6	160.9	171.5	170.5
C3-C6-H5′/C:6	148.4	170.3	161.2	158.7	159.6	159.1
C3-C6-H4′/C:5	127.6	146.6	163.9	165.6	108.8	111.7
C6-C3-H4′/T:18	135.9	132.2	128.9	110.8	136.1	143.8
C6-C3-H1′/T:18	129.3	128.9	137.3	107.4	129.0	134.5
C6-C3-H5″/C:19	128.6	132.0	133.9	132.7	124.4	121.3

and the DNA-binding site are for the most part unchanged from the I_out model. However, during the equilibration phase of the molecular dynamics run, the thiobenzoate turned and tilted so that its $C6^{iv}$-methyl sets deep in the minor groove close to the deoxyribose of C:7, near C1′ of C:7, and the $C5^{iv}$-I bond is parallel to the floor of the minor groove. The iodine moved away from the C:7-G:15 base pair and into the plane of the C:8-G:14 base pair and is the closest calicheamicin atom to the T:9-A:13 base pair. Accompanying the relocation of the thiobenzoate is the movement of the rhamnose sugar away from the floor of the minor groove. It settled down near the lower strand of the DNA where its $C2^{v}$-hydroxyl hydrogen bonds with O2P of A:16. The reorganization of the thiobenzoate is presumably due to steric crowding and electrostatic replusion between the 2-amino groups of G:17 and G:18 and the $C6^{iv}$-methyl and C^{iv}-iodine of the thiobenzoate. The crystal structures of *p*-iodobenzontrile and the 1:1 iodoform/quinoline complex illustrate the attractive interaction between iodine and the electronegative sp^1 or sp^2 nitrogen (88) and suggests that an aromatic iodine has a positive partial charge. The partial charge on the iodine of iodiobenzene is predicted to be +0.02, +0.12, and +0.12 by PM3, MNDO, and MNDO/3 (MOPAC 6.0) (116,117), respectively. While this model proved to be stable, it does not provide an explanation for the 5′-TCCT sequence specificity beyond the shape complementarity between the DNA helix and groove structure and the drug. The lack of the exocyclic C2-amino group on adenine reduces both the steric hindrance (119) and electrostatic potential (120) for A-T base pairs near the floor of the DNA minor groove. This suggests that the structural and electrostatic characteristics of the 5′-TTTT–binding site (69) are more suitable for the binding of calicheamicin when its iodine is turned into and near the floor of the minor groove (104).

The I_out model suggests that when the appropriate edge of the thiosugar, thiobenzoate, and rhamnose sets near the floor of the minor groove of the 5′-TCCT/3′-AGGA, they act as anchors to the 3′-A, GG, and A bases of the preferred binding/cleavage site, respectively. However, this part of the carbohydrate-thiobenzoate tail does not appear to affect the conformation or binding orientation of the core, hydroxylamino sugar, and ethylamino sugar. This is apparent from the lack of perturbation to the predicted cleavage pattern exhibited by the different models (Tables 5 and 6). These results suggest that the thiobenzoate is the DNA anchor. It determines 50% of the preferred binding site and may be partly responsible for holding the thiosugar and rhamnose in place for the determination of the remainder of the binding domain.

The core, hydroxylamino sugar, and ethylamino sugar residues of calicheamicin, like esperamicin C (66,78), esperamicin D (66), and calicheamicin T (69), bind with the DNA almost exclusively via the DNA backbone. The orthogonal relationship between the thiosugar and the hydroxylamino sugar is very similar to that found in the crystal structure of the dihydrocalicheamicin pseudoaglycon (13) and our esperamicin models (78). The NO-glycosidic link between the hydroxylamino and thiomethyl sugars appears to serve two important roles. It functions as an extended linker, which permits the thiosugar, thiobenzoate, and rhamnose fragment to read the DNA minor groove (imparting sequence specifity) and at the same time allows the core to be positioned for the abstraction of DNA hydrogens. Additionally, the NO-glycosidic link permits the conformation of the hydroxylamino-thiomethyl disaccharide to adopt an energy minima in which the two residues are orthogonal to one another. This minima is stabilized by the 4'NH and C1'''O5''' antiparallel dipole (121). The hydroxylamino sugar lies flat in the mouth of the minor groove, one to two water layers above the floor of the groove. Its C3'-hydroxyl group hydrogen bonds with O2P of C:7, while its methyl group (C6') sets nearly equidistant from C4' of G:17 and C5' of T:18 and points at the T:18 phosphate group. The unusual binding orientation of the hydroxylamino sugar may be partially responsible for the wider minor groove (note P_C:7-P_T:18 distance, Fig. 22c), which in turn allows the esperamicin and calicheamicin COREs to achieve binding positions in the minor groove that are suitable for simultaneous hydrogen abstraction from each strand of the DNA.

The core and hydroxylamino sugar (in both the calicheamicin and esperamicin models) float one to two water layers above the floor of the minor groove and only directly interact with the DNA backbone. The spine of hydration that runs between the floor of the minor groove and the core and hydroxylamino sugar interacts with the drug and DNA in a specific manner that stabilizes the complex and may assist in the positioning of the core for highly efficient DNA hydrogen abstraction. The nature of the spine of hydration that runs along the minor groove of DNA has been shown to be sequence dependent (122,123). The modeling studies along with the cleavage affinity experiments suggest that the sequence specificity observed for the esperamicins and calicheamicins is partly due to the drug's ability to read the DNA groove structure or inducible structure (69) as well as the spine of hydration that runs along the minor groove floor (78). DNA footprinting studies carried out on the aryl tetrasaccharide portion of calicheamicin (102,103) supports this hypothesis. The removal of the bulky CORE from calicheamicin should allow the hydroxylamino sugar to slip deeper into the minor groove of DNA sequences with "normal" or energetically noninducible wider grooves. This should not change the sequence specificity, which is predominantly selected for by the aryl tetrasaccharide tail, but should allow additional sequences to be occupied.

X. SUMMARY

The enediyne class of natural products are an extremely interesting group of structurally diverse molecules, which derive their antitumor activity by causing single- and/or double-strand DNA breaks. The synthetic, biophysical, and structural studies that have resulted from their discovery have produced new synthetic methodologies and increased our understanding of different mechanisms of activation and DNA cleavage by carbon-centered radicals. The DNA affinity cleavage experiments and modeling studies have provided insights into the process of molecular recognition. Additionally, the molecular dynamic simulations have demonstrated the flexible and dynamic nature of DNA and shown how the unique structure, stereochemistry, and substitution pattern of each enediyne gives it the required conformation and dynamic freedom about that conformation to dance with its biological host. The knowledge gained to date has provided invaluable insights into the process of molecular recognition, particularly between polysaccharides and DNA and into the organizational requirements for effective site-specific cleavage of DNA by aryl diradicals. These insights and new methodologies are paving the way for the design and preparation of novel DNA-binding antitumor and antiviral drugs.

REFERENCES

1. M. Konishi, H. Ohkuma, K.-I. Saitoh, and H. Kawaguchi, *J. Antibiot., 38,* 1605 (1985).
2. K. S. Lam, S. Forenza, J. A. Veitch, D. R. Gustavson, J. Golik, and T. W. Doyle, *Novel Microbial Products for Medicine and Agriculture* (Nash, C. H., Hunter-Cevera, J. C., Cooper R., Eveleigh, D. E., and Hamill, R. eds.), William C. Brown, Dubuque, IA, Vol. 32: 261–274, 1993.
3. J. Golik, J. Clardy, G. Dubay, G. Groenewold, H. Kawaguchi, M. Konishi, B. Krishnan, H. Ohkuma, K. I. Saitoh, and T. W. Doyle, *J. Am. Chem. Soc., 109,* 3461 (1987).
4. J. Golik, G. Dubay, G. Groenewold, H. Kawaguchi, M. Konishi, B. Krishnan, H. Ohkuma, K. I. Saitoh, and T. W. Doyle, *J. Am. Chem. Soc., 109,* 3462 (1987).
5. J. Golik, J. A. Beutler, P. Clark, J. Ross, J. Roach, W. B. Lebherz III, and G. Muschik, Applied U.S. Patent USSN323648 (1989).
6. J. Goli, H. Wong, D. M. Vyas, and T. W. Doyle, *Tetrahedron Lett., 30,* 2497 (1989).
7. M. D. Whitman, R. L. Halcomb, S. J. Danishefsky, J. Golik, and D. M. Vays, *J. Org. Chem., 55,* 1979 (1990).
8. J. Golik, T. W. Doyle, G. VanDuyne, and J. Clardy, *Tetrahedron Lett., 43,* 6149 (1990).
9. R. L. Halcomb, M. D. Whitman, S. H. Olson, S. J. Danishefsky, J. Golik, H. Wong, and D. M. Vyas, *J. Am. Chem. Soc., 113,* 5080 (1991).
10. J. Golik, H. Wong, B. Krishnan, D. M. Vyas, and T. W. Doyle, *Tetrahedron Lett., 32,* 1851 (1991).
11. J. Golik, B. Krishnan, T. W. Doyle, G. VanDuyne, and J. Clardy, *Tetrahedron Lett., 41,* 6049 (1992).
12. M. D. Lee, T. S. Dunne, M. M. Siegal, C. C. Chang, G. O. Morton, and D. B. Borders, *J. Am. Chem. Soc., 109,* 3464 (1987).

13. M. D. Lee, T. S. Dunne, C. C. Chang, G. A. Ellestad, M. M. Siegel, G. O. Morton, W. J. McGahren, and D. B. Borders, *J. Am. Chem. Soc., 109,* 3466 (1987).

14. M. D. Lee, J. K. Manning, D. R. Williams, N. A. Kunk, R. T. Testa, and D. B. Borders, *J. Antibiot., 42,* 1070 (1989).

15. M. D. Lee, T. S. Dunne, C. C. Chang, M. M. Siegel, G. O. Morton, G. A. Ellestad, W. J. McGahren, and D. B. Borders, *J. Am. Chem. Soc., 114,* 985 (1992).

16. M. Konishi, H. Ohkuma, K. Matsumoto, T. Tsuno, H. Kamei, T. Miyaki, T. Oki, H. Kawaguchi, G. D. VanDuyne, and J. Clardy, *J. Antibiot., 42,* 1449 (1989).

17. M. Konishi, H. Ohkuma, T. Tsuno, T. Oki, G. D. VanDuyne, and J. Clardy, *J. Am. Chem. Soc., 112,* 3715 (1990).

18. D. R. Langley, T. W. Doyle, and D. L. Beveridge, *J. Am. Chem. Soc., 113,* 4395 (1991).

19. Y. Tokiwa, M. Miyoshi-Saitoh, H. Kobayashi, R. Sunaga, M. Konishi, T. Oki, and S. Iwasaki, *J. Am. Chem. Soc., 114,* 4107 (1992).

20. I. H. Goldberg, *Acc. Chem. Res., 24,* 191 (1991).

21. I. Edo, M. Mizugaki, Y. Koide, H. Seto, K. Furihata, N. Otake, and N. Ishida, *Tetrahedron Lett., 26,* 331 (1985).

22. O. D. Hensons and I. H. Goldberg, *J. Antibiot., 42,* 761 (1989).

23. O. D. Hensons, J. L. Giner, and I. H. Goldberg, *J. Am. Chem. Soc., 111,* 3295 (1989).

24. A. G. Myers, P. J. Proteau, and T. M. Handel, *J. Am. Chem. Soc., 110,* 7212 (1988).

25. P. C. Dedon and I. H. Goldberg, *Biochemistry, 31,* 1909 (1992).

26. P. C. Dedon, Z.-W. Jiang, and I. H. Goldberg, *Biochemistry, 31,* 1917 (1992).

27. E. Adjadj, E. Quiniou, J. Mispelter, V. Favaudon, and J.-M. Lhoste, *Eur. J. Biochem., 203,* 505 (1992).

28. K. S. Lam, G. A. Hesler, D. R. Gustavson, A. R. Crosswell, J. M. Veitch, S. Forenza, and K. Tomita, *J. Antibiot., 44,* 472 (1991).

29. S. J. Hofstead, J. A. Matson, A. R. Malacko, and H. Marquardt, *J. Antibiotic., 45,* 1250 (1992).

30. S. J. Hofstead, J. A. Matson, K. S. Lam, S. Forenza, J. A. Bush, and K. Tomita, U.S. Patent 5,001,112 (March 9, 1991).

31. J. E. Leet, D. R. Schroeder, S. J. Hofstead, J. Golik, K. L. Colson, S. Huang, S. E. Klohr, T. W. Doyle, and J. A. Matson, *J. Am. Chem. Soc., 114,* 7946 (1992).

32. J. E. Leet, U.S. Patent 5,143,906 (Sept. 1, 1992).

33. J. E. Leet, J. Golik, S. J. Hofstead, J. A. Matson, A. Y. Lee, and J. Clardy, *Tetrahedron Lett., 33,* 6107 (1992).

34. J. E. Leet, D. R. Schroeder, D. R. Langley, S. J. Hofstead, J. Golik, K. L. Colson, S. Huang, S. E. Klohr, M. S. Lee, T. W. Doyle, and J. A. Matson, *J. Am. Chem. Soc., 115,* 8432 (1993).

35. J. Hu, Y.-C. Xue, M. Xie, R. Zhang, T. Otani, Y. Minami, Y. Yamada, and T. Marunaka, *J. Antibiotic, 41,* 1575 (1988).

36. T. Otani, Y. Minami, T. Marunaka, R. Zhang, J. Hu, and M.-Y. Xie, *41*, 1580 (1988).

37. Y. Minami, K.-I. Yoshida, R. Azuma, M. Saeki, and T. Otani, *Tetrahedron Lett.*, *34*, 2633 (1993).

38. K.-I. Yoshida, Y. Minami, R. Azuma, M. Saeki, and T. Otani, *Tetrahedron Lett.*, *34*, 2637 (1993).

39. M. Hanada, H. Ohkuma, T. Yonemoto, K. Tomita, M. Ohbayashi, H. Kamei, T. Miyaki, M. Konishi, H. Kawaguchi, and S. Forenza, *J. Antibiot.*, *44*, 403 (1991).

40. D. R. Schroeder, K. L. Colson, S. E. Klohr, N. Zein, D. R. Langley, M. S. Lee, J. A. Matson and T. W. Doyle, (maduropeptin chromophore) (1994).

41. G. J. Quigley, A. H.-J. Wang, G. Ughetto, G. van der Marel, J. van Boom, and A. Rich, *Proc. Natl. Acad. Sci. USA*, *77*, 7204 (1980).

42. A. H.-J. Wang, G. Ughetto, G. J. Quigley, and A. Rich, *Biochemistry*, *26*, 1152 (1987).

43. M. H. Moore, W. N. Hunter, B. L. d'Estaintot, and O. Kennard, *J. Mol. Biol.* *206*, 693 (1989).

44. C. A. Frederick, L. D. Williams, G. Ughetto, G. van der Marel, J. H. van Boom, A. Rich, and A. H.-J. Wang, *J. Biochemistry*, *29*, 2538 (1990).

45. T. P. Lockart, P. B. Comita, and R. G. Bergman, *J. Am. Chem. Soc.*, *103*, 4082 (1981).

46. R. G. Bergman, *Acc. Chem. Res.*, *6*, 25 (1973).

47. P. Magnus, S. Fortt, T. Pitterna, and J. P. Snyder, *J. Am. Chem. Soc.*, *112*, 4986 (1990).

48. K. C. Nicolaou, G. Zuccarello, Y. Ogawa, E. J. Schweiger, and T. Kumazawa, *J. Am. Chem. Soc.*, *110*, 4866 (1988).

49. J. P. Snyder, *J. Am. Chem. Soc.*, *111*, 7630 (1989).

50. J. P. Snyder and G. E. Tipsword, *J. Am. Chem. Soc.*, *112*, 4040 (1990).

51. J. P. Snyder, *J. Am. Chem. Soc.*, *112*, 5367 (1990).

52. S. Stinson, *C&EN*, *May 28*, 22 (1990).

53. B. H. Long, J. Golik, S. Forenza, B. Ward, R. Rehfuss, J. C. Dabrowiak, J. J. Catino, S. T. Musial, K. W. Brookshire, and T. W. Doyle, *Proc. Natl. Acad. Sci. USA*, *86*, 2 (1989).

54. B. R. Brooks, R. E. Bruccoleri, B. D. Olafson, D. J. States, S. Swaminathan, and M. Karplus, *J. Comput. Chem.*, *4*, 187 (1983).

55. M. Boldt, G. Gaudiano, M. J. Haddadin, and T. H. Koch, *J. Am. Chem. Soc.*, *111*, 2283 (1989).

56. D. L. Kleyer and T. H. Koch, *J. Am. Chem. Soc.*, *106*, 2380 (1984).

57. M. Boldt, G. Guadiano, and T. H. Koch, *J. Am. Chem. Soc.*, *52*, 2146 (1987).

58. M. Boldt, G. Guadiano, M. J. Haddadin, and T. H. Koch, *J. Am. Chem. Soc.*, *110*, 3330 (1988).

59. J. Fisher, B. R. J. Abdella, and K. E. McLane, *Biochemistry*, *24*, 3562 (1985).

60. T. Shiraki and Y. Sugiura, *Biochemistry*, *29*, 9795 (1990).

61. N. Zein, A. M. Sinha, W. J. McGahren, and G. A. Ellestad, *Science*, *240*, 1198 (1988).

62. H. Kishikawa, Y.-P. Jiang, J. Goodisman, and J. C. Dabrowiak, *J. Am. Chem. Soc., 113,* 5434 (1991).

63. Y. Sugiura, T. Shiraki, M. Konishi, and T. Oki, *Proc. Natl. Acad. Sci. USA, 87,* 3831 (1990).

64. T. Shiraki and Y. Sugiura, *Biochemistry, 29,* 9795 (1990).

65. H. Kishikawa, Y.-P. Jiang, J. Goodisman, and J. Dabrowiak, *J. Biophys. J. (Meeting Abstract), 57,* 260 (1990).

66. Y. Sugiura, Y. Uesawa, Y. Takahashi, J. Kuwahara, J. Golik, and T. W. Doyle, *Proc. Natl. Acad. Sci. USA, 86,* 7672 (1989).

67. P. B. Dervan, *Science, 232,* 464 (1986).

68. N. Zein, M. Poncin, R. Nilakatan, and G. A. Ellestad, *Science, 244,* 697 (1989).

69. S. Walker, R. Landovitz, W.-D. Ding, G. A. Ellestad, and D. Kahne, *Proc. Natl. Acad. Sci. USA, 89,* 4608 (1992).

70. J. W. Kozarich, L. Worth Jr., B. L. Frank, D. F. Christner, D. E. Vanderwall, and J. Stubbe, *Science, 245,* 1396 (1989).

71. Y. Uesawa, J. Kuwahara, and Y. Sugiura, *Biochem. Biophys. Res. Commun., 164,* 903 (1989).

72. Y. Uesawa and Y. Sugiura, *Biochemistry, 30,* 9242 (1991).

73. M. Lu, Q. Guo, B. Krishnan, J. Golik, I. E. Rosenberg, T. W. Doyle, and N. R. Kallenbach, *J. Biomol. Struct. Dyn., 9,* 285 (1991).

74. M. Lu, Q. Guo, and N. R. Kallenbach, *Crit. Rev. Biochem. Mol. Biol., 27,* 157 (1992).

75. D. F. Christner, B. L. Frank, J. W. Kozarich, J. Stubbe, J. Golik, T. W. Doyle, I. E. Rosenberg, and B. Krishnan, *J. Am. Chem. Soc., 114,* 8763 (1992).

76. M. Lu, Q. Guo, and N. R. Kallenbach, *J. Biomol. Struct. Dynm., 9,* 271 (1991).

77. T. Shiraki, M. Uesugi, and Y. Sugiura, *Biochem. Biophys. Res. Commun., 188,* 584 (1992).

78. D. R. Langley, J. Golik, B. Krishnan, T. W. Doyle, and D. L. Beveridge, *J. Am. Chem. Soc., 116,* 15 (1994).

79. P. A. Wender, R. C. Kelly, S. Beckham, and B. L. Miller, *Proc. Natl. Acad. Sci. USA, 88,* 8835 (1991).

80. M. G. Cardozo and A. J. Hopfinger, *Mol. Pharmacol., 40,* 1023 (1991).

81. M. G. Cardozo and A. J. Hopfinger, *Biopolymers, 33,* 337 (1993).

82. A. Maxam and W. Gilbert, *Methods Enzymol., 65,* 499 (1980).

83. I. H. Goldberg, *Free Radical Biol. Med., 3,* 41 (1987).

84. J. Stubbe and J. W. Kozarich, *Chem. Rev., 87,* 1107 (1987).

85. H. Sugiyama, C. Xu, N. Murugesan, and S. M. Hecht, *Biochemistry, 27,* 58 (1988).

86. D. S. Sigman, *Acc. Chem. Res., 19,* 180 (1986).

87. L. S. Kappen, C. Chen, and I. H. Goldberg, *Biochemistry, 27,* 4331 (1988).

88. R. C. Hawley, L. L. Kiessling, and S. L. Schrieber, *Proc. Natl. Acad. Sci. USA, 86,* 1105 (1989).

89. J. J. De Voss, C. A. Townsend, D.-W. Ding, G. O. Morton, G. A. Ellestad, N. Zein, A. B. Tabor, and S. L. Schreiber, *J. Am. Chem. Soc., 112,* 9669 (1990).

90. J. J. Hangeland, J. J. De Voss, J. A. Heath, C. A. Townsend, W. Ding, J. S. Ashcroft, and G. A. Ellestad, *J. Am. Chem. Soc., 114,* 9200 (1992).

91. B. L. Frank, L. Worth Jr., D. F. Christner, J. W. Kozarich, J. Stubbe, L. S. Kappen and I. H. Goldberg, *J. Am. Chem. Soc., 113,* 2271 (1991).

92. L. S. Kappen, I. H. Goldberg, B. L. Frank, L. Worth Jr., D. F. Christner, J. W. Kozarich, and J. Stubbe, *Biochemistry, 30,* 2034 (1991).

93. L. S. Kappan and I. H. Goldberg, *Biochemistry, 22,* 4872 (1983).

94. A. Ichikawa, T. Kuboya, T. Aoyama, and Y. Sugiura, *Biochemistry, 31,* 6784 (1992).

95. W. D. Wilson and I. G. Lopp, *Biopolymers, 18,* 3025 (1979).

96. Q. Guo, N. C. Seeman, and N. R. Kallenbach, *Biochemistry, 28,* 2355 (1989).

97. J. M. Kean, S. A. White, and D. E. Draper, *Biochemistry, 24,* 5062 (1985).

98. N. Zein, W. J. McGahren, G. O. Morton, J. Ashcroft, and G. A. Ellestad, *J. Am. Chem. Soc., 111,* 6888 (1989).

99. M. A. Warpehoski and L. H. Hurley, *Chem. Res. Toxicol., 1,* 315 (1988).

100. M. Chatterjee, K. D. Cramer, and C. A. Townsend, *J. Am. Chem. Soc., 115,* 3374 (1993).

101. J. Drak, N. Iwasawa, D. Danishefsky, and D. M. Crothers, *Proc. Natl. Acad. Sci. USA, 88,* 7464 (1991).

102. J. Aiyar, S. J. Danishefsky, and D. M. Crothers, *J. Am. Chem. Soc., 114,* 7552 (1992).

103. K. C. Nicolaou, S.-C. Tsay, T. Suzuki, and G. F. Joyce, *J. Am. Chem. Soc., 114,* 7555 (1992).

104. D. R. Langley, T. W. Doyle, and D. L. Beveridge, *Tetrahedron Lett., 50,* 1379 (1994).

105. D. M. J. Lilley and E. Palecek, *EMBO J., 3,* 1187 (1984).

106. T. Friedmann and D. M. Brown, *Nucleic Acids Res., 5,* 615 (1978).

107. S. Walker, K. G. Valentine and D. Kahne, *J. Am. Chem. Soc., 112,* 6428 (1990).

108. QUANTA, *Parameter Handbook, Release 3.0,* 4 (1990).

109. K. C. Nicolaou, Y. P. Hong, W.-M. Dai, Z.-J. Zeng, and W. Wrasidlo, *J. Chem. Soc. Chem. Commun.,* 1542 (1992).

110. Y. Sugiura, T. Arakawa, M. Uesugi, T. Shiraki, H. Ohkuma, and M. Konishi, *Biochemistry, 30,* 2989 (1991).

111. J. J. De Voss, J. J. Hangeland, and C. A. Townsend, *J. Am. Chem. Soc., 112,* 4554 (1990).

112. R. A. Lerner and S. J. Benkovic, *BioEssays, 9,* 107 (1988).

113. S. Neidle, L. H. Pearl, P. Herzyk, and H. M. Berman, *Nucleic Acids Res., 16,* 8999 (1988).

114. S. Kirkpatrick, C. D. Gelatt, and M. P. Vecchi, *Science, 220,* 671 (1983).

115. A. T. Brunger, G. M. Clore, A. M. Gronenborn, and M. Karplus, *Proc. Natl. Acad. Sci. USA, 83,* 3801 (1986).

116. J. J. P. Steward, *MOPAC, A Semi-Empirical Molecular Orbital Program, QCPE.,* 455 (1983).

117. F. J. Seiler, *MOPAC 6.0* (1990).

118. G. M. Clore, A. M. Gronenborn, A. T. Brunger, and M. Karplus, *J. Mol. Biol., 186,* 435 (1985).

119. L. H. Hurley and F. Leslie Boyd, *Ann. Rep. Med. Chem.*, *22*, 259 (1987).
120. R. Lavery, B. Pullman, and S. Corbin, *Nucleic Acids Res.*, *9*, 6539 (1981).
121. S. Walker, D. Yang, and D. Kahne, *J. Am. Chem. Soc.*, *113*, 4716 (1991).
122. H. R. Drew and R. E. Dickerson, *J. Mol. Biol.*, *151*, 535 (1981).
123. M. L. Kopka, A. V. Fratini, H. R. Drew, and R. E. Dickerson, *J. Mol. Biol.*, *163*, 129 (1983).

14

Biological Properties of Esperamicin and Other Enediyne Antibiotics

Anna Maria Casazza
Bristol-Myers Squibb Pharmaceutical Research Institute,
Princeton, New Jersey

Susan L. Kelley
Bristol-Myers Squibb Pharmaceutical Research Institute,
Wallingford, Connecticut

I. INTRODUCTION

Enediynes are novel cytotoxic agents, which have recently attracted the attention of several investigators because of their extremely high potency and their novel and specific mechanism of action. Most of the scientific papers and reviews published on this class of compounds deal with their chemical and mechanistic properties, whereas little attention has been given to the biological activity, which is of fundamental importance for putative anticancer agents. In this chapter, we will summarize the data so far available for the most relevant enediynes on the cytotoxic activity against in vitro tumor cells and the antitumor activity in vivo against various experimental tumor models.

II. NEOCARZINOSTATIN

Neocarzinostatin (zinostatin) is the first enediyne antibiotic reported in the literature (1), and it is the only enediyne molecule that has received approval for the clinical treatment of cancer, in particular for liver carcinoma in Japan. It consists of a enediyne core and an associated protein, with MW of approximately 10,000 (Fig. 1). In vitro studies have shown that the neocarzinostatin chromophore is responsible for the effects observed in cell-free systems, as well as in vitro cell cultures.

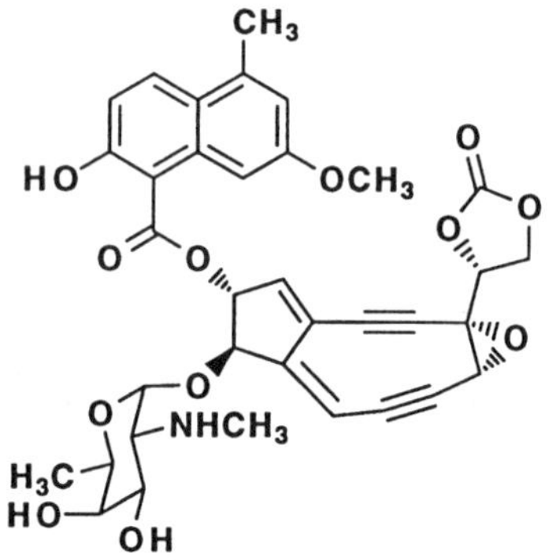

**Neocarzinostatin
Chromophore**

Figure 1 Chemical structure of neocarzinostatin.

Early studies (2) conducted using IP administration showed that neocarzinostatin was active in mice against the L1210 and the SN-36 mouse leukemias, and against solid tumor models, such as the ascitic sarcoma 180, the Ehrlich carcinoma, and the B16 melanoma, without any evidence of schedule dependency. In some of these early studies, conducted using different lots of material, the active doses varied from 12.5 (q1d × 6) to 200 mg/kg/day (3). In L1210 leukemia the optimal dose after IP administration varied from 60 to 200 mg/kg/treatment (4); no activity against SC L1210 leukemia was seen after IV administration, indicating limited distribution of the drug through the body. These high doses may have been tolerated by animals because these studies were conducted using a crude form of the compound.

Other than these early investigations, very little has been published on the in vivo antitumor activity of neocarzinostatin. Recent experiments have been performed using SMANCS, which consists of polystyrene-co-maleic acid conjugated with neocarzinostatin. This compound was designed to increase the local delivery of the cytotoxic moiety to the tumor. The in vivo effects of SMANCS were compared to those of neocarzinostatin against rat mammary tumors induced by DMBA (5). In this study, rats were treated with SMANCS q5d × 3, IV, starting when the tumors were palpable. Both compounds were able to inhibit tumor growth, at doses of 0.3 mg/kg/treatment, however, SMANCS produced a tumor inhibition of 90%, whereas neocarzinostatin treatment resulted in an inhibition of only 54%, probably not biologically significant. The doses used in this study are extremely low, and the results suggest that delivery of neocarzinostatin via conjugation to a polymer can result in increased antitumor effect.

Along this line, a very recent report describes the antitumor effect of an immunoconjugate of neocarzinostatin with monoclonal antibody A7 against pancreatic cancer (6). In this study, the immunoconjugate, administered directly in the tumor, showed a greater antitumor activity than the free compound.

The chemical synthesis of the neocarzinostatin chromophore has been reported (7), but no data are available on the biological activity in vivo of the isolated chromophore. Such data are important to assess if the neocarzinostatin chromoprotein has any role in the biological activity of this molecule.

III. CALICHEAMICIN γ_1^I

The calicheamicins (Fig. 2) were discovered in the mid-1980s and were immediately recognized to have extremely high potency both in vitro and in in vivo assays (8). In these preliminary studies, calicheamicins were active against murine tumors at doses from 0.5 to 1.5 µg/kg. As observed for neocarzinostatin, no extensive reports have been published on the biological activity of calicheamicins. Recently (9,10), the in vivo antitumor effects of calicheamicin linked to monoclonal antibodies directed towards tumor-associated antigens have been reported. These immunoconjugates are active in vivo against human tumor xenografts. The lysine-linked conjugate of N-acetyl calicheamicin γ_1^I with the humanized version of the internalizing monoclonal antibody CTM01, directed against a polymorphic epithelial murine antigen, at the maximal tolerated dose (MTD) induced complete regressions of a human ovarian carcinoma xenografted in nude mice. This specific delivery approach can increase the antitumor activity of this class of compounds by reducing the toxic effects against normal tissues and allowing appropriate drug concentrations to be reached in the tumor tissue.

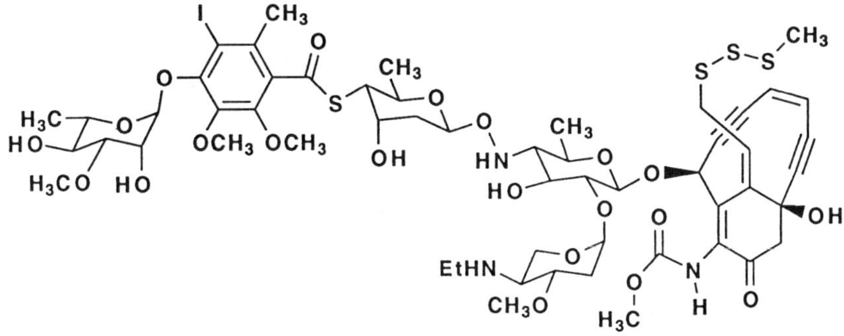

Figure 2   Chemical structure of calicheamicin γ_1^I.

IV. ESPERAMICIN A$_1$

Esperamicin A$_1$ (BMY-21875) was isolated in 1985 (11). Chemical characterization was completed in 1987 (Fig. 3) (12), and the mechanism of action of esperamicin A$_1$ at the DNA level was reported in 1989 (13).

In vitro cytotoxicity assays revealed that esperamicin A$_1$ was extremely potent, with IC$_{50}$s, after 72-hour exposure, ranging from 1.5 to 4.5 ng/ml in four tumor lines tested and of 13.5 ng/ml in the Moser human colon carcinoma line (14). Several studies were performed to evaluate the antitumor activity of this compound; optimal results are summarized in Table 1.

The antitumor activity in vivo was tested against a panel of mouse tumors transplanted IP or IV (14). Reproducible activity was observed at tolerated doses against P388 leukemia and L1210 leukemia, transplanted IP (IP treatment) or IV (IV treatment). Increase in life span ranged from 52 to >200% in the IP P388 tumor model, from 25 to 194% in the IV P388 tumor model, and from 29 to 80% in the L1210 model. Cures were observed in some experiments. In the IP leukemia models, several schedules of treatment were tested: single treatment, daily treatment for 5 or 9 days, and intermittent (every 3 or 4 days) treatment. In terms of potency, optimal (nontoxic) doses ranged from 0.6 µg/kg/treatment (daily administration) to 30 µg/kg/treatment (single or intermittent administration). These observations confirmed that the high potency observed in vitro was predictive of an exceptional potency in vivo.

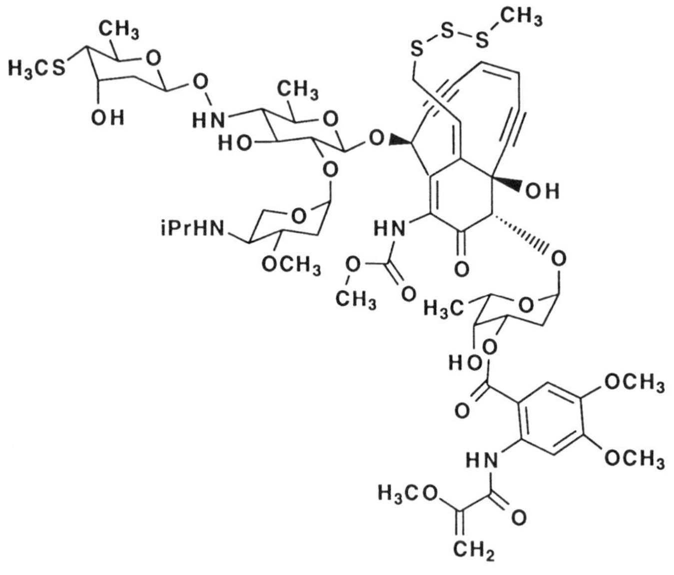

Figure 3 Chemical structure of esperamicin A$_1$.

Table 1 Optimal Antitumor Effects of Esperamicin A_1 in Preclinical Models

Tumor, route of transplant	Route of treatment	Range of optimal % increase lifespan	Optimal % tumor growth inhibition	Optimal tumor growth delay (days)
Mouse leukemias				
P388, IP	IP	52– $\geqslant$ 200		
P388, IV	IV	25–194		
L1210, IP	IP	29–80		
L1210, IV	IV	75		
Mouse solid tumors				
B16, IP	IP	43–110		
B16, SC	IP	46	41	3.5
B16, SC	IV	33–86	41–89	3.0–6.0
Lewis lung ca, IP	IP	186		
M109, IP	IP	64–100		
M109, SC	IP	64–200		
M 5076, IP	IP	56		3.8
C 26, IP	IP	21–76		
C 26, SC	IP	no effect		3.3
Human tumors				
MX-1, src	IP		83–88	

Solid mouse tumor models were also investigated. When administered IP, esperamicin A_1 was very active against several of these tumors transplanted IP, producing, at tolerated doses, optimal increases in life span of 110% in the B16 melanoma model, 186% in the Lewis lung carcinoma model, 100% in the M109 lung carcinoma model, 56% in the M5076 reticulum cell sarcoma model, and 76% against the colon 26 carcinoma model. When the tumor was transplanted SC and the compound was administered IV or IP, activity was maintained against the B16 and the M109 models, but not against the colon 26 carcinoma.

The first study of the antitumor activity of esperamicin A_1 against human tumors was performed against the MX-1 human mammary carcinoma transplanted under the renal capsule (14). Administered IP, esperamicin A_1 was able to inhibit tumor growth at optimal doses of 0.64 and 5 μg/kg/treatment in two separate experiments. These results showed that esperamicin A_1 was active against a broad spectrum of preclinical tumor models of murine and human origin and against tumors located distal to the point of drug administration.

Further experiments were performed using additional human carcinomas transplanted SC in nude mice (15). The MTD of esperamicin A_1 was lower in athymic mice than in immunocompetent mice and when the compound was administered

IV rather than IP. In addition, the toxicity of esperamicin A_1 was dependent upon the schedule of administration. At a given cumulative dose, esperamicin A_1 was more toxic when administered by repeated injections or on a more consolidated schedule than when administered in a single injection or on a less consolidated schedule. At tolerated doses, esperamicin A_1 was active against the H2981 and the LX1 human lung carcinomas transplated SC in athymic mice: optimal activity was observed with a single administration of 3–4 µg/kg, IV.

From these studies it appears that the best schedule for the treatment of subcutaneously transplanted human tumor xenografts with esperamicin A_1 was the single IV treatment (15). Similarly, in the leukemia tumor models, therapeutic results were in general superior when esperamicin A_1 was administered in a single treatment than when repeated injections were given (14). However, in the ascitic solid tumor models tested, consecutive daily treatments at very low doses were more effective than intermittent treatments with higher doses/treatment (14). These observations suggest that the optimal schedule of treatment of esperamicin A_1 is dependent on the route of administration or on the histological type of the tumor.

Toxicological evaluation of esperamicin A_1 confirmed its potency: in acute lethality tests conducted in mice, the single LD_{50} (dose at which 50% mortality occurs) was only 13 µg/m^2. Similar studies performed using a five-daily dosing schedule revealed an LD_{50} of 1.8 µg/m^2/day (R. A. Buroker, unpublished results). Qualitative assessment of toxicity in mouse, rat, and dog models revealed that the compound caused dose-related myelosuppression, which was reversible but frequently delayed beyond the "usual" time of peak marrow suppression from cytotoxic agents (14 days after dosing). The major nonhematological toxicities were phlebitis, fever, and liver dysfunction, manifested by histological changes and enzyme abnormalities, and renal dysfunction, characterized by proteinuria, elevations of serum indices of glomerular filtration, and histological changes consistent with nephrosis.

Esperamicin A_1 was selected for clinical development on the basis of its antitumor activity against distal site solid tumor models and very high potency. Given the extreme potency in preclinical studies, and the observation that esperamicin A_1 has very limited aqueous solubility and readily adsorbs to glass and plastic, the formulation chosen consisted of only 5 µg of drug with 20 mg lactose as excipient in each clinical vial, and the reconstitution vehicle was 40% ethanol in 5% dextrose in water.

Based upon the results of preclinical toxicology studies, the initial design of the Phase I trials for esperamicin A_1 incorporated a 6-week observation period between doses in any individual patient. After safety data were accumulated to support shorter course lengths, repeat doses at 4-week intervals were also evaluated.

Phase I human studies of esperamicin A_1 were initiated in 1988, using two schedules of drug administration. In the single-dose trials (16–18), the starting dose was 1/10 the mouse single dose LD_{10}, or 1.0 $\mu g/m^2$, administered every 4–6 weeks. Groups of at least three patients with advanced malignancies were treated at each dose level, and doses were escalated to a maximum of 10 $\mu g/m^2$. In this trial, toxicities included asymptomatic decreases in blood pressure, fever, chills, nausea, vein irritation at the injection sites, myelosuppression, hepatic dysfunction, and proteinuria. Cumulative delayed hepatotoxicity with hepatic necrosis and death was observed in one patient who received three courses of treatment at the 7 $\mu g/m^2$ dose level. The dose-limiting toxicity was hepatotoxicity, since courses could not be repeated in a timely fashion due to persistence of mild to moderate elevations of serum hepatic enzymes at esperamicin A_1 doses above 5 $\mu g/m^2$.

A Phase I study using a five-daily dosing schedule was also conducted (16,19). The starting dose was approximately 1/10 the mouse five-daily dose LD_{10}, or 0.15 $\mu g/m^2/day \times 5$, administered at 4-week intervals. Doses were escalated up to 2.4 $\mu g/m^2/day \times 5$. Toxicities included asymptomatic hypotension, fever, nausea, phlebitis, myleosuppression, proteinuria, and mild elevations of hepatic enzymes. The dose-limiting toxicity was delayed and prolonged bone marrow suppression, occurring in patients at the 1.8 $\mu g/m^2/day$ dose level and above. Since the acute toxicity spectrum of fever, chills, and decreased blood pressure was less problematic at the five-daily dosing schedule, this schedule was recommended for subsequent Phase II efficacy trials, using a dose of 1.0 $\mu g/m^2/day \times 5$.

Phase II clinical efficacy trials were initiated in 1992 at esperamicin A_1 dosage of 1.0 $\mu g/m^2/day$ on days 1–5, repeated every 4–6 weeks. Studies are underway to assess the antitumor activity of esperamicin A_1 in patients with carcinoma of the kidney, colon, lung, and pancreas and in patients with malignant melanoma. Toxicity reported in these studies include myelosuppression, notably delayed or cumulative thrombocytopenia, hepatic disfunction, and fatigue. Preliminary results do not suggest meaningful antitumor activity.

V. KEDARCIDIN

Kedarcidin (BMY 40935; NSC 646276) is a chromoprotein (MW 12,400) produced by a novel actinomycete in culture and isolated on the basis of its cytotoxicity in vitro (20,21). The chemical structure of the kedarcidin chromophore has been recently reported (22) and is shown in Figure 4.

Kedarcidin is highly cytotoxic in vitro, with IC_{50}s of 0.6–8 ng/ml in various cell lines (20). In a panel of 60 human tumor lines at the National Cancer Institute, kedarcidin showed, in one out of two experiments, higher potency against leukemia cell lines than against the other tumor types tested (D. Lednicer, personal communication), confirming its large spectrum of cytotoxic activity in vitro.

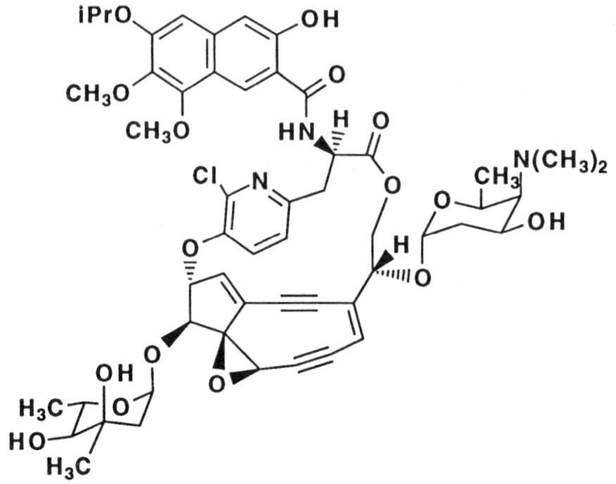

Figure 4 Chemical structure of the kedarcidin chromophore.

Administered IP to mice with IP-implanted murine P388 or L1210 leukemias or with IP B16 melanoma, kedarcidin increased the life span of the animals 40–100%. In these experiments, kedarcidin confirmed its extreme potency in vivo: optimal doses ranged from 30 μg/kg/treatment when the compound was given daily for 5 days to 8 μg/kg/treatment when treatment was prolonged for 9 consecutive days (21).

IP treatment with kedarcidin was also effective against the B16 melanoma transplanted SC, producing a tumor growth delay of 10 days, an increase in life span of 76% (21). In addition, IP-administered kedarcidin was able to inhibit by 80% the growth of two sublines of the human HCT116 colon adenocarcinoma transplanted under the kidney capsule, one sensitive and one resistant to topoisomerase II–interacting agents, such as etoposide or doxorubicin, because of low levels of topoisomerase II (20).

Subsequent studies showed that the isolated chromophore (BMY-46280) is also very potent in vitro, with IC_{50} of 1 nM against the HCT 116 human colon carcinoma cells (N. Zein and W. Solomon, unpublished results). The kedarcidin chromophore showed an interesting selectivity in its interaction with DNA (23). Data on its activity against a panel of different tumor cell lines are not available at this time and would be of interest to better understand if in vitro selectivity against particular DNA sequences can translate in ability to affect particular tumor types more than others.

The chromophore was approximately as active as the chromoprotein against the murine P388 leukemia transplanted IP or IV, producing T/C% values from 141 to 214%, after IP or IV administration at doses of 0.1–1.6 mg/kg/injection. Of

Table 2 Antitumor Activity In Vivo of Kedarcidin and Kedarcidin Chromophore

Tumor/ Implant	Schedule	Kedarcidin Chromoprotein		Kedarcidin Chromophore	
		O.D. (mg/kg/treatment)	T/C % [T-C]	O.D. (mg/kg/treatment)	T/C % [T-C]
M109 IP	5, IP	4	156	1	131
M109 SC	5, 9, 13, IV	1	[8.3]	0.25	[7]
M5076 IP	5, IP	2	138	1	138
M5076 SC	1, 9, 13, IV	1	[3.8]	0.5	[3.5]

interest was the observation of no loss of in vivo activity against two P388 sublines selected for resistance to doxorubicin and to mitomycin C through drug pressure (W. C. Rose et al., unpublished observation).

Unpublished results from our laboratories (A. Crosswell et al., to be published) also showed that the chromophore had an antitumor activity comparable to that of the chromoprotein against several experimental in vivo tumor models and maintained its high potency in vivo. Some of these preliminary results are summarized in Table 2. Both molecules, administered IP or IV at optimal doses from 0.25 to 4 mg/kg/treatment, were active against the IP or SC transplanted M109 murine lung adenocarcinoma, whereas modest or no activity was seen against the murine M5076 reticulum cell sarcoma. In comparison with esperamicin A_1, the kedarcidin chromophore is therefore similarly active against mouse leukemias and against the M109 mouse lung adenocarcinoma, but it is less toxic and can be administered at higher doses. This lower toxicity could make this compound more manageable than esperamicin A_1 for clinical trials.

It has been recently shown that the kedarcidin apoprotein, which lacks any detectable chromophore, cleaves proteins selectively (24). This unexpected result has drawn new light into the possible mechanism of action of natural enediynes. The kedarcidin apoprotein was found to selectively cleave specific proteins, with preference for histones, suggesting a role of the apoprotein not only in the delivery of the kedarcidin chromophore to the DNA, but also in facilitating the DNA-cutting effect of the chromophore. The consequences of this additional mechanism as regards the biological activity of kedarcidin are not yet understood. The isolated chromophore maintained approximately the same activity as the chromoprotein in the tumor models tested, however a more extensive range of studies could reveal biological differences still unexplored.

VI. DYNEMICINS

Dynemicin A is an antitumor antibiotic discovered in the fermentation broth of a new *Micromonospora* strain and chemically characterized (as its denomination

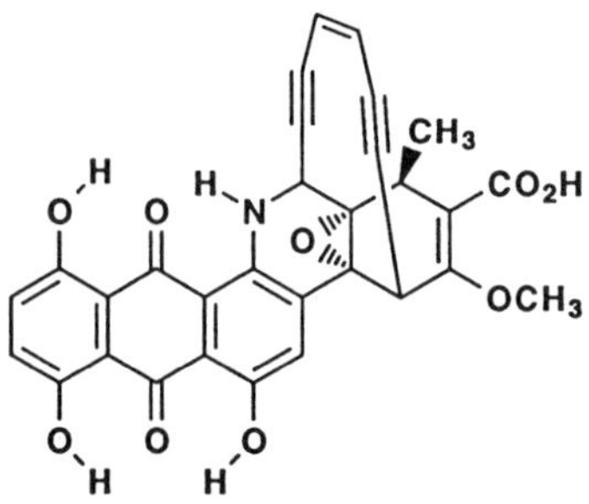

Dynemicin A

Figure 5   Chemical structure of dynemicin A.

says) by the presence of an enediyne and an anthraquinone group (Fig. 5). Both dynemicin A and its triacetate exhibited marked cytotoxic activity against human and mouse tumor cells in vitro, with IC_{50}s of about 4–5 ng/ml. No drop in activity was observed against a multiple drug–resistant cell variant (25), an interesting observation for an anthraquinone-containing compound. In vivo, dynemicin A administered IP produced a treated/control percentage (T/C%) of 135 at 1 mg/kg/injection (q1d $\times$ 3) against IP P388 leukemia and of 159 at 1 mg/kg/injection (91d $\times$ 9) against IP B16 melanoma.

Dynemicins O, P, and Q were subsequently isolated from the fermentation broth of the same *Micromonospora* strain (26). Chemical studies showed that these novel compounds do not contain the enediyne moiety. Though they maintain cytotoxic activity against in vitro tumor cells, their potency is markedly lower than that of dynemicin A, confirming that the enediyne group is the one that confers the extreme potency to dinemycin A. Unfortunately, no in vivo data are available for these compounds. A comparison of the antitumor activity in vivo of dynemicin O, P, and Q with that of dynemicin A could give information on the role played by the enediyne group on the in vivo biological effects.

VII. MADUROPEPTINS

Antitumor antibiotics isolated from cultures of *Actinomadura madurae* have been denominated maduropeptins (27). These compounds are acidic chromopeptides with MW of around 22,500, and their chromophore portion has been characterized as an enediyne compound (Fig. 6).

Maduropeptin C does not have any in vitro cytotoxic activity and was not tested in vivo. Maduropeptins A_1, A_2, and B are highly cytotoxic in vitro against B16

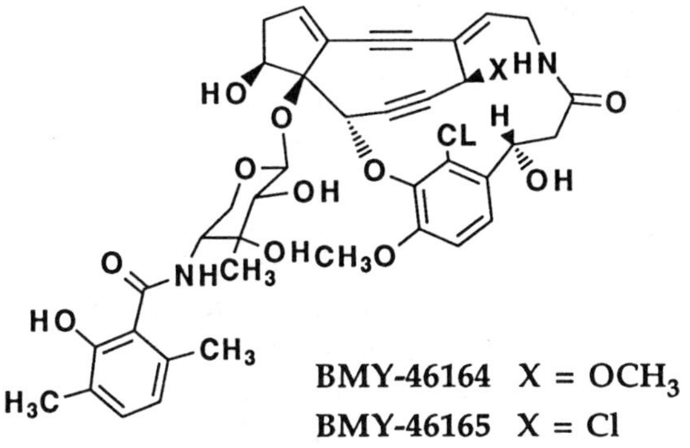
HO
O
O
OH
O
CL
H
XHN
O
OH
O
NHCH3
OH
CH3O
HO
CH3
H3C
BMY-46164 X = OCH3
BMY-46165 X = Cl
Maduropeptin
Chromophore

Figure 6 Chemical structure of maduropeptins.

mouse melanoma cells and HCT116 human colon carcinoma cells, with IC_{50}s of 7–160 nM. In vivo, these compounds, administered IP q1d × 3, are active against IP-transplanted P388 leukemia and exhibit a very high potency, in agreement with the in vitro data. Maduropeptin A_1 produced a T/C% of 165 at 0.06 mg/kg/day; maduropeptin A_2 a T/C% of 155 at 0.02 mg/kg/day; and maduropeptin B a T/C% of 235 at 0.3 mg/kg/day. Because of its extreme potency and good activity in the P388 leukemia model, maduropeptin A_1 was selected for further studies and compared to neocarzinostatin against IP P388 leukemia and against the B16 melanoma transplated under the renal capsule (src). As summarized in Table 3, maduropeptin A_1 was as active as neocarzinostatin at doses approximately 50–100 lower (27).

Table 3 Antitumor Activity of Maduropeptin A_1 Against B16 Melanoma

Tumor	Schedule of treatment	Compound	O.D. (mg/kg/injection)	T/C%	% Inhibition tumor growth
IP P388	q1dx5	Maduropeptin A_1	0.006	180	
		neocarzinostatin	0.5	210	
src B16	q1dx5	Maduropeptin A_1	0.02		97
		neocarzinostatin	1.0		84

VIII. SYNTHETIC ENEDIYNES

In the course of an extensive investigation of the structure-activity relationships of modified enediynes, a synthetic program was initiated at Bristol-Myers Squibb (28,29). Out of several compounds synthesized and tested for biological activity, one seemed of particular interest: BMY-46108, a simple core mimic of the natural product esperamicin A_1 (Fig. 7) (29).

Even if less potent than esperamicin A_1, this compound retains very high in vitro potency, with an IC_{50} of 0.1 μM against the human carcinoma cell line HCT116 (29). This compound was subjected to an extensive in vivo investigation (W. C. Rose et al., to be published) in comparison with other known enediyne compounds. In terms of potency, BMY-46108 was active at doses of 5–10 mg/kg/treatment, being therefore less potent than the other enediynes that, like esperamicin A_1 and the kedarcidin chromophore, lack the apoprotein. The antitumor activity at the optimal dose of BMY-46108 in comparison with the other enediynes is summarized in Table 4. BMY-46108 retained very good in vivo activity against both IP-transplanted and SC-transplanted tumors, after IP or IV administration. In particular, BMY-46108 was the most active enediyne against IP tumors (P388, B16, and M5076).

Of interest are recent results regarding the mechanism of action of BMY-46108 (29). In addition to its expected effect on DNA, BMY-46108 was shown to produce protein damage, in the form of protein agglomeration, at concentrations that could be relevant to the mechanism of action of the drug. The relative contribution of the DNA-damaging effect versus the effect on proteins towards the cytotoxic and antitumor activity of this molecule remains to be determined.

Another group of synthetic enediynes was prepared after the chemical structure of dinemycin A, but lacking the DNA intercalating anthraquinone moiety (30–32). These "designer" enediynes, synthesized with the aim to increase cell specificity, were tested in a panel of tumor cell lines of various histological origin, as well as against normal in vitro cultured cell lines (30,32). One selected compound had an IC_{50} (after 72-hour exposure) ranging from 10^{-6} to 10^{-14} M, lower than any other cytotoxic agent tested in parallel. In terms of specificity,

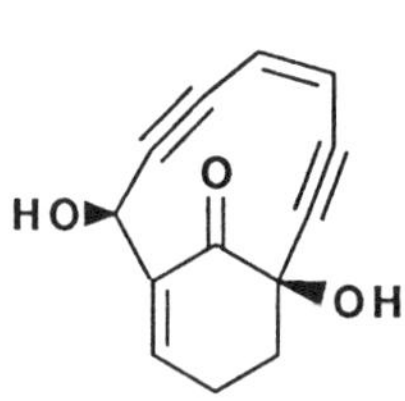

Figure 7   Chemical structure of synthetic enediyne BMY-46108.

Table 4 In Vivo Experimental Antitumor Activity of Enediynes

Compound	P388		B16		M5076		M109		A2780,
	IP/IP	IV/IV	IP/IP	SC/IV	IP/IP	SC/IV	IP/IP	SC/IV	SC/IV
Neocarzinostatin	+++		+++		+++	−	++/+++	++/+++	++
Esperamicin A$_1$	++	+++	+++	−/++[a]	++	−	++	−	
Kedarcidin chromoprotein (BMY-40935)	+++	+++	++	++	+	−	++	+	
Kedarcidin chromphore (BMY-46280)	++	+++		++	+	−	+	+	Tox
BMY-46108	++++	++	++++	−	++++	−	+	+	++

−, not active; +, ILS% = 25–40, 1LCK; ++; ILS% = 41–80, 2LCK; +++, ILS% = 81–250, 3LCK; ++++, ILS% > 250, 4LCK; Tox, toxic.

[a] Variable results.

the order of sensitivity of in vitro cell cultures to these synthetic enediynes was leukemia > human carcinomas > melanoma > normal cell lines. These in vitro results suggest a selective activity against cancer cells, in particular of the hematological type. The high sensitivity of hematological cells to cytotoxic agents is a common observation in experimental models and appears to be predictive of the elevated activity of anticancer drugs against leukemias and lymphomas in patients. This result has been attributed to the shorter doubling time or higher growth fraction of the hematopoietic tumor cells versus solid tumor or normal cells. For the synthetic enediynes here discussed, the induction of apoptosis has been evoked as the possible mechanism at the basis of the high potency against leukemia cells in vitro (32). The biochemical mechanism that brings this apoptotic effect have not been elucidated. One can speculate that apoptosis could be due to interaction of the compounds with proteins, as observed with BMY-46108, another synthetic enediyne core that lacks the DNA-targeting part of the molecule.

The actual relevance of the selectivity observed in vitro is difficult to establish, as no in vivo antitumor data have yet been reported on these synthetic compounds, to confirm that the extreme potency accompanied by the reported in vitro selectivity can translate into an in vivo therapeutic index that allows for presence of antitumor activity at nontoxic doses. The only in vivo result on these compounds reported in the literature (33) is an LD_{50} in BALB/c mice of 18–20 mg/ kg. This very low toxicity, compared to that of other enediyne molecules, suggests in vivo metabolism or inactivation and confirms the need for in vivo antitumor studies before any conclusion on the potential of cytotoxic molecules as anticancer agents can be reached.

IX. MECHANISMS OF RESISTANCE

Natural or induced resistance of cancer cells to antitumor agents is one of the major causes of the ineffectiveness of the anticancer therapy today, together with the lack of selectivity of the known drugs toward tumor cells. Therefore, several studies have been performed to characterize the profile of cross-resistance of enediynes with other known cytotoxic molecules.

An in vitro study was performed to evaluate the pattern of cross-resistance of esperamicin A_1 with other anticancer agents that interact with DNA in a panel of tumor cell lines selected through pressure in vitro. In this study, esperamicin A_1 was cross-resistant with all the agents considered, however, there was a lower level of cross-resistance with etoposide and cisplatin and a higher level of cross-resistance with doxorubicin, mitomycin C, and teniposide (34). On the contrary, dinemycin did not show multiple drug cross-resistance, and for synthetic enediyne 5 (3) no difference in activity was seen against sensitive and multiple drug–resistant T-cell leukemia. Taken together, these results suggests that enediyne chromoproteins can be sensitive to drug resistance induced by elevated P170 glycoprotein, whereas simple enediynes lacking the protein part of the molecule can be less sensitive to this mechanism. To support this suggestion, as above reported, the kedarcidin chromophore BMY 46280 was not cross-resistant with doxorubicin or mitomycin C in vivo.

Several enediynes depend for their ability to cut DNA on the activation by thiols. For example, thiols mediate the reduction of the methyl trisulfide group of calicheamicin γ_1^I after its association with the DNA minor groove, and this generates the free radicals that produce the DNA cleavage (35). Similarly, the cleavage of DNA by esperamicins is greatly accelerated in the presence of thiol compounds (13). Increased levels of intracellular thiols have been reported as the cause of resistance of cancer cells to several cytotoxic agents, including cisplatin; this could explain the cross-resistance of enediynes with cisplatin.

X.   CONCLUSIONS AND FUTURE DIRECTIONS

Enediynes are complex molecules characterized by a unique and selective mechanism of action at the DNA level. The natural enediynes have the ability to cut DNA at specific DNA sequences, and this feature has not yet been exploited in terms of directing the cytotoxic core to specific regions of relevance for the growth of cancer cells. Future studies in this direction are in progress in several laboratories and can result in compounds with specific selectivity for particular tumor types. So far, the natural enediynes that have been introduced into the clinic have shown either a limited spectrum of clinical activity (neocarzinostatin) or unpredictable toxicity (esperamicin A_1). Therefore, the major thrust in order to make enediynes successful anticancer agents is to increase their specificity, and efforts are in progress in several laboratories to obtain this goal through immunotargeting (9,10), an approach that is now giving very promising results. In fact, we have recently demonstrated (36) that conjugates between cytotoxic agents and monoclonal antibodies directed towards tumor-associated antigens can have dramatically increased antitumor activity and reduced toxicity in comparison with the unconjugated drug, with consequent marked increases in the therapeutic index.

The ability of enediynes to interact with proteins has been only recently identified using synthetic enediynes. The relevance of this biochemical effect to the biological activity of this class of compounds, in particular as regards the balance between antitumor and toxic effects, remains to be determined. In addition, the possible role of the chromoprotein in antitumor activity and toxicity of these molecules is only now starting to be explored. Finally, these molecules have been mainly investigated as far as their chemical and mechanistic properties; their full potential as biological weapons is still to be discovered.

ACKNOWLEDGMENT

Thanks are due to W. C. Rose for providing the unpublished preclinical data.

REFERENCES

1. N. Ishida, K. Miyazaki, K. Kumagai, et al., *J. Antibiot., 18,* 68 (1965).
2. S. S. Legha, D. D. Von Hoff, M. Rozencweig, et al., *Oncology, 33,* 265 (1976).
3. K. Kumagai and K. Miyazaki, *J. Antibiotic.* (Tokyo), *66,* 55 (1963).
4. W. T. Bradner and D. J. Hutchinson, *Cancer Chemoth. Rep., 50,* 79, 1966.
5. A. Kimoto, T. Konno, T. Kawaguchi, et al., *Cancer Res., 52,* 1013, 1992.
6. E. Otsuji, T. Yamaguchi, N. Yamaoka, et al., *J. Surg. Oncol., 53,* 215, 1993.
7. P. Magnus and T. Pitterna, *J. Chem. Soc. Chem. Commun., 7,* 541, 1991.
8. J. P. Thomas, S. G. Carvajal, H. L. Lindsay, et al., *Program and Abstracts,* 26th Interscience Conference on Antimicrobial Agents and Chemotherapy, New Orleans, LA, 1986, Abstract 229.
9. F. E. Durr, R. E. Wallace, P. R. Hamann, et al., NCI-EORTC Symposium on New Drugs in Cancer Therapy, Amsterdam, 1992, Program and Abstracts, p. 178.
10. L. M. Hinman, P. R. Hamann, C. F. Beyer, et al., *Proc. Am. Assoc. Cancer Res., 34,* 479, 1993.
11. M. Konishi, H. Okhuma, K. Saitoh, et al., *J. Antibiot., 38,* 1605, 1985.
12. J. Golik, J. Clardy, G. Dubay, et al., *J. Am. Chem. Soc., 109,* 3462, 1987.
13. B. L. Long, J. Golik, S. Forenza, et al., *Proc. Natl. Acad. Sci. USA, 86,* 2, 1989.
14. J. E. Schurig, W. C. Rose, H. Kamei, et al., *Invest. New Drugs, 8,* 7, 1990.
15. P. A. Trail, W. C. Rose, and A. M. Casazza, *Proc. Am. Assoc. Cancer Res., 30,* 482, 1989.
16. M. Rozencweig, L. Schacter, S. Kelley, et al., *Proceedings of the 16th International Congress on Chemotherapy* (F. Rubistein and D. Adam eds.), Jerusalem, Israel, 1989, pp. 755.1–755.3
17. C. Sessa, E. Drozd, J. Gumbrell, et al., *Proc. Am. Soc. Clin. Oncol., 9,* 66, 1990.
18. T. Melink, N. Tait, C. Engstrom, et al., *Proc. Am. Soc. Clin. Oncol., 10,* 120, 1991.
19. T. Brown, K. Harlin, G. Weiss, et al., *Proc. Am. Soc. Clin. Oncol., 9,* 72, 1990.
20. A. R. Croswell, W. C. Rose, J. L. Clark, et al., *Proc. Am. Assoc. Cancer Res., 31,* 416, 1990.
21. K. S. Lam, G. A. Hesler, D. R. Gustavson, et al., *J. Antibiot., 44,* 472, 1991.
22. J. T. Leet, D. R. Schoroeder, D. R. Langley, et al., *J. Am. Chem. Soc., 115,* 8432, 1993.
23. N. Zein, K. Colson, J. E. Leet, et al., *Proc. Natl. Acad. Sci. USA, 90,* 2822, 1993.
24. N. Zein, A. M. Casazza, T. W. Doyle, et al., *Proc. Natl. Acad. Sci. USA, 90,* 8009, 1993.
25. M. Konishi, H. Okhuma, K. Matsumoto, et al., *J. Antibiot., 42,* 1449, 1989.
26. M. Miyoshi-Saitoh, N. Morisaki, Y. Tokiwa, et al., *J. Antibiot., 44,* 1037, 1991.
27. M. Hanada, H. Ohkuma, T. Yonemoto, et al., *J. Antibiot., 44,* 403, 1991.
28. J. F. Kadow, M. M. Tun, D. M. Vyas, et al., *Tetrahedron Lett., 11,* 1423, 1992.

29. N. Zein, W. Solomon, A. M. Casazza, et al., *Biorg. Med. Chem. Lett.*, *6*, 1351, 1993.
30. K. C. Nicolau, W.-M. Dai, S.-C. Tsay, et al., *Science*, *256*, 1172, 1992.
31. K. C. Nicolau, Y. P. Hong, W.-M. Dai, et al., *J. Chem. Soc. Chem. Comm.*, *21*, 1542, 1992.
32. K. C. Nicolau, W.-M. Dai, S.-C. Tsay, et al., *Bioorg. Med. Chem. Lett.*, *2*, 1155, 1992.
33. B. Esmaeli-Azad, K. C. Nicolau, and D. W. Anderson, Fed. Am. Soc. Exp. Biology Meeting, New Orleans, LA, 1993, Abstract A 689.
34. B. H. Long, J. J. Catino, S. T. Musial, et al., *Proc. Am. Assoc. Cancer Res.*, *28*, 312, 1987.
35. N. Zein, A. M. Sinha, W. J. McGahren, et al., *Science*, *240*, 1198, 1988.
36. P. A. Trail, D. Willner, S. J. Lasch, et al., *Science*, *261*, 212, 1993.

15

Dynemicin

Masataka Konishi
Zenyaku Kogyo Company Ltd., Tokyo, Japan

Toshikazu Oki
Toyama Prefectural University, Toyama, Japan

I. INTRODUCTION

Historically, discovery of a novel antibiotic from fermentation broth by one research group may be followed by identification of the same or structurally related compounds by other research groups. This happens often and also happened
in the enediyne antibiotics.

From 1985 to 1987, the discoveries of esperamicin (1,2) and the calicheamicins
(3), a remarkable family of antibiotics, were announced by the Bristol-Myers
Squibb group and the Lederle group, respectively. About the same time, two other
groups (4,5) independently reported the isolation of what were eventually shown
to be members of the esperamicin complex. Immediately after their unusual structures and mechanism of activation were elucidated, neocarzinostatin chromophore,
the active principle of the older anticancer antibiotic neocarzinostatin, was found
to have a similar activation mechanism (6). Inspired by the structural novelty and
a fascinating mechanism of action, this family of antibiotics, now collectively
referred to as enediyne antibiotics, has been studied intensively with regard to total
chemical synthesis, mechanism of action, and DNA interaction.

Through the continued search for DNA-interacting agents among fermentation
products, the Bristol-Myers Squibb group added to the list another novel enediyne
antibiotic complex, named dynemicins, in 1989 (7). These products originated in
a rare actinomycete strain named *Micromonospora chersina* sp. nov. M956-1. It

soon became evident that dynemicin A, the major active principle of the dynemicin complex, had potent inhibitory activity against a wide range of microorganisms, especially gram-positive bacteria. It also displayed extremely strong cytotoxicity with IC_{50} values in the ng/ml range against a number of murine and human tumor cells. Extremely potent in vivo antitumor activity has been demonstrated in experimental mouse tumor models. Structural studies by spectroscopic analysis and x-ray crystallographic analysis of its triacetyl derivatives showed that dynemicin A is a new member of the enediyne antibiotic (8) family (Fig. 1). It is unique in having a bicyclo[7.3.1]-1,5-diyn-3-ene unit associated with the hydroxyanthraquinone chromophore of the classical anthracycline antibiotics. In 1990, the Institute of Microbial Chemistry reported a structural variant deoxydynemicin A as a coproduct of dynemicin A from the fermentation broth of a *M. globosa* strain (9).

II. DISCOVERY, PRODUCTION, ISOLATION, AND PHYSICOCHEMICAL PROPERTIES

As with the esperamicins and calicheamicins, the dynemicin complex was discovered by fermentation screening of rare actinomycetes as producing organisms using a prescreen for the discovery of DNA-interacting compounds. Recombination-deficient mutant strains (Rec⁻ strains) of gram-positive and gram-negative bacteria are more sensitive to DNA-damaging agents than their parent strains (Rec⁺ strains) (10). Differential assays using a Rec⁺ strain and its Rec⁻ mutant (Rec

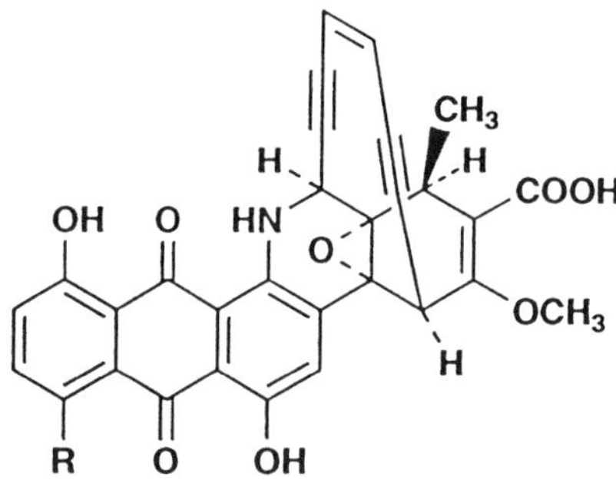

Dynemicin A   R=OH

Deoxydynemicin   R=H

Figure 1 Structures of dynemicin A and deoxydynemicin.

assay) have been used to detect chemical mutagens, but they have also proven useful as a prescreening method for DNA-damaging antitumor antibiotics. In fact, many known antitumor antibiotics such as mitomycin C, actinomycin D, and the esperamicins exhibit much stronger growth inhibition in the Rec⁻ strain of *B. subtilis* (M45 strain) than in the parent Rec⁺ strain (H17). While searching for new antitumor antibiotics using this differential assay as a prescreening system, a complex of violet-colored strongly bioactive compounds was discovered in a broth produced by a culture of a *Micromonospora* strain. The producing organism was isolated from a soil sample collected in Gujarat state, India, and thus was named *Micromonospora chersina* sp. nov. N956-1 after extensive taxonomical studies. Deoxydynemicin A was discovered together with dynemicin A in the culture broth of *M. globosa* MG-331-hF6 collected on Mt. Minobu, Yamanashi Prefecture, Japan (9). Several years before these discoveries, the Takeda and Tanabe research groups had isolated the powerful antibacterial antibiotics M-92 (11) and T-42318 (12), whose physicochemical properties were closely related to those of dynemicin A and deoxydynemicin A. The producing strains of M-92 and T-42318 were identified as *M. verruculosa* sp. nov. MCRL 0-404 and *M. papulosus* No. T-42318, respectively. Dynemicins are produced in flasks or tanks using a fermentation medium composed of cornstarch 10%, pharmamedia 0.5%, $CuSO_4 5H_2O$ 0.005%, $CaCO_3$ 0.1%, and NaI 0.00005%, pH 7.0 at 28°C with agitation (250 rpm) and aeration (120 liters/min). As with the case of the calicheamicins, a greater than 10-fold increase of antibiotic production was observed when a trace amount of sodium iodide was added to the fermentation media. The antibiotic titer reached a maximum of 0.5 ~ 1.0 µg/ml after 73–92 hours of fermentation as monitored by bioassay and HPLC (13).

To isolate the dynemicins, the cultured broth of *M. chersina* (2000 liters) was extracted with ethyl acetate with stirring. The extract was concentrated to a residue containing a large amount of antifoam (4.0 kg). HPLC analysis (Fig. 2) showed that the concentrate contained around 0.04% of dynemicin components, dynemicin A comprising 63% and dynemicin M13% of the complex. The complex was chromatographed on a column of Sephabeads SP-800 with sequential elution by 80% methanol and 50% acetone. The major bioactive fraction eluted with 50% acetone was concentrated to a residue (70.1 g) containing ca. 1% of the dynemicin complex. Trituration of the residue with methanol yielded nearly pure dynemicin A as an insoluble solid. The methanolic solution containing the aromatized dynemicins M, O, P, and Q was concentrated and chromatographed on SP-800 to roughly resolve them into individual fractions. Further purification was effected by a combination of column chromatography with various adsorbents, as illustrated in Scheme I. The final purification of the minor dynemicins O, P, and Q was achieved by preparative HPLC using ODS columns (14).

Dynemicin A is a violet amorphous solid. It is fairly soluble in dimethyl sulfoxide, dimethylformamide, and dioxane, slightly soluble in chloroform, ethyl

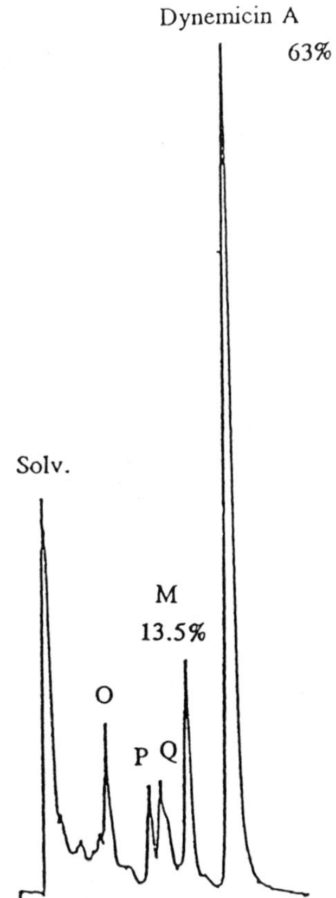

Column   :   YMC gel, A301-3, 4.6 nm I.D. x 100 mm
Mobile phase :   MeOH–0.15% KH$_2$PO$_4$, pH 3.5 (75:25, v/v)
Flow rate   :   0.8 ml/min
Detection   :   UV–595 nm

Figure 2   HPLC of dynemicin complex.

acetate, and methanol, but practically insoluble in other solvents. Upon treatment with acetic anhydride in pyridine, it yielded triacetyldynemicin A, which was crystallized as orange rods from methanol. The physicochemical properties of dynemicins A, M, O, P, and Q and triacetyldynemicin A are summarized in Table 1.

The IR spectrum of dynemicin A exhibited a broad band at 3500–3200 cm^{-1} due to hydroxyl and/or amino group and carbonyl absorptions at 1660 and 1630 cm^{-1} to be assigned to a quinone group. A marked carbonyl absorption at 1770

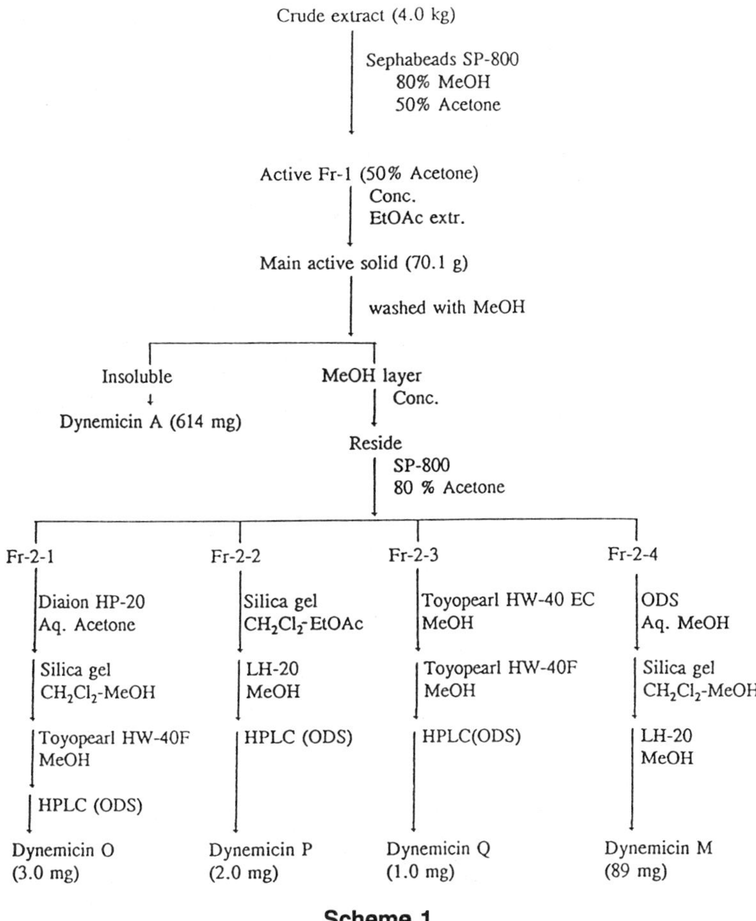

Scheme 1

cm^{-1} observed for the triacetate indicated the introduction of a phenolic acetate. The chemical shifts in the ^{1}H-NMR of dynemicin A and ^{13}C-NMR spectra of triacetyldynemicin A are analyzed in Table 2.

A complex of dynemicin A and deoxydynemicin A was extracted from cultured mycelia of *M. globosa* MG331-hF6 with methanol and enriched by solvent partition, precipitation, and Sephadex LH-20 chromatography. The two components were separated by preparative HPLC using an ODS column and DMF-0.1% $(NH_4)_2CO_3$ as the eluting solvent. Deoxydynemicin A had physicochemical and spectral properties quite similar to those of dynemicin A. The greatest differences were seen in the UV absorption and in the ^{1}H-NMR spectrum. The UV spectrum exhibited shorter absorption wavelengths with maxima at 234, 257, 393, 507,

Table 1 Physicochemical Properties of Dynemicins

	Dynemicin A	Triacetyl-dynemicin A	Dynemicin M	Dynemicin O	Dynemicin P	Dynemicin Q
Nature	Violet powder	Orange-red	Blue powder	Blue powder	Blue powder	Blue powder
M.P. (O°C, dec.)	208–210	228–231	238–240			
$[\alpha]_D^{24}$	+270° (c 0.01, DMF)	+1,300° (c 0.05, MeOH)	−2,460 (c 0.01, MeOH)			
UV$_{max}$ in MeOH(ϵ)	239 (24,900)	244 (40,100)	241 (41,700)	241 (20,600)	241 (30,700)	243 (20,800)
	282 (sh)	313 (6,700)	453 (1,500)	283 (5,900)	333 (2,630)	335 (3,070)
	569 (10,800)	482 (8,100)	589 (17,000)	335 (2,360)	586 (13,300)	588 (13,600)
	599 (10,100)		633 (17,200)	589 (11,600)	632 (14,000)	634 (13,700)
				633 (11,500)		
Molecular formula	$C_{30}H_{19}NO_9$	$C_{36}H_{25}NO_{12}$	$C_{29}H_{23}NO_9$	$C_{29}H_{23}NO_{10}$	$C_{28}H_{21}NO_9$	$C_{28}H_{19}NO_9$
FAB-MS (M+H)$^+$						
Found	538.1132	664	(M)$^+$ 529.1375	546.1334	516.1367	514.1145
Calcd	538.1138		529.1373	546.1400	516.1295	514.1138

Table 2 ^{1}H-NMR of Dynemicin A and ^{13}C-NMR of Triacetyldynemicin A (in DMSO-d_6)

Dynemicin A: R = H
Triacetyldynemicin A: = Ac

^{1}H-NMR	Chemical shift (coupling, J)	^{13}C-NMR	Chemical shift (coupling)
4-CH$_3$	1.30 (3H,d,J = 7.3)	2-C	43.8(d)
4-H	3.57 (1H,q,J = 7.3)	3-C	71.3(s)
6-OCH$_3$	3.82 (3H,s)	4-C	35.5(d)
7-H	4.78 (1H,s)	5-C	114.8(s)
2-H	5.08 (1H,d,J = 3.8)	6-C	153.3(s)
26-H	6.07 (1H,dd,J = 9.8 and 1.3)	7-C	31.4(d)
		8-C	63.2(s)
25-H	6.05 (1H,dd,J = 9.8 and 1.3)	9-C	130.1(s)
17-H	7.62 ⎫	10-C	130.0(d)
16-H	7.62 ⎭ (2H,s)	11-C	139.5(s)
10-H	8.03 (1H,s)	12-C	124.5(s)
1-NH	9.86 (1H,d,J = 4.3)	13-C	180.6(s)
		14-C	125.9(s)
11-OH	12.15 (1H,brs)	15-C	146.4(s)
15-OH	12.70 (1H,brs)	16-C	131.0(d)
18-OH	13.10 (1H,brs)	17-C	130.6(d)
		18-C	146.9(s)
5-COOH	12.30 (1H,brs)	19-C	126.1(s)
		20-C	182.7(s)
		21-C	114.7(s)
		22-C	143.8(s)
		23-C	97.3(s)
		24-C	89.6(s)
		25-C	124.4(d)
		26-C	124.2(d)
		27-C	88.9(s)
		28-C	99.4(s)
		4-CH$_3$	18.5(q)
		5-COOH	167.4(s)
		6-OCH$_3$	57.8(q)
		3 × COCH$_3$	20.6(q) × 2, 20.9(q)
			16.9(s), 169.1(s) × 2

544, and 587 nm in methanol. The ^{1}H-NMR revealed an additional aromatic proton (δ: 7.85, dd) to those of dynemicin A.

III. STRUCTURE DETERMINATION

The structure proofs for dynemicin A ($C_{30}H_{19}NO_9$) and deoxydynemicin A ($C_{30}H_{19}NO_8$), both exclusive of the absolute stereochemistry, were obtained by spectroscopic analyses and x-ray diffraction studies. Acetylation of dynemicin A in pyridine afforded a tri-O-acetyl derivative ($C_{36}H_{25}NO_{12}$), as discussed before, and diazomethane treatment a monomethyl ester derivative ($C_{31}H_{21}NO_9$). The UV spectrum of dynemicin A (λ_{max} in MeOH: 239, 282, 569, and 599) and the shift of the absorption maxima in acid (practically no shift) and in alkaline methanol (to 247, 278, 598, and 644 nm) suggested a close resemblance to those of the 1,4,6-trihydroxy- and 1,4,6,9-tetrahydroxyanthraquinone chromophores contained in anthracycline antibiotics such as ε-isorhodomycin (15) (Fig. 3).

Dynemicin A was poorly soluble in the usual NMR solvents, which hampered detailed structural analysis. However, triacetyldynemicin A (λ_{max} 244, 313, and 482 nm) was soluble enough to provide significant structural information (Table 2). ^{13}C-NMR revealed a 1,2,4,6,9-pentasubstituted anthraquinone exhibiting 14 sp^2 carbon signals at δ114.7, 124.5, 125.9, 126.1, 130.0(d), 130.1(d), 131.0, 130.6(d), 139.5, 143.8, 146.4, 146.9, 180.6, and 182.7, the last two being assigned as carbonyls and three others as proton-bearing carbons. The spectrum also disclosed four singlet carbons at δ 88.8, 89.6, 97.3, and 99.4 and two doublet carbons at δ 124.0 and 124.4 that were very similar to the characteristic carbon signals assigned to the 1,5-diyn-3-ene moieties of calicheamicin γ_1^I and esperamicin A_1. A weak absorption at 2190 cm^{-1} in the FT-IR spectrum of dynemicin A supported the presence of a triple bond. The assignment was substantiated by heteronuclear multiple-bond ^{1}H-^{13}C correlation spectroscopy experiments. Triacetyldynemicin A was analyzed by single crystal x-ray diffraction. The analysis was complicated by the crystallization of the compound in pairs of conformers and the difficulties of a phase model. After solving these problems, the structures of the two independent molecules in the asymmetric center were analyzed by a computer-generated drawing of the final x-ray experiment. They have the same overall structures with different conformations. The structure of one conformer is depicted in Figure 4 (8). The x-ray analysis determined only the relative configuration and analysis with a heavy-atom—containing derivative has not yet been successful. The structure contains a bicyclo[7.3.1]tetradeca-1,5-diyn-3-ene-8,9-epoxide system fused to a 9-amino-1,4,6-trihydroxyanthraquinone chromophore to form a heptacyclo ring system. In the crystal structure, the 1,5-diyn-3-ene ring stands perpendicular to the nearly planar anthraquinonehexahydroisoquinoline nucleus and the epoxide projects to the other side. This experiment represented the first structural determination of a natural bicyclo-enediyne system by x-ray crystallographic analysis.

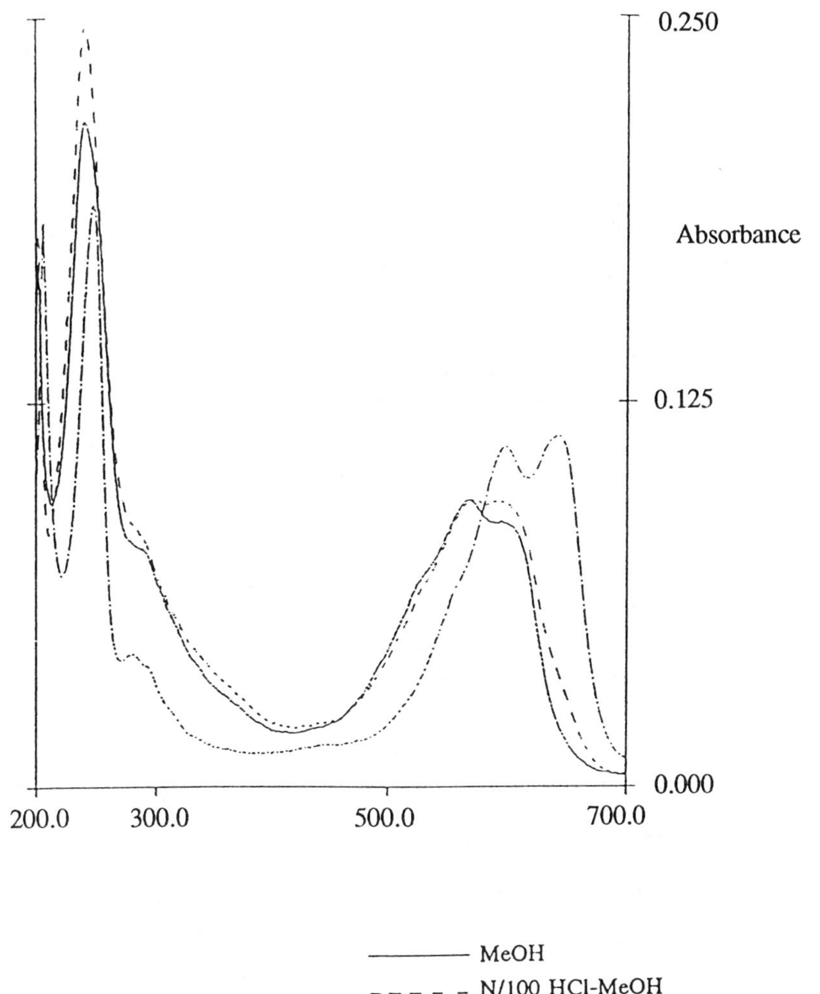

Figure 3 UV spectrum of dynemicin A.

Consistent with the proposed structure, long-range ^{1}H-^{13}C correlation (COLOC) experiments defined clear coupling between the NH and C3, C9, and C22, H-2 and C3, C8, and C-23, H-4 and C5-COOH and C6, H-7 and C3, C6, C8, C27, and C28, and H-10 and C8, C11, C12, and C22. The long-range correlations are summarized in Figure 5.

The structures of the minor components, dynemicins M ($C_{29}H_{23}NO_9$), O ($C_{29}H_{23}NO_{10}$), P ($C_{28}H_{21}NO_9$), and Q ($C_{28}H_{19}NO_9$), were established spectro-

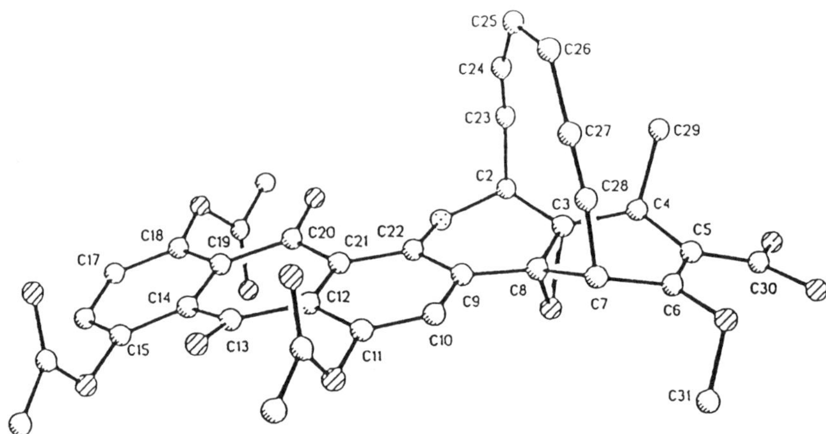

Figure 4 Computer-generated perspective drawing of x-ray model of triacetyldynemicin A.

scopically by comparison with dynemicin A. Although considerable bathochromic shifts were observed in the UV spectrum of dynemicin M, retention of a 1,4,6-trihydroxy-8,9-substituted anthraquinone chromophore in the component was evidenced by ^{13}C-NMR and other spectral data. The ^{1}H-NMR spectrum revealed four contiguous protons of a 1,2-disubstituted benzene (δ 7.10–7.60) in addition to the three aromatic protons of the anthraquinone moiety. The spectrum, however, lacked the two *cis* double bond protons (δ 6.06 and 6.09) of the 1,5-diyn-3-ene system observed in the spectrum of dynemicin A. Furthermore, two new

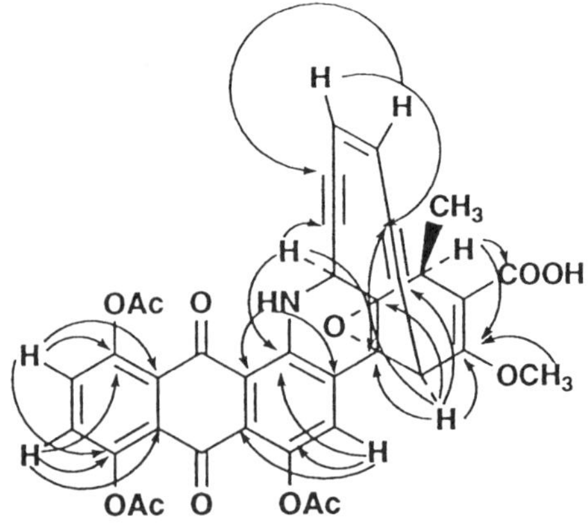

Figure 5 Long-range NMR correlations of dynemicin A triacetate.

hydroxyl proton signals (δ 5.31 and 5.95) were observed in the spectrum, indicating an opening of the epoxide of dynemicin A to a diol. In agreement with the ^{1}H-NMR, the ^{13}C-NMR of dynemicin M contained six sp^2 carbon signals (δ 126.2, 127.2, 128.2, 128.5, 135.2, and 135.6) assignable to a 1,2-disubstituted benzene in place of the diynene carbons of dynemicin A. The ^{13}C-NMR spectrum lacked the carboxylic carbon (δ 167.0) and two sp^2 carbons (δ 114.8 and 153.2) of dynemicin A and displayed a new carbonyl (δ 204.8) and a new sp^3 carbon (δ 82.7, d). These data indicated that the diyne moiety of dynemicin A was aromatized to a 1,2-substituted benzene with concomitant opening of the epoxide to diol in dynemicin A. The carboxylic acid at C5 is decarbonated to result in a C5-keto form. The NMR signal shifts of other parts fitted well with the assigned structure in Figure 6.

The UV and other spectra of dynemicins O, P, and Q are essentially the same as, or very similar to, those of dynemicin M, except that dynemicin O contains one more oxygen than dynemicin M. Its ^{3}C-NMR was similar to that of dynemicin

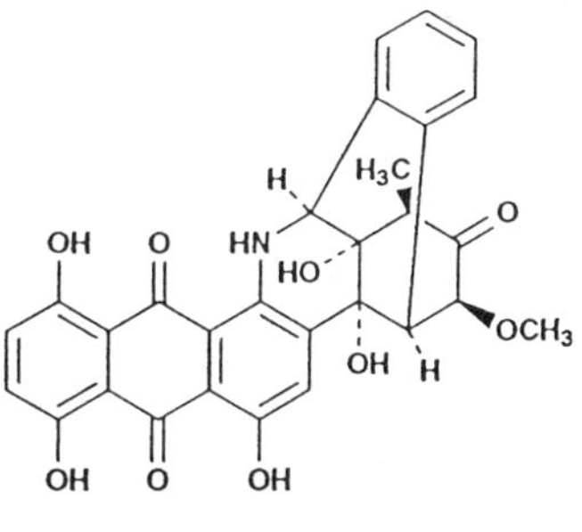

Dynemicin M

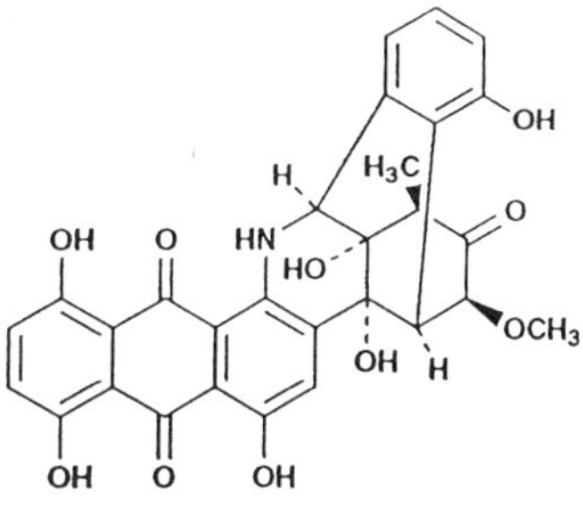

Dynemicin O

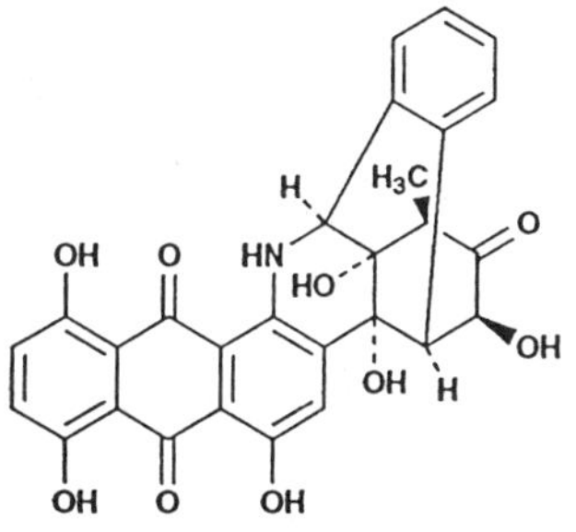

Dynemicin P

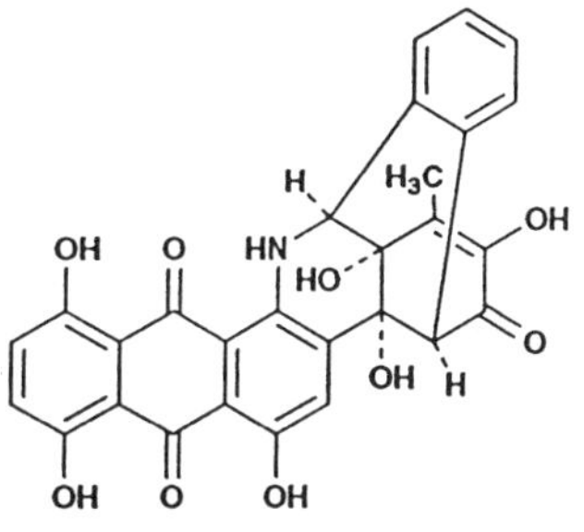

Dynemicin Q

Figure 6 Structures of the minor components, dynemicins M, O, P, and Q.

M, the difference being that one of the phenyl carbons resonated at a considerably lower field (δ 156.0). This, together with the presence of three sequential aromatic protons in ^{1}H-NMR, indicated that dynemicin O is a monohydroxyl derivative of dynemicin M. Among the three aromatic protons (δ 6.80, 6.85, and 7.10), the signal at δ 6.85 correlated with H-2 (δ 4.59) and was assigned to H-24. Since the proton was proven to be on the carbon at δ 144.8 (C24), the phenol hydroxyl was established to be on C27 (δ 156.0). A clear NOE observed between H-4 and H-6 placed the two protons diaxially with the C4-CH$_3$ and C6-OCH$_3$ being on the same side in the diequatorial orientation. The molecular formula and the spectral data of dynemicin P corresponded to desmethyldynemicin M. The ^{1}H-NMR spectrum of dynemicin P revealed the presence of a OH at C6 instead of the OCH$_3$ in dynemicin M, showing a broad doublet at δ 4.83 coupled with H-7 and a broad hydroxyl proton at δ 3.15. These data allowed des-O-methyl dynemicin M to be assigned to dynemicin P.

Dynemicin Q has a molecular formula with two fewer hydrogens than dynemicin M. Its ^{1}H-NMR lacked the quartet methine proton and the doublet methyl observed in all other dynemicin components. Instead, a singlet methyl was observed at lower field (δ 2.01), indicating that it was on a double bond. In the spectrum, the H-7 signal appeared as a singlet at low field (δ 5.28) and a hydroxyl proton as a singlet at δ 5.79. Since other parts of the molecule were quite similar to dynemicin P, dynemicin Q was determined to be an oxidized form of dynemicin P.

IV. BIOLOGICAL ACTIVITY

Dynemicin A and deoxydynemicin A possess a broad spectrum of antimicrobial activity, which is even more potent than that of esperamicins. They have minimal inhibitory concentrations of in the range of pg/ml against gram-positive bacteria, ng/ml against gram-negative bacteria, and 10 μg/ml against fungi (Table 3). Triacetyldynemicin A is significantly more active (2–8 times) than dynemicin A against all bacteria and fungi tested. Interestingly, dynemicin A cured mice infected with a lethal inoculum of *Staphylococcus aureus* Smith by intramuscular injection (PD$_{50}$: 0.13 mg/kg). Other enediyne class antibiotics did not exhibit in vivo effects, despite having marked in vitro antimicrobial activity. The most striking feature observed for dynemicins is that aromatized dynemicin M retained considerable antimicrobial activity. (MIC: 0.2–0.4 μg/ml, PD$_{50}$ vs. *S. aureus* Smith 1.8 mg/kg). This is in distinct contrast to the aromatized esperamicin X, which is virtually bioinactive.

Dynemicin A shows powerful inhibitory activity against a variety of tumor cell lines including the vincristine-resistant P388 leukemia lines (Table 4). On a molar basis, its cytotoxicity is comparable to that of esperamicins and calicheamicins and is approximately 1000–4000 times stronger than that of adriamycin. It should

Table 3 Antimicrobial Activity of Dynemicins

Organism	MIC (μg/ml)				
	A	Triacetyl A	M	O	Q
Staphylococcus aureus FDA 209P	0.000013	0.0000063	0.10	0.10	0.10
S. aureus Smith	0.000025	0.0000063	0.05	0.02	0.02
S. epidermidis D153	0.0000063	0.0000031	0.05	0.01	0.01
Micrococcus luteus PCI 1001	0.0008	0.0002	0.4	0.63	5.0
Bacillus subtilis PCI 219	0.0000063	0.0000031	0.05	0.0025	0.005
Escherichia coli NIHJ	0.05	0.0063	>10	>10	>10
Klebsiella pneumoniae D11	0.0063	0.0008	>10	>10	>10
Pseudomonas aeruginosa A9930	0.025	0.0063	>10	>10	>10
Proteus vulgaris A9436	0.0063	0.0031	>10	>10	>10
Clostridium difficile A21675	0.0063	0.0031	>10	>10	>10
Bacteroides fragilis A22693	0.2	0.1	>10	>10	>10
Candida albicans IAM 4888	12.5	0.4	>10	>10	>10
Cryptococcus neoformans D49	12.5	0.8	>10	>10	>10
Aspergillus fumigatus IAM 2530	6.3	0.1	>10	>10	>10
Trichophyton mentagrophytes D155	12.5	0.4	>10	>10	>10

Table 4 In Vitro Cytotoxicity Against Murine and Human Tumor Cells

Compound	IC$_{50}$ (ng/ml)							
	B16-F10	P388	P388/VCR	P388/ADM	HCT-116	Moser	K562	K652/ADM
Dynemicin A	4.1	0.021	0.019	0.022	0.28	0.0027	0.024	0.026
Triacetyldynemicin A	2.7	0.021	0.020	0.022	0.18	0.0040	0.019	NT
Doxorubicin	30	16	52	230	130	500	50	7,500
Mitomycin C	730	8.6	9.9	12	41	82	520	3,400

B16-F10, murine melanoma; P-388, murine leukemia; P388/VCR, vincristine-resistant P388 subline; P388/ADM, doxorubicin-resistant P388; HCT-116, human colon carcinoma; Moser, human colon carcinoma; K562, human myelogenous leukemia; K562/ADM, doxorubicin-resistant K562.

be noted that dynemicin M and other aromatized analogs also showed significant cytotoxicity, though much less so than dynemicin A. As will be discussed in a later section, the major biological activity of the enediyne antibiotics is believed to be due to DNA strand scission by the aromatic biradicals produced from the enediyne moieties. Significant biological activities specifically displayed by the aromatized dynemicins indicate that the anthraquinone moiety exerts a special role.

In antitumor tests in vivo, intraperitoneally (ip) administered dynemicin A significantly prolonged the life span of mice implanted ip with P388 and L1210 leukemias (16) (Table 5). Although the maximum T/C values were not high, dynemicin A exhibited activity over a wide dose range, with the minimum effective doses being 16–32 times lower than those of mitomycin C. Efficacy against intravenously (ip) inoculated tumors was also observed following ip administration of the drug. Similar in vivo antitumor activity was determined for triacetyldynemicin A. The aromatized dynemicin compounds appeared not to have in vivo antitumor activity.

The antitumor activity of esperamicins, calicheamicins, and neocarzinostatin is associated with the tumor cell DNA interaction. Dynemicin A strongly inhibited the incorporation of [methyl-^{3}H]-thymidine into the acid-insoluble fraction of B16 cells with an IC_{50} value of 0.0022 µg/ml, whereas the IC_{50} values for the incorporation of [2-^{14}C]-uridine and L-[4,5-^{3}H]-leucine were 8.5 and 14 µg/ml, respectively (Table 6). These results indicate that the inhibitor effect of dynemicin A on DNA synthesis is approximately 4000 and 6000 times stronger than that on RNA and protein synthesis, respectively. In contrast, dynemicin M did not show specific inhibition of DNA, RNA, and protein synthesis, indicating that the mechanism of its biological activity differs from that of dynemicin A.

V. MECHANISM OF ACTION

Together with their outstanding biological activity and unprecedented structure, the mechanisms of activation of esperamicins and calicheamicins have attracted much attention. The studies on esperamicins, calicheamicins, and neocarzinostatin chromophore have clarified several common features of their mechanisms of activation. First, they insert into the minor groove of specific DNA helices utilizing a portion of their structures. By activating their specific triggers, the enediyne cores cyclize to highly reactive aromatic diradical species under physiological conditions. The diradicals abstract hydrogen from the neighboring DNA sugar backbones, inducing either single or double strand breaks in the DNA. The unusually potent antitumor activity of these antibiotics has been ascribed to the DNA damage resulting from the above cascade.

The combination of an enediyne with a bridgehead epoxide, which prevents enediyne cyclization, led us to consider acid catalysis as a mechanism of enediyne activation in the dynemicins. In the early stage of the isolation studies when the

Table 5 Antitumor Activity Against P388 and L1210 Leukemia (IP) in Mice

Compound	Dose[a] (mg/kg/day)	P388 Leukemia		L1210 Leukemia	
		MST[b] (day)	T/C (%)	MST[b] (day)	T/C (%)
Dynemicin A	1.0	9.5	95	9.0	113
	0.5	15.5	155	9.5	119
	0.25	15.0	150	10.0	125
	0.13	14.0	140	12.0	150
	0.063	14.0	140	10.0	125
	0.031	14.0	140	10.0	125
	0.016	13.5	135	10.5	131
	0.008	12.0	120	8.5	106
	0.004	11.0	110		
Triacetyldynemicin A	1.0	11.0	110		
	0.5	13.5	135		
	0.25	13.5	135		
	0.13	12.5	125		
	0.063	12.5	125		
	0.031	13.0	130		
Mitomycin C	4.0	22.5	225	14.0	175
	2.0	15.5	155	12.5	156
	1.0	14.5	145	11.0	138
	0.5	15.0	150	10.5	131
	0.25	14.0	140	9.5	119
	0.13	11.5	115	9.0	113
Vehicle control	—	10.0		8.0	—

[a] q2d × 3, IP.
[b] Median survival time.

Table 6 Inhibition of Macromolecular Biosynthesis by Dynemicin

	IC$_{50}$ (μg/ml)		
	DNA	RNA	Protein
Dynemicin A	0.0022	8.5	14
Dynemicin L	>10	8.2	>10
Esperamicin A$_1$	0.0000017	0.013	0.17

Inhibition of incorporation of [methyl-^{3}H]-thymidine(DNA), [2-^{14}C]-uridine(RNA), and L[4,5-^{3}H]-leucine into acid-insoluble fraction of melanoma B16-F10 cells.

extraction was performed under slightly acidic conditions, two new blue components with weak activity, dynemicins L ($C_{30}H_{22}NO_9Cl$) and N ($C_{30}H_{23}NO_{10}$), were isolated. Their spectroscopic data showed that they evidently lacked the enediyne and epoxide moieties, but retained the carboxylic acid and the methoxyl on the C5-C6 double bond. Detailed NMR analysis assisted by homo- and heteronuclear correlation spectroscopy established that the 1,5-diyn-3-ene of dynemicin A had aromatized to a 1,2-substituted benzene with concomitant opening of the epoxide to yield the chlorohydrin and diol in dynemicin L and N, respectively (8). That the chlorine in dynemicin L is positioned at C8 is supported by the fact that H-7 of dynemicin L resonated at δ 4.47, 0.60 ppm lower than that of dynemicin N, whereas H-2 and H-4 of both components resonated at nearly the same fields. Further support for the structures of dynemicins L and N and the novel acid-catalyzed activation mechanism of dynemicin A were demonstrated by the rapid conversion of dynemicin A to dynemicin L followed by further gradual conversion to dynemicin N in acidic methanol (Fig. 7). Opening of the epoxide by acid and subsequent nucleophilic substitution of a chloride (or hydroxide) anion to C8 caused relaxation of the 10-membered ring, bringing C23 and C28 close enough to induce a Bergman-type aromatization. This is in contrast to neocarzinostatin chromophore, which afforded an isolable chlorohydrin upon exposure to dilute hydrochloric acid (17).

In addition to the above mechanism, the combination of the anthraquinone chromophore with the enediyne-epoxide in dynemicin A results in an activation mechanism involving anthraquinone reduction (18,19). Dynemicin A induced remarkable DNA scission in the presence of thiols, reducing agents, and visible light. One characteristic feature of DNA degradation caused by dynemicin A is the strong cleavage induction by NADPH. When dynemicin A was treated with NADPH in DMF, a new blue product (named dynemicin H) increased with a decrease in dynemicin A as monitored by HPLC (20). Dynemicin H, $C_{30}H_{23}NO_9$, exhibited UV and visible absorption spectra markedly similar to those of dynemicins M, L, and N. The presence of four contiguous protons of 1,2-dis-

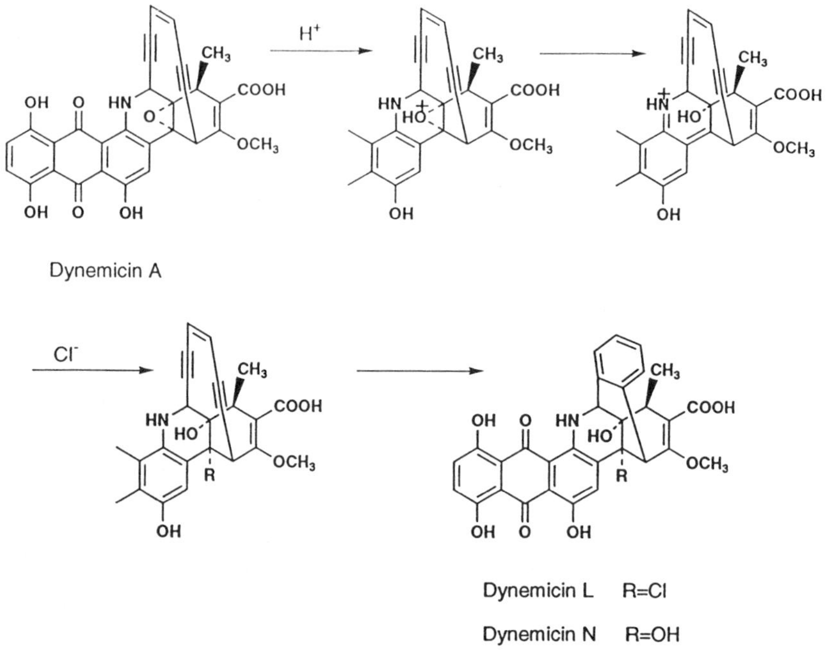

Dynemicin A

Dynemicin L   R=Cl

Dynemicin N   R=OH

Figure 7 Acid catalyzed decomposition of dynemicin A.

ubstituted benzene and three aromatic protons on the anthraquinone was demonstrated by the ^{1}H-NMR. In addition, the spectrum exhibited a new methine proton (δ 3.50, d, J = 3.0, H-8) and a hydroxyl proton (δ 5.46), the former being split by the neighboring H-7 (δ 3.96, d, J = 3.0). Therefore, dynemicin H was assigned as a C8 hydrogen analog of dynemicins L and N. Degradation of dynemicin A using ascorbate or visible light also yielded dynemicin H as the major product together with some nonisolable minor byproducts. It is of particular interest that dynemicin A showed strong DNA cleavage activity in low-energy visible light even at the 580-nm cut-off light (red light). Although esperamicin is also activated by light, only UV light is effective. The red light–induced DNA cleavage by dynemicin A apparently correlates with its characteristic anthraquinone absorption between 500 and 630 nm (21).

When the activation reaction was performed with methyl thioglycolate, a new minor product (dynemicin S, $C_{33}H_{27}NO_{11}S$) was produced together with dynemicin H (20). The physicochemical and spectroscopic data of dynemicin S were similar to those of the other aromatized dynemicins. In the NMR spectra, a new methyl (δ 3.61, s) and a methylene (δ 3.40, s) were observed and the C7-methine proton (δ 4.01) appeared as a singlet. These data allowed the assignment of the C8 thioglycolate structure to dynemicin S.

To summarize the above, reductive activation plays a major role and nucleophilic opening of the epoxide a minor role in the activation of dynemicin A with thiols, reducing agents, and light. Thus, the major degradation process appear to proceed as in Figure 8; NADPH and thiols cause two consecutive one- or two-

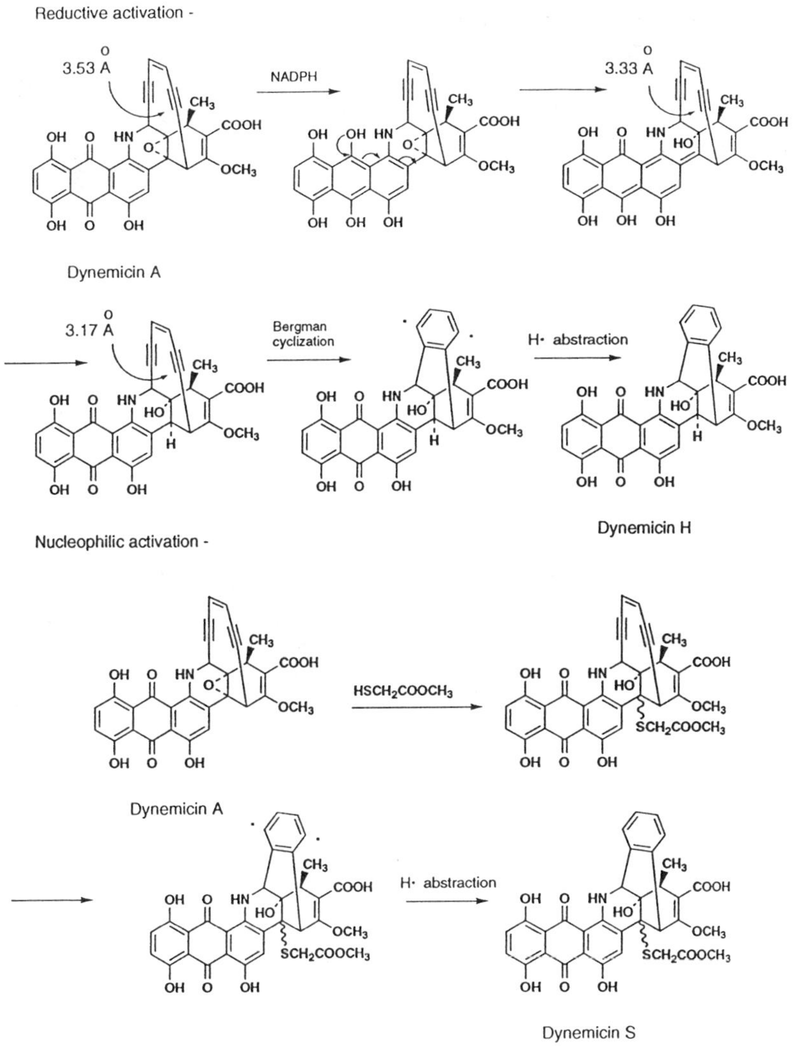

Figure 8 Reductive and nucleophilic activation of dynemicin A.

electron reductions of dynemicin A to yield a hydroquinone, which rearranges via an epoxide opening to give a semiquinone methide. Further rearrangement to quinone alcohol by protonation at C8 causes a dramatic conformational change of the molecule such that the distance between the triple bond termini is reduced from 3.54 Å in dynemicin A to 3.17 Å in the quinone alcohol (22). This induces Bergman cycloaromatization to a phenylene diradical, which can abstract hydrogen from the sugar backbone of DNA resulting in cleavage.

Having a new enediyne-epoxide conjugated with an anthraquinone, the antineoplastic action of dynemicin A was considered to be associated with intercalation by the anthraquinone and DNA scission by the biradical formed from the enediyne core (23). The fact that the aromatized dynemicins M, O, and P had no specific DNA cleavage activity but retained significant cytotoxicity supported this assumption.

In a reaction with 5′-end–labeled 128-base-pair (Sal I-Dra II) pBR322 DNA, dynemicin A preferentially cleaved the 3′ side of purine bases such as 5′-AG, 5′-GC, and 5′-AT and attacked predominantly guanine bases (Fig. 9). It is of interest that guanine is the most resistant to cleavage by esperamicins, calicheamicins, and neocarzinostatin chromophore. The histogram also demonstrated that the antibiotic very often caused breaks 3 bp apart in the two DNA strands,

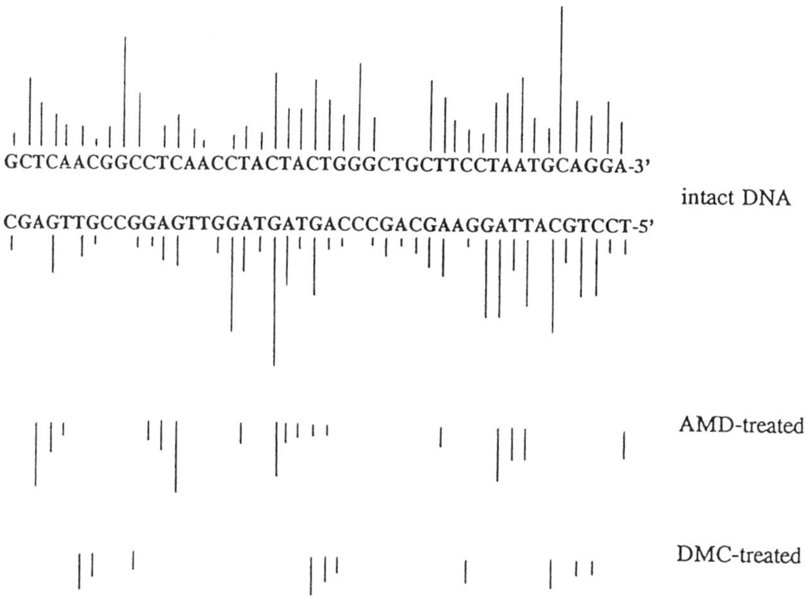

Figure 9   Histograms of DNA-cutting sites by dynemicin A for intact DNA and actinomycin D (AMD)– or distamycin A (DMC)–pretreated DNA.

which are characteristic of double strand DNA breakers. The cleavage pattern further suggested that dynemicin A interacted with the minor groove of the DNA helix. This assumption was supported by the significant alteration of the cleavage pattern by pretreatment of the DNA with distamycin A and anthramycin, typical minor groove-interacting agents. In addition, adriamycin and actinomycin D, which are DNA minor groove intercalaters, strongly inhibited dynemicin A–induced DNA cleavage. When single-stranded and double-stranded DNA substrates of the phage G4 were used for the cutting experiment, most of the preferred cleavages occurred in the double-stranded DNA and in the stem regions of the single-stranded DNA. Some cuts were also observed only on the inverted repeat sequences in the single-stranded DNA. These cuttings indicated that dynemicin A does not cleave single-stranded DNA efficiently.

To summarize the mechanism studies on dynemicin A, it first interacts with the minor groove of the DNA helix through its planar anthraquinone, after which it is activated by NADPH, thiols, reducing agents, or visible light at the anthraquinone moiety. It induces diradicals by Bergman cycloaromatization of the enediyne core and cleaves the DNA by abstraction of hydrogens from specific DNA sequences.

VI. BIOSYNTHESIS

The structure of dynemicin A has been established as a unique hybrid of an unusual bicyclo[7.3.1]-1,5-diyn-3-ene and the classical anthracycline, the former unit being similar to the core portions of esperamicins and calicheamicins. Neocarzinostatin chromophore has a bicyclo[7.3.0]dienediyne-epoxide, a core related to those of the above three antibiotics. The biosynthetic pathway of these unique compounds, particularly of their enediyne units, has been a focus of interest in relation to novel mechanisms of activation. Goldberg et al. (24) recently reported the biosynthetic origin of the carbon skelton of neocarzinostatin chromophore. In their studies using ^{13}C-labeled acetic acids as precursors, they clarified that the naphthoic acid was biosynthesized de novo from 6 moles of acetic acid linked in a head-to-tail manner. The bicyclodiynene core was produced from crepenynic acid, which in turn was derived from oleic acid. The crepenynic acid was cleaved at C4-C5 and C17-C18, and the resulting 14-carbon unit cyclized to the neocarzinostatin chromophore skelton. They also speculated in the paper that the esperamicin and calicheamicin cores were also derived from crepenynic acid through cleavage at a different position.

Recent studies, however, have shown that esperamicin A_1 is not derived from crepenynic acid (see Chapter 12). Iwasaki et al. (25) elucidated the origin of all the carbon units in dynemicin A using several labeled precursors. Their first experiment using the ^{14}C-labeled precursors, acetate and methionine, revealed that they were incorporated into dynemicin A. Thus *Micromonospora chersina* M956-

1 was fermented in the presence of [1-^{13}C]- and [2-^{13}C]-enriched acetic acids and [methyl-^{13}C]-L-methionine. The resulting dynemicin A were analyzed by ^{13}C-NMR spectrometry. The results indicated that [methyl-^{13}C]-L-methionine was incorporated only in C31-OCH$_3$ and [1-^{13}C]- and [2-^{13}]C-acetate–enriched 14 and 15 carbons, respectively, of dynemicin A, as shown in Figure 10. Among the assigned enrichment profile, two sets of neighboring dynemicin A carbons were proven to be derived from the same acetic acid carbon atoms: C5 and COOH from the methyl carbon, and C8 and C9 from the carboxyl carbon of acetic acid. This leads to the conclusion that the bicyclo[7.3.1]diynene unit and the anthraquinone unit were biosynthesized separately from two heptaketides and later assembled. The carboxylic acid linked to C5 was not biosynthesized as part of the cyclodiynene polyketide, rather it was derived from a separate acetic acid condensed at C5. The former assumption indicates that the bioactive core moiety of dynemicin A should also be classified as a bicyclo[7.3.1]diynene such as esperamicins and calicheamicin rather than as a tricyclo system. The latter hypothesis could be supported by the fact that all of the naturally occurring aromatized dynemicin components isolated lacked the carboxylic acid unit at C5. Further biosynthesis studies including incorporation of ^{13}C-double-labeled acetic acid shed light upon these matters and clarified the complete biosynthetic pathway of dynemicin A as outlined in Figure 10.

VII. SUMMARY

With their unusual chemical, biological, and mechanistic properties, the diynene antibiotics have captured the interest of a variety of research scientists interested in antitumor drugs, particularly DNA-cutting antitumor agents. Extensive studies on these antibiotics have made considerable progress in understanding how they work to kill tumor cells. The unique triggering mechanism of these antibiotics, followed by biradical formation of their enediyne cores and of the DNA recognition with their appended functionalities has suggested the potential of these molecules as novel DNA-cleaving and anticancer agents.

Among these diynene antibiotics, dynemicin A is particularly interesting because of its unique enediyne and classical antitumor anthracycline core assembly. In contrast to esperamicin X and Z and other aromatized analogs, dynemicins M, O, and P, which lack the enediyne functionality, still possess antimicrobial and cytotoxicity activity. This may reflect the unique role of the anthraquinone moiety in the biological activity of dynemicins. It has been reported that a basic amino group is highly desirable for the activation of the enediyne antibiotics (26). The 1-NH of dynemicin A is not basic due to conjugation with the quinone, and thus dynemicin A is the only enediyne antibiotic without a basic amino functionality.

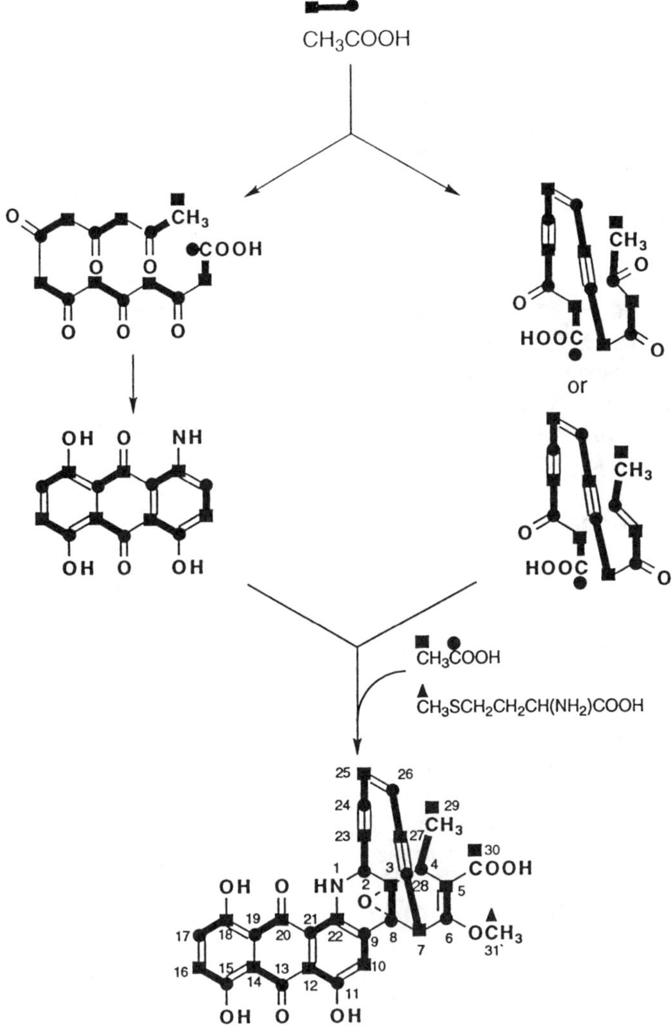

Figure 10 Biosynthetic pathway of dynemicin A.

Consequently, dynemicin A is considered to be a particularly appropriate candidate for chemical modification approaches to a new anticancer agent.

It should be noted that two antibiotics, M-92 and T-42318, reported in 1976 and 1984, respectively, were described to possess very similar chemical and biological properties to those of dynemicins. Their structural studies have not been reported.

REFERENCES

1. M. Konishi, H. Ohkuma, K. Saitoh, H. Kawaguchi, J. Golik, G. Dubay, G. Groenewold, B. Krishnan, and T. W. Doyle, *J. Antibiotics.*, *38*, 1605 (1985).
2. J. Golik, G. Dubay, G. Groenewold, H. Kawaguchi, M. Konishi, B. Krishnan, H. Ohkuma, K. Saitoh, and T. W. Doyle, *J. Am. Chem. Soc.*, *109*, 3462 (1987).
3. M. D. Lee, T. S. Dunne, C. C. Chang, G. A. Ellestad, M. M. Siegel, G. O. Morton, W. J. McGahren, and D. B. Borders, *J. Am. Chem. Soc.*, *109*, 3466 (1987).
4. S. Kiyoto, M. Nishizawa, H. Terano, H. Kohsaka, H. Aoki, H. Imanaka, Y. Kawai, I. Uchida, and M. Hashimoto, *J. Antibiotics.*, *38*, 840 (1985).
5. R. H. Bunge, T. R. Hurley, T. A. Smitka, N. E. Willmer, A. J. Brankiewicz, C. E. Steinman, and J. C. French, *J. Antibiotics, 37*, 1566 (1984).
6. A. G. Myers, *Tetrahedron Lett.*, *28*, 4493 (1897).
7. M. Konishi, H. Ohkuma, K. Matsumoto, T. Tsuno, H. Kamei, T. Miyaki, T. Oki, H. Kawaguchi, G. D. VanDuyne, and J. Clardy, *J. Antibiotics, 42*, 1449 (1989).
8. M. Konishi, H. Ohkuma, T. Tsuno, T. Oki, G. D. Vanduyne, and J. Clardy, *J. Am. Chem. Soc.*, *112*, 3715 (1990).
9. K. Shiomi, H. Iinuma, H. Naganawa, M. Hamada, S. Hattori, N. Nakamura, T. Takeuchi, and Y. Iitaka, *J. Antibiotics, 43*, 1000 (1990).
10. T. Kada, K. Tutikawa, and Y. Sadaie, *Mutation Res.*, *16*, 165 (1972).
11. K. Tani and T. Takaishi, *J. Antibiotics, 35*, 1437 (1982).
12. K. Hatano, T. Hasegawa, E. Higashide, M. Izawa, and M. Asai, Japan Patent 5279 (1984), Feb. 3, 1984.
13. M. Konishi, H. Ohkuma, K. Matsuomoto, K. Saitoh, T. Miyaki, T. Oki, and H. Kawaguchi, *J. Antibiotics, 44*, 1300 (1991).
14. M. Miyoshi, N. Morisaki, Y. Tokiwa, S. Iwasaki, M. Konishi, K. Saitoh, and T. Oki, *J. Antibiotics, 44*, 1037 (1991).
15. T. Oki, A. Yamamoto, Y. Matsuzawa, T. Takeuchi, and H. Umezawa, *J. Antibiotics, 33*, 1331 (1980).
16. H. Kamei, Y. Nishiyama, A. Takahashi, Y. Obi, and T. Oki, *J. Antibiotics, 44*, 1306 (1991).
17. E. Edo, H. Sato, K. Saito, Y. Akiyama, M. Kato, M. Mizugaki, Y. Koide, and N. Ishida, *J. Antibiotics, 39*, 535 (1986).
18. M. S. Semmelhack, J. Gallaher, and D. Cohen, *Tetrahedron Lett.*, *31*, 1521 (1990).
19. J. P. Synder and G. E. Tipsword, *J. Am. Chem. Soc.*, *112*, 4040 (1990).
20. Y. Sugiura, T. Arakawa, M. Uesughi, T. Shiraki, H. Ohkuma, and M. Konishi, *Biochemistry, 30*, 2989 (1991).
21. T. Shiraki and Y. Sugiura, *Biochemistry, 29*, 9795 (1990).
22. D. R. Langley, T. W. Doyle, and D. L. Beveridge, *J. Am. Chem. Soc.*, *113*, 4395 (1991).
23. Y. Sugiura, T. Shiraki, M. Konishi, and T. Oki, *Proc. Natl. Acad. Sci. USA, 87*, 3831 (1990).

24. O. D. Hensens, J. Giner, and I. H. Goldberg, *J. Am. Chem. Soc., 111,* 3295 (1989).
25. Y. Tokiwa, M. Miyoshi, H. Kobayashi, R. Sunaga, M. Konishi, T. Oki, and S. Iwasaki, *J. Am. Chem. Soc., 114,* 4107 (1992).
26. N. Zein, M. Poncin, R. Nilakantan, and G. A. Ellestad, *Science, 244,* 697 (1989).

16

Neocarzinostatin: Chemical and Biological Basis of Oxidative DNA Damage

Irving H. Goldberg and Lizzy S. Kappen
Harvard Medical School, Boston, Massachusetts

I. INTRODUCTION

Neocarzinostatin (NCS), the first bicyclic enediyne antitumor antibiotic with DNA-damaging properties to be described, belongs not only to a superfamily of agents containing enediyne structures but also to a superfamily of macromolecular protein antibiotics. It was only after it was appreciated that the active component of the macromolecular complex was a small, nonprotein chromophore that it was possible to begin to understand its interaction with DNA in molecular terms. These studies, in conjunction with those on the related calicheamicin/esperamicin agents, have uncovered novel mechanisms of DNA deoxyribose damage in which a diradical species of the active drug acts as a sequence-specific, bistrand-reactive agent. NCS has also proven to be a useful chemical reagent in the study of specific DNA damage mechanisms and of the role of dioxygen or its substitute in these processes. This chapter will summarize both the chemical and biological basis of its action as an antitumor agent and the properties that make it valuable as a biochemical tool in the study of DNA microstructure.

II. NEOCARZINOSTATIN: THE HOLOANTIBIOTIC

NCS was initially identified as a simple protein (MW = 11,100) (1,2), capable of inhibiting DNA synthesis and inducing DNA degradation in cells (3). The antibiotic protein could be purified by column chromatography of crude preparations of a nondialyzable ammonium sulfate fraction of culture filtrates of *Streptomyces carzinostaticus* var. F-14, which had been passed through a kaolin-celite column (4). The biologically active component of NCS, however, is a labile nonprotein chromophore (NCS-Chrom) that is tightly bound ($K_D \sim 10^{-10}$ M) to its apoprotein (MW = 11,100) (5–9). Suspicion of the presence of a nonprotein component possessing biological activity derived from several types of data. For one, it was found that the in vitro DNA-cleaving activity of the drug was enhanced, rather than inhibited, by agents, such as urea or organic solvents (10), that cause proteins to unfold or denature. Further, holo-NCS was found to have UV-visible absorption in the 300–360 nm range, beyond that expected for chromophoric amino acids (11). Finally, removal of this chromophoric material by chromatography on Amberlite XAD-7 or its destruction by irradiation at 360 nm resulted in total loss of biological activity (11). The inactive, chromophore-free form of NCS had an isoelectric point (pI) of 3.2, compared with that of native NCS of 3.3. The more acidic material, corresponding to the apoprotein, had previously been postulated to be a biosynthetic precursor of native NCS, based on its kinetics of formation and disappearance in culture filtrates of *S. carzinostaticus* var. F-14 (12,13). The difference between the active and inactive materials, however, was attributed to an amino acid change. It is now clear that addition of the nonprotein chromophore to the apoprotein is responsible for the appearance of a biologically active substance (11). These results also explain an earlier observation that NCS covalently bound to agarose is cytotoxic, a finding originally attributed to its acting at the cell membrane (14). The demonstration that the holoantibiotic consists of two components also agrees with early antibiotic isolation work, where the original strain of *S. carzinostaticus* was found to produce two components ("carzinostatin complex"), at least one of which was too labile to permit further characterization (15). This difficulty led to the isolation of variant F-14, which produced an agent, termed neocarzinostatin, as a "single entity" of greater potency (1). It remains unclear how the "carzinostatin complex" and neocarzinostatin differ.

NCS-Chrom has been presumed to reside in a hydrophobic cleft in the apoprotein (16–19), where it is shielded from degradation (Fig. 1). Recent NMR studies on holo-NCS have, in fact, detected the nonprotein chromophore and showed that it is tightly enwrapped by the β-barrel structure of the apoprotein, which provides it a protective hydrophobic environment (20). Conformational differences between the holo- and apo-forms appear to be associated with NCS-Chrom release. In aqueous solution at neutral pH (room temperature) the isolated chromophore is totally degraded in a few seconds, whereas it is stable for hours when complexed with its apoprotein (7). Other related antitumor protein antibiotics that cleave DNA (21,22), macromomycin (auromomycin) and actinoxanthine, possess primary and secondary protein structures homologous with NCS (23–25),

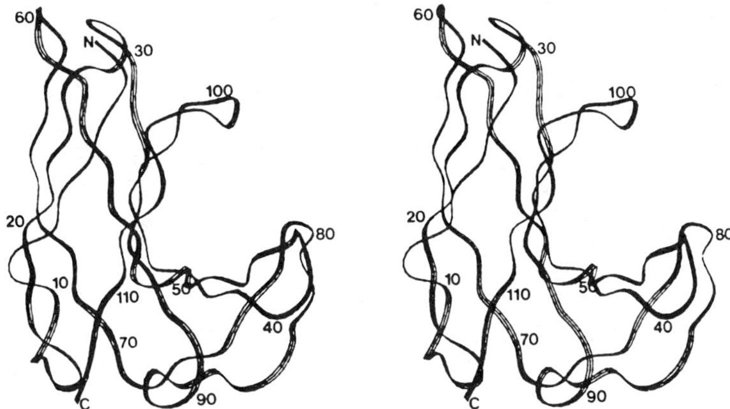

Figure 1 Stereo ribbon picture of the holo-NCS backbone by x-ray crystallography (Sieker and Ramanadham, unpublished experiments). N and C indicate the amino and carboxyl termini, respectively. (From Ref. 18.)

but their nonprotein chromophoric substances appear to be different, although they are incompletely studied. A recently discovered DNA-cleaving protein antibiotic C-1027, which has a nonprotein chromophore with at least partial structural similarity with that of macromomycin, is one of the most potent antitumor agents known (26,27). The interaction between NCS chromophore and apoprotein appears to be specific, since the NCS apoprotein is far better in protecting NCS-Chrom from degradation than the apoproteins of the other members of the family of protein antibiotics, although all appear to be significantly better than serum albumin (7). Circular dichroism and absorption spectroscopic titrations of NCS-Chrom and apoprotein show that the final complex consists of a one-to-one mixture of the two components (9).

III. CHEMICAL STRUCTURE OF NCS-CHROM AND ITS ACTIVATION

The major species (form A) of NCS-Chrom consists of three main subunits that are important in its ability to complex with DNA: a 5-methyl-7-methoxy-naphthoate, a 2,6-dideoxy-2-methylaminogalactose (N-methylfucosamine), and an interconnecting C_{12}-subunit bearing a cyclic carbonate and an epoxide (28-36). The C_{12}-subunit consists of a strained bicyclo[7.3.0] dodecadienediyne system (Scheme I) with two acetylenic bonds in a nine-membered ring (33). This unique structure has been supported by biosynthetic studies (37) and chemical synthesis (38,39). Two analogs of NCS-Chrom epoxide, the chlorohydrin and the diol monomethyl ether, have been prepared; the latter is inactive, although it can bind

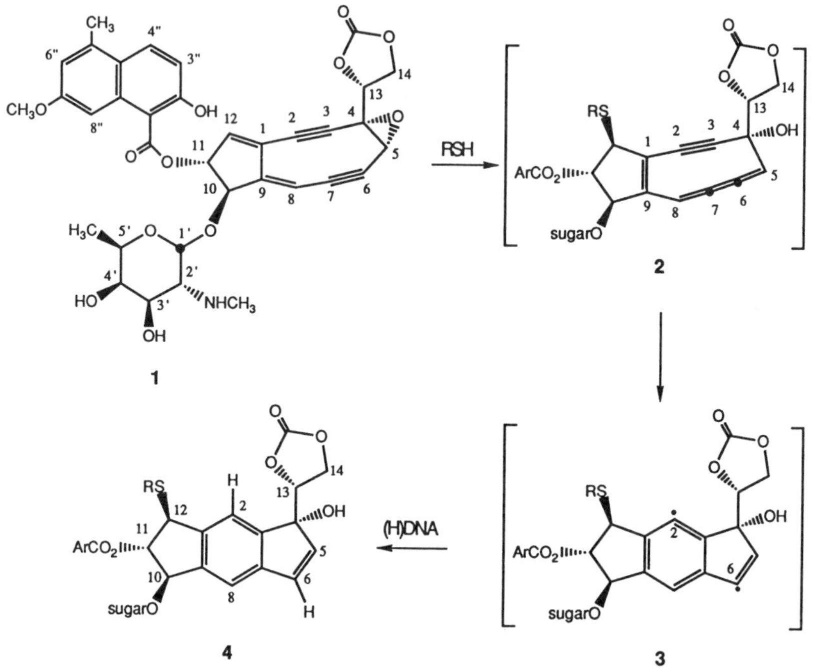

Scheme I Proposed mechanism of NCS-Chrom activation and action

to DNA, while the former is about half as active as the parent epoxide in various systems (40). The hydrogen bromide adduct of NCS-Chrom has been found to be biologically active and more stable than the epoxide and chlorohydrin to heat and UV light (41). Two other forms of NCS-Chrom, resulting from alteration in the cyclic carbonate (1,3-dioxolan-2-one) moiety have been identified: form C, the methyl ester, results from storage of NCS-Chrom A in methanol in the presence of sodium acetate, whereas form B, the open diol decarboxylation product, is an authentic natural product present in the material used clinically at the level of 10% of form A (9,29). Forms B and C possess 5% and 80%, respectively, of the activity of form A for inhibition of growth or DNA synthesis in HeLa cells; all three forms appear to be equivalently active in DNA scission in vitro. It is possible that form B is less active against cells because of diminished uptake.

Forms A, B, and C possess essentially identical absorption, CD, MCD, and fluorescence spectra (9,42). There is a single blue fluorescence emission maximum at 430 nm with excitation maxima at 270 and 340 nm. The biological activity of NCS-Chrom decreases spontaneously in aqueous neutral solution in parallel with an increase in 490 nm fluorescence (excitation at 380 nm). This inactive, intensely yellow fluorescing material has been isolated by HPLC (form D) (see Note Added in Proof). Although superoxide free radical is produced during the spontaneous degradation of NCS-Chrom, there is no evidence that it participates in the DNA damage reaction (43). An intensely blue fluorescent product forms upon addition of mercaptan to NCS-Chrom; this is associated with absorption hypochromicity between 270 and 330 nm and an increased absorption between 330 and 400 nm (42). A study of the kinetics of the fluorescence increase of NCS-Chrom A, B, and C in the presence of methylmercaptan shows a mean lifetime, τ, of A < C < B, the same relative order as the rate of hydrolytic decomposition at neutral pH. Thus forms C and B appear to be somewhat less reactive and more stable than form A.

Biosynthetic studies on NCS-Chrom A (37) have shown that the *N*-methyl of the fucosamine and the *O*-methyl of the naphthoate moieties are derived from methionine via S-adenosylmethionine and the cyclic carbonate carbonyl from carbonate. Acetate incorporation results show that the C_{12} naphthoic acid ring is derived from hexaketide. The C_{14} cyclic carbonate/bicyclo[7.3.0] dodecadienediyne ring system appears to be derived from a minimum of eight head-to-tail coupled acetate units (a linear C_{18} polyketide precursor) via the oleate-crepenynate biosynthetic pathway for polyacetylates.

It was suspected for some time that the active form of NCS was a radical species (44). DNA strand breakage and base release were found to occur in vitro provided that a cofactor, such as a thiol or borohydride, was included in the reaction (8,44,45). Evidence for the generation of free radicals upon NCS activation by thiol was provided by electron spin resonance spectroscopy, although identification of the type of radical was not possible (46,47). Thiol activation involved adduction and marked rearrangement of the chromophore structure (30), in association with major spectral changes (6). The finding that thiol-activated NCS-Chrom abstracted ^{3}H into the drug from C-5′ of deoxyribose of thymidylate residues in DNA (48,49) led to the proposal that the nucleophilic addition of thiol to NCS-Chrom converted the drug into a diradical species that was responsible for the abstraction reaction (49). With the elucidation of the NCS-Chrom structure and the demonstration that other enediyne antibiotics, esperamicin/calicheamicin (50–53), can be made to undergo a thiol-induced Bergman-type aromatization (54) to form a 1,4-benzene diradical, Myers (55), in assigning the structure of the chromophore-thiol adduct from the ^{1}H-NMR and MS data of Hensens et al. (30), proposed the mechanism for NCS-Chrom activation shown in Scheme I. Nucleophilic attack by thiol at C-12 in *trans* configuration to the naphthoate at C-11 (36) and epoxide ring opening generate a cumulene intermediate [2] (56), that cyclizes to form an indacene diradical with radical centers at C-2 and C-6 [3]. Spectral evidence for the cumulene intermediate was obtained; its $t_{1/2}$ (–70°C) = 1.5 hours. The bicyclic dienediyne core and a leaving group at C-5 (epoxide or halogen group) (40) are required for diyl formation.

Reaction with thiol or borohydride involves β-face attack at C-12, *trans* to the naphthoate at C-11 (36). The stereospecificity with which thiol nucleophilic substitution at C-12 occurs suggested involvement of an ionic thiolate species in triggering the formation of the initial intermediate, the cumulene adduct (36). This is consistent with the finding that DNA damage increases with increasing pH (43,57) and that $NaBH_4$ can substitute for thiol (30,58–60). Support for this mechanism of thiol activation comes from recent studies showing that the rates of activation of NCS-Chrom in the presence of DNA by various thiols approximates a Brønsted relation (β = 0.43, r^2 = 0.86), indicating that the basicity/nucleophilicity of the thiol is important in NCS activation (61). Recently, evidence has been presented that the aminoglycoside facilitates thiolate formation, and thus NCS-Chrom activation, by participation of its amino group as an internal base (62). An NCS-Chrom analog lacking the aminoglycoside moiety was found to be inert to methyl thioglycolate in organic solvent, unless triethylamine was included in the reaction. Based on these results, Myers suggested that NCS-Chrom bound to or close to the DNA exists in a hydrophobic environment comparable to that in the organic solvent, and its amino moiety provides base assistance for thiolate formation. This would also explain why the drug is not activated in an aqueous environment at physiological pH, where the amino function would be protonated. In addition, there appears to be a contribution to NCS-Chrom activation from the affinity of the thiol for DNA, since there is a correlation between the concentration of thiol producing maximal DNA damage and the apparent ability of the thiol to "bind" to DNA by hydrophobic and electrostatic interactions (61).

The resulting diradical species then either abstracts hydrogen from DNA to form the reduced chromophore [4] (Scheme I) or hydrogen from some other source (exchangeable or carbon-bound) to form the same product. This formulation is supported by experiments showing that in the absence of DNA, deuterium is incorporated from borodeuteride in deuteriated solvent into C-12, C-6, and C-2 of NCS-Chrom, whereas in its presence deuterium is incorporated only into C-12 and protium into C-6 and C-2 (60). These results indicate that DNA is the source of hydrogen atom donation to the two radical centers at C-6 and C-2 of NCS-Chrom. Interestingly, it was found in these studies that solvent contributes a hydrogen to C-2/C-6, in addition to the hydrogen from the borohydride. In this system both C-2 and C-6 appear to have the ability to accept hydrogen either from solvent or from the borohydride, suggesting that the radical at C-2/C-6 is in equilibrium with a 2,6-dipolar resonance form. The transient difference in electronegativity at C-2 and C-6 could result from intramolecular electron transfer and result in facilitation of addition of polar reagents such as hydride and water.

Although thiol (or borohydride) stimulates DNA damage more than 1000-fold, NCS-Chrom cleaves DNA in its absence, and this reaction is favored at acidic pH (43), suggesting that the initiating event is due to acid-induced opening of the epoxide. Evidence has recently been found for another mechanism of NCS-Chrom aromatization. It was observed that the aerobic treatment of NCS-Chrom with very low concentrations of thiol (1.5×10^{-5} M) in methanolic acetic acid leads to the formation of the indacene 12-oxo derivative (63). It was proposed that the ketone derivative is produced by hydroperoxy radical (formed by reaction of dioxygen and thiol) attack at C-12 of NCS-Chrom. Interestingly, in the process of hydroperoxide homolysis of the radical intermediate, it was suggested that the benzylic hydrogen at C-12 undergoes an intramolecular shift to C-2. Finally, it has been found that NCS-Chrom can also be activated by carboxyl radical, an electron donor generated from x-ray radiolysis of nitrous oxide–saturated formate buffer (64,65).

The source of hydrogen atoms abstracted by the thiol-activated drug into C-2 and C-6 in the absence DNA appears to be complex and has some important mechanistic implications. It has been found that at low ratios of thiol to drug (2–8 equ), such as used in DNA-cleaving reactions, there was little, if any, incorporation of exchangeable hydrogen into the chromophore (28,30,36,60), raising the possibility that a nonexchangeable carbon-bound hydrogen atom of the thiol (either that α to the sulfur or one on an NH_2-substituted carbon of glutathione) might be abstracted into one of the radical centers of the chromophore (60). Evidence for this possibility has recently come from experiments using glutathione labeled with carbon-bound deuterium (66). In these studies direct evidence of hydrogen atom abstraction from the carbon α to the sulfur of drug-bound thiol into the C-2 position of the drug was obtained. When a racemic mixture of γ-L-glutamyl-DL-cysteinylglycine with deuterium replacing both hydrogens on the α carbon was used to activate NCS-Chrom, it was found that deuterium (20–30%) was incorporated only into C-2 of the L-form adduct in a mixture of the isomers. The finding that deuterium is incorporated selectively into the C-2 position of the L form of the thiol-drug adduct suggests that the steric geometry of the thiol, which donates the hydrogen, is relatively fixed in its relationship to the drug, thus favoring an internal transfer from the attached L-form thiol at C-12. These results have been confirmed in experiments where the D- and L-form adducts have been separated and each analyzed by ^{1}H-NMR (194). A similar intramolecular hydrogen atom transfer has been observed by Wender and Tebbe (67) using a monocyclic analog of NCS-Chrom. Consistent with these studies are recent experiments by McAfee and Ashley (68) showing deuterium isotope effects on DNA damage in which NCS-Chrom is activated by [2-^{2}H$_2$]-thioglycolate (see Sec. V.D.1).

The relative ease of transfer of a carbon-bound hydrogen atom from the adducted thiol or from the C-12 position to the radical center at C-2 could account for the predominance of single-strand (SS) over double-strand (DS) lesions, since this would lead to the conversion of a bifunctional molecule into a monofunctional one. This could also account for the finding that abstraction of deuterium from C-5′ exclusively by the radical center at C-6 of the chromophore occurs when

SS break formation predominates (69). It is also possible that different reactivities of the two radicals of activated NCS-Chrom could favor cleavage on one strand over the other. The radical center at C-6 may have significant carbene character by virtue of its relationship to the C5-C6 double bond, thus changing the C-6 radical from a planar orientation with the ring system to one in which the radical is in an orbital perpendicular to the plane of the rings and in the π-systems (J. P. Snyder, personal communication). An altered orientation of this sort could affect the positioning of the radical relative to the deoxyribose hydrogens, in addition to the effect that carbene abstraction of a sugar proton could have on the NCS-Chrom cleavage spectrum.

IV. NCS-CHROM INTERACTION WITH DNA

Since there is no physical evidence of interaction of native NCS or its apoprotein with DNA, it was obvious that dissociation of the chromophore from the protein and its association with DNA must precede DNA cleavage (6–8,70). Advantage has been taken of the very tight binding of NCS-Chrom to apoprotein to follow the kinetics of dissociation of intercalated drug from the DNA (71). The addition of apoprotein, at an equimolar concentration to the chromophore, to a NCS-Chrom–poly(dA-dT) complex results in the abstraction of the chromophore from the poly(dA-dT) (thus avoiding the use of detergent to induce dissociation), so as to permit measurement of the rate of dissociation (0.75 s^{-1}). Recent studies (61) show that NCS-Chrom is activated by thiol after it binds to DNA. This does not necessarily mean that it is the bound form itself that reacts with the activating nucleophile. It is quite possible that the drug recently reversibly dissociated from the DNA is activated by the thiol and that it is this species that seeks out the sequence-specific site (see Sec. V.D.1).

NCS-Chrom binding to duplex DNA is a two-step process (71). External binding is followed by intercalation of the chromophore between adjacent base pairs. Drug binding causes the DNA helix to unwind by 21° and lengthen by 3.3 Å for each bound chromophore molecule (72). Electric dichroism measurements showed that the naphthoate portion of the chromophore, corresponding to absorbance transitions between 315 and 385 nm (the range over which the naphthoate moiety absorbs), is oriented approximately parallel to the DNA bases, in accord with its being the intercalating moiety. Equilibrium and stopped-flow kinetic studies on the reversible interaction between NCS-Chrom and DNA indicate that the chromophore binds in the minor groove of B-DNA, since bulky groups in the major groove of DNA failed to interfere with NCS-Chrom binding, whereas minor groove-specific agents, such as the antibiotics netropsin and distamycin, blocked drug binding (73). Of interest is the finding that these latter antibiotics differentially block the DNA damage reaction, with abasic site formation being more resistant than direct strand breaks (73). As will be discussed later, abasic site formation occurs in sequences containing G and C residues, whereas most strand breaks involve sequences rich in T and A residues, which are strong netropsin- and distamycin-binding sites.

Spectroscopic, thermodynamic, and ^{31}P-NMR studies (74) show that the binding of NCS-Chrom to polynucleotides differs qualitatively, as well as quantitatively, depending on base sequence, leading to the conclusion that microheterogeneity in the B-DNA structure due to sequence determines the nature of NCS-Chrom binding. Further, differences in binding parameters and in enthalpy of binding of NCS-Chrom to poly(dG-dC) and poly(dI-dC) suggest that the 2-NH_2 group of guanine in the minor groove of DNA affects chromophore binding. Most of the information on the base sequence requirements for drug-DNA interaction, however, comes from DNA cleavage experiments, which will be described later. NCS-Chrom binds duplex DNA with a $K_D \sim 10^{-6}$ M with an overall preference for DNA rich in T and A residues (6). Spectroscopic titrations indicate a tight binding site that is saturated at $r_b = 0.125$ chromophore molecule/nucleotide (four base pairs per site) and another at $r_b = 0.25$ (two base pairs per site) (72,73). Only the latter site is found in synthetic polynucleotides, such as poly(dA-dT) (73,74).

Based on these data and the results of mechanistic studies, a model was proposed for the NCS-Chrom–DNA complex in which the active portion (bicyclic enediyne) of the chromophore is positioned in the minor groove of DNA, with which it makes important hydrophobic and other contacts, by intercalation of the naphthoate moiety and electrostatic interaction of the positively charged amino sugar moiety due to the negative potential of the minor groove (42). Aromatization of the enediyne to the diyl after binding to the DNA (see later) leads to hydrogen atom abstraction from deoxyribose carbons—C-5′, C-1′, and C-4′—strategically situated in the DNA minor groove near the radical centers on NCS-Chrom.

V. CHEMISTRY OF DNA DAMAGE

The main lesions induced in DNA by NCS-Chrom consist of strand breaks, abasic sites, and drug-deoxyribose adducts. A duplex structure is required for DNA damage generation (59,75). Whereas abstraction of hydrogen by the NCS-Chrom radical from one of the deoxyribose carbons, to generate a carbon-centered radical on the DNA sugar, does not require oxygen (49), the expression of most types of DNA damage is oxygen dependent (44,76). The sugar peroxyl radicals formed by dioxygen addition subsequently undergo a series of degradative steps to give rise to the final damage products. Among the factors that determine the type of lesions are the structure of the thiol, the nature of the nucleotide attacked, and the DNA sequence and its local microstructure.

A. Damage Due to 5′-Hydrogen Atom Abstraction

Early studies on the in vitro DNA scission reaction revealed that NCS-Chrom produced primarily SS breaks and that, although there was *base* specificity, there was little evidence of *sequence* specificity (75,77,78). About 75% of the breaks were at T residues (T > A >> C > G). The break at a T residue consisted of a DNA fragment with 3′-phosphate (79) and 5′-thymidine 5′-aldehyde ends (80,81). This novel lesion resulted from the selective abstraction of a hydrogen atom by the activated drug from C-5′ of the deoxyribose of thymidylate in DNA (Scheme II, reaction b) (48,49). Using $^{18}O_2$, it was found that the oxygen of the 5′-aldehyde is derived entirely from dioxygen, not H_2O (82), consistent with reaction c, in which dioxygen adds to the carbon-centered radical at C-5′ to form a peroxyl radical species that, following reduction by thiol, results in the formation of nucleoside 5′-aldehyde and strand breaks (reaction e). (For the possible involvement of a chromophore-deoxyribose adduct in this process, see Sec. V.E.1.) This mechanism accounts for more than 80% of the breaks due to 5′-chemistry and is consistent with kinetic studies (83) showing that the initial reaction of the chromophore with a single molecule of thiol (reaction a) occurs in the absence of dioxygen and that drug activation is rapidly followed by the uptake of 1 mole of O_2 per mole of chromophore and the subsequent utilization of at least an additional sulfhydryl group, which occurs only in the presence of dioxygen.

Fewer than 20% of the breaks are actually single-nucleoside gaps with phosphate moieties at each end (81). The mechanism of generation of this lesion requires further clarification, although the observed products are compatible with reactions f and g (Scheme II) in which the peroxyl radical species converts to an oxy radical, which undergoes β-fragmentation with cleavage between C-4′ and C-5′ to generate a 3′-formlyphosphate–ended fragment (84). It remains to be determined, however, how the peroxyl radical intermediate converts to the oxy radical species. Although simple peroxyl radicals can dimerize to form tetroxide intermediates to lose dioxygen and produce alkoxy radicals (85), steric constraints in the case of DNA might be expected to limit the use of this mechanism to damage involving the two strands of duplex DNA (see discussion of bistranded lesions below). The 3′-formylphosphate–ended DNA fragment, an energy-rich formyl donor, either spontaneously hydrolyzes to form formate (86) and a 3′-phosphate–ended fragment (reaction g) or donates its formyl moiety to an available nucleophile (84). The four-carbon product derived from the deoxyribose has recently been identified (87). Kawabata et al. (87) have proposed that a Criegee-type rearrangement of a hydroperoxide intermediate at C-5′ results in the cleavage between C-4′ and C-5′. It is difficult, however, to invoke a Criegee-type mechanism in the absence of metal involvement or acidic conditions (88), unless the methylamino group of the chromophore sugar serves as a proton donor.

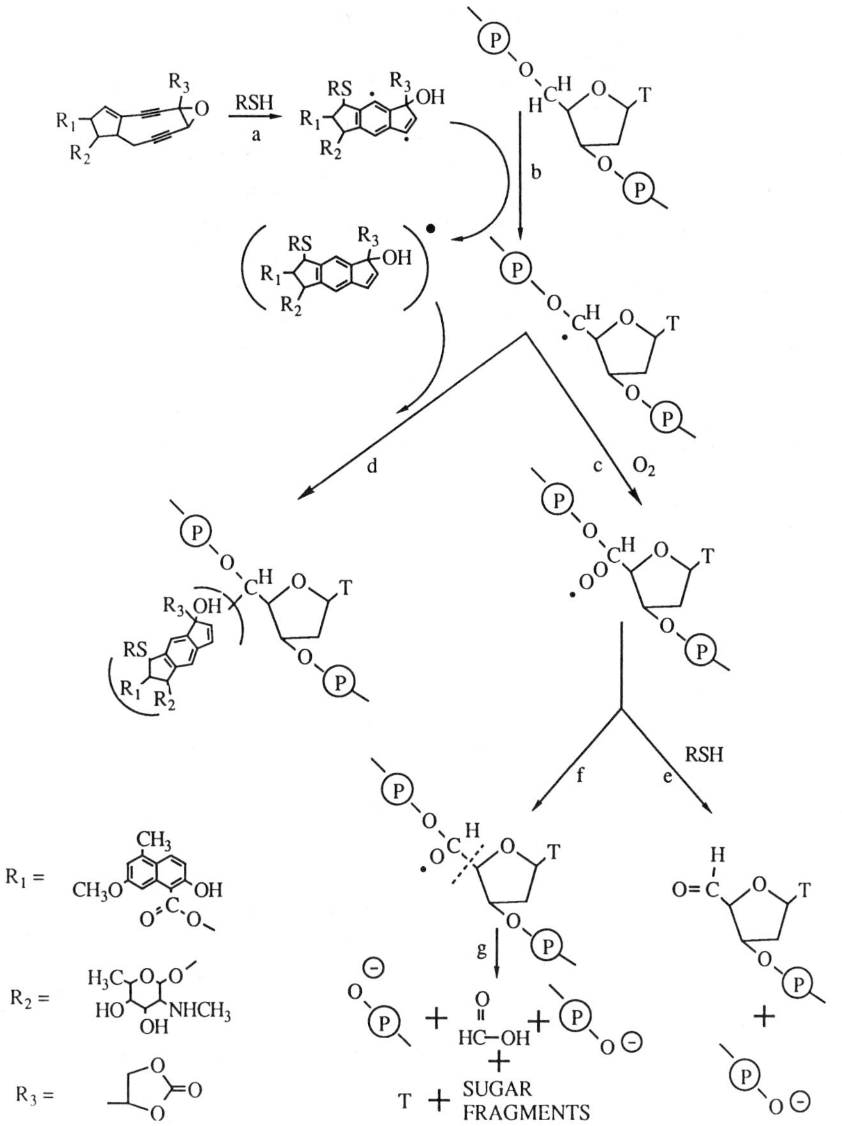

Scheme II Proposed mechanism of NCS-Chrom-induced damage at C-5′ of deoxyribose of thymidylate in DNA.

B. Substitution of Nitroimidazoles for Oxygen

The radiation sensitizer misonidazole substitutes for dioxygen in NCS-Chrom–induced DNA damage (Scheme III) (84,89). The effectiveness of various nitroimidazoles as oxygen substitutes in this reaction is correlated with their electron affinity, as measured by their one-electron reduction potentials, and is inversely related to the concentration of thiol used to activate the drug. Single-nucleoside gaps with phosphate moieties at each end are the main lesions under these conditions. Despite the difference in the relative distribution of the final damage products, abstraction of a 5'-hydrogen atom by the thiol-activated drug to form a carbon-centered radical on C-5' of deoxyribose is a common initial step in both the dioxygen- and misonidazole-dependent reactions. With misonidazole the formation of formate or its derivative (following transfer to available nucleophiles) is the major reaction, and the nitroaromatic compound appears to undergo reduction in the nitro group to the nitroso level (84). This reaction is dependent on the presence of DNA, indicating the involvement of a nascent form of DNA damage in the process and ruling out a direct action of activated NCS-Chrom on the misonidazole to generate a species that reacts with the DNA.

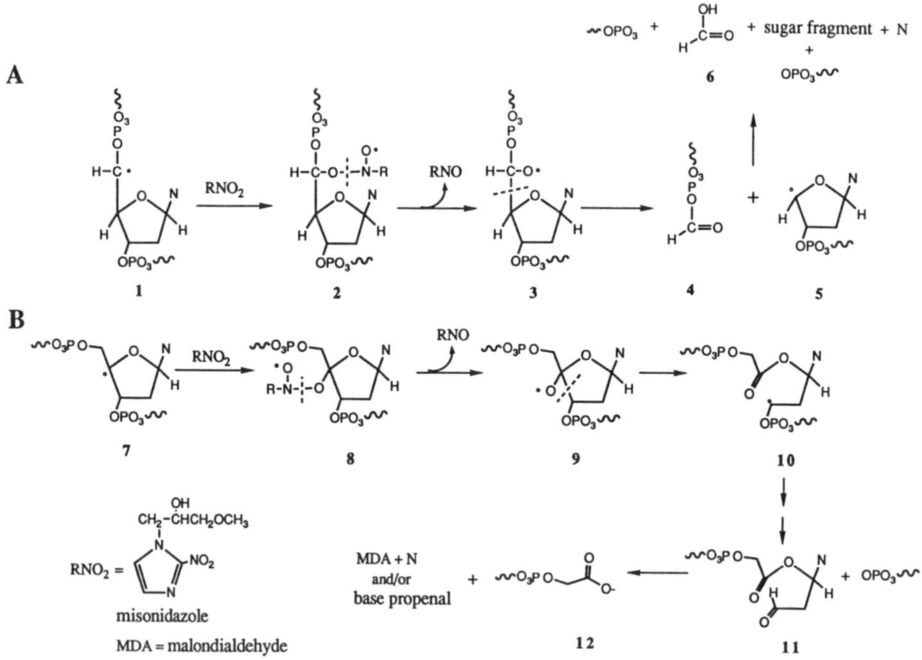

Scheme III   Proposed mechanism of involvement of misonidazole in NCS-Chrom-induced damage at C-5' and C-4'.

These results suggest a mechanism (Scheme III, A) (84) in which the carbon-centered radical at C-5' [1], generated by hydrogen atom abstraction by activated NCS-Chrom, reacts with the nitro group of misonidazole (RNO_2) to form a nitroxide radical adduct intermediate [2]. Precedence of the formation of such intermediates comes from studies on the addition of carbon-centered radicals to the oxygen of the nitro group of tetranitromethane and nitrobenzenes (90,91). The generation of adducts of this type have also been described in radiation-sensitization reactions with pyrimidines and their derivatives (91). The ease of formation of such adducts depends on the one-electron redox potential of the nitro compound (90,91), in agreement with the results showing a similar relationship for NCS-induced DNA damage (89). The adduct can undergo a fragmentation reaction (92) to form an oxy radical [3] and the nitroso reduction product of misonidazole, a two-electron process. Oxy radicals undergo β-fragmentation reactions (85), resulting in cleavage between C-5' and C-4' to form 3'-formylphosphate–ended DNA [4] and other fragments from the remaining four carbons of deoxyribose [5]. Formyl group hydrolytic release (or transfer to an available nucleophile) from the labile formylphosphate-ended DNA results in the formation of a gap with phosphates at both ends. Strong support for this novel mechanism, involving cleavage of the oxygen-nitrogen bond comes from ^{18}O studies in which the carbonyl oxygen of the formate was shown to come exclusively from the nitro group oxygen of misonidazole (93).

C. Lesions Due to C-1' and C-4' Attack

Abstraction of hydrogen atoms from the C-1' and C-4' positions generates abasic sites and, in the case of C-4' attack, also strand breaks and probably accounts for the biologically most important lesions. Abstraction of a hydrogen atom from C-1' by NCS-Chrom in the presence of dioxygen leads to the formation of an abasic site consisting of a 2'-deoxyribonolactone moiety (Scheme IV) with intact phosphodiester linkages (94). Direct evidence for hydrogen atom abstraction from C-1' comes from experiments in which deuterium replaced hydrogen at C-1' of the target residue (C in AGC; see later) (95). A deuterium isotope selection (k_H/k_D) of ~4 was determined from alkali-induced cleavage patterns on DNA-sequencing gels. Peroxyl radical formation at C-1', resulting from dioxygen addition to the carbon-centered radical, results in the formation of 2'-deoxyribonolactone with base release. Another reaction predominantly associated with attack at C-1', which is incompletely characterized, is found when NCS-Chrom is activated by carboxyl radical (65).

The chemistry of deoxyribose damage due to hydrogen atom abstraction at C-4' is somewhat more complicated, since two products, a strand break having a 3'-phosphoglycolate–ended DNA fragment and an abasic site consisting of a 4'-hydroxylated sugar moiety, are generated in the reaction (Scheme IV). The former

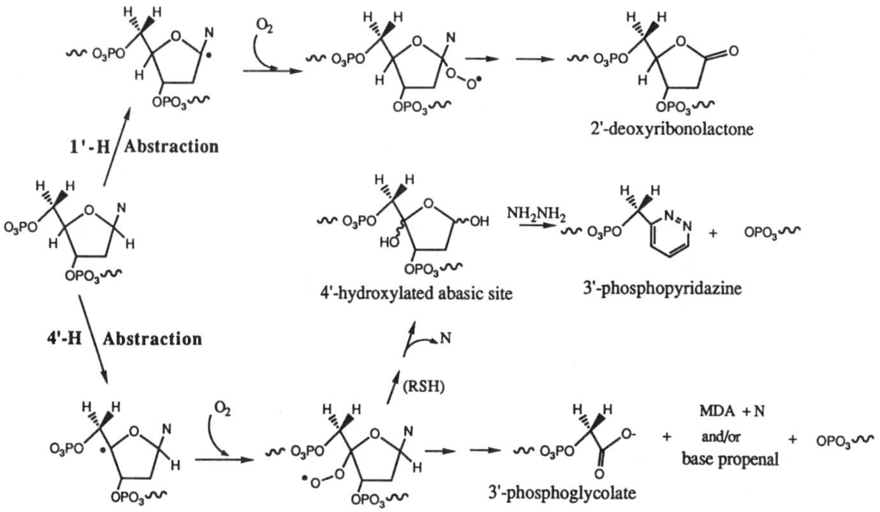

Scheme IV   Proposed mechanisms of NCS-induced chemistry at C-1′ and C-4′.

product is detected on DNA-sequencing gels by having a mobility slightly faster than that of the Maxam-Gilbert 3′-phosphate–ended marker, whereas the latter product is detected as a slower-moving band after reaction with hydrazine to form the 3′-phosphopyridazine derivative. These are the same products resulting from the action of bleomycin (88,96). Evidence that NCS-Chrom attacks C-4′ of T residues in DNA first came from studies showing the formation of the 4′-hydroxylation abasic product, but with very little (<3%), if any, 3′-phosphoglycolate with the self-complementary hexamer CGTACG (97). Experiments with DNA restriction fragments and synthetic oligonucleotides provided evidence for the partitioning of a 4′-peroxyl radical intermediate between the 4′-hydroxylated abasic product and significant amounts of the 3′-phosphoglycolate–ended fragment at the T residue of a GT step (98,99). As will be detailed later in a discussion of the formation of DS lesions, this partitioning is dependent on the thiol used as activator/reductant. The involvement of mainly 4′ chemistry at this site (also a small amount of 5′ chemistry) was confirmed by the finding of a substantial deuterium isotope effect ($k_H/k_D \sim 4$) at C-4′ for the formation of both reaction products, suggesting a common precursor for each (99). Further, the relative extent of abstraction of either a 4′- or 5′-hydrogen atom was found to be modulated by deuteriation at either position, indicating the ability of the radical species of the drug to shuttle between the two closely situated attack sites based on isotope selection effects.

Although the 4′ chemistry associated with the action of both NCS-Chrom and bleomycin leads to the formation of the same 4′-hydroxylated abasic site and 3′-phosphoglycolate–ended DNA fragment, it is clear that their mechanisms are different (see Ref. 100 for a more detailed comparison with the bleomycin mechanism). Dioxygen (or misonidazole) is required in the formation of the abasic lesion with NCS-Chrom (99) but not with bleomycin (88). Further, the Criegee-type rearrangement, proposed to precede the generation of 3′-phosphoglycolate by bleomycin, is very unlikely to occur with NCS-Chrom, since a metal, acting as a Lewis acid, is not involved in NCS-Chrom action. Also, hydrazine (and to a lesser extent borohydride) appears to react with an intermediate in 3′-phosphoglycolate formation by NCS-Chrom to prevent its conversion to the final product (101); hydrazine, however, fails to block 3′-phosphoglycolate formation by bleomycin (P. C. Dedon, L. S. Kappen, and I. H. Goldberg, unpublished data). In fact, it has been possible to calculate a $t_{1/2} = 12$ minutes for the formation of 3′-phosphoglycolate–ended fragments by NCS-Chrom by exploiting the hydrazine reaction (101). Recent preliminary experiments with borohydride have led to the partial characterization of a NCS-Chrom–induced precursor of the 3′-phosphoglycolate–ended fragment, resulting from cleavage between C3′ and C4′, that has properties consistent with structure **11** (Scheme III, B) or its abasic degradation product, suggesting the possibility of an oxy radical mechanism in its formation, in analogy with the misonidazole-dependent reaction (Z.-W. Jiang and I. H. Goldberg, unpublished data). Since in the bleomycin reaction the oxygen of the hydroxyl group of the 4′-hydroxylation product is, by contrast with NCS, derived from solvent and not dioxygen (102), it was of interest to determine the effect of misonidazole as a dioxygen substitute in the formation of the products of 4′ chemistry by NCS-Chrom. It was found that not only does misonidazole substitute for dioxygen in the NCS reaction, but the amount of 3′-phosphoglycolate relative to 4′-hydroxylation product was increased about 3.5-fold (99,101). A likely mechanism for misonidazole involvement at C-4′ (Scheme III, B), based on analogy with its reaction at C-5′ (Scheme III, A), involves nitroxide radical adduct [**8**] formation at the radical-center at C-4′ [**7**], followed by cleavage between the nitrogen and oxygen to generate an oxy radical intermediate [**9**]. Although this intermediate can be reduced by thiol to the abasic 4′-hydroxylation product, the favored reaction appears to involve cleavage between C-3′ and C-4′ to produce a radical at C-3′ [**10**]. This intermediate undergoes degradation to form the 3′-phosphogycolate–ended DNA fragment [**12**], presumably via **11**. To obtain the same product in the dioxygen-dependent reaction, one can invoke a related scheme, involving an oxy radical at C-4′, possibly derived from a tetroxide adduct intermediate formed by condensation of two peroxyl radicals. Tetroxide formation between peroxyl radicals of separate strands of polyuridylic acid has been proposed to account for chain cleavage due to ionizing radiation (85). Such an intermediate forming between the two strands of duplex DNA could account for the sugar damage products (101), without the need to invoke a Criegee-type reaction (for proposed model, see Sec.V.D.2.).

D. Sequence-Specific Bistranded DNA Lesions

Whereas SS lesions occur mainly as breaks due to 5′ chemistry or to a much lesser degree as abasic sites due to 4′ chemistry, DS lesions (DS break or abasic site with a closely opposed SS break) involve a mixture of chemistry (5′ and 1′ or 4′) at a staggered lesion site. A single molecule of the diradical species of NCS-Chrom, appropriately situated in the minor groove of duplex DNA, can abstract available carbon-bound hydrogen atoms of the deoxyribose units on the complementary DNA strands. DS lesions are sequence specific and appear to be more important than SS lesions in terms of mutagenicity and cytotoxicity. SS breaks due to NCS are rapidly repaired in mammalian cells, whereas persistent DS breaks are associated with cell killing (103).

1. *Lesion at AGC · GCT Sites*

The first DS lesion to be identified consists of an apyrimidinic abasic site due to 2′-deoxyribonolactone formation (1′ chemistry) (Scheme IV) at the C̲ residue of the sequence AGC̲ · GC̲T and a direct strand break due to 5′-nucleoside 5′-aldehyde formation (5′ chemistry) at the T̲ residue two nucleotides to the 3′ side on the complementary strand (Fig. 2) (59,94,104,105). Since virtually every abasic site at the C̲ residue is accompanied by a direct strand break at the T̲ residue on the complementary strand (105), it appears that it occurs as part of a bistranded lesion resulting from the concerted action of the two radical centers at C-2 and C-6 of a single NCS-Chrom molecule. However, because there are more strand breaks at the T̲ residue than abasic sites at the C̲ residue (59,69), it is evident that all strand breaks are not necessarily part of a bistranded lesion. The importance of local DNA microstructure in the generation of the abasic site at the C̲ residue is shown by the finding that substitution of an I residue, which lacks a 2-amino group on the base, for the G residue of AGC̲ markedly reduces abasic

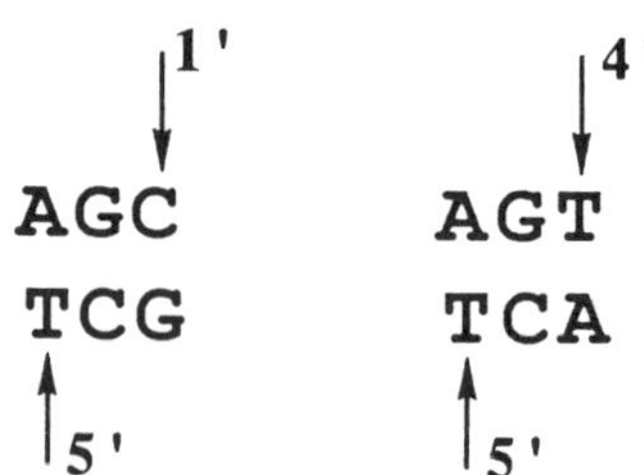

Figure 2 Main chemistry of sequence-specific bistranded lesions.

site formation, whereas placement of an I residue opposite the C̲ residue enhances (4- to 5-fold) abasic site formation in oligodeoxynucleotides (59). Interestingly, the latter base replacement eliminates the deuterium isotope effect on abasic site formation at the C̲ residue (95). This is the expected result, if the enhanced reaction is due to an increase in the relative rate of hydrogen atom abstraction by the activated drug versus its dissociation from the DNA. Further, such a consideration may be the basis for the significant variation in isotope effects observed at different sites in the DNA, in particular, for those involving chemistry at C-5′, where the values vary from 1.0 to 2.6 (95,98,99).

The nature of the thiol used as the activator/reductant is critical in determining the extent of formation of the bistranded lesion at AGC̲ · GC̲T̲; glutathione is superior to 2-mercaptoethanol or dithiothreitol (59,104). Since the size, shape, and charge of the activated drug will differ depending upon the particular thiol, these differences might be expected to result in change in binding to the DNA minor groove as well as in the orientation of the diradical species for attack on the DNA deoxyribose. The question thus arises as to the exact nature of the drug species that seeks out the sequence-specific DNA attack site. Because of the importance of the adducted thiol in this process, it is possible that the initial intermediate resulting from thiol adduction, the cumulene derivative, is this species and not the native NCS-Chrom. The estimated $t_{1/2}$ of the cumulene derivative is about 0.5 sec at 37°C (56,62), which is relatively long compared to the rate determined for the binding of native NCS-Chrom to DNA and comparable to the rate of dissociation of the intercalated complex (71), suggesting that the cumulene derivative may bind rapidly to the specific attack site before it is converted into the diradical form, the DNA-damaging species. Further, as noted earlier, the ability of the adducted thiol to donate a carbon-bound hydrogen atom to the radical at C-2 will also influence the extent of bistranded lesion formation.

Molecular model building based on energy minimization and molecular dynamics simulations has led to a proposal for the activated NCS-Chrom-AGC̲ · GC̲T̲ complex in which the radical center at C-6 abstracts a hydrogen atom from C-5′ of the T̲ residue (3.31 Å) and C-2 abstracts a hydrogen atom from C-1′ of the C̲ residue (4.10 Å) (Fig. 3) (106). The naphthoate moiety of NCS-Chrom is intercalated between the A:T and G:C base pairs, and the positively charged amino sugar is attracted by the negative potential of the DNA minor groove so as to place the indacene diradical in the DNA minor groove, projecting towards the 3′ end of the (+) strand. The intercalated naphthoate adds the equivalent of a base pair to the interaction site so that separation of the lesions on each strand by two rather than three (as with the nonintercalating calicheamicin) (107) base pairs represents the shortest distance across the DNA minor groove. The glutathione adduct at C-12 of the chromophore appears to force the radical center at C-2 deeper into the minor groove so as to facilitate attack at C-1′ of the C̲ residue, perhaps accounting for the increased formation of the abasic lesion with this thiol.

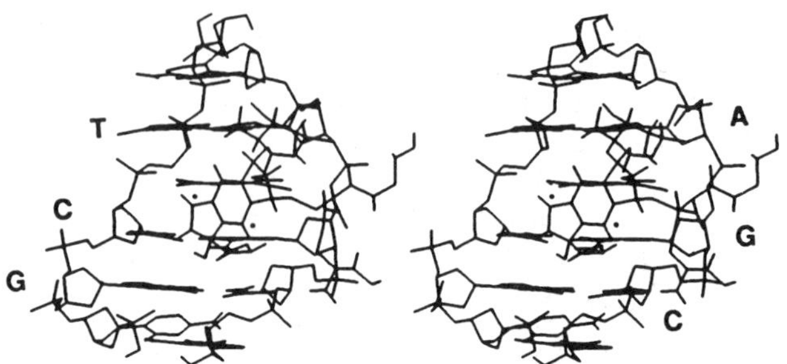

Figure 3 Stereo drawings of optimized structure of reacted form of NCS-Chrom complexed with AGC·GCT-containing oligodeoxynucleotide. C-2 and C-6 of NCS-Chrom are labeled with dots. Glutathione is attached to C-12. (Adapted from Ref. 106.)

To corroborate the model and to further clarify the underlying mechanism, the C-5′ position of the T residue was labeled with deuterium, and its incorporation into the spent NCS-Chrom was analyzed by ^{1}H-NMR (69). These studies showed that the deuterium was incorporated selectively into C-6 of the chromophore, as predicted. Of the two prochiral hydrogen atoms at C-5′ of deoxyribose, it is expected that H_S, the one projecting into the minor groove, is the one abstracted by the drug. The model is further supported by recent experiments showing that deuterium from C-1′ of the C residue is selectively abstracted by C-2 of NCS-Chrom (195). The observation that the alkali-dependent lesion at the C of AGC in an oligodeoxynucleotide was stimulated 1.5-fold when [2-^{2}H$_2$]-thioglycolate was used to activate NCS-Chrom (68) is also consistent with the proposed model, since the radical at C-2 of the chromophore, for geographic reasons, should be the recipient of the internally donated hydrogen from the adducted thiol. These experiments, however, can also be interpreted to indicate that the hydrogen from the adducted thiol quenches not the radical at C-2 of the chromophore, but (or in addition to) the DNA deoxyribose-centered radical. These experiments are further complicated by the finding that the sequence-independent total damage was enhanced 2-fold when [2-^{2}H$_2$]-thioglycolate was used. Since ^{2}H on the α-carbon of glutathione is not abstracted by C-6 (66), it appears that the 2-fold ^{2}H isotope effect on total DNA damage observed by McAfee and Ashley (68) is due to intermolecular quenching of the radical on the DNA. These two different types of experiments, however, should be repeated with the same thiol. The experiments by Chin and Goldberg (66) with NCS-Chrom and those of Wender and Tebbe (67) with the NCS-Chrom analog in which the C-2 of the chromophore (or its equivalent) abstracts hydrogen from the α-carbon of the thiol are consistent with the proposal that the radical center at C-2 is required for bistranded lesion formation, since without attack at the C̲ of AGC̲ (or at the T̲ of AGT̲, see below) by C-2 of NCS-Chrom only single-stranded lesions, due to C-6 attack, result.

The finding that direct cleavage at the T̲ residue exceeds abasic site formation at the C̲ residue, however, raises the possibility that deueterium abstraction from C-5′ of the T̲ residue by the radical center C-6 is in part due to a different mode of drug-DNA binding that leads only to direct SS breaks. However, the number of SS breaks that are not part of a bistranded lesion decreases dramatically when an I residue is placed opposite the C̲ of AGC̲ (S. M. Meschwitz and I. H. Goldberg, unpublished data), consistent with the increase in abasic lesions at the C̲ residue that are part of a bistranded lesion. The SS break lesion could be due either to a different binding mode or to the same mode that leads to the bistranded lesion but with abasic site formation being less efficient for either chemical or geometric reasons. If a different energetically allowable binding mode is involved in SS break formation, such as intercalation at the G:C · C:G step with the diradical core extending towards the 5′ end of the (+) strand (106), it is still necessary that C-6 of the activated drug attack C-5′ of the T̲ residue, since there is no detectable deuterium incorporation at C-2 (69). In this case the diradical core would have to be rotated so that it is almost perpendicular to the helix axis, resulting in a distance of 3.47 Å between C-6 of the drug and C-5′ of the T̲ residue. This model resembles that proposed by Chen et al. (108) before the structure of the activated form of NCS-Chrom was known.

2. *Lesion at AGT · ACT Sites*

Until recently the mechanism involved in the formation of DS breaks was unclear. Whereas in mammalian cells the ratio of SS to DS breaks was on the order of 5:1 (103), in vitro the ratio was 30–50:1 (57,61,109). The latter values gave rise to the conjecture that DS breaks result from the near-random (except as influenced by base selectivity) placement of SS breaks at closely opposed sites and that DS breakage as a discrete event occurred rarely, if at all. The paradox existing between the in vivo and in vitro data was resolved once it was appreciated that the difference in ratios of SS:DS breaks might be related to the fact that glutathione is the thiol in vivo and 2-mercaptoethanol was used in vitro. In fact, when glutathione was used in vitro the SS:DS ratio was found to be about 5:1 (and falls to 2:1 when abasic lesions are included) (61,109). Further, the number of DS breaks increased sevenfold. The role played by a particular thiol was further emphasized when a number of different thiols varying in structure and charge were studied for their ability to induce DS lesions in supercoiled DNA (61). It was found that thiols possessing a carboxylate moiety produce larger quantities of bistranded DNA lesions than their esterified or noncarboxylate-containing congeners. In fact, 2-hydroxythiophenol–activated NCS-Chrom rarely, if ever, generated a DS lesion, although SS lesions were produced. It is possible that aromatic thiols interfere with DS-lesion formation either by steric means or by intramolecular quenching of the radical at C-2 of the drug.

Analysis of a number of restriction fragments for NCS-induced DS-cleavage sites revealed that DS breaks were sequence specific and that most of the lesions involved the T residue of a GT step (101,109). DS breaks contained a two-base-pair stagger in the 3′ direction to the cleavage sites on each strand and occurred at sequences containing a GT step, in particular at the T residue of AGT · ACT (Fig. 2). Detailed analysis of the DS break chemistry induced by glutathione-activated NCS-Chrom at a model AGT · ACT in an AP-1 transcription factor–binding site showed that 89% of the DS DNA damage at the T of AGT was due to C-4′ hydrogen atom abstraction and 11% to C-5′ hydrogen atom abstraction (101). The latter is associated exclusively with the formation of a gap bounded by 3′- and 5′-phosphate ends, presumably formed via the formylphosphate mechanism. Of the 89%, 66% was in the form of the 4′-hydroxylated abasic site and 23% in 3′-phosphoglycolate–ended fragment. The break at the T of ACT on the complementary strand was more than 90% due to 5′ chemistry, generating mainly thymidine 5′-aldehyde. The involvement of different chemistry at the staggered sites of the DS lesion is analogous to the bistranded lesion found at AGC · AGT and suggests that each radical center on NCS-Chrom reacts mainly with either C-4′ of AGT or C-5′ ACT to produce the bistranded lesion. It has, in fact, been recently found that C-6 of the chromophore selectively abstracts hydrogen from C-5′ of ACT (S. M. Meschwitz and I. H. Goldberg, unpublished data), compatible with a model similar to that proposed for AGC · GCT. SS breaks (direct and indirect) contained virtually no glycolate but a substantial amount of 4′-hydroxylated abasic site. The chemistry of the DS lesion varied with the thiol, so that the lesion associated with dithiothreitol had virtually no glycolate (but substantial 4′-hydroxylated product) and 2-hydroxythiophenol produced essentially no DS lesions. From these results it is clear that different thiols lead to different partitioning of a 4′-chemistry intermediate; in general thiols possessing greater reducing ability result in less glycolate formation. DNA sequence also influences the reaction resulting from 4′ chemistry. Deuterium isotope effects at C-4′ varied from 2.4 to 5.5 at different GT steps (98). Further, as was noted earlier with AGC · GCT, substitution of I for G in AGT markedly diminishes the 4′ chemistry at the T residue (99).

It is especially interesting that in the presence of dioxygen 3′-phosphoglycolate–ended fragment formation appears to be limited to DS breaks and that whatever 5′ chemistry occurs at this same site (T of AGT) goes via the formylphosphate pathway (f, g, Scheme II). In the presence of misonidazole (anaerobic conditions), however, not only is glycolate relatively increased in the DS lesion, but there is even substantial formation in SS breaks (101). These results suggest that misonidazole, in effect, acts as the equivalent of the complementary DNA strand, forming the nitroxide radical adduct at C-4′ of deoxyribose on one strand, while in the dioxygen reaction the peroxyl radical lesions on the T residues of each of the strands of AGT · ACT form a tetroxide bridge between

C-4' of AG$\underline{T}$ and C-5' of AC$\underline{T}$ (Scheme V). The tetroxide decays to form sugar products on each strand either via oxy radical formation or a concerted reaction (110). This formulation is consistent with model building showing that the tetroxide can form between deoxyribose residues staggered three base pairs in a 3' direction, the equivalent of which occurs in NCS-Chrom–mediated bistranded lesions (P. C. Dedon and I. H. Goldberg, unpublished data). Further, such an intermediate may be favored at a GT · AC step because of its extremely narrow and deep minor groove (111). This model would explain the findings that significant quantities of 3'-phosphoglycolate are found only in bistranded lesions and that the 5' chemistry found at the $\underline{T}$ of AG$\underline{T}$ follows predominantly the formylphosphate pathway, presumably via an oxy radical intermediate.

3. *NCS-Chrom as a Sensitive Probe of Minor Groove Heterogeneity*

The ability of NCS-Chrom to act as a sequence-specific bistrand-reactive agent derives from its DNA-binding moieties and the bifunctional nature of its active species. Full elucidation of the role played by the adducted thiol in complex formation with DNA will require separation of the activator from the reductant properties of the nucleophile. The precise chemistry carried out on each strand from the DNA minor groove, however, is determined to a considerable extent by the DNA microstructure at the sites of reaction. Hydrogen atoms at C-5', C-1', and C-4' are all readily accessible to the diradical lying in the minor groove (106), but it is, to a considerable degree, the local geometry that determines whether SS or DS lesions ensue and whether C-1' or C-4' is a component of the bistranded lesion. The two types of bistranded lesions (Fig. 2) result from different chemical mechanisms, depending on whether a C or a T residue is 3' to a G residue.

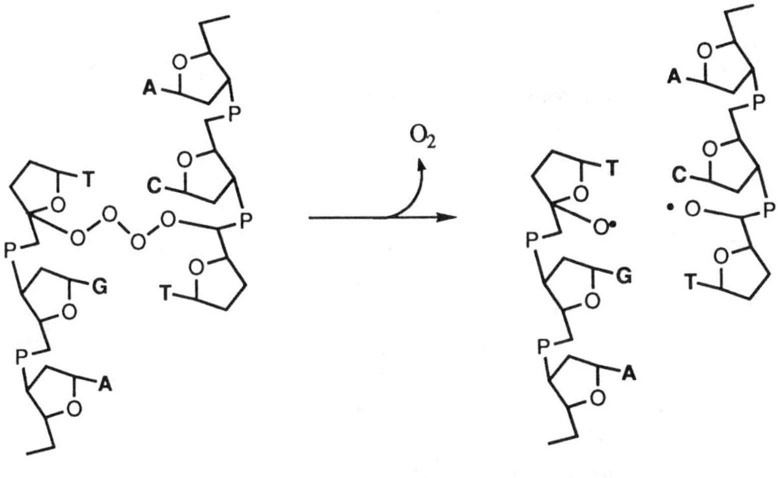

Scheme V Tetroxide bridge model for NCS-Chrom-mediated bistranded lesions (101).

Further, the omission of a 2-NH$_2$ group from either strand at the site of interaction has profound effects on DS lesion formation (59). In addition, recent work has shown that changes in DNA microstructure induced by stable base pair mismatches can lead to switching of DNA sugar attack sites. In these experiments, a wobble G · T mismatch 5′ to the C of AGC in an oligodeoxynucleotide duplex results in switching of the chemistry of attack at the C from 1′ to 4′ (112). This effect has been attributed to the displacement of the guanine of the G·T mispair into the minor groove of DNA (112), as shown earlier by single-crystal x-ray analysis (113). Since C1′ lies deeper in the minor groove than C4′, it seems likely that protrusion of guanine keeps the drug in a more superficial position in the minor groove so that it attacks C1′ poorly, but is better situated for reacting with C4′. Further, a G · A mismatch 3′ to the T of AGT markedly increases the 1′ chemistry at the T residue (114). On the other hand, a G · T mismatch 5′ to the T of this sequence leads to a substantial increase in 4′ chemistry at the attack site without generating 1′ chemistry. This intimate relationship between DNA microstructure and the chemistry of NCS-Chrom–induced damage makes this agent a potentially useful probe in the study of the nature and function of particular DNA microstructures. It must be emphasized, however, that while such effects are usually perceived as being sequence related, it is actually the local *geometry* of the formed complex that is the critical determinant. In fact, it has been found that cleavage of DNA by NCS-Chrom is especially prominent immediately 3′ to a single-base bulge on the opposite strand, *independent of the sequence involved* (115). Given the diversity of structures with which it interacts, it is possible that the drug contributes to the binding process by inducing the appropriate geometrical configuration of the DNA at the site of binding.

E. NCS-Chrom–Deoxyribose Adducts

In addition to causing DNA strand breaks and abasic sites, NCS-Chrom forms novel covalent adducts with the DNA sugar. These adducts are of two types: labile (116,117) and stable (118,119).

1. *Labile Adducts*

Quantitatively, the chromophore-DNA adduct is a minor lesion; only 1 in 50 chromophore molecules forms a DNA adduct under optimal conditions. The predominant labile adduct recovered from nuclease digests of NCS-Chrom–treated poly(dA-dT) · poly(dA-dT) in the presence of 2-mercaptoethanol and dioxygen is a compound with the structure chromophore-d(TpApT) in which the attached chromophore rendered both phosphodiester bonds refractory to endonuclease S1. This adduct fragment was completely hydrolyzed at pH 12, releasing adenine, 3′-dTMP, and 5′-dTMP. At pH 7, the adduct fragment slowly released chromophore and 3′-dTMP with parallel kinetics, leaving a modified d(ApT), which was cleaved by snake venom phosphodiesterase to yield 5′-dTMP and a modified deoxyadenosine. These hydrolysis patterns, which are unlike those of any previously characterized base or phosphotriester DNA adduct, indicate the presence of an altered deoxyadenosine sugar with chemical properties similar to those of thymidine 5′-aldehyde. The modified deoxyadenosine was identified as deoxyadenosine 5′-aldehyde by a series of chemical derivatizations. The formation of adducts containing a modified deoxyribose suggests that deoxyribose is the site of covalent chromophore attachment. Support for such a possibility comes from experiments in which this compound was subjected to mild acid hydrolysis to release free adenine and to snake venom exonuclease (pH 6.5) treatment to release 5′-TMP so as to leave, in both cases, adducts of slightly altered chromatographic mobility. These results eliminate adenine and 5′-dTMP as possible sites of covalent chromophore attachment. In addition, electrophoresis studies indicate that the adduct is not a phosphotriester. These data suggest that NCS-Chrom is covalently attached to the C-5′ of deoxyadenosine in some labile structure that breaks down at neutral pH to deoxyadenosine 5′-aldehyde and free chromophore. The chemistry of this structure remains to be elucidated, but its properties suggest the possibility of its role as an intermediate in strand break formation (see Scheme I in Ref. 120 for some possibilities).

2. *Stable Adducts*

A similar but much more stable adduct species has also been isolated, again with structure chromophore-d(TpApT). Dithiothreitol is much more effective in producing the stable adduct than is 2-mercaptoethanol. Acid hydrolysis of the adduct released free adenine, as well as both 3′-dTMP and 5′-dTMP, leaving a compound that contained only chromophore and the deoxyadenosine sugar moiety. These results clearly indicate the formation of a covalent linkage between chromophore and deoxyribose in DNA. Formation of this adduct shows an oxygen dependence that is the inverse of that seen for nucleoside 5′-aldehyde formation, that is, the yield of adduct is maximal under anaerobic conditions. This apparent competition between DNA sugar oxidation and adduct formation suggests that the two lesions share a common precursor. A chromophore-induced carbon-centered radical on the deoxyribose, which could react by addition with the same chromophore molecule to form the stable covalent adduct or with O_2 to form the peroxyl radical intermediate, would be the most logical candidate for such a precursor (see below). A minor stable adduct with the structure chromophore-d(ApTpA) has also been isolated (S. Lee and I. H. Goldberg, unpublished data).

The resistance of both labile and stable types of chromophore-oligonucleotide adducts to further nuclease digestion suggested that the adducts block exonucleolytic digestion of the DNA and that the sequence specificity of adduct formation might then be determined by mapping the adducts as exonuclease termination sites in defined-sequence DNA. A 5′-end–labeled DNA restriction fragment was treated with NCS-Chrom under anoxia in the presence of dithiothreitol, conditions known to maximize the formation of chromophore-deoxyribose adducts. Under conditions where unmodified DNA was digested to completion, chromophore-treated DNA was highly resistant to digestion by exonuclease III plus the $3' \rightarrow 5'$ exonucleolytic activity of T4 DNA polymerase and partially resistant to digestion by exonuclease III plus snake venom exonuclease. The electrophoretic mobilities of the products of exonucleolytic digestion indicated that (1) digestion by exonuclease III or T4 polymerase terminated one nucleotide before the nucleotide containing the adduct; (2) the remaining nucleotide directly adjacent to the adduct (3' side) could be removed by snake venom phosphodiesterase, but at a slow rate; (3) the covalently linked chromophore decreased the electrophoretic mobilities of the digestion products by the equivalent of approximately three nucleotides; and (4) adducts formed under anaerobic conditions occurred at the same nucleotide positions as the strand breaks formed under aerobic conditions (at T and, to a lesser extent, A residues). The site of adduct formation was further identified by isolating the adduct-containing fragments on a sequencing gel and then subjecting it to the chemical cleavage reactions. The close similarity in sequence specificity of adducts and strand breaks suggests that a common form of nascent DNA damage may be a precursor to both lesions. Again, a chromophore-induced free radical on the deoxyribose, subject to competitive fixation by addition reactions with either oxygen or chromophore, is the most likely candidate for such a precursor.

Adducts on the sugar in DNA are novel DNA damage products. Most adducts of nucleic acids are on the base or phosphate (121). In the case of RNA only, an adduct of dimethylbenzanthracene is found on the 2'-hydroxyl of the ribose (122). It is clear that C-5' in DNA must first be converted into a radical center by NCS-Chrom before a suitable site is generated for adduct formation. Any agent capable of inducing carbon-centered deoxyribose radicals could, in principle, also lead to deoxyribose adduct formation as a result of addition reactions between these radicals and other molecules, including other nucleic acids, proteins, drugs, or intramolecularly with its own base (see below). Bulky adducts on DNA sugars obviously could not be removed by repair glycosylases, and it seems unlikely, although not impossible, that the DNA would be recognized by polymerases as a normal substrate. Further, the phosphodiester bonds of adduct-containing DNA sugars appear to be relatively resistant to a variety of nucleases. While the physiological consequences of NCS-Chrom–DNA adducts remain to be determined, they appear not to act as significant premutagenic lesions (123), but their effect on DNA replication and transcription has not yet been studied.

A reaction entirely analagous to stable NCS-deoxyribose adduct formation occurs when DNA is γ-irradiated, especially under anaerobic conditions. The cycloaddition products 8,5'-cyclo-2'-deoxyadenosine (124), 8,5'-cyclo-2'-deoxyguanosine (125), and 5',6-cyclo-5,6-dihydrothymidine (126) have been identified recently in γ-irradiated DNA. These products result from the intramolecular cyclization between C-5′ of deoxyribose and C-8 of the purine or C-6 of the pyrimidine, following hydrogen atom abstraction from C-5′ by radiation-generated hydroxyl radicals. Instead of the carbon-centered radical at C-5′ reacting with a well-positioned drug, as in the case of NCS, it reacts with its own base to form the cycloaddition product.

VI. ACTION OF NCS IN MAMMALIAN CELLS

Early studies from several laboratories using holo-NCS showed that DNA is its target in a wide variety of mammalian cells. NCS causes inhibition of DNA synthesis (127–131) and breakdown of cellular DNA (45,132–136). It appears that the breakage of cellular DNA by the drug is the primary event that leads to inhibition of DNA synthesis and cytotoxicity (130). Further, NCS induces preferential cleavage of an actively transcribed gene (137) and in nuclei causes breaks in the linker region, resulting in the release of nucleosomes (138,139). At low levels NCS selectively inhibits initiation of DNA synthesis, whereas at high concentrations chain elongation is also inhibited (131,140). The quantitative correlation obtained between NCS-induced inhibition of replicon initiation and the generation of sufficient strand breakage to relax domains of supercoiling in mammalian DNA (target size of about 10^9 daltons) suggests that a single event, presumably a strand break, is adequate to disrupt DNA structure sufficiently to interrupt replicon initiation (140).

Ataxia telangiectasia (AT) fibroblasts that are hypersensitive to ionizing radiation are also hypersensitive to NCS and exhibit reduced inhibition of DNA synthesis (140–144). Also, NCS has been found to enhance the sensitivity of several mammalian cell lines to x-irradiation in proportion to the capabilities of the cells to repair sublethal damage (145). NCS induces repair synthesis in cells (103,146–149) and in isolated nuclei (150). The lethal effect of NCS on mammalian cells is potentiated by caffeine, an agent that inhibits postreplication repair (151,152). Also, the cell cycle effects of NCS are suppressed by caffeine (153). Interestingly, in contrast to *E. coli* (154) and mammalian cells (155), the nucleotide excision repair system appears to be involved in the repair of DNA damaged by ionizing radiation (156) and NCS (157) in *Neurospora crassa*. In human cells, repair is of the "small patch" type for both x-rays and NCS (155). DNA polymerase β is primarily responsible for repair synthesis induced by NCS (158). Also, both γ-radiation and NCS cause similar metabolic changes in mammalian cells in association with the activation of poly-(adenosine diphosphate ribose) polymerase (159,160). Low levels of NCS cause a block in the G_2 phase of the cell cycle (129,161) and produce chromosomal aberrations in CHO cells (161,162) but not sister chromatid exchanges (SCE) (162). Induction of chromosomal aberrations, with poor stimulation of SCE, by NCS was also found in human lymphocyte cultures (163). However, increased SCE due to NCS (and bleomycin) has recently been reported for several lines of AT-derived lymphoblastoid cells (144).

Isolated NCS-Chrom possesses the full biological activity of the native drug in inhibiting DNA synthesis and inducing DNA strand scissions (7,8,164). NCS-Chrom interacts irreversibly with HeLa cells at 0°C so as to inhibit subsequent DNA synthesis at 37°C (7). The mechanism of DNA damage by NCS in mammalian cells appears to be the same as in the in vitro reaction. As is the case for the in vitro reaction, there is a thiol requirement for DNA damage in cells, since depletion of cellular glutathione results in lower toxicity, mutagenesis (165,166), and DNA strand breakage (164). Additional evidence for the involvement of thiol in the cellular action of NCS comes from the finding that adjunctive treatment of neuroblastoma cells with NCS and 6-mercaptodopamine, a thiol-containing dopamine analog, specifically enhances NCS toxicity for these cells (167). Presumably, selective targeting of toxicity for neuroblastoma cells is achieved by utilizing the dopamine uptake mechanism enriched in these cells. Interestingly, one of the effects of NCS in this cell line is the induction of morphological differentiation (168).

The products of DNA damage by NCS in the in vitro reaction and in the cells appear to be the same (164). In DNA isolated from NCS-treated HeLa cells, nucleoside 5′-aldehyde, measured after its reduction to the 5′-hydroxyl group as the polynucleotide kinase-dependent incorporation of ^{32}P from $[\gamma\text{-}^{32}P]ATP$, accounts for at least 30–45% of the drug-generated 5′ ends. The distribution of the ^{32}P representing nucleoside aldehyde (77% in TMP and the rest in AMP >> CMP > GMP) is in close agreement with that obtained for in vitro damage. Further, DNA-sequencing experiments using the highly reiterative 340-base-pair alphoid DNA fragment isolated from NCS-treated cells gives a cleavage pattern similar to that produced in the in vitro reaction (164).

Whether the holo-NCS enters the cell and then releases the chromophore at the site of its action or the chromophore is released at the cell surface to be carried inside remains unsettled. As noted earlier, prior to the recognition of the chromophore as the active component, Lazarus et al. (14) used holo-NCS, covalently bound to agarose, to study its effect on the growth of human leukemic cells. These studies are now interpreted to indicate that NCS-Chrom released at the cell surface can be taken up by cells. Further, pretreatment of cells with NCS-Chrom at 0°C leads to biological effects at 37°C, indicating binding of NCS-Chrom to the cells at the lower temperature (7). These studies clearly show that apoprotein is not required for chromophore uptake but do not settle the question as to whether holo-NCS is ordinarily taken up intact when cells are treated with the drug. Holo-NCS uptake into cells has been studied using either ^{14}C-labeled or fluorescein-labeled antibiotic (169,170). In each case evidence for uptake of the protein-label into the cell, as well as into the nuclei, was presented. While these studies are compatible with the cellular uptake of holo-NCS, they do not eliminate the possibilities that the observed cellular label is in a fragment of the protein or that the nonprotein chromophore was taken up separately at the cell surface. On the other hand, NCS-Chrom appears to be excreted by multidrug-resistant cells via the active efflux mechanism associated with the P-glycoprotein (171).

VII. CLINICAL ASPECTS

NCS has seen limited clinical use, mainly in Japan, because of limited effectiveness and significant toxicity, especially allergic reactions due to the administration of a foreign protein, apo-NCS. It has been used against acute leukemia and certain solid tumors (stomach, colon, kidney, and bladder) with variable results (172–175).

Recent efforts have been directed to making the agent more selective in its toxicity. Along these lines it has been shown that NCS coupled to immunoglobulin (176–178), monoclonal antibody (179–181), or transferrin (182) retains its biological activity and is directed to a specific target cell. In these studies antibody is covalently linked to the NCS apoprotein, obviating inactivation of the nonprotein chromophore and the need for cleavage of a covalent bond for its uptake into the cell. This approach offers avenues for achieving selective elimination of tumor or antibody-producing cells. Other efforts have been directed to synthesizing drug forms with more favorable pharmacological properties such as the conjugation of holo-NCS with a copolymer of styrene-maleic acid anhydride (smancs) (183,184). There have been recent clinical studies in which these forms of holo-NCS have been used in cancer chemotherapy with some success (180,185,186).

VIII. MUTAGENIC LESIONS

NCS-induced mutagenesis in bacteria is SOS-dependent, requiring *recA* and *umuC* functions in *Escherichia coli* and pKM101, the mutagenesis enhancing plasmid, in *Salmonella typhimurium* (187,188). NCS generates 6-thioguanine–resistant HGPRT mutants of CHO cells (162). In yeast NCS is active in reverting several nonsense mutants; a *rad52* strain shows lower survival but no change in the mutation frequency (189). In *Neurospora crassa* NCS induces forward mutations in an excision repair–deficient strain (157).

NCS-induced nonsense mutations in the *lacI* gene of *Escherichia coli* include all types of substitutions, with GC to AT transitions being the most frequent (190). The spectrum was dominated by a hotspot in the *ochre21* position, which is the only AGC site in the gene at which a GC to AT transition is monitorable in vitro (104). Further, a correlation was found between the frequency of GC to AT transitions seen in vivo and the incidence of abasic sites at C residues in AGC sequences found in *lacI* DNA restriction fragment treated with NCS-Chrom in vitro (104). In the cI gene of lambda phage an unusually high proportion of the mutants, particularly GC to AT transitions, occurred at the same trinucleotide sequence (191). These lesions are 10-fold more likely to occur at the C residue in AGC sequences than at other G:C base pairs.

Since the abasic (apyrimidinic) site at AGC is virtually always accompanied by a strand break two nucleotides to the 3′ side on the opposite strand, it is this staggered bistranded lesion that is the premutagenic lesion leading to GC to AT transitions. Although abasic sites (generally apurinic lesions) have been noted before to be mutagenic, this conclusion has been reached mainly on the basis of the generation of such lesions in SS DNAs, where the simple abasic site acts as a noncoding lesion (192). This would be expected to be much less likely for an abasic site lesion in DS DNA. The bistranded lesion produced by NCS, however, may be inherently more mutagenic due to the break on the complementary strand. Because of the closely opposed break, there is probably a loss of the duplex character of the DNA at the abasic lesion site. This may account for the finding that various apurinic/apyrimidinic (AP) endonucleases appear to be less effective in placing an endonucleolytic break at the abasic lesion (104). Further, such a nick would, in effect, lead to the formation of a DS break at this site, a potentially lethal lesion. Rather, it seems likely that repair of the direct strand break at the T of GCT on the complementary strand occurs first, resulting in the formation of a small repair patch, exposing the abasic site as a single noncoding lesion. Filling in of the patch results in the insertion of a wrong base opposite the abasic site. Since base insertion is nonrandom and follows the specificity A > T > G > C in frequency of incorporation (192), one would predict that substitutions would occur at G:C base pairs with a frequency GC to AT > GC to TA > GC to CG. Analysis of the pattern of mutations occurring at the G:C site of AGC · GCT fulfills this prediction (191). With the reestablishment of the duplex structure, the abasic site is removed but replaced by a base coded for by the mutagenized lesion on the complementary strand. A mutagenic lesion has thus been generated without replicating the DNA. The same considerations apply to the bistranded lesion at AGT · ACT, consisting of an abasic site at the T of AGT due to 4′ chemistry and a direct strand break at the T of ACT. In this case, however, insertion of an A residue opposite the abasic site eventuates in a T-residue replacement for the abasic site—a mutationally silent lesion. For this reason, the abasic site at the T of AGT is probably less active in mutagenesis than that at the C of AGC (123). Bistranded lesions of this type, possessing an abasic site on one strand and a direct strand break within a few nucleotides on the other strand, may be of general significance as premutagenic lesions due to other modalities of formation, including ionizing radiation. It seems possible that for abasic lesions to be strongly premutagenic, they must be accompanied by a closely opposed break, either a direct strand break or one generated by AP endonucleolytic cleavage of a nearby apurinic lesion on the complementary strand.

IX. CONCLUDING REMARKS

Neocarzinostatin has proven to be a remarkably useful reagent in the study of the chemistry of oxidative DNA deoxyribose damage by agents working via free radical mechanisms (193). The exact lesions NCS-Chrom generates in the minor groove of DNA are determined not only by the location of each of the two radical centers on the indacenediyl moiety but by their positioning in relation to accessible attack sites at C-5′, C-1′, and C-4′ of the deoxyribose moieties on each strand of duplex DNA. It has been shown that even small changes in DNA sequence and functional groups in the minor groove or the presence of strategically situated stable base pair mismatches will have profound effects in determining deoxyribose attack sites. Additionally, the structure of the active form of the drug, as influenced by the nature of the adducted thiol used as the drug activator, influences the types of damage produced, especially as reflected in the ratios and structures of the single- and double-stranded lesions. Also, the reducing property of the thiol importantly affects the partitioning of the lesions resulting from 4′ chemistry. By manipulating these various elements, it is possible to obtain considerable information on the local geometry of the drug interaction site on the DNA.

It has also been possible with NCS to study the chemical mechanisms whereby nitroaromatic radiation sensitizers substitute for dioxygen in generating DNA damage lesions. These studies have, in addition, helped to clarify the mechanisms involved in the oxygen-dependent reaction. Support for the involvement of oxy radical species of deoxyribose in such reactions and for a mechanism of peroxyl radical decay via a tetroxide bridge between complementary strands comes from such studies. Further, these and related experiments have revealed clear mechanistic differences between NCS-Chrom and bleomycin in the formation of DNA sugar degradation products resulting from 4′ chemistry, even though the initial intermediate, the 4′-carbon–centered radical produced by hydrogen from abstraction, is the same.

Finally, the identification of staggered bistranded lesions, involving an abasic site on one strand and a nearby strand break on the other, has revealed a novel mutagenic mechanism in which mutagenesis occurs during the repair process, not during replication. This type of lesion may be generally important in the conversion of abasic sites, formed by other means, into mutagenic lesions.

Although NCS may see limited use in cancer chemotherapy, it has already served an important role as the prototypic agent of two superfamilies of antitumor antibiotics, especially in the elucidation of the chemistry of DNA deoxyribose damage and in defining the influence of DNA conformational changes on this damage. Further, the biological consequences of the DNA lesions generated, in particular those involving abasic sites and closely opposed strand breaks, may be far-ranging and provide an important model for other types of DNA-damaging modalities.

ACKNOWLEDGMENT

This work was supported by Grant CA44257 from the National Institutes of Health.

Note Added in Proof: NCS-Chrom undergoes spontaneous activation, in the absence of thiol, to a diradical species that cleaves site-specifically at a DNA bulge containing more than a single nucleotide (196-199). Drug activation is base-catalyzed and results from the stereoselective intramolecular nucleophilic attack of the enolate at C-1″ of the naphthoate moiety at C-12 of the chromophore (see Scheme I for numbering) to form a 5-membered spirolactone. This novel reaction is presumably accompanied by epoxide ring opening to generate the cumulene intermediate, which then undergoes a Bergman-type rearrangement to the 2,6-diradical. The DNA bulge conformation is essential for the subsequent quenching of the radical at C-2 by C-8″ of the naphthoate to form the final drug product. Without DNA or with a DNA lacking the specific bulge structure this reaction does not occur; instead the radical at C-2 is quenched by solvent. It appears then that the DNA bulge induces a conformational change in the diradical species to enable selective intramolecular quenching of the C-2 radical. This represents a new role for DNA, as an effector–molecule in a chemical reaction. In addition to revealing unexpected mechanisms of drug activation and of DNA conformation involvement in drug product formation, these studies extend the usefulness of NCS-Chrom as a probe of unusual nucleic acid structures.

REFERENCES

1. N. Ishida, K. Miyazaki, K. Kumagai, and M. Rikimaru, *J. Antibiot., 18,* 68 (1965).

2. J. Meinehofer, H. Maeda, C. B. Glaser, J. Czombos, and K. Kuromizu, *Science, 178,* 875 (1972).

3. Y. Ono, Y. Watanabe, and N. Ishida, *Biochim. Biophys. Acta., 119,* 46 (1966).

4. T. S. A. Samy, J.-M. Hu, J. Meienhofer, H. Lazarus, and R. K. Johnson, *J. Natl. Cancer Inst., 58,* 1765 (1977).

5. M. A. Napier, B. Holmquist, D. J. Strydom, and I. H. Goldberg, *Biochem. Biophys. Res. Commun., 89,* 635 (1979).

6. L. F. Povirk and I. H. Goldberg, *Biochemisry, 19,* 4773 (1980).

7. L. S. Kappen and I. H. Goldberg, *Biochemistry, 19,* 4786 (1980).

8. L. S. Kappen, M. A. Napier, and I. H. Goldberg, *Proc. Natl. Acad. Sci. USA, 77,* 1970 (1980).

9. M. A. Napier, B. Holmquist, D. J. Strydom, and I. H. Goldberg, *Biochemistry, 20,* 5602 (1981).

10. L. S. Kappen and I. H. Goldberg, *Biochemistry, 18,* 5647 (1979).

11. M. A. Napier, L. S. Kappen, and I. H. Goldberg, *Biochemistry, 19,* 1767 (1980).

12. M. Kikuchi, M. Shoji, and N. Ishida, *J. Antibiot., 27,* 766 (1974).

13. M. Maeda and K. Kuromizu, *J. Biochem.*, (Tokyo) *81*, 25 (1977).

14. H. Lazarus, V. Raso, and T. S. A. Samy, *Cancer Res.*, *37*, 3731 (1977).

15. J.-I. Shoji, *J. Antibiot. Ser. A.*, *14*, 27 (1961).

16. K. Saito, Y. Sato, E. Edo, M. Akiyama, Y. Y. Koide, N. Ishida, and M. Mizugaki, *Chem. Pharm. Bull.*, *37*, 3078 (1989).

17. E. Adjadj, J. Mispelter, E. Quiniou, J.-L. Dimicoli, V. Favaudon, and J.-M. Lhoste, *Eur. J. Biochem.*, *190*, 263 (1990).

18. M. L. Remerowski, S. J. Glaser, L. C. Sieker, T. S. A. Samy, and G. P. Drobny, *Biochemistry*, *29*, 8401 (1990).

19. X. Gao and W. Burkhart, *Biochemistry*, *30*, 7730 (1991).

20. H. Takashima, S. Amiya, and Y. Kobayashi, *J. Biochem.*, *109*, 807 (1991).

21. L. S. Kappen, I. H. Goldberg, and T. S. Samy, *Biochemistry*, *18*, 5123 (1979).

22. L. S. Kappen, M. A. Napier, I. H. Goldberg, and T. S. A. Samy, *Biochemistry*, *19*, 4780 (1980).

23. T. S. A. Samy, K. S. Hahn, E. J. Modest, G. W. Lampman, H. T. Keutman, H. Umezawa, W. C. Herlihy, B. W. Gibson, S. A. Carr, and K. Biemann, *J. Biol. Chem.*, *258*, 183 (1983).

24. V. Z. Pletnev, A. P. Kuzin, S. D. Trakhanov, and P. V. Kostetsky, *Biopolymers*, *21*, 287 (1982).

25. P. Van Roey and T. A. Beerman, *Proc. Natl. Acad. Sci. USA*, *86*, 6587 (1989).

26. Y.-S. Zhen, X.-Y. Ming, B. Yu, T. Otani, H. Saito, and Y. Yamada, *J. Antibiot.*, *42*, 1294 (1989).

27. Y. Sugimoto, T. Otani, S. Oie, K. Wierzba, and Y. Yamada, *J. Antibiot.*, *43*, 417 (1990).

28. G. Albers-Schonberg, R. S. Dewey, O. D. Hensens, J. M. Liesch, M. A. Napier, and I. H. Goldberg, *Biochem. Biophys. Res. Commun.*, *95*, 1351 (1980).

29. M. S. Napier, I. H. Goldberg, O. D. Hensens, T. R. S. Dewey, J. M. Liesch, and G. Albers-Schonberg, *Biochem. Biophys. Res. Commun.*, *100*, 1703 (1981).

30. O. D. Hensens, R. S. Dewey, T. M. Liesch, M. A. Napier, R. A. Reamer, J. L. Smith, G. Albers-Schonberg, and I. H. Goldberg, *Biochem. Biophys. Res. Commun.*, *113*, 538 (1983).

31. M. Shibuya, K. Toyooka, and S. Kubota, *Tetrahedron Lett.*, *25*, 1171 (1984).

32. E. Edo, S. Katamine, F. Kitame, N. Ishida, Y. Koide, G. Kusano, and S. Nozoe, *J. Antibiot.*, *33*, 347 (1980).

33. E. Edo, M. Mizugaki, Y. Koide, H. Seto, K. Furihata, N. Otake, and N. Ishida, *Tetrahedron Lett.*, *26*, 331 (1985).

34. E. Edo, Y. Akiyama, K. Saito, M. Mizugaki, Y. Koide, and N. Ishida, *J. Antibiot.*, *39*, 1615 (1986).

35. A. G. Myers, P. J. Proteau, and T. M. Handel, *J. Am. Chem. Soc.*, *110*, 7212 (1988).

36. O. D. Hensens and I. H. Goldberg, *J. Antibiot.*, *42*, 761 (1989).

37. O. D. Hensens, J.-L. Giner, and I. H. Goldberg, *J. Amer. Chem. Soc.*, *111*, 3295 (1989).

38. P. A. Wender, J. A. McKinney, and C. Mukai, *J. Am. Chem. Soc.*, *112*, 5369 (1990).

39. A. G. Myers, P. M. Harrington, and E. Y. Kuo, *J. Am. Chem. Soc.*, *113*, 694 (1991).
40. S. H. Lee and I. H. Goldberg, *Mol. Pharmacol.*, *33*, 396 (1988).
41. E. Edo, Y. Akiyama, K. Saito, M. Mizugaki, Y. Koide, and N. Ishida, *J. Antibiot.*, *41*, 1272 (1988).
42. M. A. Napier and I. H. Goldberg, *Mol. Pharm.*, *23*, 500 (1983).
43. D.-H. Chin and I. H. Goldberg, *Biochemistry*, *25*, 1009 (1986).
44. L. S. Kappen and I. H. Goldberg, *Nucleic. Acids Res.*, *5*, 2959 (1978).
45. T. A. Beerman and I. H. Goldberg, *Biochem. Biophys. Res. Comm.*, *59*, 1254 (1974).
46. E. Edo, S. Iseki, N. Ishida, T. Horie, G. Kusano, and S. Nozoe, *J. Antibiot.*, *33*, 1586 (1980).
47. R. P. Sheridan and R. K. Gupta, *Biochem. Biophys. Res. Comm.*, *99*, 213 (1981).
48. R. L. Charnas and I. H. Goldberg, *Biochem. Biophys. Res. Comm.*, *122*, 642 (1984).
49. L. S. Kappen and I. H. Goldberg, *Nucleic Acids Res.*, *13*, 1637 (1985).
50. J. Golik, J. Clardy, G. Dubay, G. Groenewald, H. Kawaguchi, M. Konishi, B. Krishnan, H. Ohkuma, K.-I. Saitoh, and T. W. Doyle, *J. Am. Chem. Soc.*, *109*, 3461 (1987).
51. J. Golik, G. Dubay, G. Groenewald, H. Kawaguchi, M. Konishi, B. Krisnan, H. Ohkuma, K.-I. Saitoh, and T. W. Doyle, *J. Am. Chem. Soc.*, *109*, 3462 (1987).
52. M. D. Lee, T. S. Dunne, C. C. Chang, G. A. Ellestad, M. M. Siegel, G. O. Morton, W. J. McGahren, and D. B. Borders, *J. Am. Chem. Soc.*, *109*, 3466 (1987).
53. M. D. Lee, T. S. Dunne, M. S. Marshall, C. C. Chang, G. O. Morton, and D. B. Borders, *J. Am. Chem. Soc.*, *109*, 3464 (1987).
54. R. G. Bergman, *Acc. Chem. Res.*, *6*, 25 (1973).
55. A. G. Myers, *Tetrahedron Lett.*, *28*, 4493 (1987).
56. A. G. Myers and P. J. Proteau, *J. Am. Chem. Soc.*, *111*, 1146 (1989).
57. R. Poon, T. A. Beerman, and I. H. Goldberg, *Biochemistry*, *16*, 486 (1977).
58. I. H. Goldberg, T. Hatayama, L. S. Kappen, M. A. Napier, and L. F. Povirk, in *Molecular Actions and Targets for Cancer Chemotherapeutic Agents* (A. C. Sartorelli, J. S. Lazo, and J. R. Bertino, eds.), Academic Press, N.Y., 1981, pp. 163–191.
59. L. S. Kappen, S.-Q. Chen, and I. H. Goldberg, *Biochemistry*, *27*, 4331 (1988).
60. D.-H. Chin, C.-H. Zeng, C. E. Costello, and I. H. Goldberg, *Biochemistry*, *27*, 8106 (1988).
61. P. C. Dedon and I. H. Goldberg, *Biochemistry*, *31*, 1909 (1992).
62. A. G. Myers, P. M. Harrington, and B.-M. Kwon, *J. Am. Chem. Soc.*, *114*, 1086 (1992).
63. T. Tanaka, K. Fugiwara, and M. Hirama, *Tetrahedron Lett.*, *31*, 5947 (1990).
64. V. Favaudon, *Biochimie*, *65*, 593 (1983).
65. V. Favaudon, R. L. Charnas, and I. H. Goldberg, *Biochemistry*, *24*, 250 (1985).
66. D. H. Chin and I. H. Goldberg, *J. Am. Chem. Soc.*, *114*, 1914 (1992).
67. P. A. Wender and M. J. Tebbe, *Tetrahedron Lett.*, *32*, 4863 (1991).

68. S. E. McAfee and G. W. Ashley, *Nucleic Acids Res., 20,* 805 (1992).
69. S. M. Meschwitz and I. H. Goldberg, *Proc. Natl. Acad. Sci. USA, 88,* 3047 (1991).
70. G. Jung and W. Kohnlein, *Biochem. Biophys. Res. Commun., 98,* 176 (1981).
71. D. Dasgupta, D. S. Auld, and I. H. Goldberg, *Biochemistry, 24,* 7049 (1985).
72. L. F. Povirk, N. Dattagupta, B. C. Warf, and I. H. Goldberg, *Biochemistry, 20,* 4007 (1981).
73. D. Dasgupta and I. H. Goldberg, *Biochemistry, 24,* 6913 (1985).
74. D. Dasgupta and I. H. Goldberg, *Nucleic Acids Res., 14,* 1089 (1986).
75. T. Hatayama, I. H. Goldberg, M. Takeshita, and A. P. Grollman, *Proc. Natl. Acad. Sci. USA, 75,* 3603 (1978).
76. R. M. Burger, J. Peisach, and S. B. Hoywitz, *J. Biol. Chem., 253,* 4830 (1978).
77. M. Takeshita, L. S. Kappen, A. P. Grollman, M. Eisenberg, and I. H. Goldberg, *Biochemistry, 20,* 7599 (1981).
78. S. H. Lee and I. H. Goldberg, *Biochemistry, 28,* 1019 (1989).
79. L. S. Kappen and I. H. Goldberg, *Biochemistry, 17,* 729 (1978).
80. L. S. Kappen, I. H. Goldberg, and J. M. Liesch, *Proc. Natl. Acad. Sci. USA, 79,* 744 (1982).
81. L. S. Kappen and I. H. Goldberg, *Biochemistry, 22,* 4872 (1983).
82. D.-H. Chin, S. A. Carr, and I. H. Goldberg, *J. Biol. Chem., 259,* 9975 (1984).
83. L. F. Povirk and I. H. Goldberg, *J. Biol. Chem., 258,* 11763 (1983).
84. D.-H. Chin, L. S. Kappen, and I. H. Goldberg, *Proc. Natl. Acad. Sci. USA, 84,* 7070 (1987).
85. C. von Sonntag, C., in *The Chemical Basis of Radiation Biology*, Taylor & Francis, New York, 1987, pp. 57–93.
86. T. Hatayama and I. H. Goldberg, *Biochemistry, 19,* 5890 (1980).
87. H. Kawabata, H. Takeshita, T. Fujiwara, H. Sugiyama, T. Matsuura, and I. Saito, *Tetrahedron Lett., 30,* 4263 (1989).
88. J. Stubbe and J. W. Kozarich, *Chem. Rev., 87,* 1107 (1987).
89. L. S. Kappen and I. H. Goldberg, *Proc. Natl. Acad. Sci. USA, 81,* 3312 (1984).
90. V. Jagannadham and S. Steenken, *J. Am. Chem. Soc., 106,* 6542 (1984).
91. S. Steenken and V. Jagannadham, *J. Am. Chem. Soc., 107,* 6818 (1985).
92. M. J. Perkins and P. B. Roberts, *J. Chem. Soc. Perkin, II,* 297 (1974).
93. L. S. Kappen, T. R. Lee, C.-C. Yang, and I. H. Goldberg, *Biochemistry, 28,* 4540 (1989).
94. L. S. Kappen and I. H. Goldberg, *Biochemistry, 28,* 1027 (1989).
95. L. S. Kappen, I. H. Goldberg, S. H. Wu, J. Stubbe, L. Worth, and J. W. Kozarich, *J. Am. Chem. Soc., 112,* 2797 (1990).
96. L. Giloni, M. Takeshita, F. Johnson, C. Iden, and A. P. Grollman, *J. Biol. Chem., 256,* 8608 (1981).
97. I. Saito, H. Kawabata, T. Fujiwara, H. Sugiyama, and T. Matsuura, *J. Am. Chem. Soc., 111,* 8302 (1989).
98. B. L. Frank, L. Worth, Jr., D. F. J. Christner, J. W. Kozarich, J. Stubbe, L. S. Kappen, and I. H. Goldberg, *J. Am. Chem. Soc., 113,* 2271 (1991).
99. L. S. Kappen, I. H. Goldberg, B. L. Frank, L. J. Worth, D. F. Christner, J. W. Kozarich, and J. Stubbe, *Biochemistry, 30,* 2034 (1991).

100. P. C. Dedon and I. H. Goldberg, *Chem. Res. Toxicol., 5,* 311 (1992).

101. P. C. Dedon, Z.-W. Jiang, and I. H. Goldberg, *Biochemistry, 31,* 1917 (1992).

102. L. E. Rabow, G. H. McGall, J. Stubbe, and J. W. Kozarich, *J. Am. Chem. Soc., 112,* 3203 (1990).

103. T. Hatayama and I. H. Goldberg, *Biochim. Biophys. Acta, 563,* 59 (1979).

104. L. F. Povirk and I. H. Goldberg, *Proc. Natl. Acad. Sci. USA, 82,* 3182 (1985).

105. L. F. Povirk, C. W. Houlgrave, and Y.-H. Han, *J. Biol. Chem., 263,* 19263 (1988).

106. A. Galat and I. H. Goldberg, *Nucleic Acids Res., 18,* 2093 (1990).

107. N. Zein, A. M. Sinha, W. J. McGahren, and G. A. Ellestad, *Science, 240,* 1198 (1988).

108. K.-X. Chen, N. Gresh, and B. Pullman, *Nucleic Acids Res., 15,* 2175 (1987).

109. P. C. Dedon and I. H. Goldberg, *J. Biol. Chem., 265,* 14713 (1990).

110. C. von Sonntag and H.-P. Schuchmann, *Int. J. Radiat. Biol., 49,* 1 (1986).

111. M. Gochin and T. L. James, *Biochemistry, 29,* 11172 (1990).

112. L. S. Kappen and I. H. Goldberg, *Proc. Natl. Acad. Sci. USA, 89,* 6706 (1992).

113. W. N. Hunter, T. Brown, G. Kneale, N. N. Anand, D. Rabinovich, and O. Kennard, *J. Biol. Chem., 262,* 9962 (1987).

114. L. S. Kappen and I. H. Goldberg, *Biochemistry, 31,* 9081 (1992).

115. L. D. Williams and I. H. Goldberg, *Biochemistry, 27,* 3004 (1988).

116. L. F. Povirk and I. H. Goldberg, *Proc. Natl. Acad. Sci. USA, 79,* 369 (1982).

117. L. F. Povirk and I. H. Goldberg, *Nucleic Acids Res., 10,* 6255 (1982).

118. L. F. Povirk and I. H. Goldberg, *Biochemistry, 23,* 6304 (1984).

119. L. F. Povirk and I. H. Goldberg, *Biochemistry, 24,* 4035 (1985).

120. I. H. Goldberg, *Free Radical Biol. Med., 3,* 41 (1987).

121. B. Singer and J. T. Kusmierek, *Ann. Rev. Biochem., 51,* 655 (1982).

122. K. Frenkel, D. Grunberger, H. Kasai, H. Komura, and K. Nakanishi, *Biochemistry, 20,* 4377 (1981).

123. L. F. Povirk and I. H. Goldberg, *Biochimie, 69,* 815 (1987).

124. A. F. Fuciarelli, G. G. Miller, and J. A. Raleigh, *Radiat. Res., 104,* 272 (1985).

125. M. Dizdaroglu, *Biochem. J., 238,* 247 (1986).

126. A. A. Shaw and J. Cadet, *Int. J. Radiat. Biol., 54,* 987 (1988).

127. M. Homma, T. Koida, T. Saito Koide, I. Kamo, M. Seto, K. Kumagai, and N. Ishida, *6th Int. Congr. Chemotherap., 2,* 410 (1970).

128. H. Sawada, K. Tatsumi, M. Sasada, S. Shirakawa, T. Nakamura, and G. Wakisaka, *Cancer Res., 34,* 3341 (1974).

129. T. Ebina, K. Ohtsuki, M. Seto, and N. Ishida, *Eur. J. Cancer, 11,* 155 (1975).

130. T. A. Beerman and I. H. Goldberg, *Biochim. Biophys. Acta, 475,* 281 (1977).

131. T. Hatayama and M. Yukioka, *Biochim. Biophys. Acta., 740,* 291 (1983).

132. K. Tatsumi, T. Nakamura, and G. Wakisaka, *Gann, 65,* 459 (1974).

133. K. Ohtsuki and N. Ishida, *J. Antibiot., 28,* 143 (1975).

134. D. S. R. Sarma, S. Rajalakshmi, and T. S. A. Samy, *Biochem. Pharmacol., 25,* 789 (1976).

135. R. Ishida, T. Nishimoto, and T. Takahashi, *Cell Structure and Function, 4,* 235 (1979).

136. D. E. Berry and J. M. Collins, *Cancer Res., 40,* 2405 (1980).
137. R. P. Beckmann, M. J. Agostino, M. M. McHugh, R. D. Sigmund, and T. A. Beerman, *Biochemistry, 26,* 5409 (1987).
138. M. T. Kuo and T. S. A. Samy, *Biochim. Biophys. Acta, 518,* 186 (1978).
139. T. A. Beerman, G. Mueller, and H. Grimmond, *Molec. Pharmacol., 23,* 493 (1983).
140. L. F. Povirk and I. H. Goldberg, *Biochemistry, 21,* 5857 (1982).
141. Y. Shilo and Y. Becker, *Cancer Res., 42,* 2247 (1982).
142. Y. Shilo, E. Tabor, and Y. Becker, *Biochem. Biophys. Res. Commun., 110,* 483 (1983).
143. R. W. Babilon, K. J. Soprano, and E. E. Henderson, *Mutation Res., 146,* 79 (1985).
144. M. J. Li and Y. Shiraishi, *Mutation Res., 230,* 167 (1990).
145. S. Antoku and S. Kura, *Int. J. Radiat. Biol., 58,* 613 (1990).
146. K. Tatsumi, T. Sakane, H. Sawada, S. Shirakawa, T. Nakamura, and G. Wakisaka, *Gann, 66,* 441 (1975).
147. M. Sasada, H. Sawada, T. Nakamura, and H. Uchino, *Gann, 69,* 407 (1978).
148. W. H. Hittelman and M. Pollard, *Cancer Res., 42,* 4584 (1982).
149. W. L. Kuo, R. E. Meyn, and C. W. Haidle, *Cancer Res., 44,* 1748 (1984).
150. L. S. Kappen and I. H. Goldberg, *Biochim. Biophys. Acta, 520,* 481 (1978).
151. M. Sasada, H. Sawada, T. Nakamura, and H. Uchino, *Gann, 67,* 447 (1976).
152. K. Tatsumi, M. Tashima, S. Shirakawa, T. Nakamura, and H. Uchino, *Cancer Res., 39,* 1623 (1979).
153. S. Iseki, T. Ebina, and N. Ishida, *Cancer Res., 40,* 3786 (1980).
154. K. Tatsumi and H. Nishioka, *Mutation Res., 48,* 195 (1977).
155. K. Tatsumi, K. K. Bose, K. Ayres, and B. S. Strauss, *Biochemistry, 19,* 4767 (1980).
156. M. E. Schupbach and F. J. deGerres, *Mutation Res., 81,* 49 (1981).
157. W. G. DeGraff, *Mutation Res., 128,* 127 (1984).
158. M. R. Miller and D. N. Cinault, *J. Biol. Chem., 257,* 46 (1982).
160. P. M. Goodwin, P. J. Lewis, M. I. Davies, C. J. Skidmore, and S. Shall, *Biochim. Biophys. Acta., 543,* 576 (1978).
161. Y. Sawada, N. L. Reichenback, C. C. Cross, and Suhadolnik, *J. Antibiot., 35,* 119 (1982).
160. A. P. Rao and P. N. Rao, *J. Natl. Cancer Inst., 57,* 1139 (1976).
162. W. W. Au, J. P. O'Neill, W. Wang, H. E. Luippold, and R. J. Preston, *Teratogen. Carcinogen. Mutagen., 4,* 515 (1984).
163. K. Psaraki and N. A. Demopoulos, *Mutation Res., 204,* 669 (1988).
164. L. S. Kappen, T. E. Ellenberger, and I. H. Goldberg, *Biochemistry, 26,* 384 (1987).
165. W. G. DeGraff and J. B. Mitchell, *Cancer Res., 45,* 4760 (1985).
166. W. G. DeGraff, A. Russo, and J. B. Mitchell, *J. Biol. Chem., 260,* 8312 (1985).
167. N. F. Schor, *J. Clin. Invest., 89,* 774 (1992).
168. N. F. Schor, *J. Pharmacol. Exp. Therapeut., 249,* 906 (1989).
169. H. Maeda, S. Aikawa, and A. Yamashita, *Cancer Res., 35,* 554 (1975).

170. J. Takeshita, H. Maeda, and K. Koike, *J. Biochem., 88,* 1071 (1980).

171. Y. Miyamoto and H. Maeda, *Jpn. J. Cancer Res., 82,* 351 (1991).

172. S. S. Lagha, D. D. Von Hoff, M. Rozencweig, D. Abraham, M. Slavik, and M. Muggia, *Oncology, 33,* 256 (1976).

173. H. Maeda, S. Sakamoto, and J. Ogata, *Anti-microb. Agents Chemother., 11,* 941 (1977).

174. Y. Kinami, H. Miyazaki, F. Koyama, M. Noguchi, K. Konishi, N. Furukawa, and Y. Nishida, *J. Jpn. Soc. Cancer Ther., 10,* 502 (1975).

175. I. Satake, K. Tari, M. Yamamoto, and H. Nishimura, *J. Urol., 133,* 87 (1985).

176. D. L. Urdal and S. Hakomori, *J. Biol. Chem., 255,* 10509 (1980).

177. I. Kimura, T. Ohnoshi, T. Tsubota, Y. Sato, T. Kobayashi, and S. Abe, *Cancer Immunol. Immunother., 7,* 235 (1980).

178. T. Sasaki, E. Tamate, T. Muryoi, O. Takai, and K. Yoshinaga, *J. Immunol., 142,* 1159 (1989).

179. G. Luders, W. Kohnlein, C. Sorg, and J. Bruggen, *Cancer Immunol. Immunother., 20,* 85 (1985).

180. T. Takahashi, T. Yamaguchi, K. Kitamura, H. Suzuyama, M. Honda, T. Yokota, H. Kotanagi, M. Takahashi, and Y. Hashimoto, *Cancer, 61,* 881 (1988).

181. U. Gottschalk, A. Maibucher, H. Menke and W. Kohnlein, *J. Antibiot., 63,* 1051 (1990).

182. Y. Kohgo, H. Kondo, J. Kato, K. Sasaki, N. Tsushima, T. Nishisato, M. Hiryama, K. Fujikawa, N. Shintani, Y. Mogi, and Y. Niitsu, *Jpn. J. Cancer Res., 81,* 91 (1990).

183. H. Maeda, M. Ueda, T. Morinaga, and T. Matsumoto, *J. Med. Chem., 28,* 455 (1985).

184. T. Oda and H. Maeda, *Cancer Res., 47,* 3206 (1987).

185. S. Noda, S. Konno, J. Tanaka, M. Yamada, and N. Yoshitake, *Anticancer Res., 10,* 709 (1990).

186. M. Kobayashi, K. Imai, S. Sugihara, H. Maeda, T. Konno, and H. Yamanaka, *Urology, 37,* 288 (1991).

187. E. Eisenstadt, M. Wolf, and I. H. Goldberg, *J. Bacteriol., 144,* 656 (1980).

188. D. Denklau, R. Stahl, and W. Kohnlein, *Z. Naturforsch, 44,* 791 (1989).

189. E. Mousstachhi and V. Favaudon, *Mutation Res., 104,* 87 (1982).

190. P. L. Foster and E. Eisenstadt, *J. Bacteriol., 153,* 379 (1983).

191. L. F. Povirk and I. H. Goldberg, *Nucleic Acids Res., 14,* 1417 (1986).

192. L. A. Loeb, *Cell, 40,* 483 (1985).

193. I. H. Goldberg, *Accounts Chem. Res., 24,* 191 (1991).

194. D.-H. Chin and I. H. Goldberg, *Biochemistry, 32,* 3611 (1993).

195. S. M. Meschwitz, R. G. Schultz, G. W. Ashley, and I. H. Goldberg, *Biochemistry, 31,* 9117 (1992).

196. L. S. Kappen and I. H. Goldberg, *Science, 261,* 1319 (1993).

197. L. S. Kappen and I. H. Goldberg, *Biochemistry, 32,* 13138 (1993).

198. O. D. Hensens, G. L. Helms, D. L. Zink, D.-H. Chin, L. S. Kappen, and I. H. Goldberg, *J. Am. Chem. Soc., 115,* 11030 (1993).

199. O. D. Hensens, D.-H. Chin, A. Stassinopoulos, D. L. Zink, L. S. Kappen, and I. H. Goldberg, *Proc. Natl. Acad. Sci. USA, 91,* 4534 (1994).

17

The Clinical Effects of Neocarzinostatin and Its Polymer Conjugate, SMANCS

Hiroshi Maeda

Kumamoto University School of Medicine, Kumamoto, Japan

I. INTRODUCTION

A comprehensive review of neocarzinostatin (NCS) appeared more than 10 years ago (1), and its second-generation drug, NCS-polymer conjugate (SMANCS) is now attracting strong clinical interest.

Despite the extremely potent biological activity of NCS in vitro or in experimental animals, its clinical use is very limited. Japanese Pharmacopeia (or FDA) permits its use for cancers in digestive organs including stomach, pancreas, and liver, for cancers of the urinary bladder and brain, and for leukemia. It is not used outside of Japan clinically. The reason for its limited use is its potent toxicity, particularly bone marrow toxicity, e.g., leukocytopenia and thrombocytopenia, perhaps because of non–tumor-selective delivery. A high toxicity means the chemotherapeutic index (ratio of maximum tolerable dose/minimum effective dose) is very small and tumor targeting efficiency is very low (1–3). NCS has, however, a very high renal clearance rate, similar to low molecular weight substances described later, and surprisingly it is absorbed by the urinary bladder tissue from urine and routed back into the general circulation (4).

One can overcome the pharmacological drawbacks of NCS by conjugating it with appropriate polymers (5–12). When conjugated with a biocompatible polymer, NCS becomes a completely different drug and clinical efficacy is greatly increased (6–10). The great clinical potential, particularly by arterial administra-

363

tion, appears to depend on its extremely high biological activity and the high tumor-targeting efficiency of the conjugate. This almost tumor-selective targeting was accomplished to an unprecedented extent by arterial administration with oily formulation, as described later. Since the total injectable amount is rather limited by means of arterial injection of oily formulation, extremely high biological activity of the drug is a prerequisite for this method. Arterial injection of poly(*s*tyrene-co-*m*aleic *a*cid)–NCS conjugate (SMANCS) solubilized in lipid contrast medium (Lipiodol)–abbreviated SMANCS/Lipiodol is now approved by the Japanese government as the first-choice treatment for liver cancer, which is one of the most difficult and most abundant types of tumors in the world.

II. PHARMACOLOGICALLY UNIQUE CHARACTERISTICS OF NCS AND SMANCS

Although the molecular size of NCS, 12 kDa, is very large when compared with conventional drugs (mostly less than 1 kDa), in vivo behavior of NCS is almost the same as conventional low molecular weight drugs in view of renal clearance and plasma half-life ($t_{1/2}$). We have found its plasma half-life to be about 1.9 minutes in mice (4,8–10,13,14). It is also degraded by proteolytic enzymes in serum or plasma because various protease inhibitors inhibit inactivation of NCS in vitro (15).

SMANCS is a conjugate of two chains of poly(styrene-co-maleic acid) (SMA) and NCS in which SMA has a mean molecular mass of 1.6 kDa and half of the carboxy groups are esterified with *n*-butanol (5,6,8–10) and the mean molecular mass of SMANCS is 16 kDa. In vitro stability of SMANCS in blood or in serum or plasma is about 10 times higher than that of NCS (8,9). Among the four different SMA derivatives, i.e., the free carboxylate form, ethylester-, methylcellosolve-, or *n*-butyl-ester of maleyl residues, we found that *n*-butyrate half ester had the best blood/plasma stability in vitro and albumin-binding property (8,10,16). SMANCS behaves in vivo, however, as if it had a molecular size close to 80 kDa because it binds with plasma albumin noncovalently (16).

SMANCS is not cleared into urine via the kidney but into bile (17), and $t_{1/2}$ is about 10 times longer than NCS in vivo in mice (8–10,13,14). A similar result is observed in humans (9).

III. SUBCELLULAR SITE OF ACTION: INTERNALIZATION INTO CELLS

A. NCS

Details of the molecular mechanisms of NCS on DNA are documented elsewhere in this book. We have investigated the subcellular sites of action of NCS and SMANCS. Our results, utilizing fluorescein isothiocyanate (FITC)–conjugated or

[^{14}C]-labeled NCS, showed that NCS was taken up into the cytosol and nucleus of cancer cells (18–21). This phenomenon of intracellular uptake of NCS was initially observed by autoradiography of [^{14}C]-NCS–treated intact cells. [^{14}C]-NCS was prepared by succinylation of two amino groups (Ala 1 and Lys 20). It remained active, and its molecular size was not altered (20). Furthermore, by utilizing the FITC-NCS and fluorescence polarization techniques, we have elucidated that its molecular size after its incorporation remained almost constant (19). These data, however, are in disagreement with a speculation that NCS acts on cell membranes or on the outside membrane of cells (22–24). To clarify this point, we compared the effect of NCS on four different states of DNA: (1) naked DNA (colicin E_1 plasmid), which has neither membrane nor DNA-bound chromatin proteins; (2) DNA with chromatin proteins (of burst cell), which lacks cell membrane; (3) intact viable lymphoblastoid cells, which are known to take up NCS quite rapidly, but which possess a membrane barrier that protects DNA from a direct attack by NCS; (4) normal lymphocytes, which incorporate NCS very slowly, but in which DNA is protected by both cellular and nuclear membranes (18–20). The result clearly showed that NCS degraded the DNA states in the following order: (1) > (2) > (3) > (4). This indicates that direct access by NCS is required for its action on DNA. Separate studies with an *E. coli* mutant that is hypersensitive to NCS and lacks membrane protein support this interpretation (25). A need for intracellular incorporation was confirmed in other lymphoid cells in which treatment by NCS at 4°C did not show any effect after washing and necessity for internalization was confirmed (26). The results also indicate that an endocytotic process is required for its action (27).

There are a few studies on NCS effects on cell microtubules. NCS appears to affect microtubules of cells in culture at high lethal concentrations (50% effective concentration: 20 µg/ml, almost 100-fold higher than that for DNA) (23).

B. SMANCS

The binding of NCS and SMANCS to cultured cells was studied, and the latter was found to exhibit a remarkably increased association constant to tumor cells. From time course analyses, it was found that binding of the fluorescein-labeled protein drugs to HeLa cells was time dependent and proceeded rapidly at 37°C during the initial 30 minutes, reaching equilibrium after 2 hours (28).

In the presence of 100-fold molar excess of unlabeled NCS, the binding of SMANCS was inhibited, as was that of NCS. These results suggested that the binding of NCS or SMANCS to HeLa cells was mediated by a specific receptor or binding site on the cell surface, and most of the SMANCS also bound to the same receptor. Furthermore, the amount of cell-bound SMANCS was increased about 20-fold as compared to NCS. The increase of binding activity of SMANCS to cells was examined by Scatchard plot analysis for the number of binding sites and apparent association constant (K_a) to HeLa cells. The results are summarized

Table 1   Association Constant (K_a) and Number of Binding Sites of NCS and SMANCS evaluated from Scatchard plot analysis

Cells	Drugs	Temp. (°C)	K_a ($\times 10^{-4} M^{-1}$)	No. of binding sites per cell ($\times 10^{-7}$)
HeLa	NCS	0	1.97	0.68
		37	0.53	3.20
	SMANCS	0	20.38	1.68
		37	13.39	4.48

Source: Ref. 28, 29.

in Table 1. No significant differences between NCS and SMANCS in the number of binding sites could be demonstrated. However, K_a values of SMANCS were 13.4 ($\times 10^4 M^{-1}$), while that of neocarzinostatin was $0.5 \times 10^4 M^{-1}$, 27-fold lower (28,29). Similar results were obtained using another tumor cell line, WISH, in culture (28,29). These facts indicate that the binding affinity and the rate of internalization of SMANCS into HeLa cells are greatly increased by conjugating an appropriate polymer. This result was also substantiated by the biological activity (inhibition of colony formation) for the conjugate, which required a much shorter exposure time (5 min) to the cells than the parental drug (NCS) (>80 min) to kill 80% of the tumor cells in culture, respectively (28,29).

The rate of internalization was more than 10 times greater at pH 4.5 than at pH 7.5 for SMANCS, perhaps because protonation of carboxylate confer hydrophobicity, thus higher affinity to membrane lipid of cells (29). It is generally considered that tumor tissue is more acidic than normal tissue. Therefore, this evidence favors an idea that hydrophobic polyanion conjugates are more likely to be taken up more effectively by tumor cells than by normal cells, particularly in in vivo settings. Thus, SMANCS has another prominent aspect at the subcellular level.

In conclusion, we have determined that both NCS and SMANCS need to be internalized into the target tumor cells in order to exert their action, i.e., degradation of DNA and inhibition of DNA synthesis, or cell death. This finding is concordant with the fact that their active principle "enediyne" chromophore must be inside cells to react with DNA.

IV.   TOXICITY AND SIDE EFFECTS

The lethal dose 50% (LD_{50}) for NCS ad SMANCS in animals is shown in Table 2. Although LD_{50} of SMANCS given intravenously (IV) is approximately 1

Table 2 Acute Toxicity and Antimicrobial Activity OF NCS and SMANCS

Animal	Route of administration (single injection)	LD$_{50}$ (mg/kg)	
		NCS[a]	SMANCS[b]
A. Acute toxicity			
mouse	IV	1.61[a] (1.0)[b]	3.4[b]
	IP	1.94[a] (1.3)[b]	4.6[b]
	PO	~1000.0	—
rat	IV	1.13 (<0.65)[c]	1.0[c]
	IP	0.94	1.3[c]
	PO	≥300	—
rabbit	IV	0.96	—

B. Antimicrobial activity (agar plate diffusion method)[b]		
Test bacteria	Minimal inhibitory concentration (μg/ml)	
Micrococcus luteus	0.01	0.03

[a] From Ref. 1.
[b] From Ref. 6.
[c] From Ref. 17.

mg/kg (1,6), 0.3 mg/kg given every fifth day three times was tolerated and showed significant antitumor effect in rats (31). Angiotensin II–induced hypertension (100 → 150 mmHg) chemotherapy showed less toxicity at this dose (32). There seems to be some difference in the manifestation of toxicity of NCS and SMANCS. At the dose above LD$_{50}$ of SMANCS, i.e., 1.35–2.80/kg bolus IV, anemia, emaciation, piloerection, ataxic gait, decreased locomotor activity, loss of hair, bradypnea, and soft stool were observed. Proneness and occasionally nasal and peritoneal bleeding were also observed (17).

Electron microscopic observation of tumor tissue after SMANCS treatment at the therapeutic dose showed extensive degeneration and encapsulation accompanying fatty degeneration 30 days after drug administration, which were not observed in the group treated with NCS (31). In the blood vessels of the SMANCS-treated tumors we frequently observed deposition of platelets, fibrin clot, and thrombi together with leakage of blood cells out of vascular bed (31).

In conclusion, early clinical signs of toxicity of NCS and SMANCS are hematological (Tables 3, 4). Preliminary phase I data showed that a daily dose of SMANCS at 2 mg/60 kg of body weight by slow IV infusion did not produce any remarkable toxicity during a 3-week period. Slow IV infusion of 4 mg/day/60 kg body weight resulted in a decrease in the counts of white blood cells and/or platelets after 3 consecutive weeks, although this effect was reversible.

Table 3 Hematological Toxicity of Neocarzinostatin in Humans

	Schedule of one course	
	bolus, 1 mg IV daily × 7, followed by 1 week intermission[a]	IV continuous infustion 6 mg/24 hr, × 5 consecutive days[b]
No. of courses (total dose, mg)	4 (24)	5 (30)
Total dose per day (mg)	1	6
WBC (per μl)	3300 (median value)	<4000 23/33, <2000 10/33
Platelet counts (per μl × 10^6)	2.8 (median value)	<0.1 26/32, <0.5 13/32
Fall of hemoglobin (>1.5/dl)	Insignificant	16/30

[a] From Ref. 2.
[b] From Ref. 3.

V. ROUTES OF ADMINISTRATION

NCS, which is soluble only in water, is usually administered via IV route, although the intravesical route for bladder cancer (2,30), and intracerebral compartment for intraspinal/cranial dissemination of brain tumor using Ommaya's reservoir (35–37) are used. For the treatment of brain tumor via these routes of administrations, the extremely short half-life became a definite advantage (35–37). Intraarterial (IA) injection has been used less frequently for liver and pancreatic cancers, which has resulted in fewer side effects.

SMANCS can be used as an aqueous injection via the IV or IA route. But more interestingly, we have developed its lipid formulation using lipid contrast medium [Lipiodol^R] (a product of Laboratoire Guerbet, Paris, France), or medium-chain triglyceride, both usually at 1 mg/ml. This oily formulation SMANCS/Lipiodol was possible because of the highly lipophilic nature of SMANCS, although it cannot be given intravenously. SMANCS/Lipiodol has shown unprecedented tumor-targeting effects when given via tumor-feeding arteries resulting in a tumor/blood ratio of more than 2000 (39,40). Thus, very little systemic toxicity is observed because the drug distributed was very low in normal tissue other than tumor. In addition, it will release the drug (SMANCS) very slowly for a period of weeks, and thus definite antitumor effects can be seen even by a single administration. This means the intervals between administrations will be very long. Table 5 shows clinical data to support this notion.

Furthermore, SMANCS/Lipiodol can visualize tumor images clearly because of the predominant localization of Lipiodol (containing SMANCS) in tumor tissue. Thus, dosage (or intratumor deposition) can be semi-quantified by x-ray images such as CT scan since presence of SMANCS depends upon the amount of Lipiodol (41–43).

Table 4 General Side Effects of Neocarzinostatin in Humans

Side effects	IV infusion, 2–4 mg/day, 4–6 days[a] (%)	IV infusion, 2–4 mg/day, 4–6 days[b] (%)	1 mg bolus, IV in 20 sec[c] (%)	6 mg IV infusion continuous for 24 hr for 5 successive days[d] (%)
Anorexia or stomatitis	50.0	} 33.0	87.5	19.2
Nausea	42.3		57.5	46.2
Vomiting	11.5	—	2.5	30.7
Dullness	11.5	16.6	—	—
Fever and/or chills	9.6	12.5	0	24.2
Cutaneous eruption	3.8	8.3	5	9.6
Cardiac stimulation	3.8	—	—	—
Hepatic dysfunction	17.3	Insignificant (GPT, AL-P, LDH)	0	23.1
Hemorrhage	1.9	—	0	—
Shock	1.9	—	—	—
Phlebitis or cellulitis at IV site	—	—	2.5	21.1
No. of cases	55	20	40	52

[a] From Ref. 33.
[b] From Ref. 34.
[c] From Ref. 1, 30.
[d] From Ref. 3.

Table 5 Effect of NCS against Bladder Cancer[a]

Tumor grade	Total no. of patients	No. of cases[b] (%)				
		+++	++	+	±	−
II	28	0 (0)	15 (53.6)	8 (28.6)	4 (14.3)	1 (3.6)
III	10	2 (20.0)	4 (40.0)	1 (5.8)	2 (10.0)	1 (5.0)

[a] Based on 38 evaluable cases with transitional cell carcinoma.
[b] +++, disappearance of tumor; ++, reduction of tumor size more than 50%; +, reduction of tumor size less than 50%; ±, tumor stabilization; −, tumor growth continued.
Source: Ref. 2, 30.

Oily formulation or macromolecular drug in aqueous milieu can be administered via intracavitary injection, such as into the pleural or peritoneal cavity, for the control of carcinomatosis, and we found that the lipid formulation or macromolecular drugs remain in the compartment 20–30 times longer at higher concentration than the aqueous formulation, and thus, free-floating tumor cells can be completely eradicated after one or several administrations in a period of a week or so (44). This observation is also valid for human peritoneal and pleural carcinomatoses (Kimura, M., Konno, T. and Maeda, H., unpublished observation).

VI. OILY FORMULATION OF SMANCS IN LIPIODOL (SMANCS/LIPIODOL)

SMANCS has much higher lipid permissibility than NCS. A solution of SMANCS in lipid contrast medium, Lipiodol is prepared by taking advantage of this lipophilic character. Lipiodol is iodinated ethylester of poppy seed oil, $\rho = 1.37$, and iodine content is 37% (w/w). Initially, higher molecular weight SMA polymer (mean molecular weight of 6.5 kDa vs. 1.55 kDa of present form)–NCS conjugate was prepared (5), which was completely soluble in Lipiodol. However, the present pharmaceutical grade of SMANCS consists of much lower molecular weight SMA (1.55 kDa) because of ease of purification, although it is only slightly soluble for Lipiodol. A slow release of SMANCS from Lipiodol, for a period of several weeks after a single injection, eliminates frequent injections. In vitro experiments showed its retention in Lipiodol to be more than 10% after about 96 hours (8), which means more than 100 µg/ml, or more than 2000-fold higher than minimal effective concentration is retained in this lipid (45).

As a result of the imaging capability of SMANCS/Lipiodol, the determination of a rational dosing regimen became possible, as stated above. Accordingly, one can avoid excessive and unnecessary drug administration and definite anticancer effects can be achieved with few side effects. Accounts of tumor visualization or imaging under x-ray systems and diagnostic values have been reviewed previously (38–43).

In this connection it should be mentioned that extremely high biological activity of enediyne antitumor agents becomes very critical. The reason is that in a given tissue or organ, it is only possible to deposit Lipiodol to a limited, although selective, degree, i.e., no more than 15–20% of tissue weight in animal experiments. However, injected doses in the tumor can be as high as 70% at 15 minutes after IA injection in a rabbit model, although the injectable amount is limited (40).

Although the oily formulation can provide the most selective delivery of the drug to the target tumor, its density will be no more than a few percent (w/w) of the tissue weight in a clinical setting. Thus, drug concentration will be diluted 30–100 times. The usual concentration of SMANCS in Lipiodol is 1000 μg/ ml; it will theoretically become available to the tumor tissue at 10–30 μg/ml. This value is very close to the observed values (41). This concentration is still about 100- to 1000-fold higher than the minimal inhibitory concentration (MIC) required to kill tumor cells (45). In contrast, other anticancer agents, e.g., 5-fluorouracil or cisplatin, are known to have much higher concentrations for minimum inhibitory concentration, and thus the carrier lipid needs to contain a very high concentration, e.g., 10% (w/w) or more, of Lipiodol in order to attain effective concentration against cancer cells, which is almost impossible. The usual IV dose of cisplatin and 5-fluorouracil is 100 mg/m^2 or more in humans, while that of SMANCS is 2 mg/m^2. This means, for example, that 100 mg of a polar drug in 5 ml of lipid is difficult to achieve, while 2 mg of SMANCS can be readily formulated.

Many low molecular weight anticancer compounds can be washed out rapidly and are difficult to maintain at high concentrations in tumor tissue, while macromolecular drugs are well retained (see below). Therefore, the highly potent bioactivity of enediyne compounds is ideal for this type of administration. Many experimental data support the notion that macromolecular substances and lipids are highly permeable to tumor blood vessels and leak into tumor interstitium but that they are not so in normal tissue. Furthermore, they are also not readily cleared from tumor tissue by the lymphatic systems. This phenomenon is called the *enhanced permeability and retention* (EPR) effect of macromolecules and lipids in solid tumor. It is attributed to the architectural and pathophysiological differences between blood vessels in tumor tissue versus normal tissue (8–11,13,14, 32,46,57).

One last advantage of the lipid formulation of SMANCS is its increased stability in lipids, which may be attributed to the lack of access of water and hydrolytic enzymes for hydrolysis (46,47).

Table 6 Summary of Clinical Trial of Neocarzinostatin for Brain Tumor

Case no.	Age and sex	Previous treatment	Diagnosis	Surgical procedure	Radiation	Neocarzinostatin	Follow-up (months) and outcome
1	13 M		Pineal germinoma	V-P shunt	local 4600 r head 1050 spine 450	ventricle 0.041 mg intrathec 0.091	26, full activity
2	26 M		Pineal germinoma	V-P shunt Ommaya	head 3000 local 2000	ventricle 0.104 intrathec 0.191	26, full activity
3	3M		Medulloblastoma	Partial removal V-P shunt Ommaya	head 1000 local 2350 spine 600	ventricle 0.364	6, expired
4	10 M	craniectomy and radiation, 1977 (7000 r)	Medulloblastoma recurrent	V-P shunt Ommaya	head 3000 local 2000 spine 3000 neck 4500	ventricle 0.304 cisternal 0.060	12, expired
5	14 F		Medulloblastoma	Subtotal removal Torkildsen Ommaya	head 4050 local 3000 spine 750	ventricle cisternal intrathec total 0.940	17, full activity
6	12 M	craniectomy & radiation, 1977 (5100 r)	Medulloblastoma	Ommaya	head 3000 local 2000 spine 2880	ventricle 0.950 intrathec 0.110	15, full activity

7	14 M		Medulloblastoma	Total removal V-P shunt Ommaya	head 2050 local 2700 spine 3000	ventricle 0.180 intrathec 0.120 perfusion 1.310	2, full activity
8	11 F	craniotomy and radiation, 1976 (4700 r)	Astrocytoma dissemination	Torkildsen V-P shunt Ommaya		ventricle 0.970 cisternal 0.970 intrathec 0.720	7, full activity with OPD treatment
9	66 M	laparotomy stomach cancer	Meningeal carcinomatosis	Ext. drainage Ommaya V-P shunt		perfusion 0.385	2, expired
10	59 F	laparotomy stomach cancer	Meningeal carcinomatosis	Ext. drainage V-P shunt		perfusion 1.000 intrathec 0.040	6, temporarily well and expired
11	9 M	crainotomy and radiation, 1975 (4000 r)	Glioblastoma recurrent	Partial removal Ommaya in cyst	local 3450	intracyst 0.066	34, full activity
12	26 M	biopsy and radiation, 1978 (5000 r) Me-CCNU 340 mg	Glioblastoma recurrent	Cranioplasty Partial removal Ommaya in cyst	local 5000	intracyst 0.640	14, fair

Summary: Total cases, 12; 7 cases response, (+); 2 cases response, (±); 3 cases, no response. V-P, venticular-peritoneal.
Source: Ref. 35.

VII.   CLINICAL EFFECTS OF NCS AND SMANCS

A.   NCS

Antitumor effect of NCS in experimental animals and humans was documented long ago (48–52). Its effect on L-1210 and Walker carcinoma has been extraordinary (50). Clinical use for urinary bladder cancer, brain tumor, and leukemia is recognized (2,30,35–37) (Table 5 and 6) but rather limited. The efficacy of NCS for brain tumor seems encouraging and is definitely positive if the dosing regimen is meticulously manipulated to attain effective therapeutic concentration while avoiding toxic concentration (35–37) (Table 6); this type of use should be worth pursuing more extensively. A unique advantage of this treatment is that free tumor cells in cerebrospinal fluid, which are difficult to remove by radiation because of their widespread nature, can be cleared completely by infusion of NCS at extremely low doses (35). We reported that brain tumor cells were very sensitive to NCS while normal glia or neural cells are rather resistant (35); glia cells tolerated 0.3 μg/ml while glioblast cells were killed at 0.005 μg/ml of NCS in vitro (37). Therefore, this method offers the alternative of total body radiation for intraspinal dissemination. Its use for leukemia may be effective (33,34), though only as a third choice.

B.   SMANCS

SMANCS has been most extensively used as SMANCS/Lipiodol, which can be administered arterially or intracavitarilly. The advantages have been described already (9,10,38,41–43). The effectiveness of this method is based on the fact that Lipiodol acts both as the targeting carrier and reservoir of the anticancer agent SMANCS.

The most well-proven clinical efficacy of SMANCS is on primary hepatoma (hepatocellular carcinoma), for which it is administered via the proper hepatic artery, the common hepatic artery, or the celiac artery. The dose and frequency of SMANCS administration differ depending upon the patient. The usual dose for hepatoma is 0.25–1.0 mg (1.0 mg dissolved in 1.0 ml of Lipiodol) per cm^2 of cut surface of tumor image in x-ray CT scan (42,43). The interval may be every 4–6 weeks during the initial 6 months. The results, shown in Table 7, are extraordinary since there is no reliable therapy for this tumor at a very advanced stage. Overall response rate is 90%. Metastatic liver cancer may require more frequent drug administrations, and 2 mg/ml Lipiodol may be preferable. Combination with 5-fluorouracil seems to be more effective.

The result with lung cancer seems to be very good, although the number is too small for generalization (Table 7). Lung cancers are most frequently fed by the bronchial artery, and selective access of a catheter to the bronchial artery is required. Further access of the catheter into the interior of the lobe is not easy.

Table 7 Effect of SMANCS/Lipiodol Given Arterially Against Primary Hepatoma and Lung Cancer

A. Change in tumor size and tumor marker (AFP)[a] in hepatoma (percent of patients)

Change	size[b]	AFP[a]
Reduction		
Total	91.9	91.1
100%	6.0	7.0
100–50%	51.0	52.0
50–30%	31.0	16.0
<30%	12.0	25.0
No change	2.7	1.8
Enlarged	5.4	7.1

B. Change in tumor size in lung cancer given via the bronchial artery[c]

Change in size	No. of cases	%
Reduction		
>70%	10/12	83.3
50–70%	2/12	16.7
Unchanged	0/12	0
Enlarged	0/12	0

[a] Only α-fetoprotein (AFP)–positive patients are applicable. In this study 86% are AFP positive. SMANCS/Lipiodol was administered 2–4 times. Most of patients were inoperable because they were too advanced.
[b] Compared with tumor size before treatment. 100% means complete disappearance.
[c] Caution needs to be taken to avoid affecting the spinal artery with contrast medium (Lipiodol). These patients were stage III or IV.

The branching point to the bronchial artery is occasionally near the spinal artery, which may be vulnerable to the contrast agent Lipiodol, and could result in paralysis if excessive Lipiodol flows in. More details of lipid formulation are described in Ref. 46.

The survival rates of treated patients with hepatoma are shown in Figure 1. When patients have little or no liver cirrhosis (classified as Child's A group) and tumor is confined within one segment of the liver, their survival rate can be 90% even after 5 years, although continued monitoring and treatments may be needed during this period, e.g., intraarterial injection once a year.

Clinical efficacy of the aqueous formulation of SMANCS in human tumors still needs to be established, although preliminary results for lung cancer are known

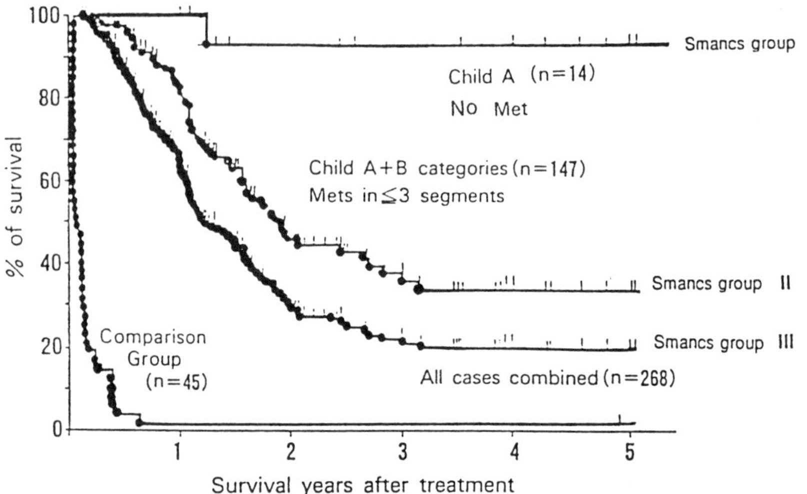

Figure 1 Survival of patients with unresectable hepatocellular carcinoma (primary liver cancer) treated with intraarterial administration of SMANCS/Lipiodol. Child A, hepatoma patients with mild liver cirrhosis; Child B, moderate/intermediate degree of cirrhosis; Child C, severe cirrhosis with jaundice and/or ascites, sometimes dying even without tumor. Intrahepatic spread of tumor or metastasis to other organs resulted in poorer prognosis. Met, metastasis to other segment of the liver.

(56). An important rationale for the high expectation of aqueous SMANCS is that it exhibits a high tumor accumulation, which is explained by EPR effect or by pathophysiological differences in tumor blood vessel and normal vessels (8–10,13,14,57) (Figs. 2 and 3). To enhance this effect further, angiotensin II–induced hypertension chemotherapy during the infusion of SMANCS would be more beneficial, namely, twice the amount of drug delivered to the tumor tissue than without hypertension and a decrease in accumulation in the bone marrow and the intestine (32). This also awaits clinical verification.

C. Side Effects

Despite the remarkable clinical effects of SMANCS/Lipiodol, the side effects are rather mild and easily tolerable (Table 8). This fact may also be attributed to the tumor-selective targeting.

VIII. CONCLUSION

An enediyne-containing protein antitumor agent, NCS is highly active against tumor cells, but its very rapid plasma clearance or short life in vivo in addition

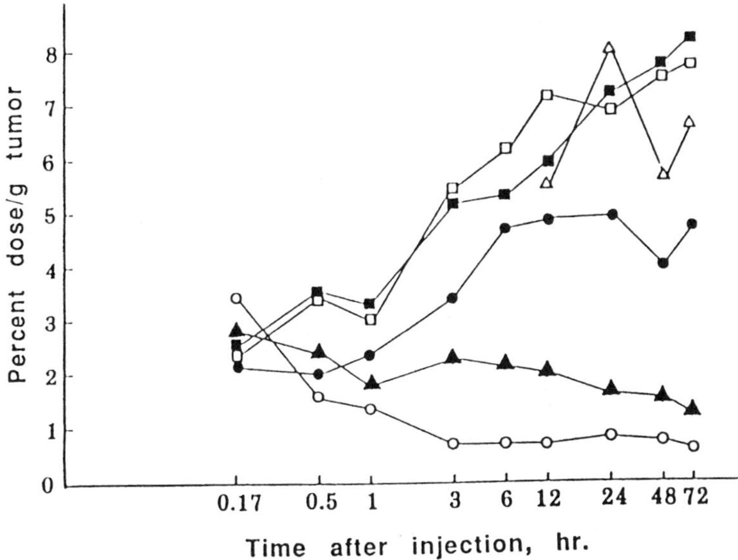

Figure 2 Intratumor accumulation of proteins with different sizes injected intravenously. All proteins were labeled with ^{51}Cr via the chelating agents DTPA (diethylenetriaminepentaacetic acid): □, bovine serum albumin; ■, mouse serum albumin; Δ, mouse IgG; ●, SMANCS; ▲, ovomucoid (29 kDa); and ○, neocarzinostatin (12 kDa). (From Ref. 13.)

to potent myelosuppressive toxicity resulted in its limited use in the clinical setting. Meticulously manipulated clinical skillfulness and dosing regimens will make it more useful against brain tumor or cerebrospinal dissemination of tumor cells. Intravesical use against bladder cancer warrants further exploration. Earlier reports on its effect against leukemia, particularly of myelogenous origin, need to be reevaluated based on pharmacokinetic optimization for better therapeutic effect (36,53).

A second-generation drug of enediyne-containing NCS is SMANCS, which is a conjugate of NCS and a synthetic polymer of styrene-maleic acid (SMA). The clinical effect of SMANCS/Lipiodol for primary hepatoma seems unprecedented due to the extremely high targeting efficiency, deposition, slow release, long-term effect, and potent cytotoxicity to tumor but lack of toxicity to normal tissues. Tumor-image enhancement under x-ray systems is also of great benefit for diagnosis when SMANCS/Lipiodol is used. Its effect on renal cell carcinoma (41,54,55) and lung cancer (41,56) also seems promising, but this needs further research.

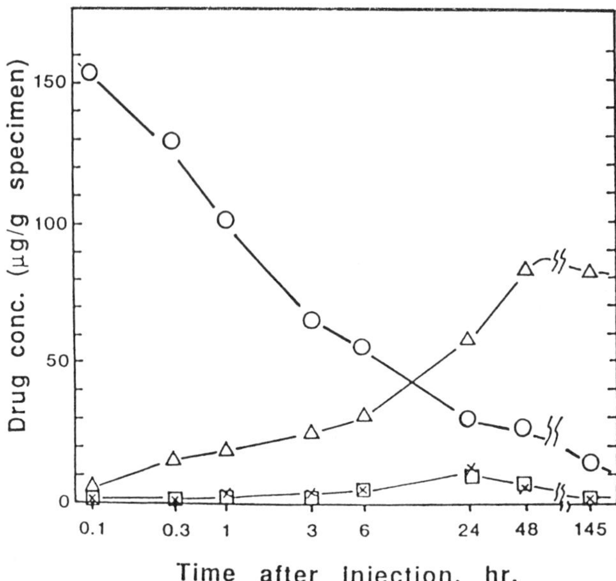

Figure 3 Clearance of Evans blue–albumin complex (a model for macromolecular drug) from blood plasma and its accumulation in the tumor tissue and the normal skin in tumor-bearing mice. Tumor S-180 (5×10^6 cells) was injected into the skin of mice, and after 7 days Evans blue was injected intravenously. The tumor became progressively blue due to the accumulation of Evans blue–albumin complex. The amounts of Evans blue–albumin complex in tissues were quantified after removal and extraction: ○, plasma; □, normal skin; ×, normal muscle; △, tumor. (From Ref. 13.)

Table 8 Side Effects of Arterial Administration of SMANCS/Lipiodol

Effect	Change	No. (%) of patients affected	Duration of effect
Fever	38–39°C	112/233 (48)	Transitory (3–10 days)
Abdominal pain		56/229 (24)	Transitory (<20 min)
Liver function			
GOT value	Elevated	52/204 (25)	Transitory
	Unchanged	130/204 (64)	
	Decreased	21/204 (10)	
GPT value	Elevated	36/204 (18)	Transitory
	Unchanged	143/204 (70)	
	Decreased	25/204 (12)	
White blood cell count	Increased	66/159 (42)	
	Unchanged	65/159 (41)	
	Decreased	28/159 (17)	Transitory

Usual dose about 3–4 mg SMANCS/3–4 ml Lipiodol given via the hepatic artery for hepatoma patients, mostly inoperable. GOT, glutamic-oxaloacetic transaminase; GPT, glutamic-pyruric transaminase.

The optimal drug concentration and viscosity of SMANCS/Lipiodol need to be established for each different tumors; renal cancer needs higher drug concentration and viscosity, whereas cancers of the stomach and lung or colon may require lower viscosity and lower concentrations than for hepatoma. In any event, the best result will require highly skillful catheterization and meticulous consideration of the dosing regimen for these drugs.

Similar to SMANCS, the advantages of hydrophobic polyanhydride conjugate of peptide hormones have been documented by Langer's group in view of their slow release, stability, and improved formulability (58).

REFERENCES

1. H. Maeda, *Anticancer Res., 1,* 175 (1981).
2. S. Sakamoto, J. Ogata, and H. Maeda, *Nishinihon J. Urol., 43,* 223 (1981).
3. T. Ohnuma, C. Nogeire, J. Cuttner, and J. F. Holland, *Cancer, 42,* 1670 (1978).
4. H. Maeda, S. Sakamoto, and J. Ogata, *Antimicrob. Agents Chemother., 22,* 941 (1977).
5. H. Maeda, J. Takeshita, and R. Kanamaru, *Int. J. Peptide Protein Res., 14,* 81 (1979).
6. H. Maeda, M. Ueda, T. Morinaga, and T. Matsumoto, *J. Med. Chem., 29,* 455 (1985).
7. H. Yamamoto, T. Miki, T. Oda, T. Hirano, Y. Sera, M. Akagi, and H. Maeda, *Eur. J. Cancer, 26,* 253 (1990).
8. H. Maeda, T. Matsumoto, T. Konno, K. Iwai, and M. Ueda, *J. Protein Chem., 3,* 181 (1984).
9. H. Maeda, *Adv. Drug Delivery Rev., 6,* 181 (1991).
10. H. Maeda, L. W. Seymour, and Y. Miyamoto, *Bioconjugate Chem., 3,* 351 (1992).
11. R. Duncan, *Anti-Cancer Drugs, 3,* 175 (1992).
12. R. Duncan, L. W. Seymour, K. B. O'Hare, P. A. Flanagan, S. Wedge, I. C. Hume, K. Ubrich, J. Strohalm, V. Subr, F. Spceafico, M. Grandi, M. Ripamonti, M. Faruo, and A. Suarato, *J. Controlled Release, 19,* 331 (1992).
13. Y. Matsumura and H. Maeda, *Cancer Res., 46,* 6387 (1986).
14. H. Maeda, Y. Matsumura, T. Oda, and K. Sasamoto, in *Protein Tailoring for Food and Medical Uses* (R. E. Feeny and J. R. Whitaker, eds.), Marcel Dekker Inc., New York, 1986, p. 353.
15. H. Maeda and J. Takeshita, *J. Antibiotics, 29,* 111 (1976).
16. A. Kobayashi, T. Oda, and H. Maeda, *J. Bioact. Compat. Polym., 3,* 319 (1988).
17. Yamanouchi Pharmaceutical Co. Ltd., Preclinical toxicity data, 1991. Tokyo, Japan.
18. H. Maeda and M. Matsumoto, *Tohoku J. Exp. Med., 128,* 313 (1979).
19. J. Takeshita, H. Maeda, and K. Koike, *J. Biochem., 88,* 1071 (1980).
20. H. Maeda, S. Aikawa, and A. Yamashita, *Cancer Res., 35,* 554 (1975).
21. S. Sakamoto, H. Maeda, and J. Ogata, *Experientia, 35,* 1233 (1979).
22. T. Ebina, K. Ohtsuki, M. Seto, and N. Ishida, *Eur. J. Cancer, 11,* 155 (1975).
23. T. Ebina and N. Ishida, *Cancer Res., 35,* 3705 (1975).
24. H. Lazarus, V. Raso, and T. S. A. Samy, *Cancer Res., 37,* 3731 (1977).

25. T. Ohishi, Y. Yamagata, and S. Udaka, *Agri. Biol. Chem., 43,* 371 (1979).
26. A. Yamashita, Y. Kitawaki, M. Miyamoto, and H. Maeda, *Immunopharmacology, 1,* 255 (1979).
27. S. C. Silverstein, R. M. Steinman, and Z. A. Cohn, *Ann. Rev. Biochem., 46,* 669 (1977).
28. T. Oda and H. Maeda, *Cancer Res., 47,* 3206 (1987).
29. T. Oda, F. Sato, and H. Maeda, *J. Natl. Cancer Inst., 79,* 1205 (1987).
30. S. Sakamoto, J. Ogata, K. Ikegami, and H. Maeda, *Eur. J. Cancer, 16,* 103 (1980).
31. A. Kimoto, T. Konno, T. Kawaguchi, T. Miyauchi, and H. Maeda, *Cancer Res., 52,* 1013 (1992).
32. C. L. Li, Y. Miyamoto, Y. Kojima, and H. Maeda, *Br. J. Cancer, 67,* 975 (1993).
33. K. Kitajima, T. Nagao, I. Takahashi, O. Kamimura, M. Toki, H. Hayashi, P. Chen, T. Naito, K. Niiya, N. Nakanishi, and H. Sanada, *Clin. Rep., 9,* 1864 (1975) (in Japanese).
34. T. Masaoka, H. Nakamura, Y. Hasegawa, H. Shibata, N. Tatsumi, T. Ueda, T. Takubo, J. Yoshitake, N. Senda, K. Kinoshita, M. Miyatake, and T. Tsubakio, *Rinsho Ketsueki, 15,* 1309 (1974) (in Japanese).
35. Y. Matsukado, H. Maeda, S. Uemura, J. Kuratsu, and H. Sonoda, *Gan to Kagakuryoho* [*Cancer and Chemotherapy*], *9,* 1933 (1982).
36. H. Maeda, Y. Sano, J. Takeshita, Z. Iwai, H. Kosaka, T. Marubayashi, and Y. Matsukado, *Cancer Chem. Pharmacol., 5,* 243 (1981).
37. H. Maeda, Y. Matsukado, Z. Iwai, S. Uemura, J. Kuratsu, J. Takeshita, and Y. Sano, *Gan to Kagakuryoho* [*Cancer and Chemotherapy*], *9,* 1040 (1982).
38. T. Konno, H. Maeda, K. Iwai, S. Tashiro, S. Maki, T. Morinaga, M. Mochinaga, T. Hiraoka, and I. Yokoyama, *Eur. J. Cancer Clin. Oncol., 19,* 1053 (1983).
39. K. Iwai, H. Maeda, and T. Konno, *Cancer Res., 44,* 2114 (1984).
40. K. Iwai, H. Maeda, T. Konno, Y. Matsumura, R. Yamashita, K. Yamasaki, S. Hirayama, and Y. Miyauchi, *Anticancer Res., 7,* 321 (1987).
41. T. Konno, H. Maeda, K. Iwai, S. Maki, S., Tashiro, M. Uchida, and Y. Miyauchi, *Cancer, 54,* 2367 (1984).
42. S. Maki, T. Konno, and H. Maeda, *Cancer, 56,* 751 (1985).
43. T. Konno and H. Maeda, in *Neoplasm of the Liver* (K. Okuda and K. G. Ishak, ed.), Springer-Verlag, New York, 1987, p. 343.
44. M. Kimura, T. Konno, T. Oda, H. Maeda, and Y. Miyauchi, *Anticancer Res. 13,* 1287 (1993).
45. T. Oda, F. Sato, H. Yamamoto, M. Akagi, and H. Maeda, *Anticancer Res., 9,* 261 (1987).
46. H. Maeda and Y. Miyamoto, in *Drug Absorption Enhancement* (A. G. de Boer, ed.), Harwood Academic Pub., Switzerland (in press).
47. S. Hirayama, F. Sato, T. Oda, and H. Maeda, *Jpn. J. Antibiotics, 39,* 818 (1986) (in Japanese).
48. H. Maeda, J. Takeshita, R. Kanamaru, H. Sato, J. Katoh, and H. Sato, *Gann, 70,* 601 (1979).
49. N. Ishida, K. Miyazaki, K. Kumagai, and M. Rikimaru, *J. Antibiotics* (Ser. A), *18,* 68 (1965).
50. W. Bradner and D. Hutchison, *Cancer Chem. Rep., 50,* 79 (1966).

51. G. Kallistratos and E. Fasske, *Folia Biochim. Biologica Graeca, 15,* 1 (1978).
52. H. Maeda, H. Ichimura, H. Satoh, and K. Ohtsuki, *J. Antibiotics, 31,* 468 (1978).
53. H. Maeda, J. Takeshita, Z. Iwai, Y. Yamanami, and S. Sakamoto, *Gan to Kagakuryoho* [*Cancer and Chemotherapy*], *6,* 96 (1979). (*in Japanese*)
54. M. Kobayashi, H. Maeda, K. Iwai, T. Konno, S. Sugihara, and H. Yamanaka, *Urology, 37,* 288 (1991).
55. S. Noda, S. Konno, J. Tanaka, M. Yamada, and N. Yoshitake, *Anticancer Res., 10,* 709 (1990).
56. H. Maeda, *J. Controlled Release, 19,* 315 (1992).
57. H. Maeda and Y. Matsumura, *Critical Rev. Ther. Drug Carrier Systems, 6,* 193 (1989).
58. E. Ron, T. Turek, E. Mathiowitz, M. Chasin, M. Hageman, and R. Langer, *Proc. Natl. Acad. Sci., 90,* 4176 (1993).

18

Synthetic Studies of the Enediyne Antiobiotics

Randall L. Halcomb
University of Colorado, Boulder, Colorado

I. INTRODUCTION

Occasionally a novel class of naturally occurring compounds is discovered which initiates an evaluation of both the capabilities and the limits of technology for contemporary organic synthesis. One such class of compounds is comprised of the extremely potent enediyne antitumor antibiotics. The highly unusual structures of these compounds present many exciting challenges to synthetic chemists and, as a result, a starburst of research activity has followed their disclosure. Furthermore, the remarkable potency and unusual mechanism of action of these drugs should provide valuable insights into the design of new therapeutic and medicinal agents.

In 1987, workers at the Bristol-Myers company and at Lederle Laboratories simultaneously reported the chemical structures of esperamicin A_{1a} [1] (1) and calicheamicin γ_1^I [2] (2), respectively (Fig. 1). The esperamicins and calicheamicins contain many common features, including a highly unsaturated aglycone sector and a carbohydrate domain. The aglycone sectors of these compounds are identical except for the oxidation state of the sp^3 carbon α to the ketone, and both contain many unique structural elements including a 3-ene-1,5-diyne fragment, a bridgehead olefin conjugated to a ketone, and an allylic methyl trisulfide.

The carbohydrate domains are no less complex. The two compounds contain a common trisaccharide core, which features a novel *O*-glycosylhydroxylamine

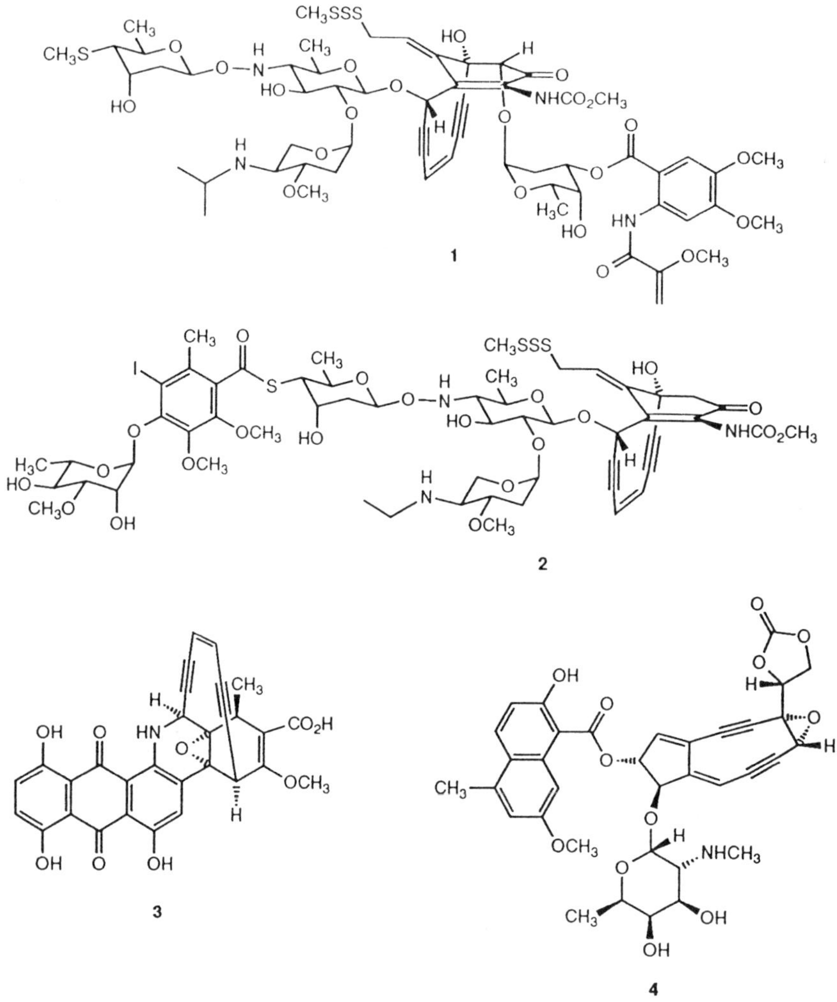

Figure 1 Structures of the enediyne antibiotics esperamicin A_{1a} (**1**), calicheamicin γ_1^I (**2**), dynemicin (**3**), and neocarzinostatin chromophore (**4**).

linkage, as well as an unusual 2,4,6-trideoxy-4-thio-allose subunit. The carbohydrate domains differ at two points. First, the secondary amine function of esperamicin bears an isopropyl group, while that of calicheamicin contains an ethyl moiety. Second, the sulfur of the thiosugar of esperamicin is "capped" by a methyl group, whereas that of calicheamicin is acylated with a hexasubstituted benzoic acid. This aromatic unit itself bears an α-L-mannosyloxy substituent *para* to the thiobenzoate linkage.

The structure of dynemicin A [3], which shares the same 3-ene-1,5-diyne unit with esperamicin and calicheamicin, was disclosed in 1989 (3). Other than the enediyne unit, dynemicin is structurally quite different from 1 and 2. The enediyne is fused onto an anthraquinone-containing pentacyclic nucleus, which itself displays a methyl group *syn* to the enediyne bridge as well as a fully substituted benzylic epoxide.

A related compound, the neocarzinostatin chromophore, 4, was isolated in 1979 (4a), however, the exact chemical structure remained unknown until more recently (4b,c). This chromophore contains a highly functionalized carbon skeleton, similar to those described earlier, which bears L-galactosamine and naphthoyl appendages. The kedarcidin chromophore, which contains a related core skeleton, was subsequently isolated (5).

Since their discovery, the enediynes have been the subject of a wide range of creative synthetic efforts by many research groups. From these studies, a wealth of information concerning the chemistry of the natural products has been obtained. Despite these efforts, these compounds have only recently begun to yield to total synthesis. Presented below is a review of the recent studies directed toward the synthesis of this group of compounds (for review, see Ref. 6).

II. CALICHEAMICIN/ESPERAMICIN AGLYCONE

It is believed that the cytotoxicity of esperamicin and calicheamicin is derived from their known ability to cleave double stranded DNA (7). The cascade of events that results in DNA damage is initiated by bioreductive cleavage of the trisulfide functionality to an allylic thiolate 5 (Scheme I) (8). This thiolate is poised to add

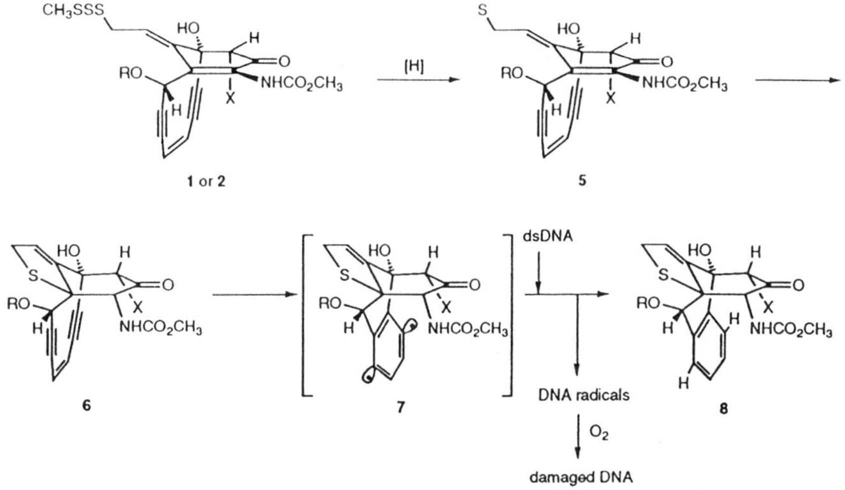

Scheme I Mechanism of DNA Cleavage by Esperamicin and Calicheamicin.

in a conjugate sense to the bridgehead enone to generate the intermediate **6**. The change in hybridization of the bridgehead carbon from sp^2 to sp^3 brings the termini of the enediyne closer together, allowing a Bergman-type (9) cycloaromatization to occur to produce the 1,4 diradical species **7**. This diradical abstracts hydrogen atoms from the carbohydrate backbone of DNA, resulting in DNA strand scission (10).

A. Methods for Introducing the Enediyne Ring and the Bridgehead Olefin

One of the most synthetically challenging aspects of the calicheamicin and esperamicin aglycones is the highly unsaturated [7.3.1] bicyclic ring system. Several strategies have been employed to introduce the enediyne bridge and the bridgehead olefin into the system, the major points of which will be detailed below (for syntheses of other related enediyne models, see Ref. 11).

Several simple cyclic enediynes were synthesized, as illustrated in Scheme II, by Nicolaou and coworkers (12). The Ramberg-Bäcklund reaction (13) of α-chlorosulfones was used to install an olefin between the two acetylenes. The stability of these enediynes as a function of ring size was subsequently evaluated. A notable example is compound **10h**, which was shown to cause double-stranded DNA cleavage (14). A similar compound, diol **10**, was synthesized using an intramolecular pinacol coupling of the corresponding dialdehyde (15).

Another method for the synthesis of cyclic enediynes, which is based on a reductive elimination, was developed by Semmelhack and coworkers (16). The cyclic diynes **14a–b**, synthesized according to Scheme III, were converted into the thionocarbonates **15a–b**. Treatment with Ni(0) effected reduction and elimination, producing the enediynes **16a–b**.

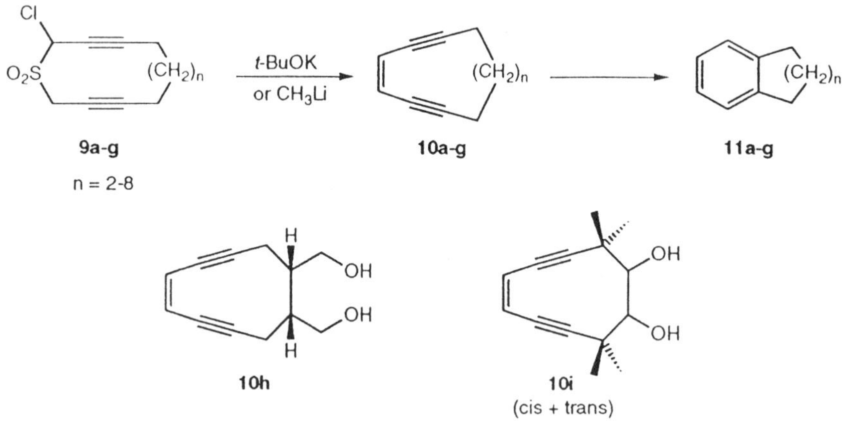

Scheme II Simple Cyclic Enediynes Synthesized by Nicolaou and coworkers (12–15).

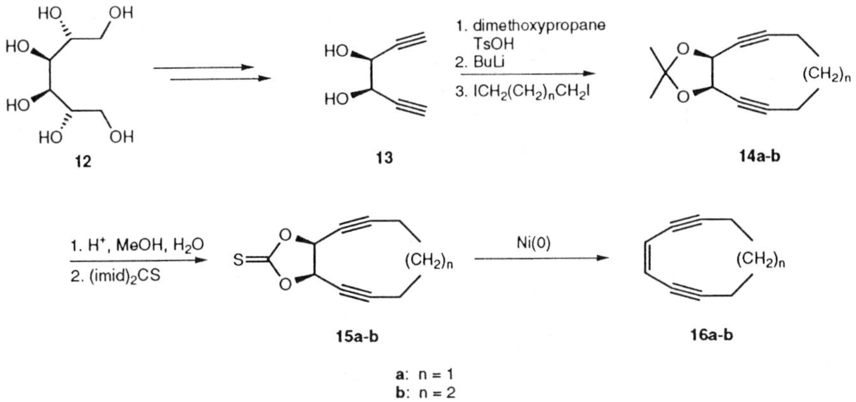

Scheme III drawing.

a: n = 1
b: n = 2

Scheme III Semmelhack's Method for Preparing Cyclic Enediynes (**16**).

Magnus and coworkers have utilized a cyclization onto a proparglyic cation equivalent, specifically a cobalt complex such as **22**, as an entry into the ring system (Scheme IV) (17). The cyclization precursor was synthesized from compound **17**, the adduct of lithium acetylide and cyclohexane-1,4-dione monoketal. A Castro-Stephans coupling (18) between the acetylene **17** and *cis*-dichloroethylene generated, after silylation, compound **19**. Following ketal cleavage, the second acetylene moiety was installed by a coupling with methyl 2-propynyl ether (**20**) under the same Pd⁰-catalyzed conditions. Chemoselective acetylene complexation of **21** with $Co_2(CO)_8$, followed by enol ether formation, produced the cobalt com-

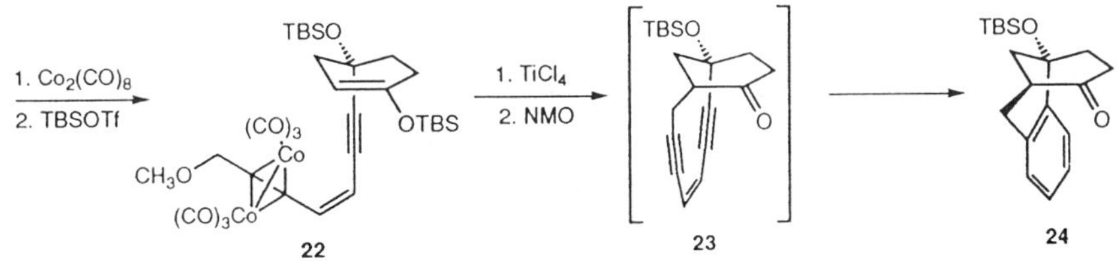

Scheme IV Use of a Propargyl Cation in the Synthesis of a Calicheamicin Model (Magnus and coworkers) (17).

plex **22**. The cyclization step was carried out under Lewis acid catalysis, and subsequent decomplexation presumably produced compound **23**, whose lability prevented isolation or characterization. This compound underwent spontaneous cycloaromatization to yield compound **24**.

This group subsequently found that the spontaneous Bergman cyclization could be suppressed by positioning a ketone at the one-carbon bridge (19). The acyclic enediyne precursor to such a compound, **29**, was synthesized from the enone **25** as shown in Scheme V using chemistry similar to that described earlier (see Scheme IV). Chemoselective complexation of the distal acetylene, Lewis acid–mediated cyclization, and decomplexation afforded compound **31**, which was relatively stable at room temperature. The bridgehead olefin could conveniently be installed from compound **31** (Scheme VI) (19). Enolization and subsequent α-selenation and oxidative elimination produced compound **33**. Alternatively, treatment of **32** with SeO_2 installed the bridgehead double bond and produced the hemiketal **34** (20). More forcing conditions effected further oxidation and afforded compound **35**. Michael addition of phenols to the enone of **33** served to trigger aromatization, thus providing **37** (Scheme VII) (21).

The same cyclization methodology, when implemented on a more highly oxidized substrate, allowed incorporation of the propargylic alcohol (Scheme VIII)

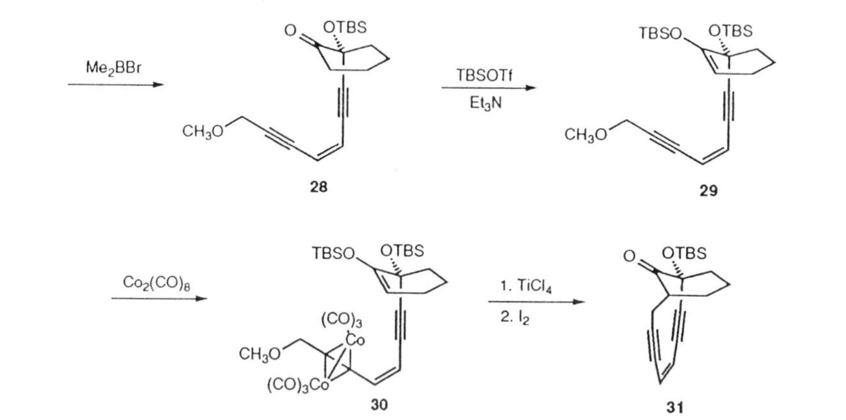

Scheme V   Synthesis of a Calicheamicin Model (Magnus and coworkers) (19).

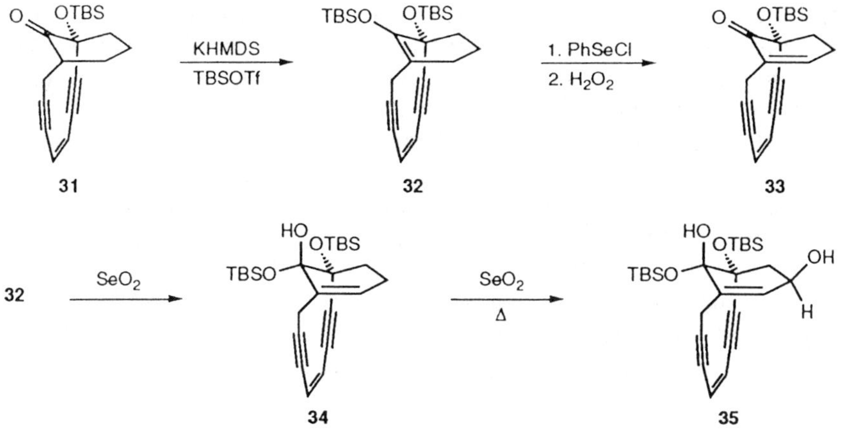

Scheme VI Introduction of a Bridgehead Olefin into the Calicheamicin Ring System (Magnus and coworkers) (19–20).

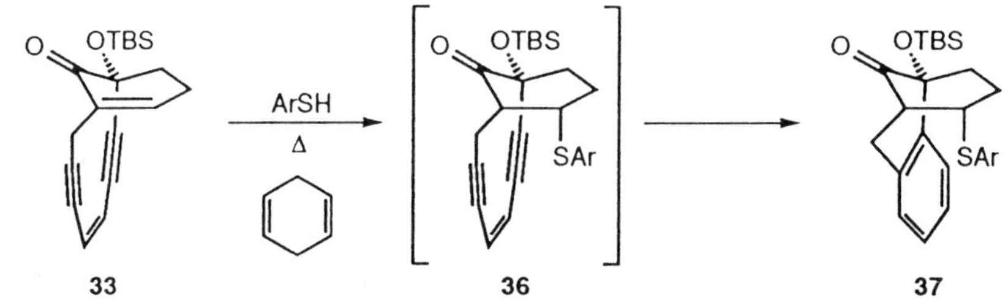

Scheme VII Activation of Model **33** by Thiols (21).

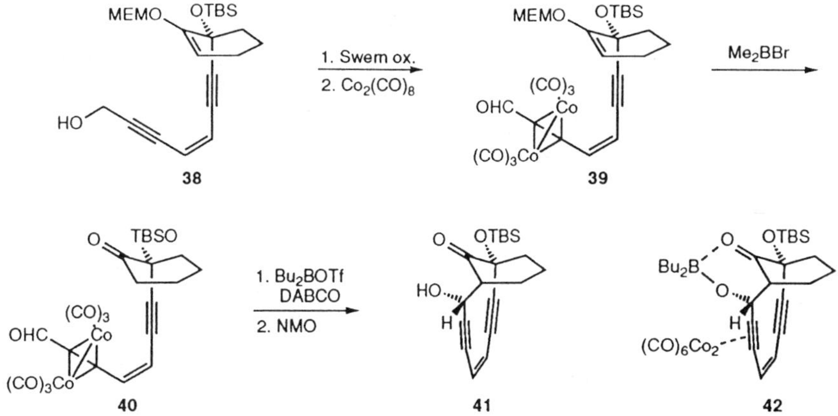

Scheme VIII Synthesis of a Calicheamicin Model via Intramolecular Aldol Reaction (22).

(22). The acyclic enediyne precursor **38** was synthesized analogously to compound **27**. Swern oxidation of **38** followed by complexation gave the dicobalt cluster **39**, and subsequent ketone deprotection provided **40**. Treatment of **40** with di-*n*-butylboron triflate followed by a decomplexing agent selectively produced compound **41**, which possessed the desired configuration at the propargylic alcohol center. The stereochemical outcome of this reaction is presumably due to the intermediacy of a chelated complex between the boron of the enolate and the aldehyde oxygen. This complex serves to direct a synclinal attack of the enolate onto the aldehyde to generate **41** via the intermediate **42** (22).

Kadow and coworkers have employed a similar strategy to incorporate both the proparglyic alcohol and the bridgehead olefin (23). Acetylide anion **46** was added to the ketone **45**, prepared as shown in Scheme IX, to provide **47**. Ther-

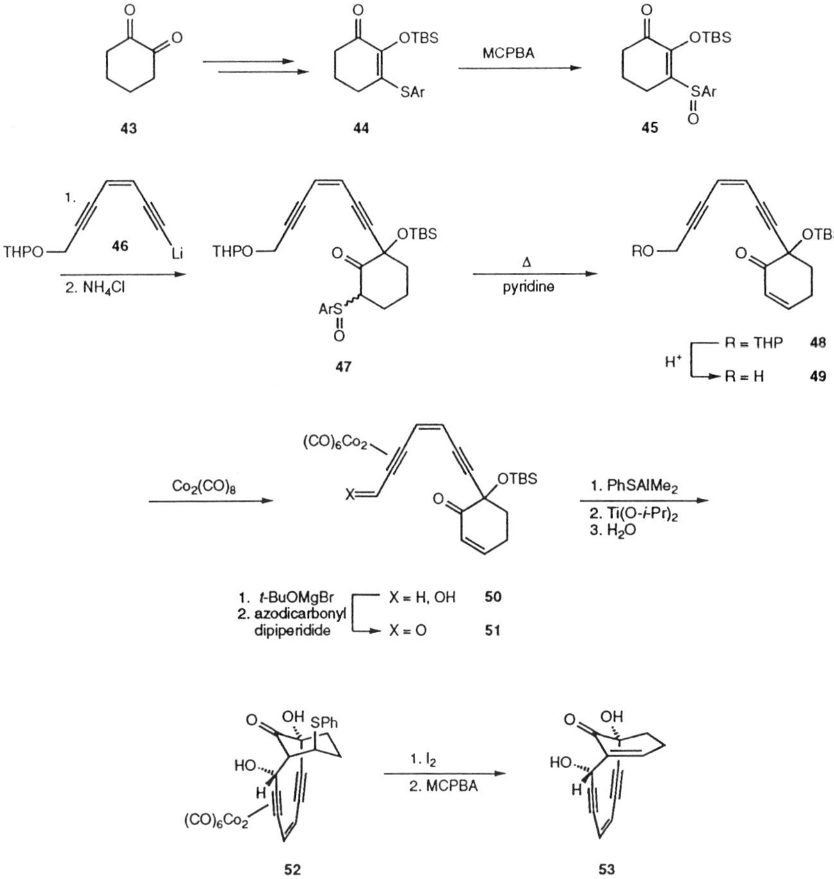

Scheme IX   Kadow's Route to an Esperamicin Model System (23).

mal elimination of the sulfoxide followed by removal of the THP group, complexation with cobalt, and oxidation gave aldehyde **51**. Conjugate addition of benzene thiolate to the enone and a subsequent in situ intramolecular aldol condensation of the intermediate enolate afforded **52**. Finally, removal of the cobalt complex with I_2 followed by oxidation of the corresponding sulfoxide and elimination gave **53**.

Syntheses of the [7.3.1] ring system based on acetylide cyclizations have been developed by two research groups. The concept behind the first, that of Danishefsky, is the addition of the dianion of hex-3-ene-1,5-diyne [**58**] (24) to a bis-electrophile (Scheme X) (25,26). The bis-electrophiles employed were ketoaldehydes such as **56**, which were generated from aromatic precursors. A key transformation in this endeavor was a Becker-Adler oxidation (27) of the phenol **54** with sodium periodate to afford the spiroepoxide **55**. In practice, it was found that a two-step procedure provided the most favorable results for the enediyne ring annulation. This entailed an initial addition of the enediyne dianion to the ketone functionality, with the cyclization onto the aldehyde effected in a separate step. The preference for chemoselective addition to the aldehyde rather than the ketone was overcome by utilizing an in situ protection of the aldehyde functionality according to the protocol of Comins (28). Treatment of **56** with lithium *N*-methylanilide resulted in addition of the amide to the aldehyde and generated the tetrahedral C-oxide-C-amino species **57**. Addition of dilithioenediyne **58** to this "protected" compound resulted in nucleophilic attack only at the ketone center. Upon quenching, the aldehyde functionality was liberated and the unstable compound **59** was isolated and subsequently silylated. The principal isomer observed was that derived from addition of the nucleophile to the face of the ketone *syn*

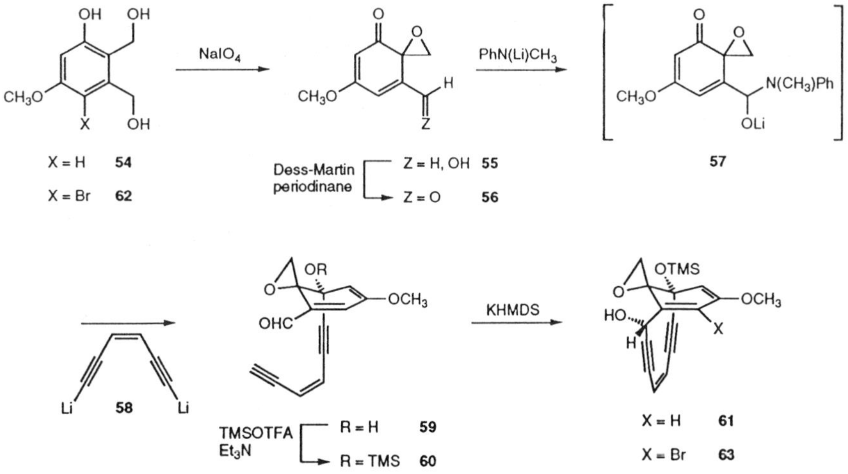

Scheme X   Danishefsky's Route to the Calicheamicin Ring System (24–26).

to the epoxide oxygen. Deprotonation of the acetylene moiety of **60** led to stereoselective anionic cyclization onto the aldehyde to generate compound **61**. The configuration of the proparglyic alcohol resulted from addition of the acetylide to the preferred *s-trans* rotamer of the enal. The spiroepoxide at the one-carbon bridge proved to be quite robust during these manipulations and effectively served to mask the functionality that was later elaborated into the allylic trisulfide (see below).

In an analogous sequence, compound **63** was synthesized from the aromatic precursor **62** (25). Compound **63** possesses a bromine to allow the introduction of the required urethane functionality and was eventually employed as an intermediate in a total synthesis of calicheamicinone (see below).

The second route based on this concept, illustrated in Scheme XI, was developed by Kende and coworkers and incorporated a similar cyclization onto an enal (29). Standard manipulations were used to transform cyclohexadiene **64** into the acetylene **66** via aldehyde **65**. Addition of a vinyl Grignard reagent to **66** followed by acidic hydrolysis yielded compound **67**, which was converted into the alcohol **68**. The remaining carbons of the enediyne unit were attached using a Castro-Stephans coupling with the chloroeneyne **69**. Deprotonation of the acetylene of

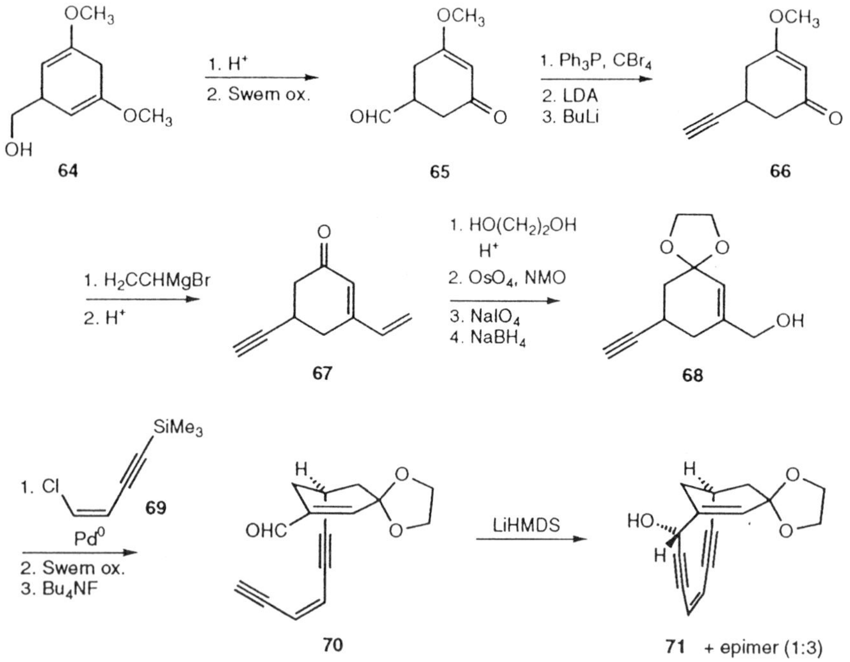

Scheme XI Kende's Approach to the Calicheamicin System (29).

70 with LiN(SiMe$_3$)$_2$ effected cyclization onto the aldehyde and provided the carbinol **71** as the minor isomer in a 1:3 mixture of epimers. The major reactive rotamer of the enal in this instance appeared to be the *s-cis*.

A conceptually different approach was undertaken by Schreiber and coworkers in which, rather than annulating the enediyne bridge onto a cyclohexane-type precursor, both rings were assembled in a single transformation, specifically an intramolecular Diels-Alder reaction (Scheme XII) (30). The substrate for the Diels-Alder reaction, **78**, was assembled from *cis*-dichloroethylene. Sequential palladium-catalyzed coupling of **18** with the two alkynes **72** and **73** produced the enediyne **74**, which was converted to the cycloaddition precursor **78**. Heating a solution of **78** in benzene selectively afforded the *para* adduct **79** rather than the desired *meta* adduct **80** (30b). Based on this observation, a *para*-type product similar to **79**, which could be rearranged to provide a formal *meta*-type cycloaddition adduct, was synthesized, thereby opening a route to the calicheamicin ring system.

The mesylate **85** (Scheme XIII) was an appropriate substrate for such a rearrangement (31). The acyclic precursor to this ring system was synthesized from compound **81**, obtained in a similar fashion to **76**. Coupling of **81** to the bromocarbonate **82** yielded the Diels-Alder substrate **83**, which was thermally cyclized to produce the [7.2.2] adduct **84**. Compound **84** was converted to the mesylate **85**, which, upon exposure to diethylaluminum chloride, underwent a pinacol rearrangement and subsequent diastereoselective acyloin shift to provide compound **87**, apparently through the intermediate **86**. The product possesses the same relative stereochemistry at the newly formed carbinol center as is found in the esperamicin aglycone.

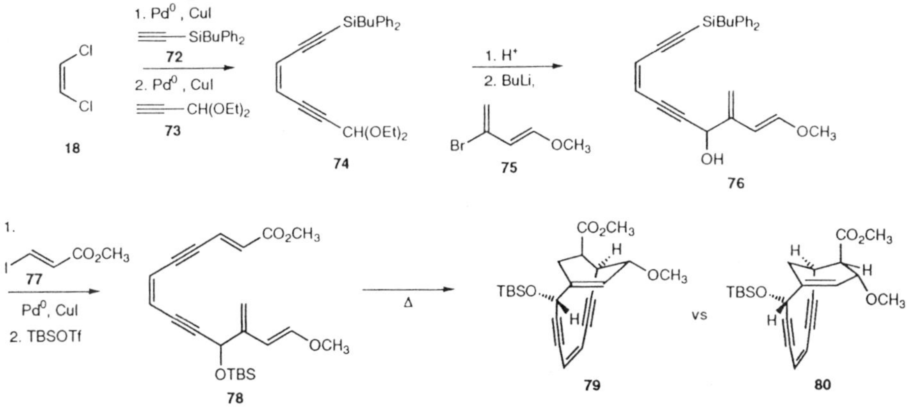

Scheme XII Intramolecular Diels-Alder Approach to the Calicheamicin Ring System (Schreiber and coworkers) (30).

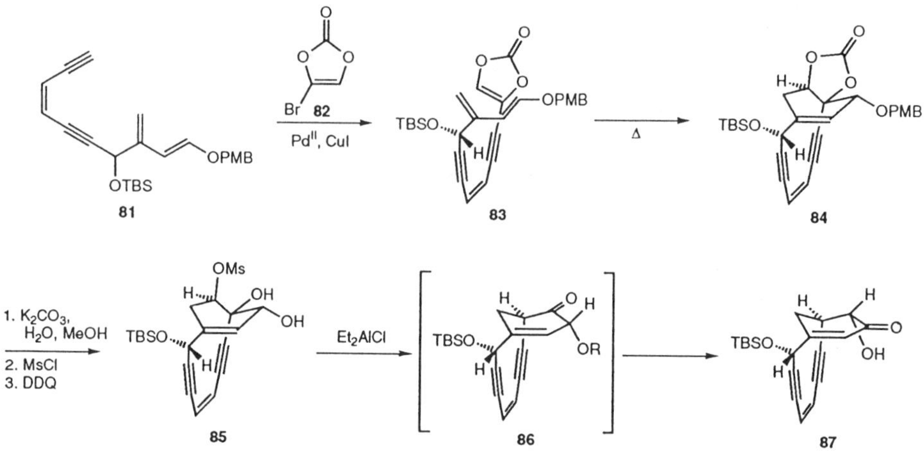

Scheme XIII   Schreiber's Second Generation Approach to the Esperamicin Ring System (31).

B.   Synthesis of Trisulfide-Containing Systems and Models for the Biomechanism

The first example of the installation of an allylic trisulfide into the calicheamicin-type ring system was accomplished by Magnus and coworkers (32). Treatment of the previously described enone **33** with the Emmons reagent **88** gave compound **89** (Scheme XIV). None of the compound having the alternate olefin geometry was observed. The cyano group was reduced to the allylic alcohol **90**, which was, in turn, converted into the thioacetate **92**. The acetate was reductively removed and the intermediate thiol was treated with the known disulfide reagent **93** to give the allylic trisulfide **94**.

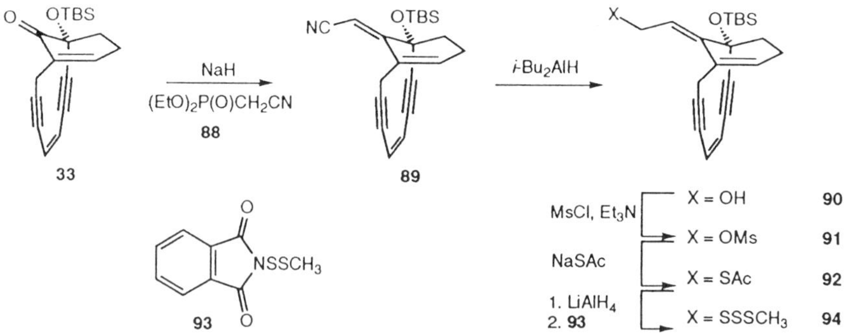

Scheme XIV   First Installation of the Allylic Trisulfide (Magnus and coworkers) (32).

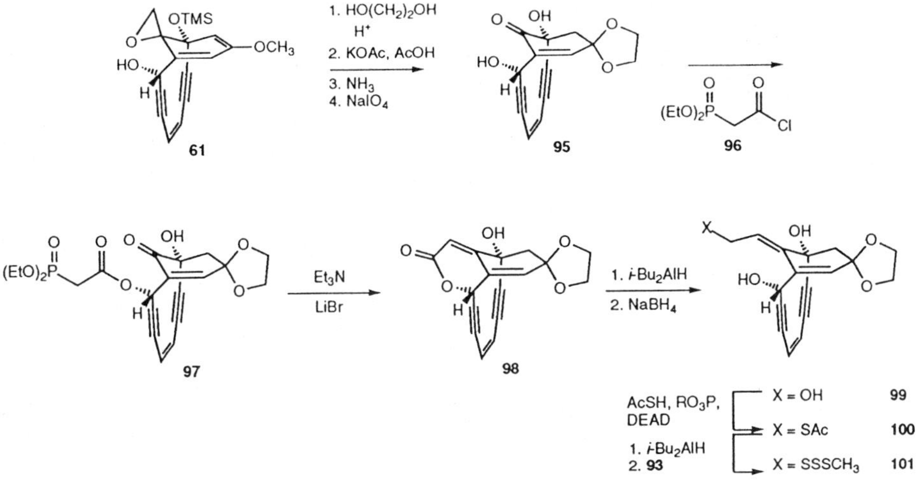

Scheme XV Danishefsky's Method for Installing the Allylic Trisulfide (33).

A somewhat different method of setting the olefin geometry was implemented by Danishefsky and coworkers (Scheme XV) (33). This plan involved installing the two carbons at the bridge with an intramolecular Emmons reaction and making use of the proparglyic alcohol to control the olefin geometry. The substrate for such a reaction, **95**, was synthesized from the previously described epoxide **61**. Acylation of the proparglyic alcohol with the acid chloride **96** provided **97**, which was cyclized with base to provide the lactone **98**. This lactone was reductively opened to give the allylic alcohol **99**, which was converted to the thioacetate **100** using a Mitsunobu reaction with thioacetic acid. The trisulfide was introduced, using a method similar to that of Magnus, by reductive deacylation followed by treatment of the resulting thiol with **93** to afford **101**.

Several model systems that mimic the mechanism of action of the natural products were synthesized by the Danishefsky group from intermediates in this sequence. Compound **102** was synthesized as shown in Scheme XVI and was shown to undergo a Bergman cyclization and to effect DNA damage upon activation with

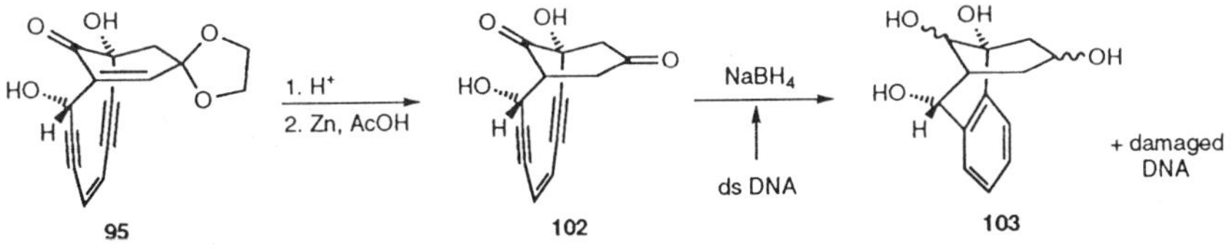

Scheme XVI DNA Cleavage by Model Enediynes (Danishefsky and coworkers) (34).

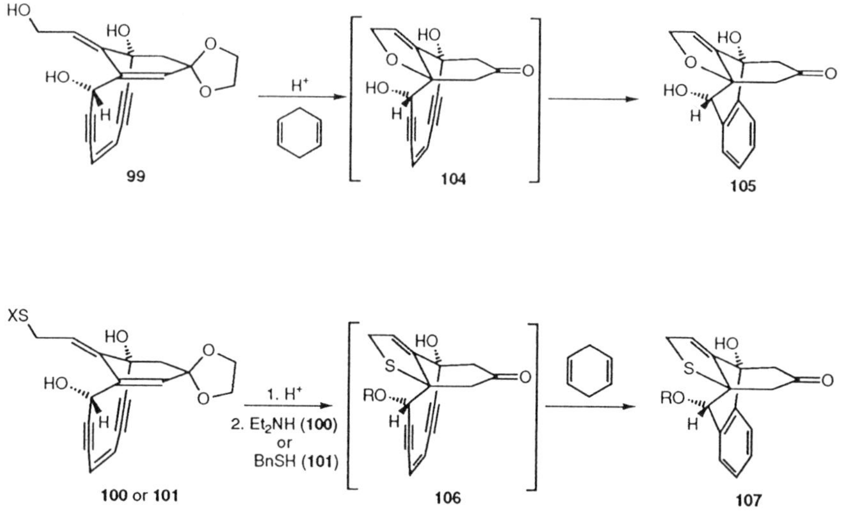

Scheme XVII First Demonstration of the Activation of Model Enediynes by Intramolecular Michael Additions (Danishefsky and coworkers) (33,35).

sodium borohydride (34). Additionally, it was shown that an alcohol as well as a thiol could add intramolecularly to the bridgehead enone of calicheamicin-type systems and thus trigger cycloaromatization (Scheme XVII) (33,35).

C. Total Syntheses of Calicheamicinone

The first total synthesis of the calicheamicin aglycone was recorded by Danishefsky (Scheme XVIII) (25,36). The synthesis proceeded from the bromide **63** (see above) and utilized the chemistry developed in the synthesis of the descarbamoyl compound **101**. Compound **63** was ketalized with ethylene glycol, and the epoxide was solvolyzed with acetic acid/potassium acetate to give compound **108**. Acetate removal and periodate cleavage, as before, provided the ketone **109**. The β-bromoenone was used to incorporate the necessary nitrogen functionality through a 1,4-addition/elimination sequence with sodium azide. Compound **110** thus produced was then acylated with the Emmons reagent **96** and subsequently treated with base to afford the lactone **111**. Reduction of the azide functionality with hydrogen sulfide produced the corresponding vinylamine which was then converted into the methyl carbamate **112**. Reductive opening of the lactone gave the allylic alcohol **113**, which was transformed into compound **115** following the protocol described earlier. Acid-catalyzed deketalization then provided racemic calicheamicinone **116**.

Routes to enantiomerically pure calicheamicinone and descarbamoyl-calicheamicinone have also been developed by Danishefsky and coworkers

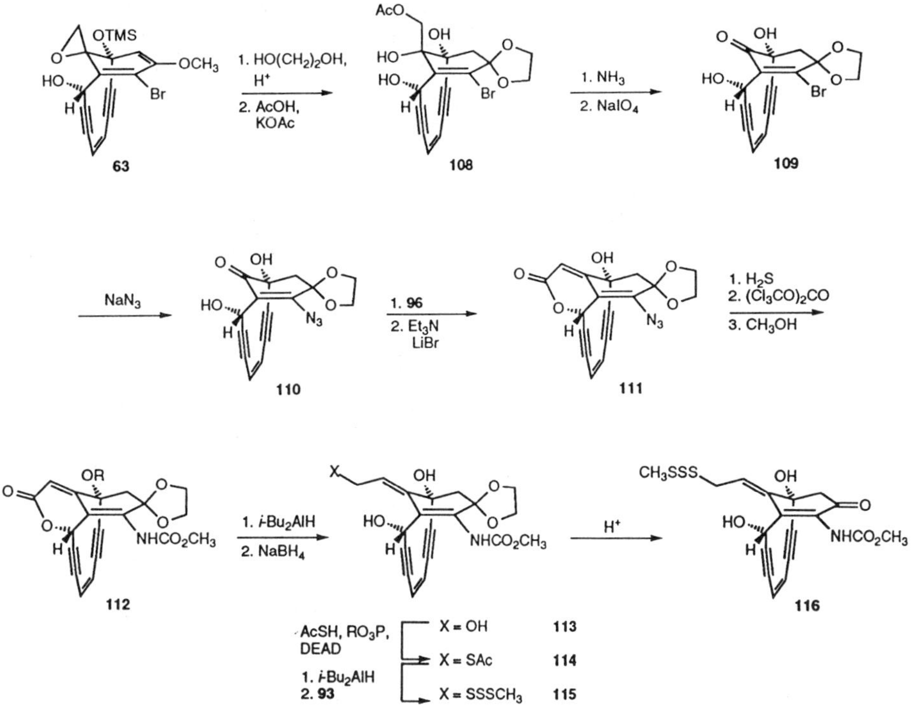

Scheme XVIII The First Synthesis of Calicheamicinone by Danishefsky and coworkers (25,36).

(Scheme XIX) (37). Asymmetry was established in the desbromo series using an enantioselective reduction of the ketone **117** to the alcohol **118**, whose conversion into the spiroepoxide **119** involved a stereospecific Becker-Adler oxidation (37a). Addition of dilithioenediyne gave compound **120**, which was subsequently elaborated into the enantiomerically pure ketone (+)-**95**. This allowed for correlation with racemic material. Although this strategy was unsuccessful in the bromo series, a resolution of the racemic intermediate **121** with *Pseudomonas* lipase PS-30, as shown in Scheme XIX, allowed for the practical, preparative-scale synthesis of both enantiomers of the synthetic intermediate **121** (37b).

An asymmetric synthesis of (-)-calicheamicinone has been achieved by Nicolaou and coworkers (38). An addition of an optically pure allylborane reagent to the tetronic acid derivative **122** (Scheme XX) was used to establish asymmetry, thus affording **123** in high optical purity. Compound **123** was converted into the oxime **124**, which, when oxidized to the corresponding nitrile oxide, underwent an intramolecular [2+3] cycloaddition to provide **125**. Conversion to the ketone **126** followed by stereoselective acetylide addition gave **127**. Removal of the MEM

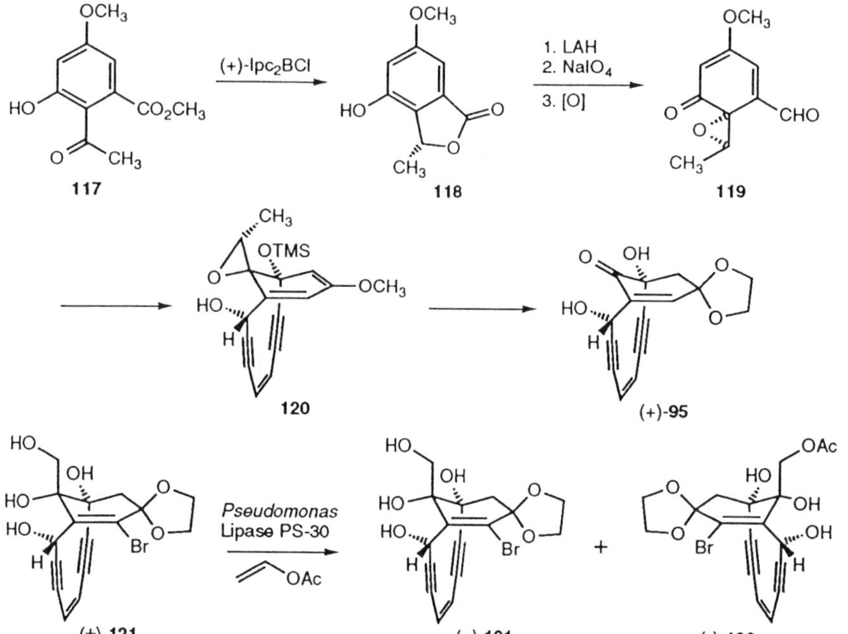

Scheme XIX Danishefsky's Route to Enantiomerically Pure Calicheamicinone (37).

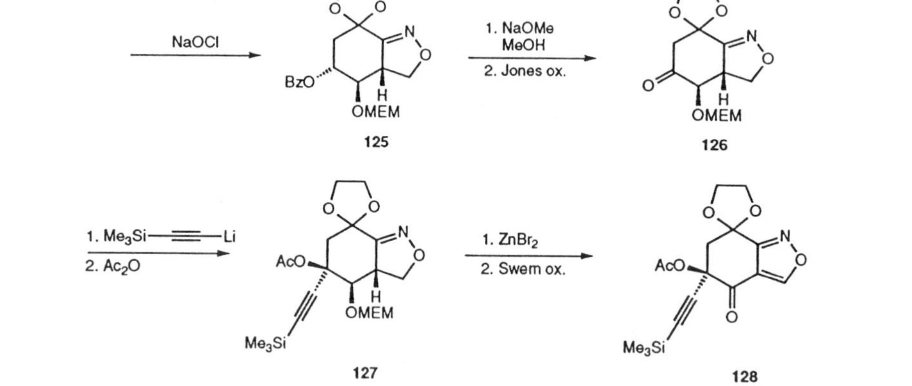

Scheme XX Nicolaou's Synthesis of (-)-Calicheamicinone (38).

blocking group and Swern oxidation provided the keto-isoxazole **128**. The formation of **128** apparently involved an in situ aerial oxidation subsequent to the Swern reaction.

The two precursor carbons to the allylic trisulfide were then introduced by a Horner-Emmons–type reaction (Scheme XXI), providing **129** as a single geometrical isomer. Compound **129** was converted into **131** after removing the C-silyl protecting group and coupling to **69**. The isoxazole moiety was reductively cleaved to give the vinylogous formamide **132**, which, after manipulation of protecting groups, was cyclized to compound **134** under basic conditions. Compound **134** possesses the incorrect stereochemistry at the secondary proparglyic alcohol cen-

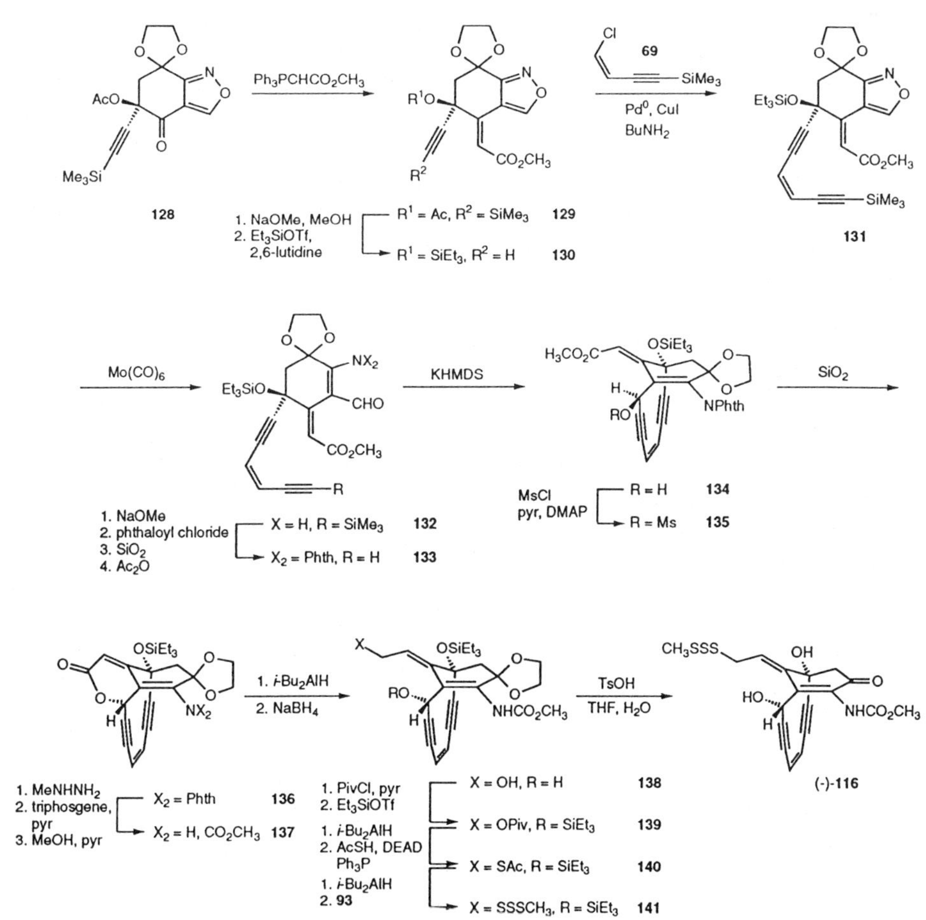

Scheme XXI   Nicolaou's Synthesis of (-)-Calicheamicinone (continued) (38).

ter, however, this was accounted for in the subsequent transformations. Compound **134** was converted into the mesylate **135**, which, when exposed to silica gel, underwent an intramolecular cyclization to give the lactone **136**. After introduction of the carbamate functionality, reductive opening of the lactone according to the Danishefsky protocol (25) provided **138**. Installation of the trisulfide moiety, and removal of the protecting groups gave (-)-calicheamicinone, (-)-**116**.

III. ESPERAMICIN/CALICHEAMICIN OLIGOSACCHARIDE DOMAINS

A growing body of evidence exists that indicates that the oligosaccharide domains of esperamicin and, particularly, calicheamicin play an important role in DNA binding prior to cleavage (7b,39). Not surprisingly, these sugar domains have become attractive targets for synthesis. The unusual hydroxylamine linkage and the previously unknown thiosugar residue are the most daunting obstacles and have been the focus of most synthetic efforts in this area.

The first synthesis of the calicheamicin aryl-tetrasaccharide fragment **142** (Fig. 2) was reported by Nicolaou and coworkers (40). This synthesis employed an interesting [3,3] sigmatropic rearrangement of a thioimidazolide to install the B-ring sulfur functionality and a reduction of an oxime to establish the hydroxylamine linkage (see below). The remaining glycosidic linkages were constructed using glycosyl fluorides.

The E-ring amino sugar (for other syntheses see Ref. 41) was synthesized from the L-serine derivative **143** (Scheme XXII) (42). The remaining carbons were introduced by reaction with an allyldi-(-)-isopinocampheylborane reagent to provide **144**. Compound **144** was further elaborated to the glycosyl fluoride **146**, which was coupled to the fucose-derived alcohol **147** under standard Mukaiyama-type conditions (Scheme XXIII) (43). The product disaccharide **148** was subsequently converted to compound **149**, the ketone component of the desired oxime intermediate.

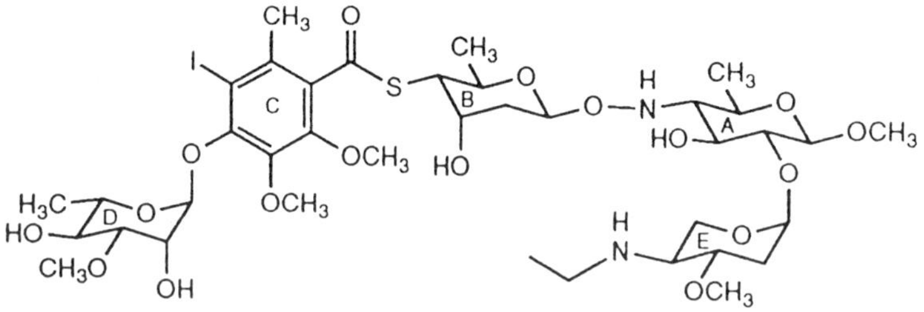

Figure 2 Structure of the aryl-tetrasaccharide of calicheamicin γ_1^I. Letters A-E refer to the numbering scheme of the individual residues.

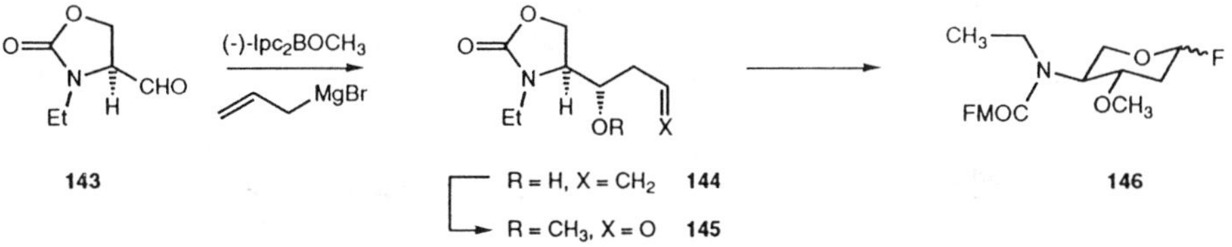

Scheme XXII Nicolaou's Synthesis of the Aminosugar of Calicheamicin (42).

The second component for oxime formation, the *O*-glycosylhydroxylamine **155**, was synthesized as shown in Scheme XXIV from the differentially protected fucal **150** (43). Notable transformations include a stereoselective reduction of **152**, with concomitant benzoyl migration and anomerization, to provide **153** and a subsequent Mitsunobu reaction at the anomeric center with *N*-hydroxyphthalimide to introduce the protected hydroxylamine functionality in the desired β configuration.

The C-D aryl glycoside subunit was synthesized from the thioglycoside **156** (Scheme XXV) (42). Compound **156** was converted, following standard protocols, to the glycosyl fluoride **157**, which was used to glycosolate the phenol **158** (44) and provide the aryl glycoside **159**. Compound **159** was further elaborated to the acyl chloride **160**.

The aryl tetrasaccharide was assembled from the three building blocks **149**, **155**, and **160** in the following manner (Scheme XXVI). The *O*-glycosylhydroxylamine **155** and the ketone **149** were condensed to provide the oxime **161**, which was converted into the thiomidazolide **163**. A thermally induced [3,3] sigmatropic rearrangement of the allylic thioimidazolide installed the sulfur in the desired configuration and provided **164**, which was elaborated to **165**.

The thiol **165** was acylated with the acid chloride **160** to give the thiolester **166** (Scheme XXVII). The silyl enol ether was cleaved and the resulting ketone was stereoselectively reduced with K-Selectride to produce the axial alcohol **167**. Following removal of all protecting groups, the oxime was reduced with $NaCNBH_3$ to provide the calicheamicin aryl-tetrasaccharide **142** along with its C-

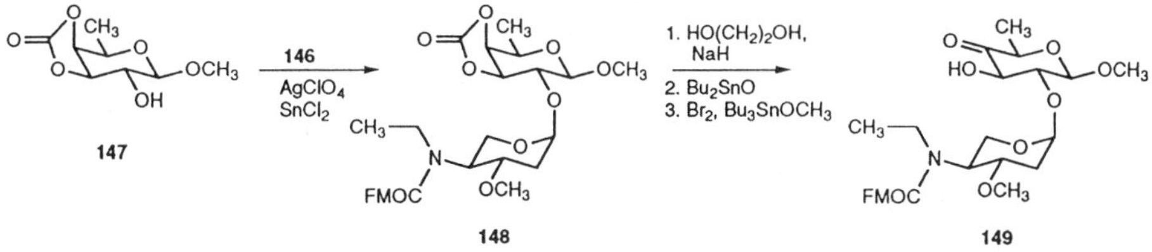

Scheme XXIII Synthesis of the AE Subunit of the Calicheamicin Oligosaccharide (Nicolaou and coworkers) (43).

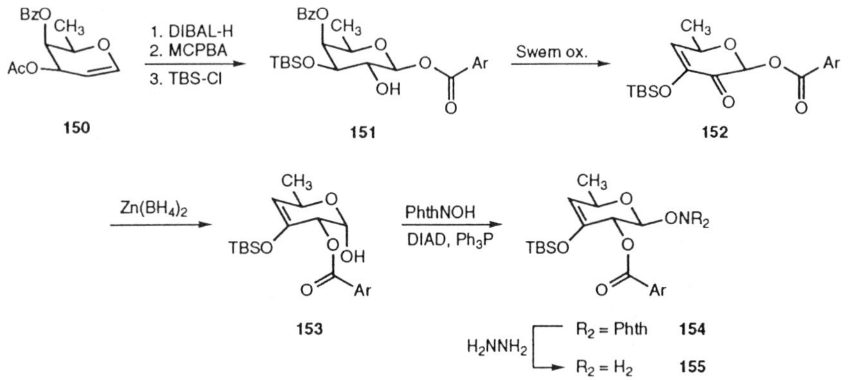

Scheme XXIV Synthesis of the *O*-Glycosylhydroxylamine Subunit of Calicheamicin (Nicolaou and coworkers) (43).

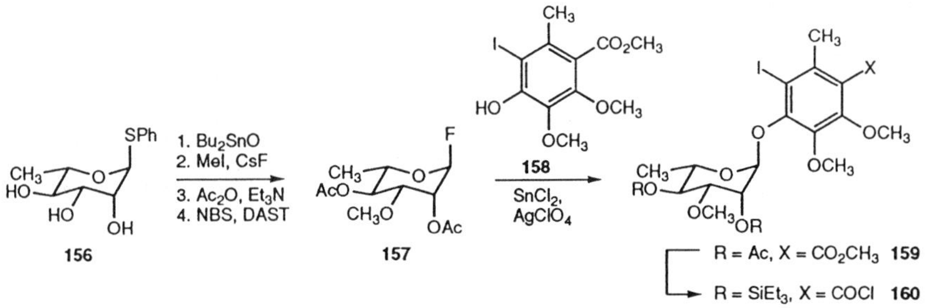

Scheme XXV Nicolaou's Synthesis of the Aryl-Glycoside Subunit of **142** (42).

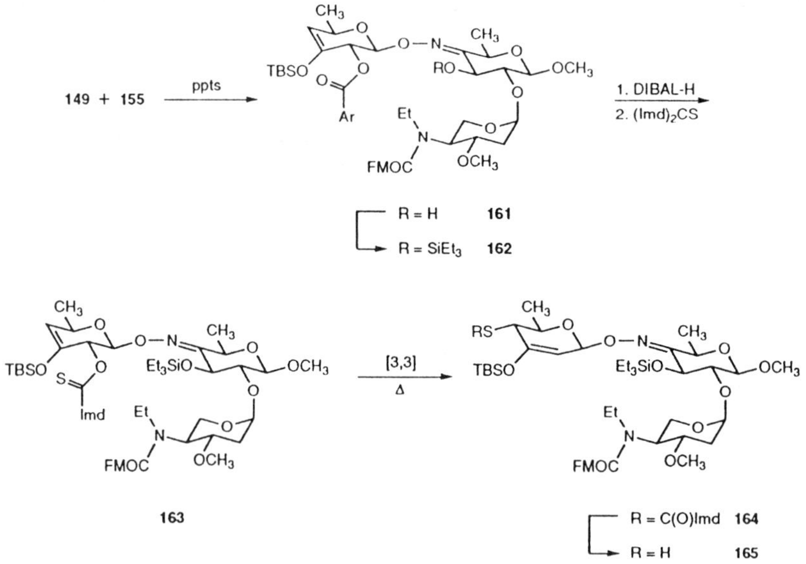

Scheme XXVI Synthesis of the Aryl-Tetrasaccharide of Calicheamicin (Nicolaou) (40).

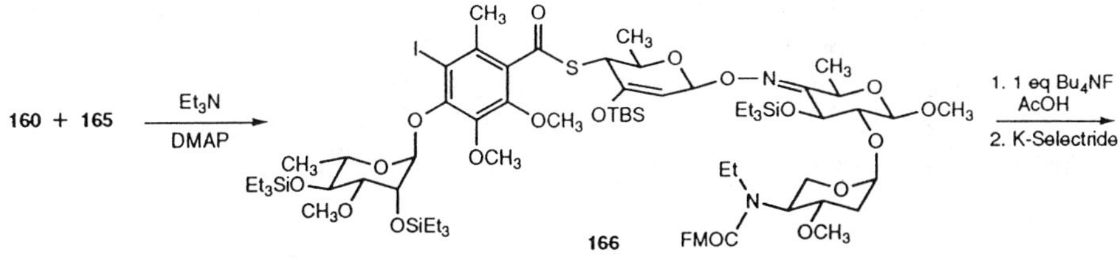

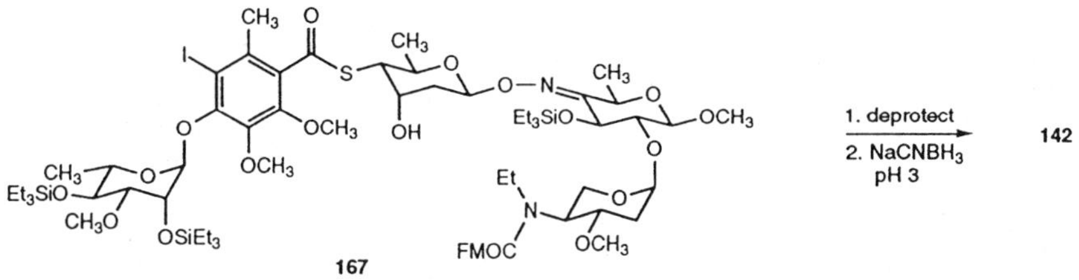

Scheme XXVII Nicolaou's Synthesis of the Calicheamicin Aryl-Tetrasaccharide (continued) (40).

4A epimer in a 1:2 ratio. Reduction conditions have been developed in other systems whereby the ratio of epimers produced at C-4A can be greatly improved to favor the desired equatorial hydroxylamine (43,45). The chemistry thus developed has also been incorporated into the synthesis of the esperamicin carbohydrate units (46).

A synthesis of the core tricyclic system of the calicheamicin aryl-tetrasaccharide was described by Kahne and coworkers (47) and relied on an S_N2 displacement of a leaving group by the anion of an *N*-(glycosyloxy)urethane to establish the hydroxylamine linkage. The glycosidic linkages were constructed using anomeric sulfoxides as coupling partners.

The E-ring residue was synthesized from the protected L-serine derivative **168** (Scheme XXVIII) (48). A hetero-Diels-Alder reaction between the aldehyde **168** and the diene **169** provided compound **170**, which was degraded by two carbons to give compound **171**. The aldehyde **171** was subsequently elaborated to the sulfoxide coupling partner **172**.

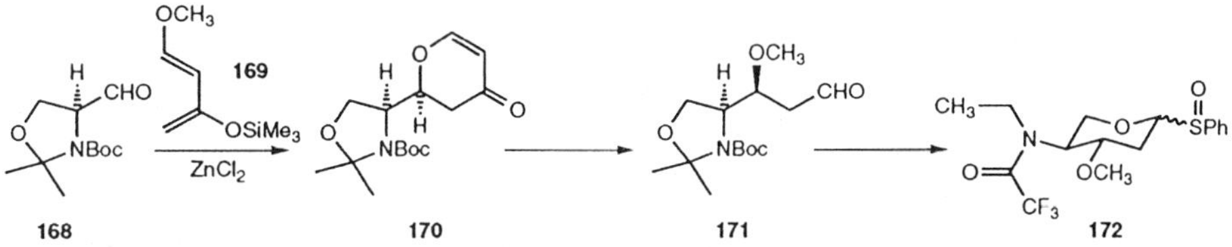

Scheme XXVIII Kahne's Synthesis of the Aminosugar of Calicheamicin (48).

The sulfoxide **172** was coupled to the stannyl ether **173** (Scheme XXIX), making use of glycosylation methodology also developed by Kahne (49) to provide the disaccharide **174**. Compound **174** was converted to the triflate **175**, which was subsequently allowed to react with the anion obtained by deprotonating **176** with NaH. After alkaline hydrolysis of the protecting groups, the calicheamicin core trisaccharide **177** was obtained.

An interesting method to synthesize hydroxylamine-linked glycosides such as that in **142** has been developed by Beau and coworkers (Scheme XXX) (50). The method involves the glycosylation of nitrone **181** with the donor **182** to give, after protecting group removal, the *O*-glycosylhydroxylamine **183**. The synthesis of nitrone **181** featured a stereoselective reduction of the cyclic oxime derivative **180** to the corresponding hydroxylamine (for other routes to related hydroxylamines, see Ref. 51.).

A synthesis of the core trisaccharide of esperamicin which is based on the use of glycals as building blocks has been developed by Danishesfky and coworkers (52). The hydroxylamine linkage was installed by displacing an axial leaving group on the disaccharide **189** with an *N*-(glycosyloxy)urethane anion. Scheme XXXI illustrates the synthesis of the disaccharide coupling partner **189**. The fucal derivative **184** was epoxidized with dimethyldioxirane and subsequently methanolyzed to provide the diol **185**. Compound **185** was selectively iodoglycosylated by glycal **186** at the equatorial hydroxyl group to provide, after further elaboration, the triflate **189**.

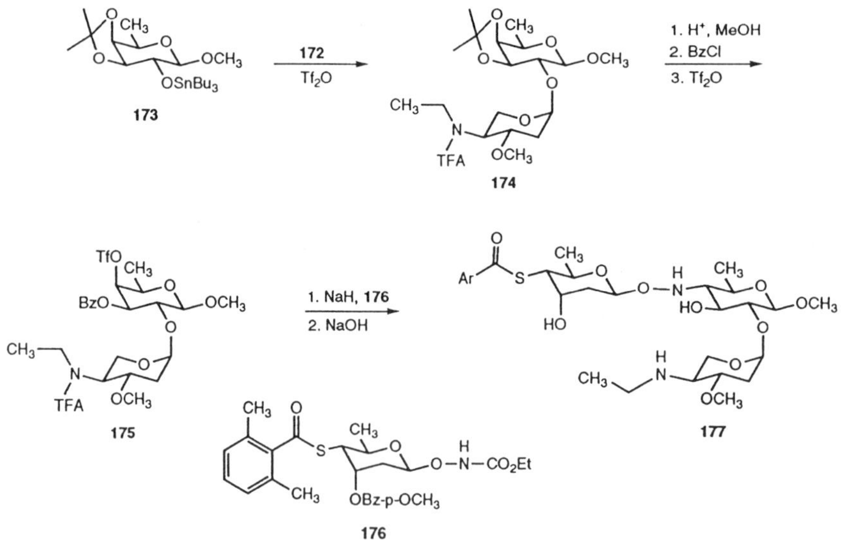

Scheme XXIX Kahne's Synthesis of the Core Trisaccharide of Calicheamicin (48).

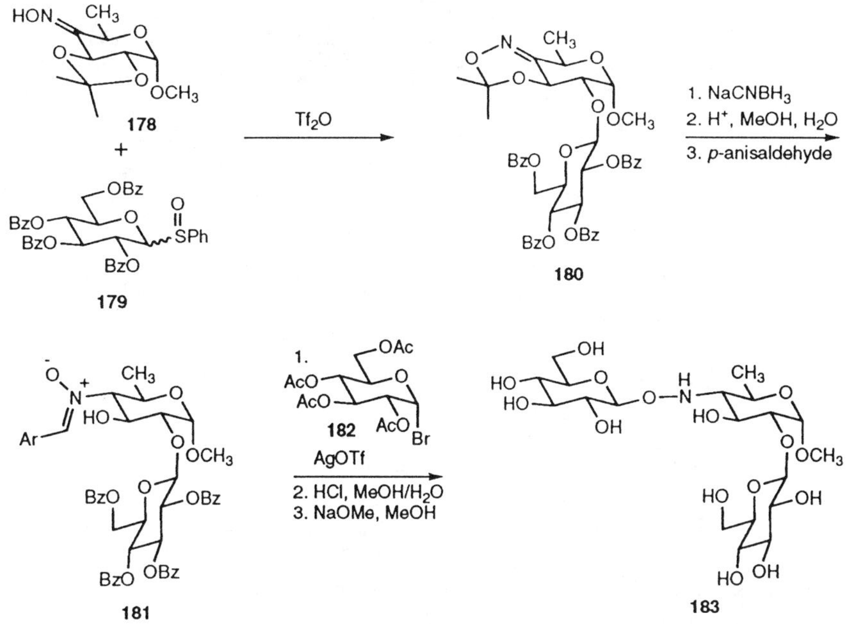

Scheme XXX Nitrone-Based Approach to the Calicheamicin Oligosaccharide (Beau and coworkers) (50).

The synthesis of the thiosugar component **197** is shown in Scheme XXXII (52–54). Key transformations include a selective oxidation of the anomeric sulfide of **193** and a subsequent [2,3] sigmatropic rearrangement of the intermediate sulfoxide to formally invert the stereochemistry of C-3 and provide compound **194**. The protected hydroxylamine functionality was introduced by treating glycal **195** with TEOC-NHOH and triphenylphosphine hydrobromide.

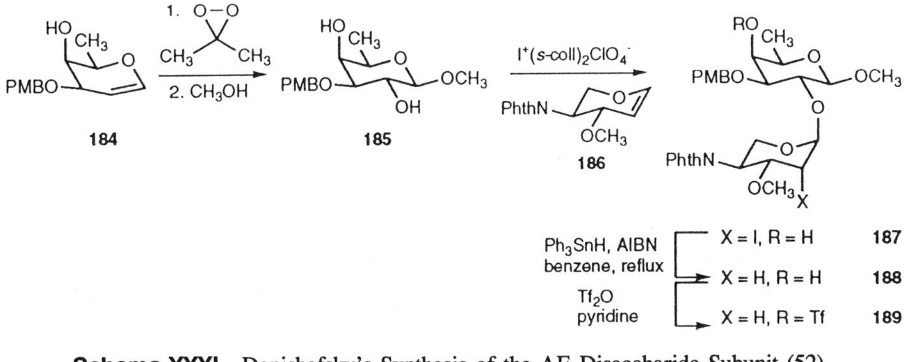

Scheme XXXI Danishefsky's Synthesis of the AE Disaccharide Subunit (52).

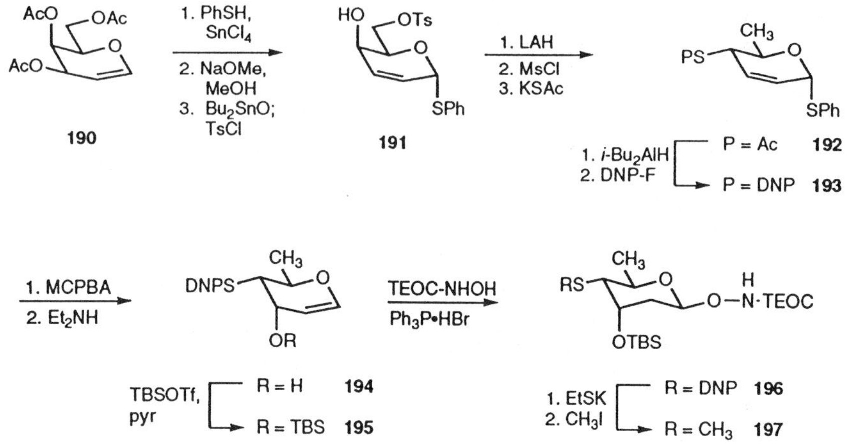

Scheme XXXII   Danishefsky's Synthesis of the *O*-Glycosylhydroxylamine (52).

Treatment of the triflate **189** with the anion of the urethane **197** provided compound **198**, which was converted to **200**, the core trisaccharide of esperamicin (Scheme XXXIII) (52). Compound **201** (Scheme XXXIV), synthesized by an analogous route, was elaborated to the rearranged trisaccharide **204**, which was correlated with material derived from degradation of esperamicin A_{1a} (55).

The Danishefsky group has expanded its route to the esperamicin trisaccharide to allow for a synthesis of the calicheamicin aryl-tetrasaccharide (56). The

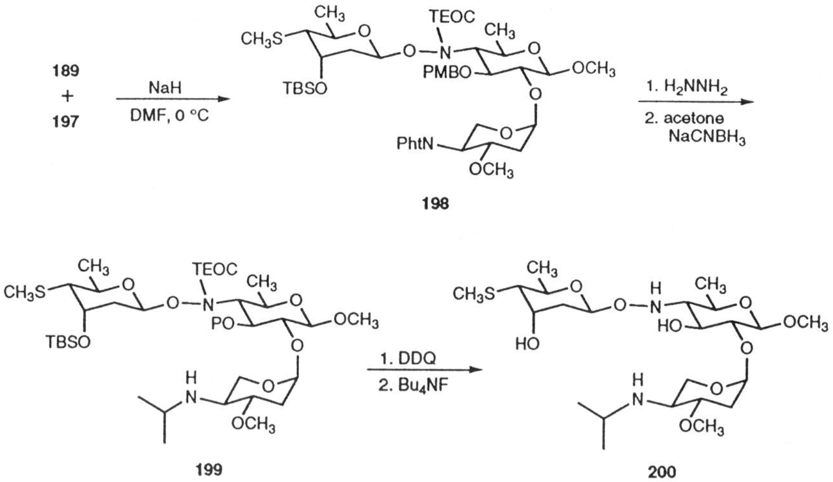

Scheme XXXIII   Danishefsky's Synthesis of the Esperamicin Trisaccharide (52).

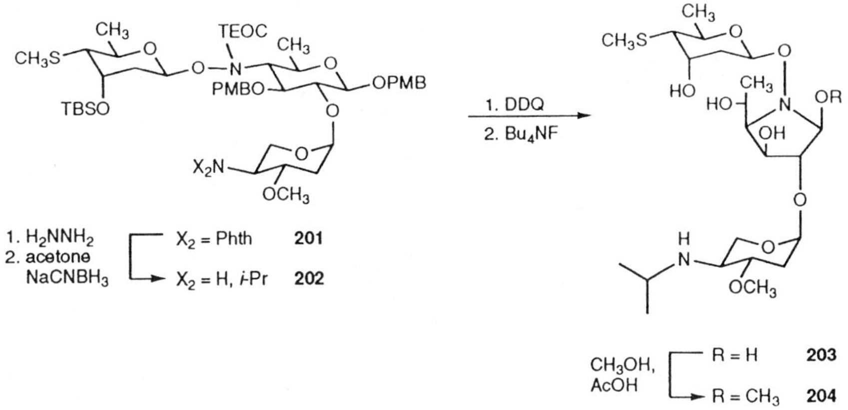

Scheme XXXIV Synthesis and Structural Corroboration of an Esperamicin Degradation Product (Danishefsky and coworkers) (52).

synthesis of **212**, the acid chloride corresponding to the C-D subunit, is shown in Scheme XXXV. A fourth glycal building block, L-rhamnal **205**, was utilized as a starting material. A Schmidt glycosylation was used to couple **208** to the phenol **209** (44). A chemoselective methoxycarbonylation, similar to that used by Nicolaou (44), served to install the methyl ester and provide **211**, which was converted into **212** (for syntheses of a related aryl glycoside, see Ref. 57). The

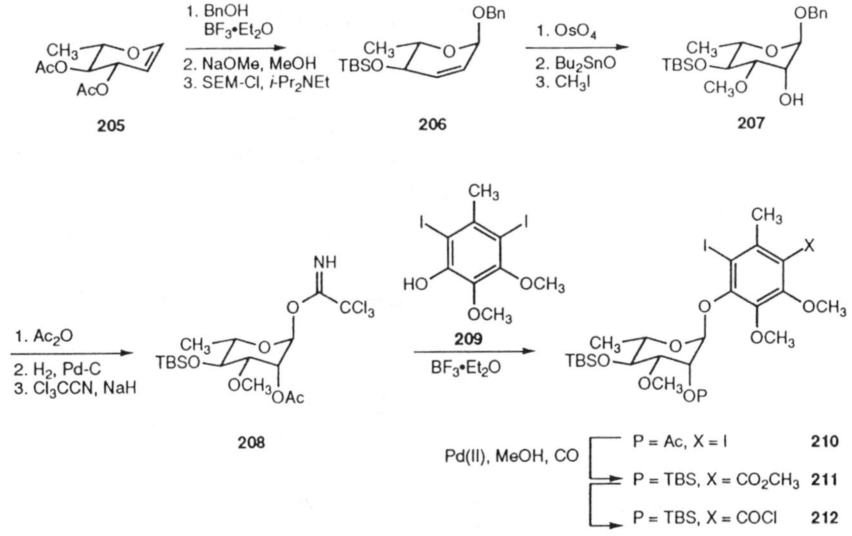

Scheme XXXV Danishefsky's Synthesis of the Calicheamicin Aryl-Glycoside Subunit (56).

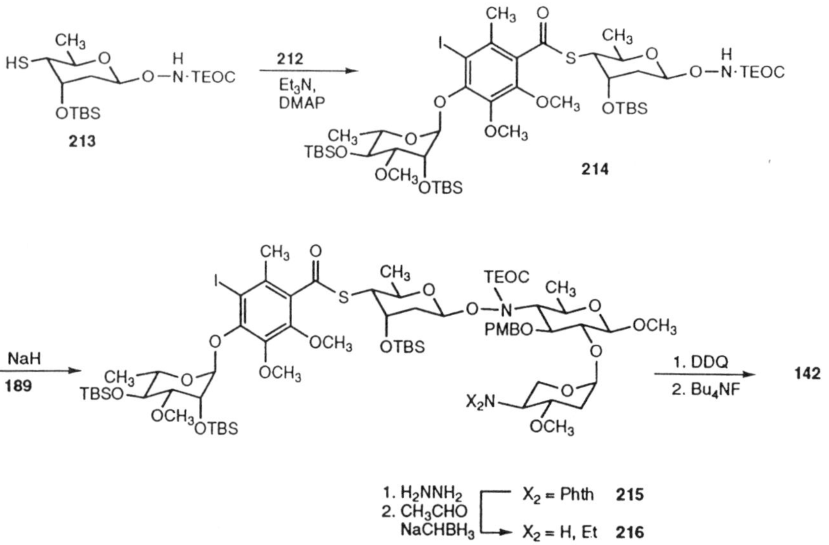

Scheme XXXVI Danishefsky's Synthesis of the Calicheamicin Aryl-Tetrasaccharide (56).

acid chloride **212** acylated the thiol **213**, obtained as previously described, to provide the thiolester **214** (Scheme XXXVI). Compound **214** was coupled to the triflate **189** to give **215**, which was subsequently elaborated into **142**.

A version of the aryl-tetrasaccharide which was activated as a glycosyl donor was synthesized by a similar route (Scheme XXXVII) (56). The carbamate **214** was elaborated, under conditions similar to those described in Scheme XXIV, to compound **217**, which was, in turn, converted into the trichloroacetimidate **218**. Compound **218** was suitably activated for coupling to glycosyl acceptors, and effectively glycosylated compound (+)-**109** (37b), an intermediate in the synthesis of calicheamicinone, to provide the glycoconjugate **219**.

IV. TOTAL SYNTHESIS OF CALICHEAMICIN

A landmark total synthesis of calicheamicin has recently accomplished by the Nicolaou group (58). Employing chemistry analogous to that developed in the synthesis of **142**, the aryl-tetrasaccharide **220**, which contains a selectively removable *ortho*-nitrobenzyl protecting group at the reducing end, was assembled (Scheme XXXVIII). After photolytic deprotection of the anomeric center, the resulting intermediate **221** was activated as the trichloroacetimidate **222**. Compound **222** was coupled to the aglycone **223** to stereoselectively provide **224**, having the β configuration at the new anomeric center. After installation of the allylic sulfur functionality, the oxime was reduced to the corresponding hydroxylamine, thus

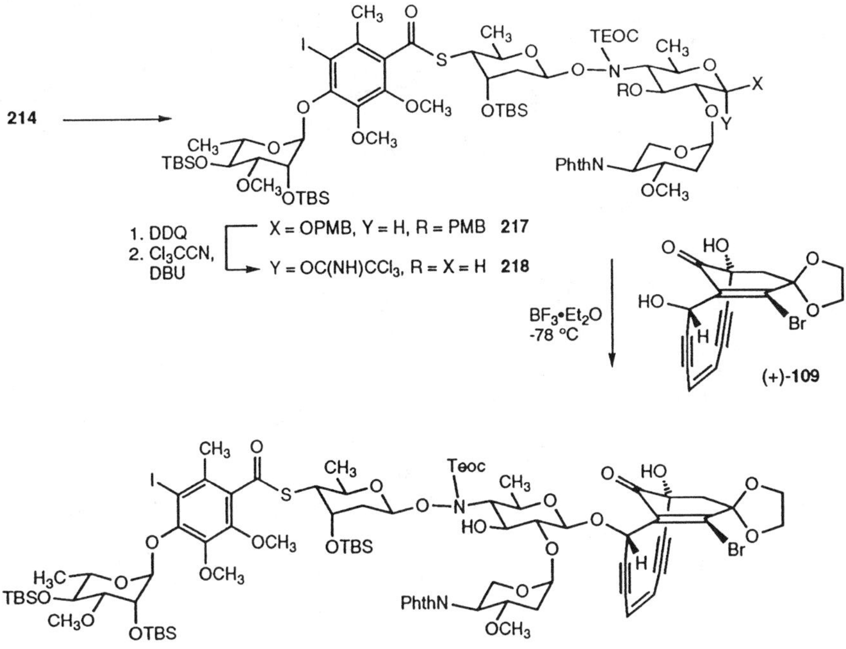

Scheme XXXVII First Glycosylation of a Calicheamicin Aglycone Model with the Full Calicheamicin Carbohydrate Domain (Danishefsky and coworkers) (56).

affording **228**. It is interesting to note that removal of the silyl protecting group from the hydroxyl vicinal to the oxime was necessary to achieve stereochemistry in the reduction step. Reprotection of **228** gave **229** (Scheme XXXIX), which was reductively deacylated and subsequently treated with **93** to provide the trisulfide-containing intermediate **230**. Finally, the protecting groups were removed to afford synthetic calicheamicin.

V. DYNEMICIN

Dynemicin cleaves double-stranded DNA by a mechanism similar to that of esperamicin and calicheamicin (59). It is postulated that an initial reduction of the quinone moiety to the hydroquinone **231** allows an epoxide ring opening to occur, providing a quinone methide–like compound such as **232** (Scheme XL) (59). Compound **232** can either suffer nucleophilic attack or be protonated to give compounds **233a** and **233b**, respectively. The relief in strain in going from **3** to **233** triggers a Bergman cyclization (9) of the enediyne unit to an aromatic 1,4-diradical **234**, which abstracts hydrogen atoms from DNA and provides compound **235**.

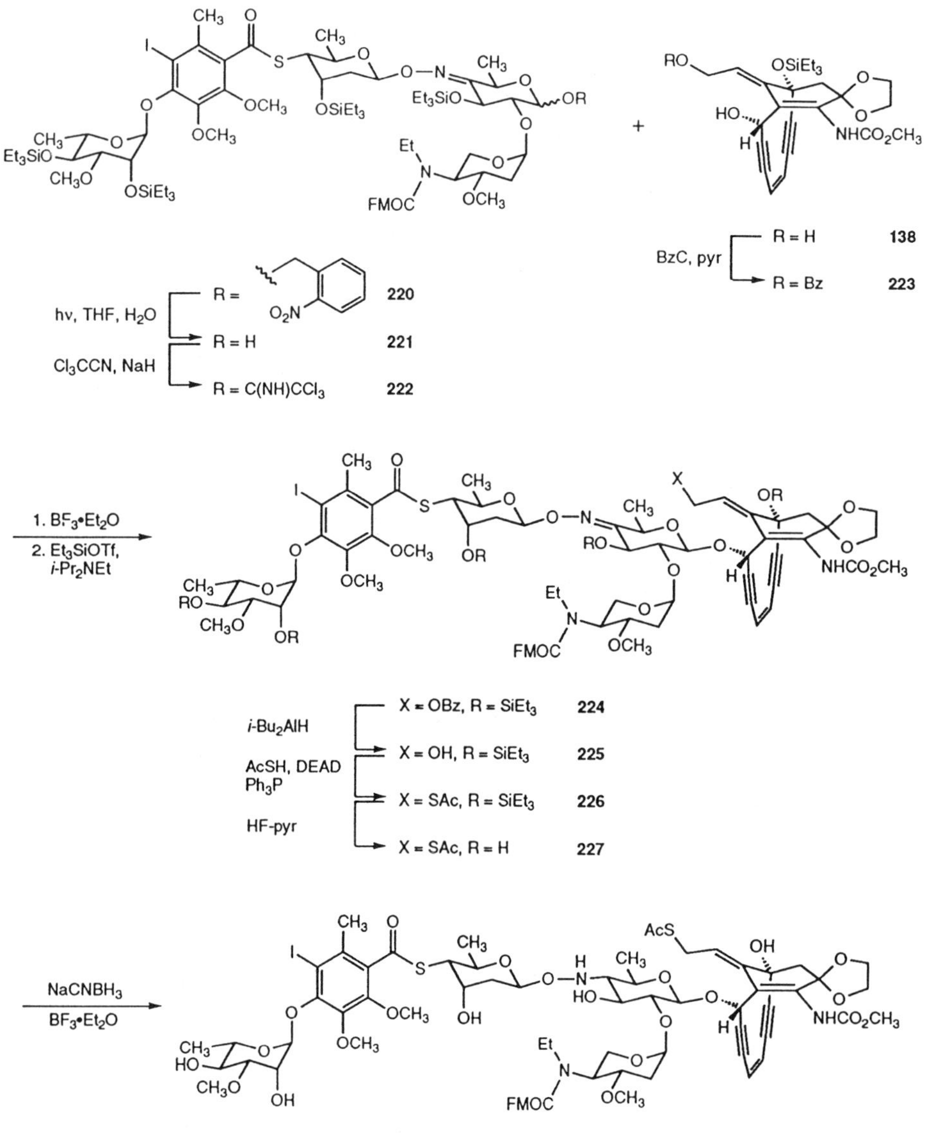

Scheme XXXVIII   Nicolaou's First Total Synthesis of Calicheamicin γ_1^I (58).

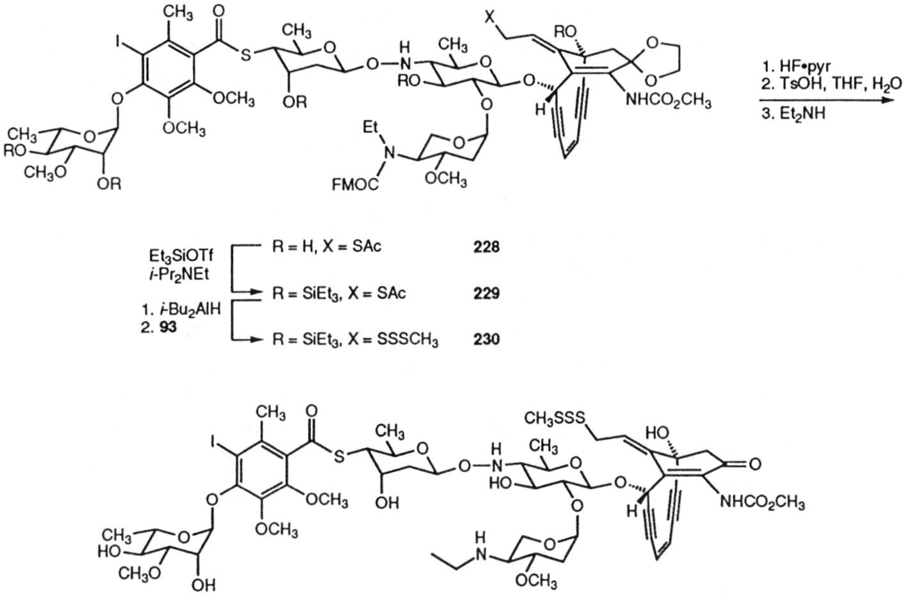

Scheme XXXIX   Nicolaou's Total Synthesis of Calicheamicin (continued) (58).

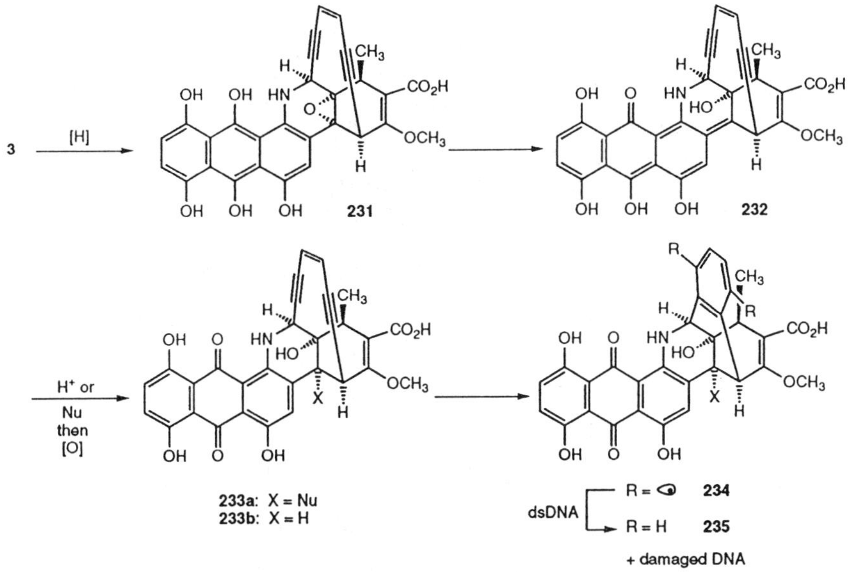

Scheme XL   Mechanism of DNA Cleavage by Dynemicin.

Several dynemicin models have been synthesized, some of which were found to mimic the biomechanism of the natural product. Three different strategies have been employed to synthesize the enediyne-containing ring system of dynemicin. One employed by Nicolaou and coworkers is illustrated in Scheme XLI (60). Acetylide addition to the *N*-acylpyridinium species derived from **236** afforded compound **237**, which was subsequently converted into the ketoepoxide **238**. Palladium-mediated coupling with **69** followed by desilylation provided compound **240**. Deprotonation of the acetylene effected cyclization onto the ketone and provided **241**, which was subsequently deoxygenated to give **242**. Compound **242** was shown to mimic the biomechanism of dynemicin upon acid-catalyzed hydrolysis of the epoxide (60). Treatment of **242** with TsOH/H$_2$O or HCl in the presence of a hydrogen atom donor produced the aromatized compound **243a** or **243b**, respectively (Fig. 3). Using analogous routes, compounds **244** and **245a–c** (Fig. 3) were synthesized (61), each of which contains a novel triggering mechanism for the cascade of events leading to Bergman cyclization and DNA cleavage (for review see Ref. 62; for synthesis and evaluation of other dynemicin models see Ref. 63).

A route to a dynemicin model system, which was also based on an anionic cyclization, was developed by the Wender group (Scheme XLII) (64). Compound **248** was synthesized from the quinoline **246** via an *N*-acylpyridinium intermedi-

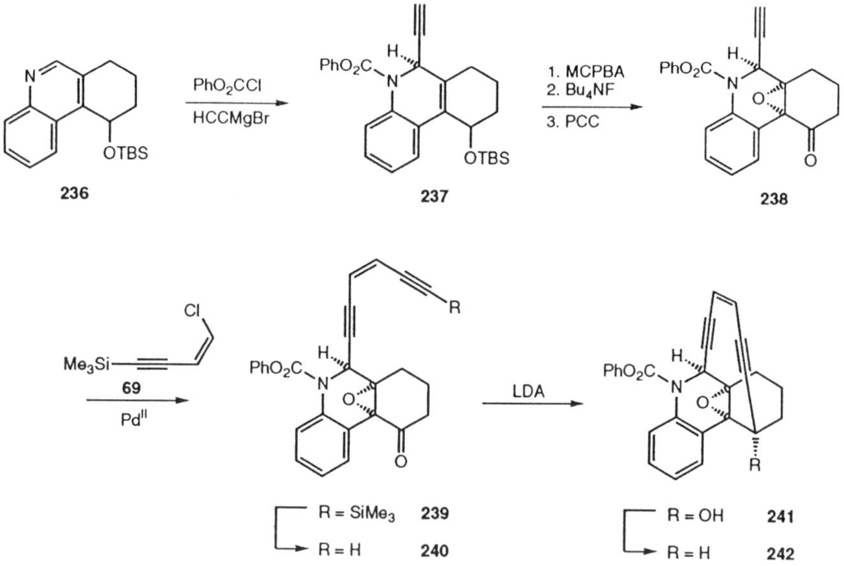

Scheme XLI Synthesis of Model Ring Systems of Dynemicin (Nicolaou and coworkers) (60).

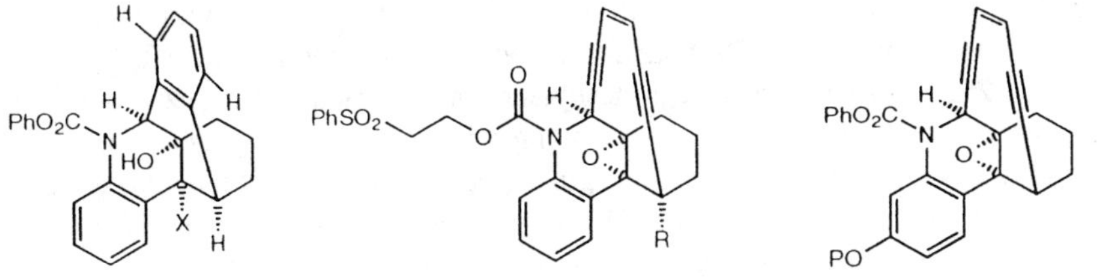

243a: X = OH
243b: X = Cl

244

P = *o*-nitrobenzyl 245a
P = Piv 245b
P = CH$_3$ 245c

Figure 3 Compounds **243a** and **243b** are the aromatized products derived from **242**. Also shown are dynemicin models that are activated under basic (**244** and **245b**), photolytic (**245a**), or oxidative and acidic (**245c**) conditions (61–62).

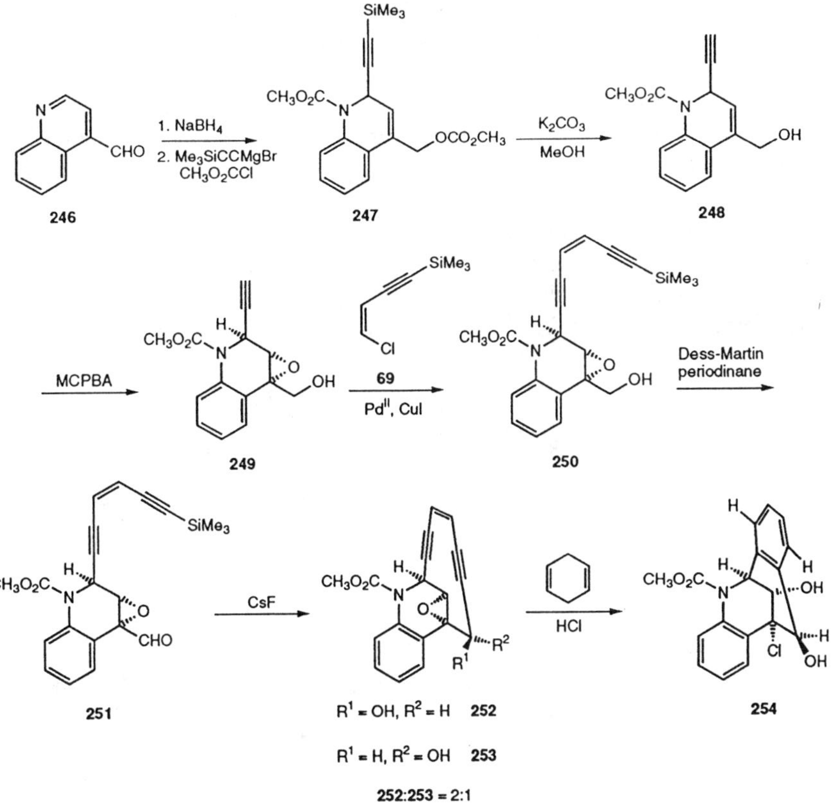

246

1. NaBH$_4$
2. Me$_3$SiCCMgBr
   CH$_3$O$_2$CCl

247

$\xrightarrow{\text{K}_2\text{CO}_3}$ MeOH

248

$\xrightarrow{\text{MCPBA}}$

249

69

Pd^{II}, CuI

250

Dess-Martin periodinane

251

$\xrightarrow{\text{CsF}}$

R^1 = OH, R^2 = H   252

R^1 = H, R^2 = OH   253

252:253 = 2:1

HCl

254

Scheme XLII   Wender's Route to the Dynemicin Ring System (64).

ate. Following installation of the epoxide, the acetylene moiety was coupled to **69** to provide compound **250**, which was converted into the aldehyde **251**. Treatment of **251** with CsF resulted in desilylation and subsequent cyclization of the acetylide intermediate to provide **252** along with its carbinol epimer **253**. Compound **252** was found to undergo Bergman cyclization in a fashion analogous to dynemicin and afford compound **254** upon epoxide cleavage.

A synthesis of a simple bicyclic model compound also based on this concept was reported by Isobe and coworkers (65). This bicyclic enediyne system, **259**, was obtained upon treatment of the aldehyde **258**, synthesized according to Scheme XLIII, which LiHMDS and CeCl$_3$.

As an example of the second strategy, Magnus and coworkers have synthesized the model compound **264** (Scheme XLIV) using chemistry similar to that employed in their calicheamicin work (see Scheme IV) (66). The key transformation was a cyclization of the enol moiety of **263** onto a propargyl cation equivalent generated by treatment compound **263** with triflic anhydride. Subsequent removal of the cobalt complex provided **264**. This substrate was found to be quite robust but underwent smooth cycloaromatization at elevated temperatures in the presence of 1,4-cyclohexadiene to give **265**.

The third strategy, which ultimately led to a total synthesis of trimethyldynemicin, was developed by Schreiber and coworkers and employed a transannular Diels-Alder reaction to generate the enediyne bridge (Scheme XLV) (67). The substrate for the Diels-Alder reaction was synthesized from the bromoquinoline **266**. A palladium-catalyzed coupling of the bromide **266** with the vinyl stannane **267** produced compound **268**. Addition of the Grignard reagent **269** to the N-acylpyridinium salt derived from reaction of **268** with methyl chloroformate afforded, after desilylation, compound **270**. Subsequent esterifica-

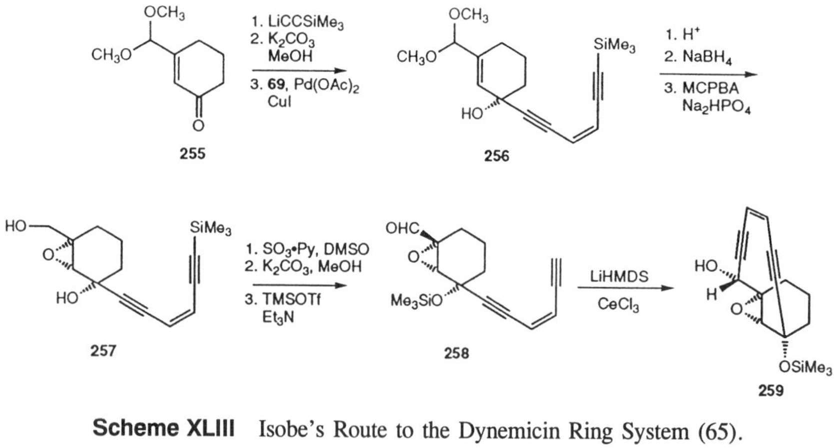

Scheme XLIII Isobe's Route to the Dynemicin Ring System (65).

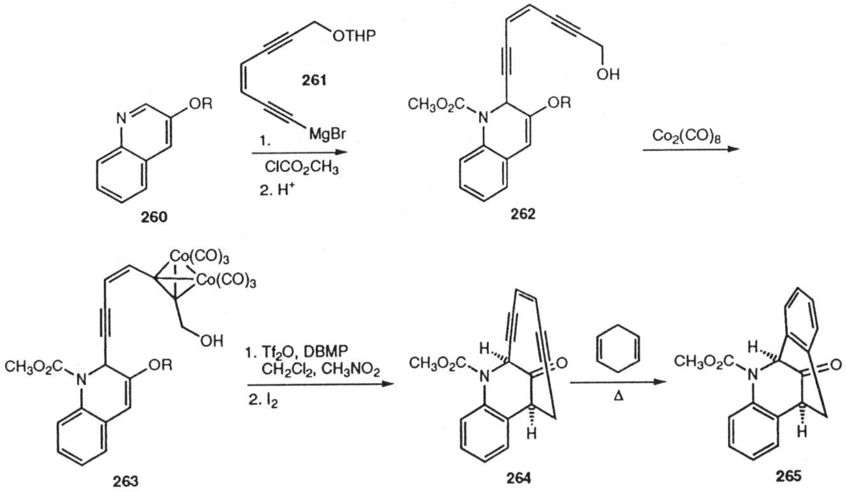

Scheme XLIV   Magnus's Route to the Dynemicin Ring System (66).

tion of the alcohol **270** with *trans*-3-bromopropenoic acid provided **272**. A palladium-mediated ring closure of **272** provided the intermediate macrocyclic lactone **273**, which spontaneously underwent the desired transannular Diels-Alder reaction to provide **274**. The same result was obtained when the order of the esterification and the final palladium-catalyzed coupling reactions was reversed. The epoxide was installed by direct epoxidation of compound **276**, which was obtained from **274** by a sequence of reactions resulting in a formal olefin migration (Scheme XLVI) (67).

A dynemicin model (**285**) containing all of the functionality except the anthraquinone moiety and having the correct stereochemistry at the methyl-bearing carbon was synthesized by extending this route (Scheme XLVII) (68). Compound **276** was epimerized at the position α to the ester and subsequently hydroxylated at the benzylic carbon to give **278**. A notable reduction of the olefin, which involved a sigmatropic rearrangement of the diazene **279** with intramolecular delivery of hydride, was then employed to generate the correct stereochemistry at the methyl stereocenter and provided **280**. The diazene **279** was generated from **278** as illustrated. The lactone ring was transformed into the vinylogous carbonate **284** via the intermediates **281–283**. Finally, treatment with MCPBA installed the epoxide and afforded **285**.

A total synthesis of dimethyl- and trimethyldynemicin (**293** and **294**, respectively) has been accomplished by Schreiber and coworkers and is summarized in Scheme XLVIII (69). The synthesis proceeded via the intermediate **286**, which was assembled using chemistry analogous to that in the previous two schemes.

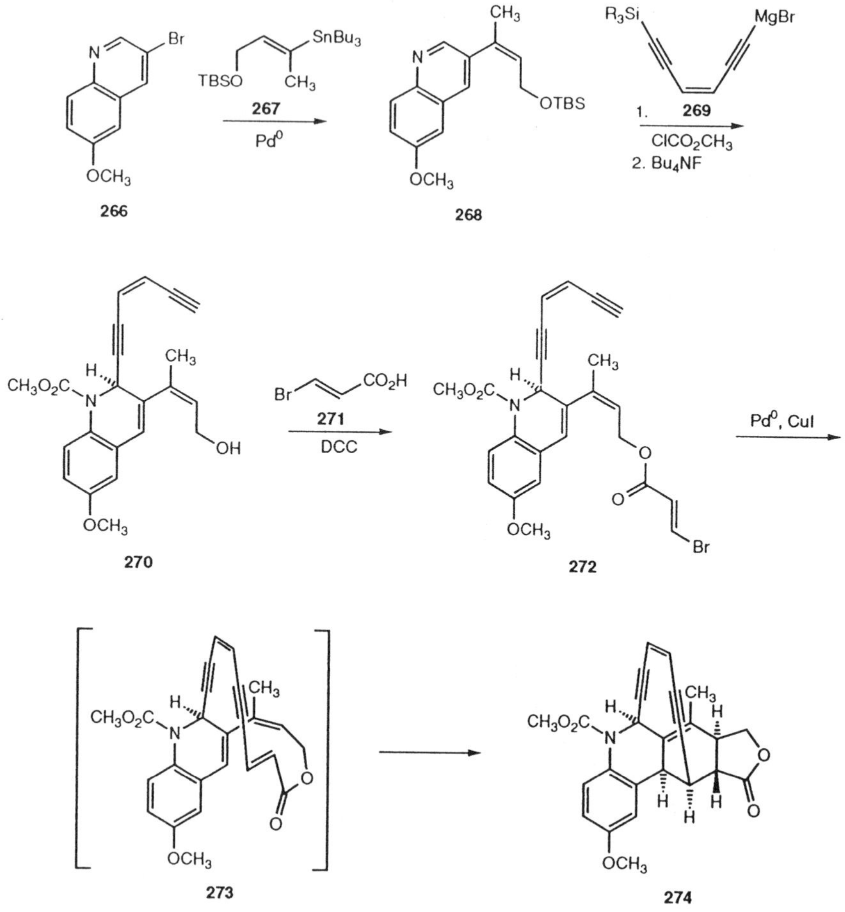

Scheme XLV Transannual Diels-Alder Route to the Dynemicin Ring System (Schreiber and coworkers) (67).

The anthraquinone precursor **288** was synthesized by treating **286** with the bromide **287** and AgOTf, followed by *O*-methylation of the enol. Benzylic reduction gave **289**, which was subsequently cyclized to give **290**. Epoxidation with MCPBA and base-induced deprotection of the nitrogen gave the epoxide **291**. Treatment of **291** with ceric ammonium nitrate then effected oxidation of the B-ring to the quinone, with concomitant demethylation, to give dimethyldynemicin **293**. The reaction apparently goes through the iminoquinone intermediate **292**. Methylation of the phenol thus produced gave trimethyldynemicin **294**, which was correlated with the same material derived from the natural product.

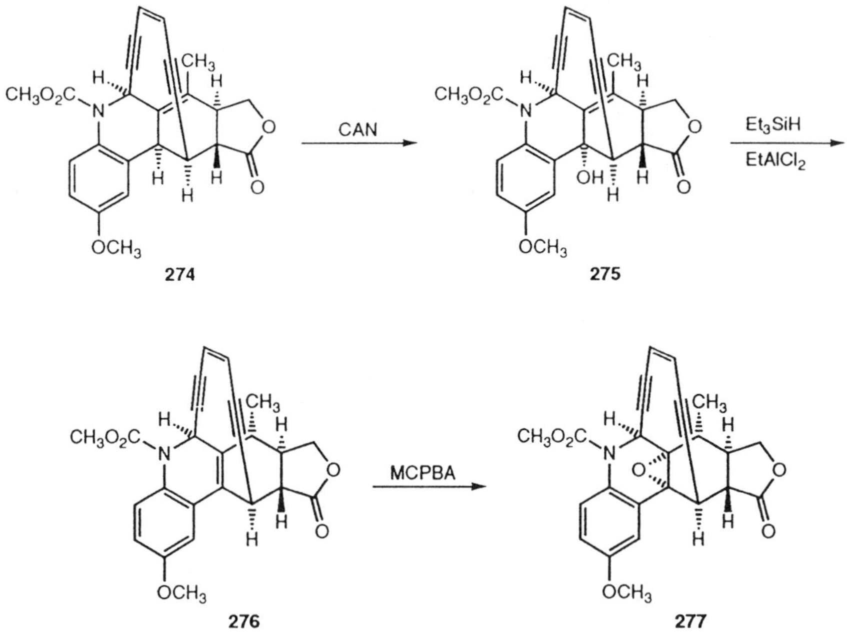

Scheme XLVI   Schreiber's Synthesis of an Advanced Dynemicin Intermediate (67).

VI. THE NEOCARZINOSTATIN CHROMOPHORE

The neocarzinostatin chromophore (NCS Chrom, **4**) cleaves double-stranded DNA by a mechanism similar to, yet distinct from, the other enediyne antibiotics. The sequence of events leading to the activated species begins with an S_N2' opening of the epoxide of NCS Chrom to give the cumulene intermediate **295** (Scheme IL) (70). This cumulene cyclizes to the diradical **296** (71), which abstracts hydrogen atoms from the DNA backbone, resulting in DNA cleavage (72). Compound **297** is the end product derived from NCS Chrom (70).

A. Synthesis of Acyclic Enyne-Allene Systems

Several simple acyclic eneyne-allene–containing compounds have been synthesized with the intent of studying the mechanism of action of NCS Chrom. Myers and coworkers have synthesized the parent (Z)-1,2,4-heptatriene-6-yne **300** from the enediyne **298** and have studied its thermal decomposition to toluene via the diradical **301** (Scheme L) (73,74).

The Myers group has also synthesized compound **308** (Scheme LI), which allows access to an acyclic enediyne system under very mild conditions (74a,75).

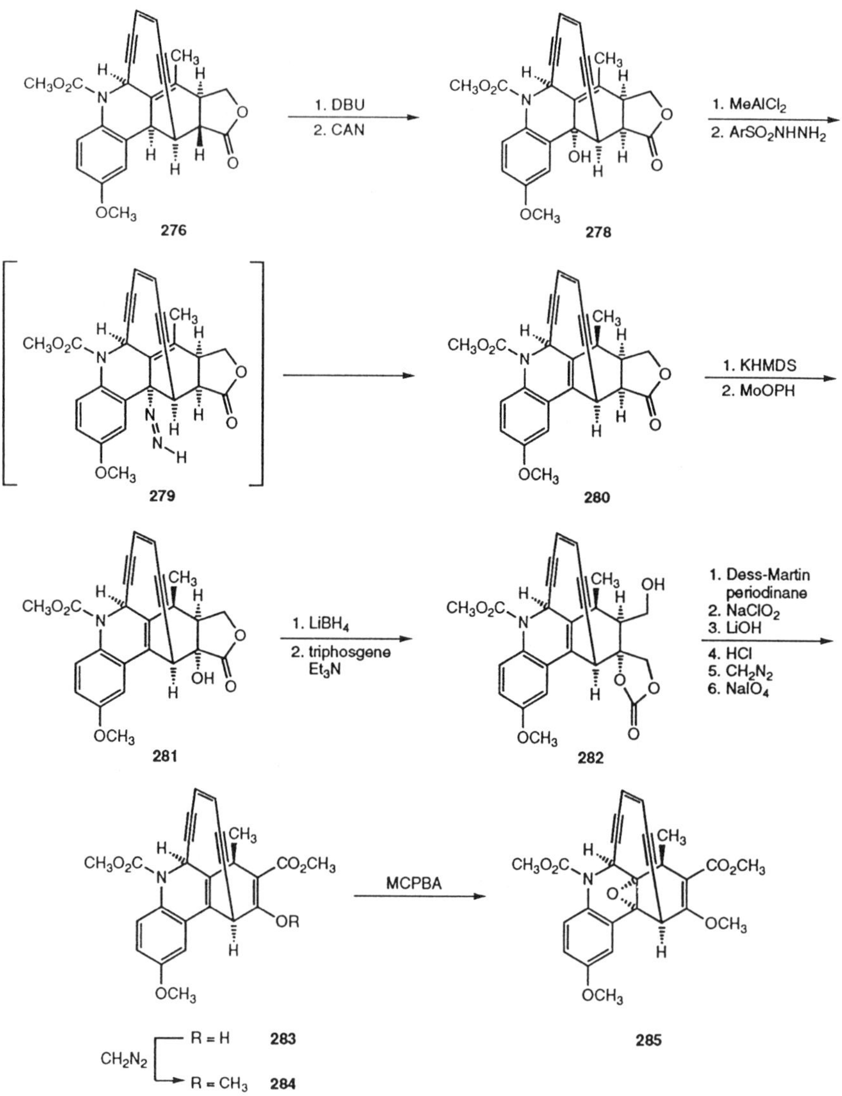

Scheme XLVII Synthesis of a Dynemicin System Containing all of the Functionality except the Anthraquinone (Schreiber and coworkers) (68).

Treatment of the thiol **308** with mild base resulted in an intramolecular S_N2' displacement of the dinitrobenzoate to provide compound **309**, which was shown to cyclize to the aromatic compound **311** via the diradical **310**.

The eneyne-allene **313** was synthesized and studied by Saito and coworkers (Scheme LII) (76). The synthesis involved a [2,3]-sigmatropic rearrangement of

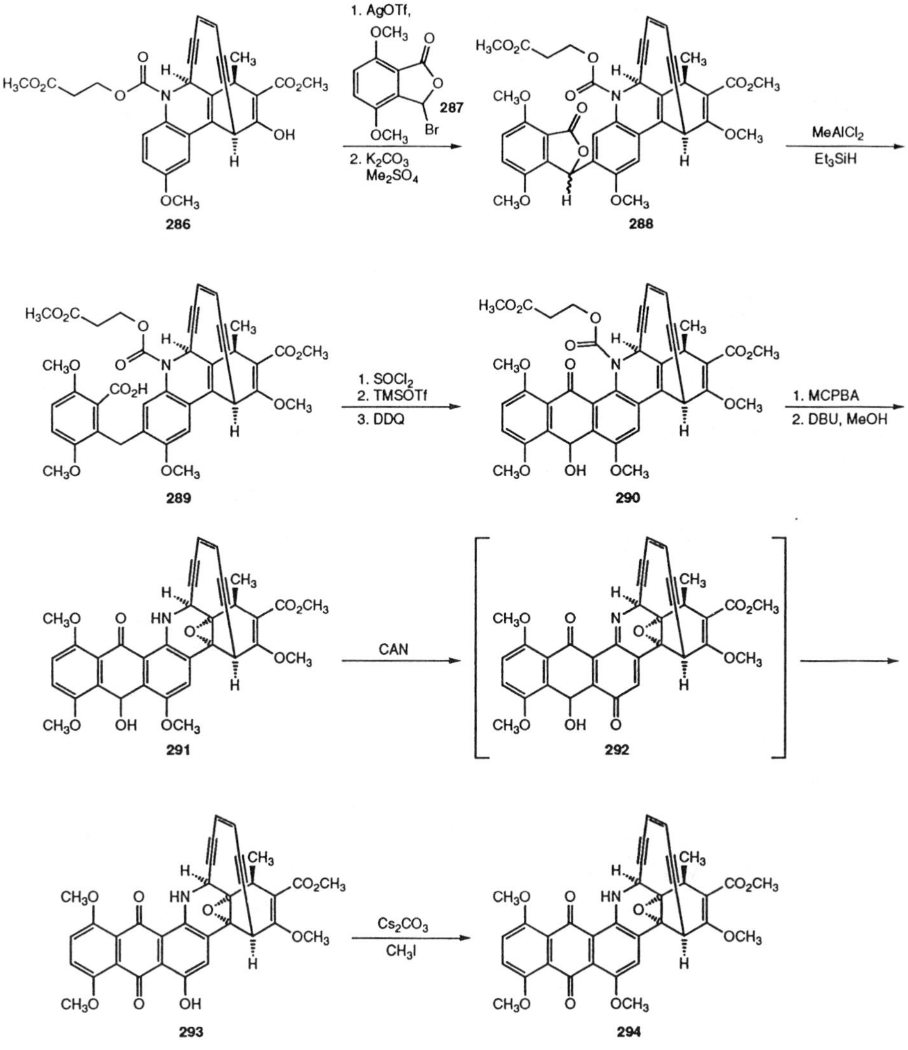

Scheme XLVIII   Schreiber's Total Synthesis of Di- and Trimethyl Dynemicin (69).

the phosphinite obtained upon treating **312** with chlorodiphenylphosphine. The resulting phosphine oxide **313** cyclized to the diradical **314** under mild conditions and ultimately provided **315**.

B.   Synthesis of Carbocyclic Core Structures

The first synthesis of a carbocyclic core structure of NCS Chrom was reported by Wender and coworkers (Scheme LIII) (77). Compound **317** was synthesized

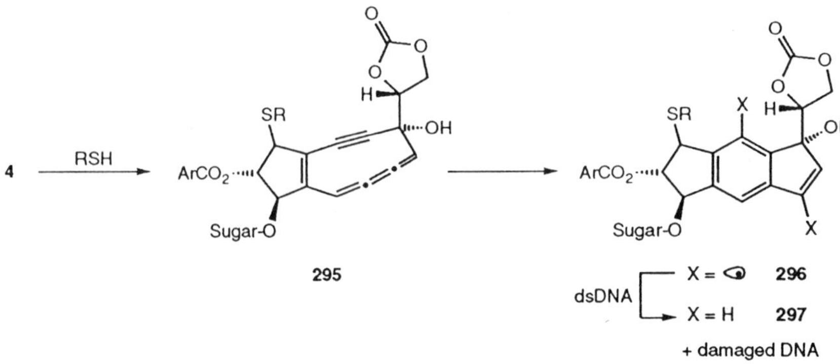

Scheme IL Mechanism of DNA Cleavage by Neocarzinostatin Chromophore.

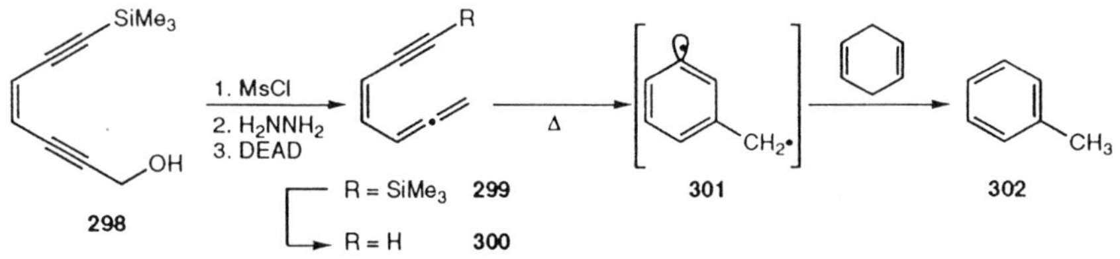

Scheme L Myers's Synthesis of the Parent Enyne-Allene Intermediate of NCS Chrom (73–74).

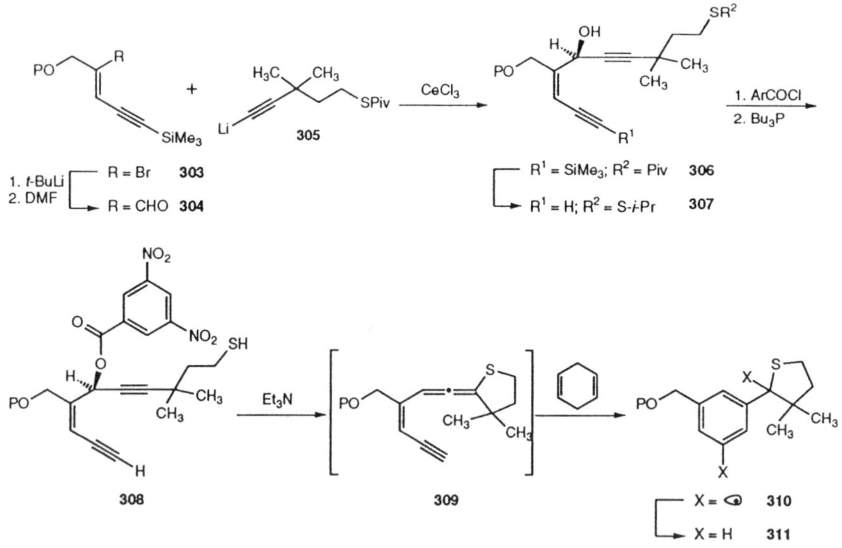

Scheme LI Synthesis and Activation of a Model for NCS Chrom (Myers and co-workers) (75).

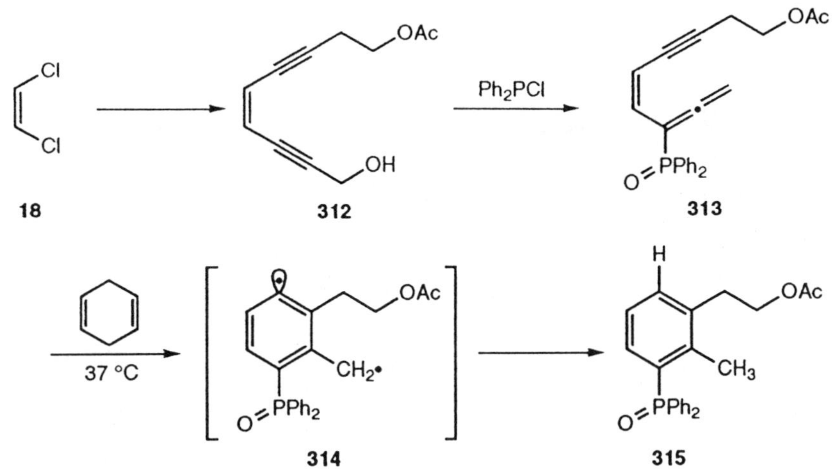

Scheme LII Saito's Synthesis and Activation of an NCS Model (76).

in a straightforward manner from the bromocyclopentenone **316** and was coupled
to *tert*-butyldimethylsilyl propargyl ether to provide, after deprotection, **318**.
Compound **318** was converted into the cyclic sulfide **319**, which was subsequently
oxidized to the sulfone **320**. Photolytic extrusion of SO_2 followed by dehydration gave the carbocyclic core **321**.

The Wender group has also synthesized a more highly functionalized core structure (Scheme LIV) (78). Compound **322** (see Scheme LIII) was coupled to the
vinyl iodide **323** to provide **324**, which was subsequently converted into the aldehyde **326**. Treatment of **326** with $CrCl_2$ resulted in an intramolecular Nozaki-
type cyclization to provide **327**. Acetylation and dehydration then gave **328**. The

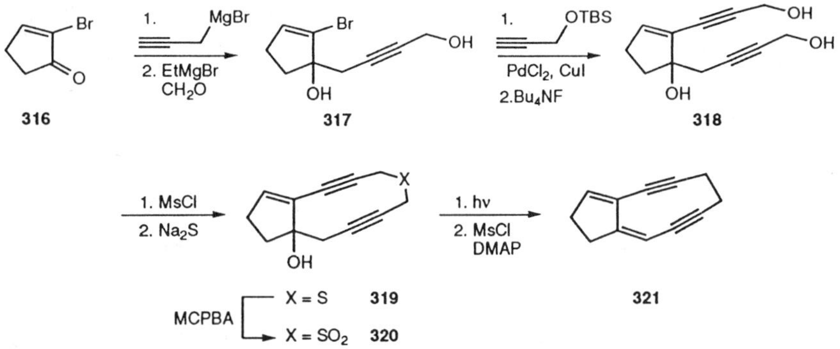

Scheme LIII Wender's Synthesis of the Diene-Diyne Core Structure of NCS Chrom
(77).

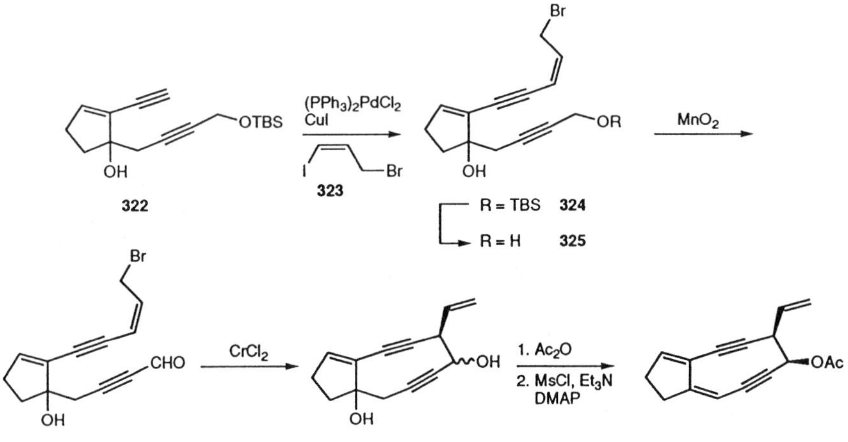

322

326 327 328

Scheme LIV Synthesis of a NCS Chrom Core Structure (Wender and coworkers) (78).

intermediate **327** was also synthesized by a sequence that involved a [2,3]-Wittig rearrangement of the cyclic ether **331** (Scheme LV).

Takahashi and coworkers have employed a similar [2,3]-Wittig rearrangement to construct the ring system (Scheme LVI) (79). Coupling of a vinyl bromide **332** with the acetylene **333** gave **334**, which was elaborated to the cyclic ether **337**.

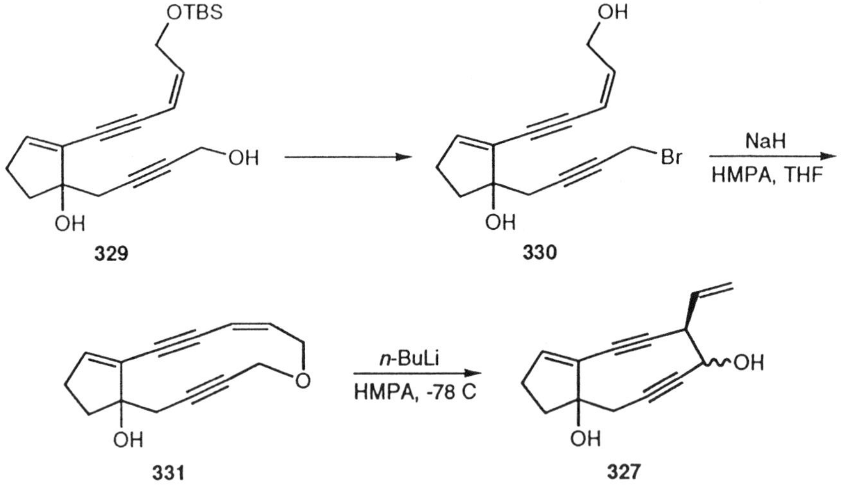

329 330

331 327

Scheme LV Route to the NCS Chrom System Based on a [2,3]-Wittig Rearrangement (Wender and coworkers) (78).

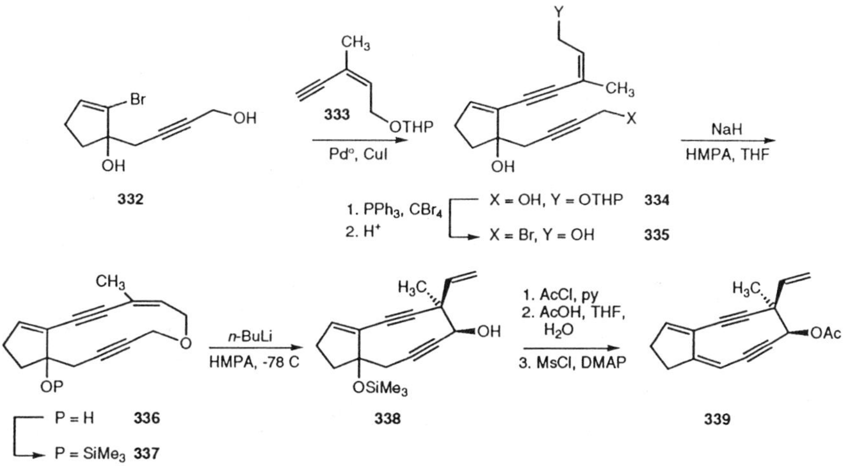

Scheme LVI   Takahashi's [2,3]-Wittig Approach to the NCS Chrom Ring System (79).

Wittig rearrangement of **337** afforded **338**, which was converted into the dienediyne **339**. In a separate study (Scheme LVII), compound **338** was transformed into the ketone **340**, which was shown to mimic the biomechanism of NCS Chrom (79). Conjugate addition of a thiol to **340** produced the cycloaromatized compound **342**, apparently through the cumulenol intermediate **341**.

An enantioselective synthesis of a core ring system was developed by the Myers group and is illustrated in Scheme LVIII (80). Their strategy involved annulation of a functionalized epoxydiyne ring onto a cyclopentanoid nucleus. The optically active epoxydiyne fragment **347** was synthesized from **346** using a Sharpless asymmetric epoxidation. Compound **346** was, in turn, synthesized from the di-

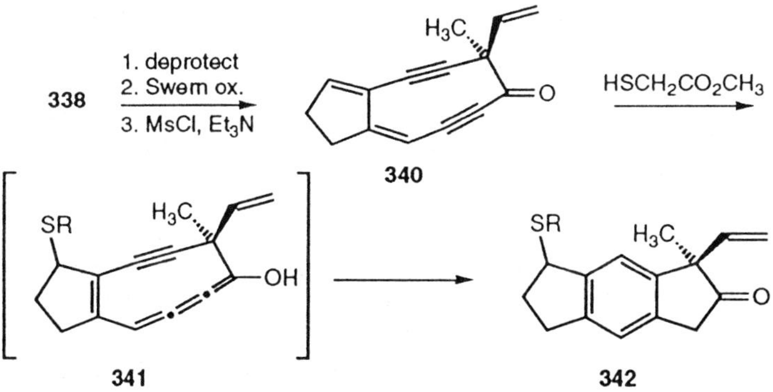

Scheme LVII   Mechanism of Activation of **388** by Thiols (Takahashi and coworkers) (79).

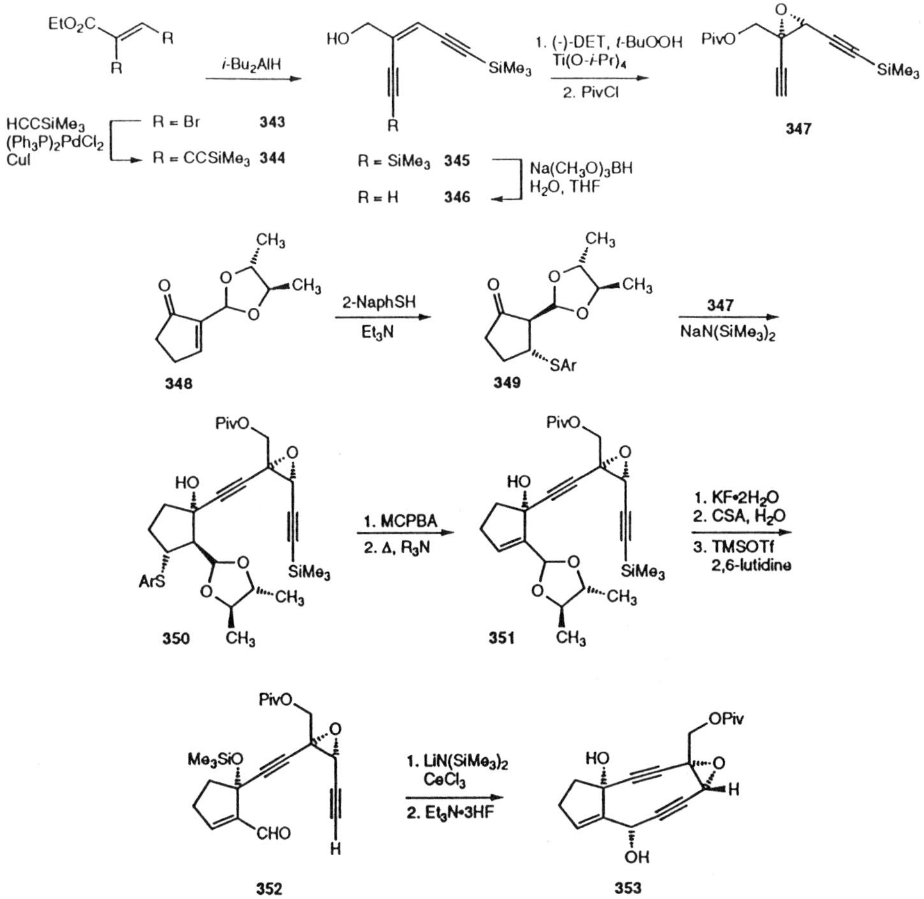

Scheme LVIII   Myers's Enantioselective Route to the NCS Chrom Ring System (80).

bromide **343** by a sequence of reactions which included a notable selective disilylation of **345**. The anion of **347** was allowed to react with the cyclopentanone **349**, obtained by Michael addition of 2-naphthalenethiol to **348**, to produce the adduct **350**. After reinstallation of the double bond, compound **351** was elaborated to the aldehyde **352**. Deprotonation of the acetylene resulted in a stereospecific cyclization onto the aldehyde and produced, after deprotection, compound **353**.

The most highly functionalized NCS Chrom core structure synthesized to date was also recorded by the Myers group (Scheme LIX) (81). Treatment of **354**, obtained similarly to **353**, with trifluoroacetic acid resulted in a suprafacial trans-

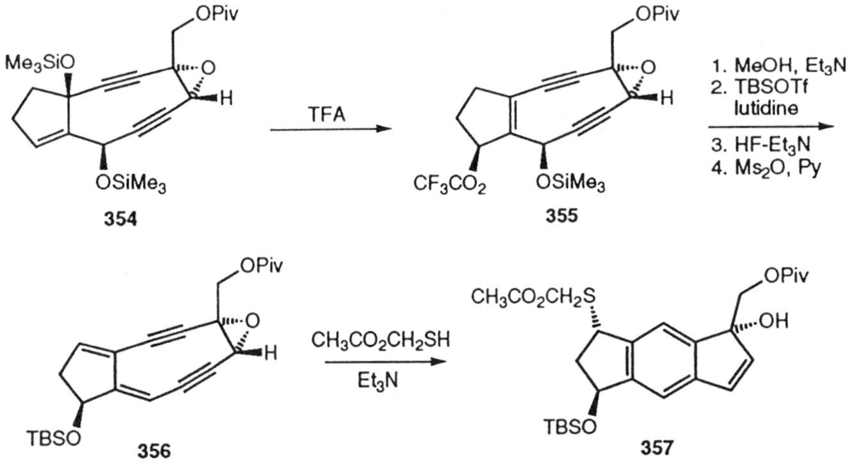

Scheme LIX Myers's Synthesis and Activation of an Advanced Model of NCS Chrom (81).

position of functionality to provide **355**. Adjustment of the protecting groups and a subsequent dehydration then afforded the epoxy dienediyne core **356**. Compound **356** was found to undergo reaction with methyl thioglycolate, in the same fashion as **4**, and provide **357**. However, unlike **4**, the presence of added base was required for reaction to occur (81).

Magnus and coworkers have developed a route to the carbocyclic system which is based on their cobalt-mediated cyclization methodology (82). The substrate for the desired cyclization, **363**, was synthesized as shown in Scheme LX. The vinyl iodide **360**, synthesized as shown, was coupled to the acetylene **361** to provide **362**. Chemoselective acetylene complexation with $Co_2(CO)_8$ and manipulation of protecting groups gave the aldehyde **363**. Intramolecular aldol reaction afforded **364** which, upon removal of the complexing metals, provided the cycloaromatized compound **366** rather than the enediyne **365**. The undesirable Bergman cyclization could be suppressed by replacing the central olefin of the enediyne appendage with an epoxide moiety, as is present in the natural product (Scheme LXI) (83). This was accomplished by a Sharpless asymmetric epoxidation of the intermediate **367**, which was synthesized analogously to **362**. The resulting epoxide **368** was converted into the aldehyde **369**, which was cyclized as before to provide the highly functionalized NCS Chrom core structure **370**.

C. Synthesis of 10-Membered Ring Analogs

Several research groups have synthesized analogs that contain a 10-membered rather than a 9-membered ring as is present in the carbocyclic core structure of the

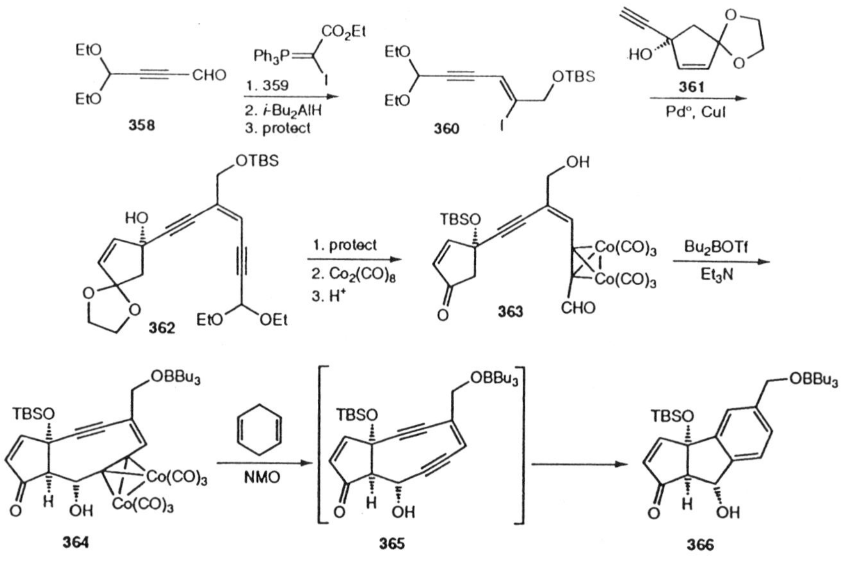

Scheme LX

Scheme LX   Magnus's Approach to the NCS Chrom Ring System (82).

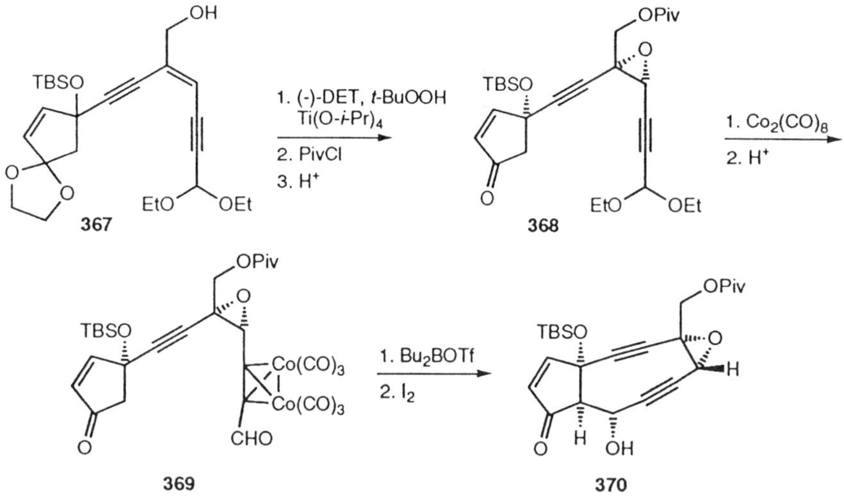

Scheme LXI   Second Approach by Magnus to the NCS Chrom Core Structure (83).

natural product. Valuable information about the mechanism of action of the natural product has been obtained from the study of these compounds.

Hirama and coworkers have synthesized ketone **376** as illustrated in Scheme LXII (84). Key transformations included reaction of the acetylide ion derived from **371** with the aldehyde **372** to provide **373** and an intramolecular coupling of the stannyl acetylene **374**. The ketone **376** was shown to react with thiols in a conjugate sense and to subsequently cyclize in a manner similar to **4** to produce **377** as a mixture of stereoisomers.

Additionally, this research group has synthesized the isomeric ketone **382** (Scheme LXIII) (85). The synthesis of **382** also features a palladium-catalyzed intramolecular coupling as a means of forming the 10-membered ring. The acetylene functionalities of ketone **382** present a different reactivity pattern from those of **376**, which was studied in some detail.

Incorporation of an asymmetric center into the ring system of **376** was accomplished by Hirama as illustrated in Scheme LXIV (86). Enantiomerically pure **383** was synthesized from the *meso* diol and was elaborated to the enone **384**. The ketone **385** was assembled from **384** using an analogous reaction sequence to that described in Scheme LXII.

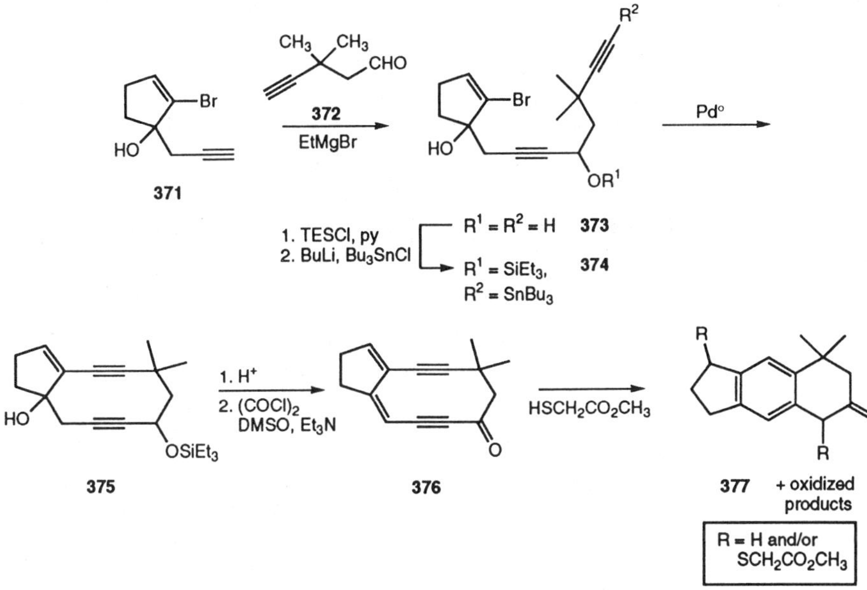

Scheme LXII Synthesis and Activation of a Ten-Membered Ring Analog of NCS Chrom (Hirama and coworkers) (84).

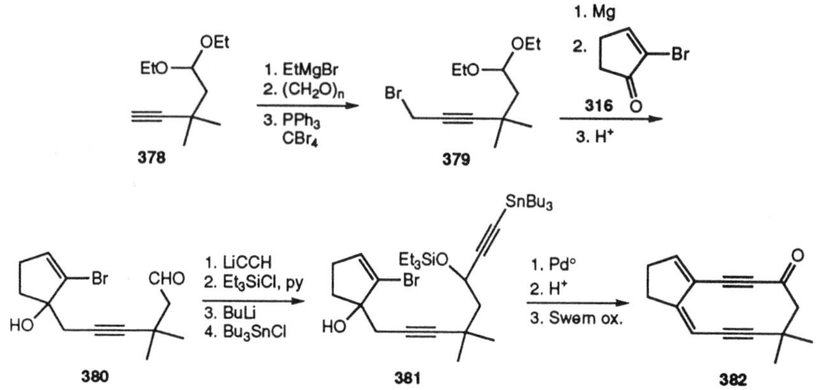

Scheme LXIII Synthesis of an Isomeric Ten-Membered NCS Chrom Analog (Hirama and coworkers) (85).

An intramolecular aldol reaction was used by Krebs and coworkers to construct the 10-membered ring analogs **390** and **392** (87). The acetal **389** was synthesized from the bromide **386** as shown in Scheme LXV. When treated with TMSOTf, compound **389** underwent intramolecular aldol condensation and subsequent β elimination to afford the enone **390**. Alternatively, compound **389** could be converted into the silyl enol ether **391**, which cyclized to the β-methoxyketone **392** upon treatment with $TiCl_4$ (for other 10-membered analogs, see Ref. 88).

D.   Synthesis of Related Functionalized 5-Membered Rings

The synthesis of two highly functionalized cyclopentene analogs of NCS Chrom that contain an acyclic dienediyne unit corresponding to the 9-membered ring have been synthesized by Terashima and coworkers (Scheme LXVI) (89). The alde-

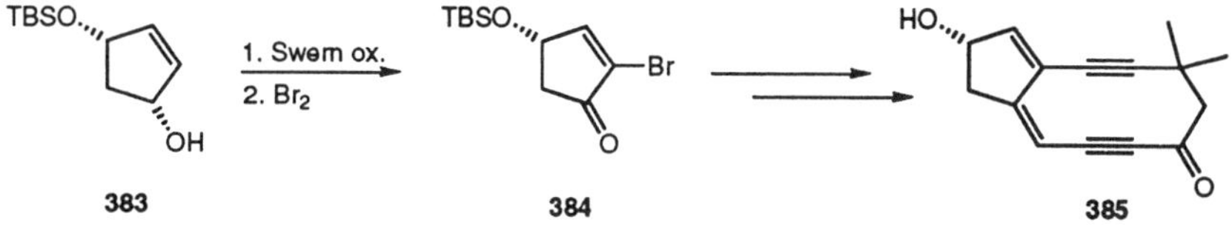

Scheme LXIV Enantioselective Synthesis of a Ten-Membered NCS Chrom Analog (Hirama and coworkers) (86).

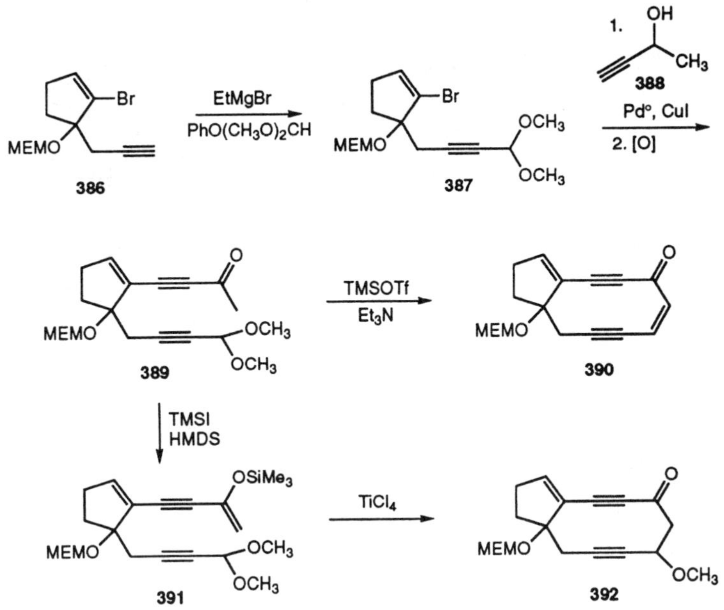

Scheme LXV Krebs's Synthesis of a Ten-Membered NCS Chrom Analog via an Intramolecular Aldol Condensation (87).

hyde **393** was elaborated to the (*E*)-enyne **394**, which could be photoisomerized to produce a 2:1 mixture of **394** and the (*Z*)-isomer **395**. Ketones **394** and **395** were converted into the enol triflates **396** and **397**, respectively. Compound **397** was coupled to the acetylene **402**, which was synthesized from the tartaric acid derivative **398**, to provide th acyclic analog **403**. Substituting the triflate **396** in the sequence for **397** led to compound **404**.

Another expedient route to a relevantly functionalized cyclopentene was reported by Suffert and coworkers (Scheme LXVII) (90). This group found that formylcyclopentanone **405** could be selectively converted into the (*Z*)-enol triflate **406**, which was subsequently transformed into the bis-triflate **407**. Treatment of **407** with Pd^{II}-Cu^{I} and 2.4 equivalents of a terminal acetylene provided **408**. Alternatively, when 1.1 equivalents of acetylene was used, reaction selectively occurred with the exocyclic triflate to provide **409**.

A strategy developed by the Nuss group is illustrated in Scheme LXVIII (91). This sequence involved a cyclization of the vinyl bromide **412**, which was synthesized from the acetylene **410**. Treatment of **412** with Pd^{0} in the presence of stannylacetylene **413** resulted in an initial cyclization of **412** to produce an inter-

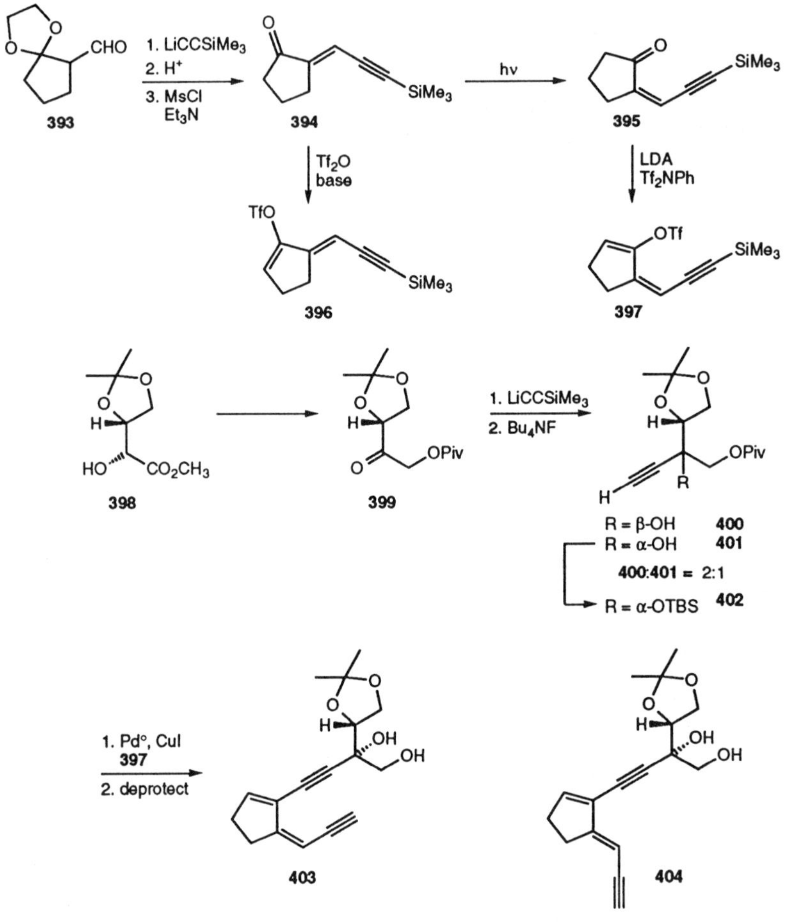

Scheme LXVI   Synthesis of Monocyclic Analogs of NCS Chrom (Terashima an co-workers) (89).

mediate vinylpalladium species, which underwent a subsequent stereospecific Stille-type coupling with **413** to give **414** (for related constructions, see Ref. 92).

A novel method to synthesize enediynes such as **419**, a compound that corresponds to the epoxydiyne of neocarzinostatin, has been developed by Petasis and coworkers (Scheme LXIX) (93). It was found that an α-silyl allenoate **415** could be deprotonated at the γ position to give the alkynyl enolate **416**. Addition of **416** to the aldehyde **417** gave the intermediate aldol product **418**, which underwent a Peterson-type olefination reaction to give **419**.

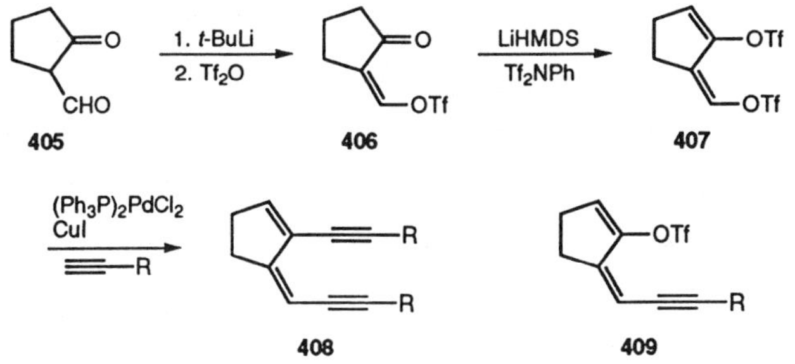

Scheme LXVII Regiocontrolled Synthesis of a Monocyclic Analog of NCS Chrom (Suffert and coworkers) (90).

VI. FUTURE PROSPECTS

A large body of knowledge concerning the chemistry of the enediyne antibiotics has been accumulated at a remarkable pace. The methodologies and strategies developed in response to the challenge of these unique structures has begun to allow access to the natural products, however, a wealth of creative synthetic pursuits are still unexplored. Additionally, many other exciting avenues in this area remain to be discovered. For example, incorporation of the novel mechanism of action of these compounds into the design of new synthetic therapeutic agents offers tremendous possibilities, and indeed this concept has begun to be realized (see also Ref. 94). It is hoped that many more members of this exciting family of compounds will soon be uncovered and that practitioners of synthetic organic chemistry can rise to the task of providing access to these structures and helping to understand the details of how these antibiotics elicit biological responses.

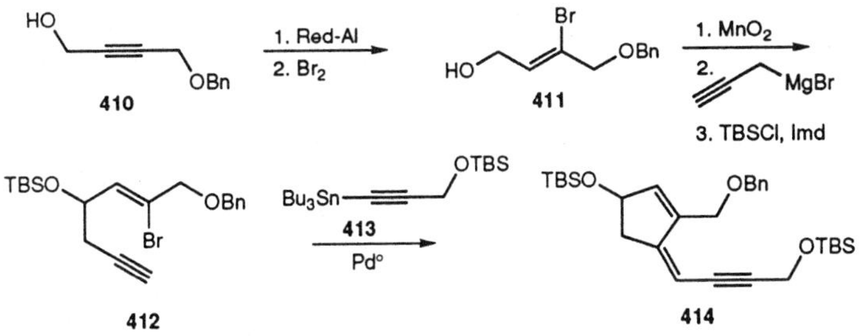

Scheme LXVIII Synthesis of an NCS Model by Intramolecular Pd-Mediated Cyclization (Nuss and coworkers) (91).

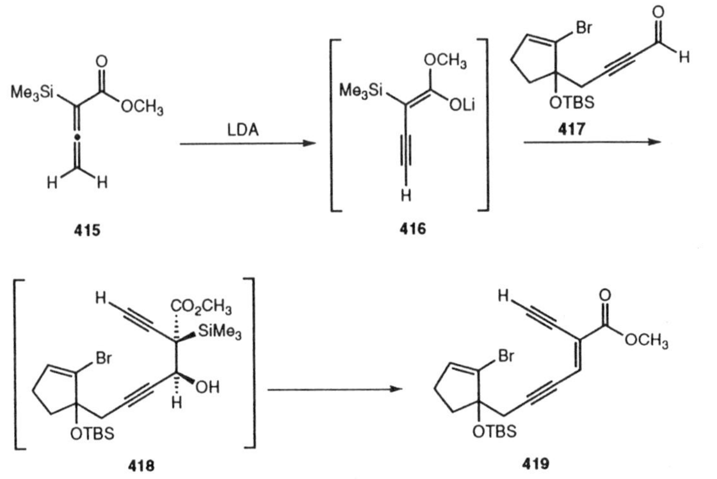

Scheme LXIX Stereocontrolled Synthesis of Enediynes Related to NCS Chrom (Petasis and coworkers) (93).

ACKNOWLEDGMENTS

This manuscript was prepared in part during the author's tenure in the laboratory of Professor Samuel J. Danishefsky (Yale University). Dr. John W. Benbow (Yale University) is thanked for many valuable comments and suggestions concerning the manuscript. Professors Andrew G. Myers (California Institute of Technology) and Stuart L. Schreiber (Harvard University) are thanked for allowing the use of results from their laboratories prior to publication.

Note Added in Proof After the submission of this manuscript, several noteworthy publications have appeared which, unfortunately, could not be discussed in detail due to time constraints. The structure of C-1027, another member of the enediyne class, was elucidated (95). The synthesis of each enantiomer of calicheamicinone (96) and a total synthesis of calicheamicin (97) were accomplished by Danishefsky and coworkers. The synthesis of the calicheamicin aryltetrasaccharide was reported by the group of Kahne (98). Nicolaou and coworkers described the synthesis of several calicheamicin derivatives with interesting biological properties (99). Roush and coworkers reported the synthesis of two monosaccharides of calicheamicin (100). Several publications pertaining to the synthesis of enediyne-containing compounds that are related to esperamicin and calicheamicin have also appeared (101). A construction of an advanced intermediate in the synthesis of dynemicin was achieved by the Danishefsky group (102).

The synthesis of other enediyne (103) and anthraquinone (104) systems related to dynemicin have also appeared. Several model systems of neocarzinostatin were assembled and studied (105).

REFERENCES

1. (a) J. Golik, J. Clardy, G. Dubay, G. Groenewold, H. Kawaguchi, M. Konishi, B. Krishnan, H. Ohkuma, K.-I. Saitoh, and T. W. Doyle, *J. Am. Chem. Soc.,* *109,* 3461 (1987). (b) J. Golik, G. Dubay, G. Groenewold, H. Kawaguchi, M. Konishi, B. Krishnan, H. Ohkuma, K.-i. Saitoh, and T. W. Doyle, *J. Am. Chem. Soc., 109,* 3462 (1987).
2. (a) M. D. Lee, T. S. Dunne, M. M. Siegel, C. C. Chang, G. O. Morton, and D. B. Borders, *J. Am. Chem. Soc., 109,* 3464 (1987). (b) M. D. Lee, T. S. Dunne, C. C. Chang, G. A. Ellestad, M. M. Siegel, G. O. Morton, W. J. McGahren, and D. B. Borders, *J. Am. Chem. Soc., 109,* 3466 (1987). (c) M. D. Lee, G. A. Ellestad, and D. B. Borders, *Acc. Chem. Res., 24,* 235 (1991). (d) M. D. Lee, T. S. Dunne, C. C. Chang, M. M. Siegel, G. O. Morton, G. A. Ellestad, W. J. McGahren, and D. B. Borders, *J. Am. Chem. Soc., 114,* 985 (1992).
3. (a) M. Konishi, H. Ohkuma, K. Matsumoto, T. Tsuno, H. Kamei, T. Miyaki, T. Oki, H. Kawaguchi, G. D. VanDuyne, and J. Clardy, *J. Antibiotics, 42,* 1449 (1989). (b) M. Konishi, H. Ohkuma, T. Tsuno, T. Oki, G. D. VanDuyne, and J. Clardy, *J. Am. Chem. Soc., 112,* 3715 (1990).
4. (a) M. A. Napier, B. Holmquist, D. J. Strydom, and I. H. Goldberg, *Biochem. Biophys. Res. Commun., 89,* 635 (1979). (b) K. Edo, M. Mizugaki, Y. Koide, H. Seto, K. Furihata, N. Otake, and N. Ishida, *Tetrahedron Lett., 26,* 331 (1985). (c) A. G. Myers, *Tetrahedron Lett., 28,* 4493 (1987).
5. (a) J. E. Leet, D. R. Schroeder, S. J. Hofstead, J. Golik, K. L. Colson, S. Huang, S. E. Klohr, T. W. Doyle, and J. A. Matson, *J. Am. Chem. Soc., 114,* 7946 (1992). (b) J. E. Leet, D. R. Schroeder, D. R. Langley, K. L. Colson, S. Huang, S. E. Klohr, M. S. Lee, J. Golik, S. Hofstead, T. W. Doyle, and J. A. Matson, *J. Am. Chem. Soc., 115,* 8432 (1993).
6. (a) K. C. Nicolaou and W.-M. Dai, *Angew. Chem. Int. Ed. Eng., 30,* 1387 (1991). (b) Nicolaou, A. L. Smith, *Acc. Chem. Res., 25,* 497 (1992).
7. (a) N. Zein, A. M. Sinha, W. J. McGahren, and G. A. Ellestad, *Science, 240,* 1198 (1988). (b) N. Zein, M. Poncin, R. Nilakantan, and G. A. Ellestad, *Science, 244,* 697 (1989). (c) Y. Sugiura, Y. Uegawa, Y. Takahashi, J. Kuwahara, J. Golik, and T. W. Doyle, *Proc. Natl. Acad. Sci. USA, 86,* 7672 (1989).
8. B. H. Long, J. Golik, S. Forenza, B. Ward, R. Rehfuss, J. C. Dabrowiak, J. J. Catino, S. T. Musial, K. W. Brookshire, and T. W. Doyle, *Proc. Natl. Acad. Sci. USA, 86,* 2 (1989).
9. (a) R. G. Bergman, *Acc. Chem. Res., 6,* 25 (1973). (b) N. Darby, C. U. Kim, J. A. Salaün, K. W. Shelton, S. Takada, and S. Masamune, *J. Chem. Soc., Chem. Commun.,* 1516 (1971).
10. (a) N. Zein, W. J. McGahren, G. O. Morton, J. Ashcroft, and G. A. Ellestad,

J. Am. Chem. Soc., 111, 6888 (1989). (b) J. J. De Voss, C. A. Townsend, W.-D. Ding, G. O. Morton, G. A. Ellestad, N. Zein, A. B. Tabor, and S. L. Schreiber, *J. Am. Chem. Soc., 112,* 9669 (1990).

11. (a) D. Schinzer and J. Kabbara, *SYNLETT,* 766 (1992). (b) C. Crévisy and J.-M. Beau, *Tetrahedron Lett., 32,* 3171 (1991). (c) H. Audrain, T. Skrydstrup, G. Ulibarri, and D. S. Grierson, *SYNLETT,* 20 (1993) (d) A. G. Myers and P. S. Dragovich, *J. Am. Chem. Soc., 114,* 5859 (1992). (e) M. E. Maier and T. Brandstetter, *Tetrahedron Lett., 33,* 7511 (1992). (f) K. N. Bharucha, R. M. Marsh, R. E. Minto, and R. E. Bergman, *J. Am. Chem. Soc., 114,* 3120 (1992). (g) P. A. Magriotis, M. A. Scott, and K. D. Kim, *Tetrahedron Lett., 32,* 6085 (1991). (h) P. A. Magriotis and K. D. Kin, *J. Am. Chem. Soc., 115,* 2972 (1993). (i) M. F. Semmelhack, T. Neu, and F. Foubelo, *Tetrahedron Lett., 33,* 3277 (1992). (j) T. Skrydstrup, H. Audrain, G. Ulibarri, and D. S. Grierson, *Tetrahedron Lett., 32,* 4563 (1992).

12. K. C. Nicolaou, G. Zuccarello, Y. Ogawa, E. J. Schweiger, and T. Kumazawa, *J. Am. Chem. Soc., 110,* 4866 (1988). (b) K. C. Nicolaou, G. Zuccarello, C. Riemer, V. A. Estevez, and W.-M. Dai, *J. Am. Chem. Soc., 114,* 7360 (1992).

13. L. A. Paquette, *Org. React., 25,* 1 (1977).

14. K. C. Nicolaou, Y. Ogawa, G. Zuccarello, and H. Katoaka, *J. Am. Chem. Soc., 110,* 7247 (1988).

15. K. C. Nicolaou, E. J. Sorenson, R. Discordia, C.-K. Huang, R. E. Minto, K. N. Bharucha, and R. G. Bergman, *Angew. Chem. Int. Ed. Engl., 31,* 1044 (1992).

16. M. F. Semmelhack and J. Gallagher, *Tetrahedron Lett., 34,* 4121 (1993).

17. (a) P. Magnus and P. A. Carter, *J. Am. Chem. Soc., 110,* 1626 (1988). (b) P. Magnus, P. Carter, J. Elliott, R. Lewis, J. Harling, T. Pitterna, W. W. Bauta, and S. Fortt, *J. Am. Chem. Soc., 114,* 2544 (1992).

18. R. D. Stephans and C. E. Castro, *J. Org. Chem., 28,* 3313 (1963).

19. P. Magnus, R. T. Lewis, and J. C. Huffman, *J. Am. Chem. Soc., 110,* 6921 (1988).

20. P. Magnus and F. Bennett, *Tetrahedron Lett., 30,* 3637 (1989).

21. P. Magnus and R. T. Lewis, *Tetrahedon Lett., 30,* 1905 (1989).

22. P. Magnus, H. Annoura, and J. Harling, *J. Org. Chem., 55,* 1711 (1990).

23. J. F. Kadow, M. M. Tun, D. M. Vyas, M. D. Wittman, and T. W. Doyle, *Tetrahedron Lett., 33,* 1423 (1992).

24. S. J. Danishefsky, D. S. Yamashita, and N. B. Mantlo, *Tetrahedron Lett., 29,* 4861 (1988).

25. J. N. Haseltine, M. P. Cabal, N. B. Mantlo, N. Iwasawa, D. S. Yamashita, R. S. Coleman, S. J. Danishefsky, and G. K. Shulte, *J. Am. Chem. Soc., 113,* 3850 (1991).

26. S. J. Danishefsky, N. B. Mantlo, D. S. Yamashita, and G. Shulte, *J. Am. Chem. Soc., 110,* 6890 (1988).

27. H.-D. Becker, T. Bremholt, and E. Adler, *Tetrahedron Lett., 12,* 4205 (1972).

28. D. L. Comins and J. D. Brown, *Tetrahedron Lett., 22,* 4213 (1981).

29. (a) A. S. Kende and C. A. Smith, *Tetrahedron Lett., 29,* 4217 (1988). (b) J. F. Kadow, M. G. Saulnier, M. M. Tun, D. R. Langley, and D. M. Vyas, *Tetrahedron Lett., 30,* 3499 (1989).

30. (a) S. L. Schreiber and L. L. Kiessling, *J. Am. Chem. Soc.*, *110*, 631 (1988). (b) S. L. Schreiber and L. L. Kiessling, *Tetrahedron Lett.*, *30*, 433 (1989).

31. F. J. Schoenen, J. A. Porco, S. L. Schreiber, G. D. VanDuyne, and J. Clardy, *Tetrahedron Lett.*, *30*, 3765 (1989).

32. (a) P. Magnus, R. T. Lewis, and F. Bennett, *J. Chem. Soc., Chem. Commun.*, 916 (1989). (b) P. Magnus, R. Lewis, and F. Bennett, *J. Am. Chem. Soc.*, *114*, 2560 (1992).

33. J. N. Haseltine, S. J. Danishefsky, and G. Shulte, *J. Am. Chem. Soc.*, *111*, 7638 (1989).

34. N. B. Mantlo and S. J. Danishefsky, *J. Org. Chem.*, *54*, 2781 (1989).

35. J. N. Haseltine and S. J. Danishefsky, *J. Org. Chem.*, *55*, 2576 (1990).

36. M. P. Cabal, R. S. Coleman, and S. J. Danishefsky, *J. Am. Chem. Soc.*, *112*, 3253 (1990).

37. (a) D. S. Yamashita, V. P. Rocco, and S. J. Danishefsky, *Tetrahedron Lett.*, *32*, 6667 (1991). (b) V. P. Rocco, S. J. Danishefsky, and G. Shulte, *Tetrahedron Lett.*, *32*, 6671 (1991).

38. (a) A. L. Smith, C.-K. Hwang, E. Pitsinos, G. R. Scarlato, and K. C. Nicolaou, *J. Am. Chem. Soc.*, *114*, 3134 (1992). (b) A. L. Smith, E. N. Pitsinos, C.-K. Hwang, Y. Mizuno, H. Saimoto, G. R. Scarlato, T. Suzuki, and K. C. Nicolaou, *J. Am. Chem. Soc.*, *115*, 7612 (1993).

39. (a) S. Walker, K. G. Valentine, and D. Kahne, *J. Am. Chem. Soc.*, *112*, 6428 (1990). (b) S. Walker, D. Yang, D. Kahne, and D. Gange, *J. Am. Chem. Soc.*, *113*, 4716 (1991). (c) J. Drak, N. Iwasawa, D. M. Crothers, and S. J. Danishefsky, *Proc. Natl. Acad. Sci. USA*, *88*, 7464 (1991). (d) J. Aiyar, S. J. Danishefsky, and D. M. Crothers, *J. Am. Chem. Soc.*, *114*, 7552 (1992). (e) K. C. Nicolaou, S.-C. Tsay, T. Suzuki, and G. F. Joyce, *J. Am. Chem. Soc.*, *114*, 7555 (1992). (f) S. Walker, J. Murnick, and D. Kahne, *J. Am. Chem. Soc.*, *115*, 7954 (1993).

40. (a) K. C. Nicolaou, R. D. Groneberg, T. Miyazaki, N. A. Stylianides, T. J. Schulze, and W. Stahl, *J. Am. Chem. Soc.*, *112*, 8193 (1990). (b) R. D. Groneberg, T. Miyazaki, N. A. Stylianides, T. J. Schulze, W. Stahl, E. P. Schreiner, T. Suzuki, Y. Iwabuchi, A. L. Smith, and K. C. Nicolaou, *J. Am. Chem. Soc.*, *115*, 7593 (1993).

41. (a) J. Golik, H. Wong, D. Vyas, and T. W. Doyle, *Tetrahedron Lett.*, *30*, 2497 (1989). (b) E. A. Mash and S. K. Nimkar, *Tetrahedron Lett.*, *34*, 385 (1993).

42. K. C. Nicolaou, R. D. Groneberg, N. A. Stylianides, and T. Miyazaki, *J. Chem. Soc., Chem. Commun.*, 1275 (1990).

43. K. C. Nicolau and R. D. Groneberg, *J. Am. Chem. Soc.*, *112*, 4085 (1990).

44. K. C. Nicolaou, T. Ebata, N. A. Stylianides, R. D. Groneberg, and P. J. Carrol, *Angew. Chem. Int. Ed. Eng.*, *27*, 1097 (1988).

45. K. C. Nicolaou, E. P. Schreiner, and W. Stahl, *Angew. Chem. Int. Ed. Eng.*, *30*, 585 (1991).

46. K. C. Nicolaou and D. Clark, *Angew. Chem. Int. Ed. Eng.*, *31*, 855 (1992).

47. D. Yang, S.-H. Kim, and D. Kahne, *J. Am. Chem. Soc.*, *113*, 4715 (1991).

48. D. Kahne, D. Yang, and M. D. Lee, *Tetrahedron Lett.*, *31*, 21 (1990).

49. D. Kahne, S. Walker, Y. Cheng, and D. Van Engen, *J. Am. Chem. Soc.*, *111*, 6881 (1989).

50. B. Toufik, J.-M. Lancelin, and J.-M. Beau, *J. Chem. Soc., Chem. Commun.*, 1494 (1992).
51. (a) M. D. Wittman, R. L. Halcomb, and S. J. Danishefsky, *J. Org. Chem., 55,* 1981 (1991). (b) H. Rainer and H.-D. Scharf, *Liebigs Ann. Chem.,* 117 (1993).
52. R. L. Halcomb, M. D. Wittman, S. H. Olson, S. J. Danishefsky, J. Golik, H. Wong, and D. Vyas, *J. Am. Chem. Soc., 113,* 5080 (1991).
53. M. D. Wittman, R. L. Halcomb, S. J. Danishefsky, J. Golik, and D. Vyas, *J. Org. Chem., 55,* 1979 (1990).
54. (a) K. Van Laak and H.-D. Scharf, *Tetrahedron Lett., 30,* 4505 (1989). (b) A. Claben and H.-D. Scharf, *Liebigs Ann. Chem.,* 183 (1993). (c) F.-Y. Dupradeau, S. Allaire, J. Prandi, and J.-M. Beau, *Tetrahedron Lett., 34,* 4513 (1993).
55. J. Golik, H. Wong, B. Krishnan, D. Vyas, and T. W. Doyle, *Tetrahedron Lett., 32,* 1851 (1991).
56. R. L. Halcomb, S. H. Boyer, and S. J. Danishesfky, *Angew. Chem. Int. Ed. Eng., 31,* 338 (1992).
57. K. Van Laak, H. Rainer, and H.-D. Scharf, *Tetrahedron Lett., 31,* 4113 (1990).
58. (a) K. C. Nicolaou, C. W. Hummel, E. N. Pitsinos, M. Nakada, A. L. Smith, K. Shibayama, and H. Saimoto, *J. Am. Chem. Soc., 114,* 10082 (1992). (b) K. C. Nicolaou, C. W. Hummel, M. Nakada, K. Shibayama, E. N. Pitsinos, H. Saimoto, Y. Mizuno, K.-U. Baldenius, and A. L. Smith, *J. Am. Chem. Soc., 115,* 7625 (1993).
59. (a) Y. Sugiura, T. Shiraki, M. Konishi, and T. Oki, *Proc. Natl. Acad. Sci. USA, 87,* 3831 (1990). (b) M. F. Semmelhack, J. Gallagher, and D. Cohen, *Tetrahedron Lett., 31,* 1521 (1990).
60. K. C. Nicolaou, C.-K. Hwang, A. L. Smith, and S. V. Wendeborn, *J. Am. Chem. Soc., 112,* 7416 (1990).
61. K. C. Nicolaou, W.-M. Dai, S. V. Wendeborn, A. L. Smith, Y. Torisawa, P. Maligres, and C.-K. Hwang, *Angew. Chem. Int. Ed. Eng., 30,* 1032 (1991).
62. K. C. Nicolaou, A. L. Smith, and E. W. Yue, *Proc. Natl. Acad. Sci. USA, 90,* 5881 (1993).
63. (a) K. C. Nicolaou, Y.-P. Hong, Y. Torisawa, S.-C. Tsay, and W.-M. Dai, *J. Am. Chem. Soc., 113,* 9878 (1991). (b) K. C. Nicolaou, Y. P. Hong, W.-M. Dai, Z.-J. Zeng, and W. Wrasidlo, *J. Chem. Soc., Chem. Commun.,* 1542 (1992). (c) K. C. Nicolaou, P. Maligres, T. Suzuki, S. V. Wendeborn, W.-M. Dai, and R. K. Chadha, *J. Am. Chem. Soc., 114,* 8890 (1992). (d) K. C. Nicolaou and W.-M. Dai, *J. Am. Chem. Soc., 114,* 8908 (1992). (e) K. C. Nicolaou, W.-M. Dai, S. C. Tsay, V. A. Estevez, and W. Wrasidlo, *Science, 256,* 1172 (1992). (f) K. C. Nicolaou, W.-M. Dai, Y. P. Hong, S.-C. Tsay, K. K. Baldridge, and J. S. Siegel, *J. Am. Chem. Soc., 115,* 7944 (1993).
64. P. A. Wender and C. K. Zercher, *J. Am. Chem. Soc., 113,* 2311 (1991). (b) T. Nishikawa, A. Ino, M. Isobe, and T. Goto, *Chem. Lett.,* 1271 (1991).
65. T. Nishikawa, M. Isobe, and T. Goto, *Synlett,* 393 (1991).
66. P. Magnus and S. M. Fortt, *J. Chem. Soc., Chem. Commun.,* 544 (1991).
67. J. A. Porco Jr., F. J. Schoenen, T. J. Stout, J. Clardy, and S. L. Schreiber, *J. Am. Chem. Soc., 112,* 7410 (1990).
68. (a) J. L. Wood, J. A. Porco, Jr., J. Taunton, A. Y. Lee, J. Clardy, and S. L.

Schreiber, *J. Am. Chem. Soc.*, *114*, 5898 (1992). (b) H. Chikashita, J. A. Porco, Jr., T. J. Stout, J. Clardy, and S. L. Schreiber, *J. Org. Chem.*, *56*, 1692 (1991).

69. J. Taunton, J. L. Wood, and S. L. Schreiber, *J. Am. Chem. Soc.*, *115*, 10378 (1993).

70. A. G. Myers, P. J. Proteau, and T. M. Handel, *J. Am. Chem. Soc.*, *110*, 7212 (1988).

71. A. G. Myers and P. J. Proteau, *J. Am. Chem. Soc.*, *111*, 1146 (1989).

72. (a) T. A. Beerman and I. H. Goldberg, *Biochem. Biophys. Res. Commun.*, *59*, 1254 (1974). (b) T. A. Beerman, R. Poon, and I. H. Goldberg, *Biochim. Biophys. Acta*, *475*, 294 (1977) (c) L. S. Kappen and I. H. Goldberg, *Nucleic Acids Res.*, *5*, 2959 (1978).

73. (a) A. G. Myers, N. S. Finney, and E. Y. Kuo, *Tetrahedron Lett.*, *30*, 5747 (1989). (b) A. G. Myers, E. Y. Kuo, and N. S. Finney, *J. Am. Chem. Soc.*, *111*, 9130 (1989).

74. (a) A. G. Myers, P. S. Dragovich, and E. Y. Kuo, *J. Am. Chem. Soc.*, *114*, 9369 (1992). (b) A. G. Myers and N. S. Finney, *J. Am. Chem. Soc.*, *114*, 10986 (1992). (c) A. G. Myers and P. S. Dragovich, *J. Am. Chem. Soc.*, *115*, 7021 (1993).

75. A. G. Myers and P. S. Dragovich, *J. Am. Chem. Soc.*, *111*, 9130 (1989).

76. R. Nagata, H. Yamanaka, E. Okazaki, and I. Saito, *Tetrahedron Lett.*, *30*, 4995 (1989).

77. P. A. Wender, M. Harmata, D. Jeffrey, C. Mukai, and J. Suffert, *Tetrahedron Lett.*, *29*, 909 (1988).

78. P. A. Wender, J. A. McKinney, and C. Mukai, *J. Am. Chem. Soc.*, *112*, 5369 (1990).

79. T. Doi and T. Takahashi, *J. Org. Chem.*, *56*, 3465 (1991).

80. (a) A. G. Myers, P. M. Harrington, and E. Y. Kuo, *J. Am. Chem. Soc.*, *113*, 694 (1991). (b) A. G. Myers, M. M. Alauddin, and M. A. M. Fuhry, *Tetrahedron Lett.*, *30*, 6997 (1989).

81. A. G. Myers, P. M. Harrington, and B.-M. Kwon, *J. Am. Chem. Soc.*, *114*, 1086 (1992).

82. P. Magnus and T. Pitterna, *J. Chem. Soc., Chem. Commun.*, 541 (1991).

83. P. Magnus and M. Davies, *J. Chem. Soc., Chem. Commun.*, 1522 (1991).

84. (a) M. Hirama, K. Fujiwara, K. Shigematu, and Y. Fukazawa, *J. Am. Chem. Soc.*, *111*, 4120 (1989). (b) M. Hirama, M. Tokuda, and K. Fujiwara, *SYNLETT*, 651 (1991).

85. K. Fujiwara, A. Kurisaki, and M. Hirama, *Tetrahedron Lett.*, *30*, 4329 (1990).

86. M. Hirama, T. Gomibuchi, K. Fujiwara, Y. Sugiura, and M. Uesugi, *J. Am. Chem. Soc.*, *113*, 9851 (1991).

87. T. Wehlage, A. Krebs, and T. Link, *Tetrahedron Lett.*, *31*, 6625 (1990).

88. (a) K. Nakatani, K. Arai, and S. Terashima, *J. Chem. Soc., Chem. Commun.*, 289 (1992). (b) K. Nakatani, K. Arai, and S. Terashima, *Tetrahedron*, *49*, 1901 (1993).

89. (a) K. Nakatani, K. Arai, N. Hirayama, F. Matsuda, and S. Terashima, *Tetrahedron Lett.*, *31*, 2323 (1990). (b) K. Nakatami, K. Arai, K. Yamada, F. Matsuda, and S. Terashima, *Tetrahedron*, *48*, 3045 (1992).

90. (a) R. Brückner, S. W. Scheuplein, and J. Suffert, *Tetrahedron Lett.*, *32*, 1449 (1991). (b) S. W. Schcuplein, K. Karms, R. Brückner, and J. Suffert, *Chem. Ber.*, *125*, 271 (1992).

91. J. M. Nuss, B. H. Levine, R. A. Rennels, and M. M. Heravi, *Tetrahedron Lett.*, *32*, 5243 (1991).

92. (a) J. M. Nuss, R. A. Rennels, and B. H. Levine, *J. Am. Chem. Soc.*, *115*, 6991 (1993). (b) S. Torii, H. Okumoto, T. Tadokoro, A. Nishimura, and M. A. Rashid, *Tetrahedron Lett.*, *34*, 2139 (1993).

93. N. A. Petasis and K. A. Teets, *Tetrahedron Lett.*, *34*, 805 (1993).

94. (a) K. C. Nicolaou, G. Skokotas, S. Furuya, H. Suemune, and D. C. Nicolaou, *Angew. Chem. Int. Ed. Eng.*, *29*, 1064 (1990). (b) K. C. Nicolaou, Y.-P. Hong, S.-C. Torisawa, and W.-M. Dai, *J. Am. Chem. Soc.*, *113*, 9878 (1991). (c) K. C. Nicolaou, E. P. Schreiner, and W. Stahl, *Angew. Chem. Int. Ed. Engl.*, *30*, 585 (1991). (d) K. C. Nicolaou, E. P. Schreiner, Y. Iwabuchi, and T. Suzuki, *Angew. Chem. Int. Ed. Engl.*, *31*, 340 (1992). (e) D. L. Boger and J. Zhou, *J. Org. Chem.*, *58*, 3018 (1993). (f) M. Tokuda, K. Fujiwara, T. Gomibuchi, M. Hirama, M. Uesugi, and Y. Sugiura, *Tetrahedron Lett.*, *34*, 669 (1993).

95. (a) Y. Minami, K.-i. Yoshida, R. Azuma, M. Saeki, and T. Otani, *Tetrahedron Lett.*, *34*, 2633 (1993). (b) K.-i. Yoshida, Y. Minami, R. Azuma, M. Saeki, and T. Otani, *Tetrahedron Lett.*, *34*, 2638 (1993).

96. J. Aiyar, S. A. Hitchcock, D. Denhart, K. K. C. Liu, S. J. Danishefsky, and D. M. Crothers, *Angew. Chem. Int. Ed. Engl.*, *33*, 855 (1994).

97. S. A. Hitchcock, S. H. Boyer, M. Y. Chu-Moyer, S. H. Olson, and S. J. Danishefsky, *Angew. Chem. Int. Ed. Engl.*, *33*, 858 (1994).

98. S.-H. Kim, D. Augeri, D. Yang, and D. Kahne, *J. Am. Chem. Soc.*, *116*, 1766 (1994).

99. (a) K. C. Nicolaou, T. Li, M. Nakada, C. W. Hummel, A. Hiatt, and W. Wrasidlo, *Angew. Chem. Int. Ed. Engl.*, *33*, 183 (1994). (b) T. Li, Z. Zeng, V. A. Estevez, K. U. Baldenius, K. C. Nicolaou, and G. F. Joyce, *J. Am. Chem. Soc.*, *116*, 3709 (1994).

100. (a) W. R. Roush and D. Gustin, *Tetrahedron Lett.*, *35*, 4931 (1994). (b) W. R. Roush and B. C. Fellows, *Tetrahedron Lett.*, *35*, 4935 (1994).

101. (a) M. F. Semmelhack, J. J. Gallagher, T. Minami, and T. Date, *J. Am. Chem. Soc.*, *115*, 11618 (1993). (b) T. Brandstetter and M. E. Maier, *Tetrahedron, 50*, 1435 (1994). (c) H. Audrain, T. Skrydstrup, G. Ulibarri, C. Riche, A. Chiaroni, and D. S. Grierson, *Tetrahedron, 50*, 1469 (1994). (d) J. F. Kadow, D. J. Cook, T. W. Doyle, D. R., Langley, K. M. Pham, D. M. Vyas, and M. D. Wittman, *Tetrahedron, 50*, 1519 (1994). (e) G. P. Roth, D. R. Marshall, J. F. Kadow, S. W. Mamber, W. C. Rose, W. Solomon, and N. Zein, *Bioorg. Med. Chem. Lett.*, *4*, 711 (1994).

102. (a) T. Yoon, M. D. Shair, S. J. Danishesfsky, and G. K. Shulte, *J. Org. Chem.*, *50*, 3752 (1994). (b) M. D. Shair, T. Yoon, and S. J. Danishesfsky, *J. Org. Chem.*, *50*, 3755 (1994).

103. (a) P. A. Wender, C. K. Zercher, S. Bechman, and E.-M. Haubold, *J. Org. Chem.*, *58*, 5867 (1993). (b) P. Magnus, S. A. Eisenbeis, W. C. Rose, N. Zein, and W. Solomon, *J. Am. Chem. Soc.*, *115*, 12627 (1993). (c) T. Nishikawa, A. Ino, and M. Isobe, *Tetrahedron, 50*, 1449 (1994). (d) T. Nishikawa and M. Isobe, *Tetrahedron, 50*, 5621 (1994).

104. (a) W.-M. Dai, *J. Org. Chem.*, *58*, 7581 (1993). (b) K. C. Nicolaou, J. L. Gross, M. S. Kerr, R. H. Lemus, K. Ikeda, and K. Ohe, *Angew. Chem. Int. Ed. Engl.*, *33*, 781 (1994).

105. (a) M. Lamothe and P. L. Fuchs, *J. Am. Chem. Soc.*, *115*, 4483 (1993). (b) T. Takahashi, H. Tanaka, Y. Hirai, T. Doi, H. Yamada, T. Shiraki, and Y. Sugiura, *Angew, Chem. Int. Ed. Engl.*, *32*, 1657 (1993). (c) K. Nakatani, S. Isoe, S. Maekawa, and I. Saito, *Tetrahedron Lett.*, *35*, 605 (1994). (d) J. Suffert and R. Brüchner, *SYNLETT, 51* (1994). (e) P. A. Wender and M. J. Tebbe, *Tetrahedron, 50*, 1419 (1994).

Index

N-Acetyl calicheamicin γ_1^I
   activity against P388 leukemia 131
   aromatic degradation products of, 63
   clonogenic assays of 133
   constituent sugars of, 63
   mass spectrum of, 62
   methanolic degradation of, 62
   multiple drug resistance, induction of,
     133, 134
N-Acetyl esperamicin D, 203
   nmr shifts of anomeric H in, 205,
     206
Actinomadura
   A. madurae, 12
   A. pulveracae, 163
     ATCC accession number of, 163
     carbohydrate utilization in, 164
   A. verrucosospora, 2
     ATCC accession numbers of, 163,
      170
     carbohydrate utilization in, 164
     effect of added polypropylene
      glycol on, 169

[Actinomadura]
   effect of carbon sources on, 167
   effect of cerulenin on growth of,
     22
   effect of halide addition on, 43,
     168–170
   effect of metal ions on, 167–168
   effect of nitrogen sources on, 167
   effect of sodium oleate on, 226
   large scale fermentation of, 176–
     180
   media development for, 165–170
   mutation studies of, 170–172
   production medium for, 169–170
   taxonomy of, 163
Actinomycetes, plasmids from, 123
Actinomycin D
   activity against Rec$^-$ and Rec$^+$
     strains, 303
Actinoxanthin
   apoprotein of, 7
     tertiary structure of, 6
   general description, 328

About the Editors

DONALD B. BORDERS is President of BioSource Pharm, Inc., Suffern, New York. Previously, he was Head of the Natural Products Chemistry Department in the Medical Research Division at Lederle Laboratories, American Cyanamid Company, Pearl River, New York. A member of the American Chemical Society, the Royal Chemical Society, the American Society of Pharmacognosy, and Sigma Xi, he is the author or coauthor of over 90 professional papers, abstracts and book chapters, and the coholder of 30 U.S. patents. Dr. Borders received the B.S. (1954) and M.S. (1958) degrees in chemistry from Indiana University, Bloomington, and the Ph.D. degree (1963) in organic chemistry from the University of Illinois, Urbana.

TERRENCE W. DOYLE is Vice President of Research at OncoRx, Inc., New Haven, Connecticut. Previously he was Executive Director of Antitumor and Natural Products Chemistry at Bristol-Myers Squibb Pharmaceutical Research Institute, Wallingford, Connecticut. He is a member of the American Chemical Society and the American Association for Cancer Research, among other organizations; serves on the editorial boards of five journals; is the author or coauthor of more than 130 professional papers, abstracts, book chapters, and reviews; and is the coholder of over 40 U.S. patents. Dr. Doyle received the B.Sc. degree (1963) in chemistry from Loyola College, Montreal, Canada, and the Ph.D. degree (1966) in organic chemistry from the University of Notre Dame, South Bend, Indiana.